SMALL ANIMAL
MEDICAL
DIAGNOSIS

SMALL ANIMAL
MEDICAL
DIAGNOSIS

SECOND EDITION

Michael D. Lorenz, B.S., D.V.M.

Diplomate, American College of Veterinary Internal Medicine—
Internal Medicine
Dean of Veterinary Medicine
College of Veterinary Medicine
Kansas State University
Manhattan, Kansas

Larry M. Cornelius, D.V.M., Ph.D.

Diplomate, American College of Veterinary Internal Medicine—
Internal Medicine
Professor of Small Animal Medicine
College of Veterinary Medicine
The University of Georgia
Athens, Georgia

With 10 Contributors

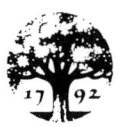

J.B. Lippincott Company   Philadelphia

Acquisitions Editor: Mary K. Smith
Assistant Editor: Anne Geyer
Production Editor: Virginia Barishek
Indexer: Maria Coughlin
Cover Designer: Tom Jackson

Production: P. M. Gordon Associates, Inc.
Compositor: Achorn Graphic Services, Inc.
Printer/Binder: R. R. Donnelley & Sons Company

Second Edition

6   5   4   3   2   1

Library of Congress Cataloging-in-Publication Data

Small animal medical diagnosis / [edited by] Michael D. Lorenz, Larry
    M. Cornelius ; with 10 contributors. — 2nd ed.
        p.   cm.
    Includes bibliographical references and index.
    ISBN 0–397–51200–7
        1. Dogs—Diseases—Diagnosis.   2. Cats—Diseases—Diagnosis.
    3. Veterinary medicine—Diagnosis.   I. Lorenz, Michael D.
    II. Cornelius, Larry M.
    SF991.S592   1993
    636.7'0896075—dc20   92–46032
                                                                    CIP

The authors and publisher have exerted every effort to ensure that drug selection and dosage set forth in this text are in accord with current recommendations and practice at the time of publication. However, in view of ongoing research, changes in government regulations, and the constant flow of information relating to drug therapy and drug reactions, the reader is urged to check the package insert for each drug for any change in indications and dosage and for added warnings and precautions. This is particularly important when the recommended agent is a new or infrequently employed drug.

*This book is dedicated to our colleagues
who have championed the problem-oriented method,
and to our many students
who have faithfully applied this method in their practice
of veterinary medicine*

CONTRIBUTORS

Dennis N. Aron, D.V.M. Diplomate, American College of Veterinary Surgeons; Assistant Professor, Department of Small Animal Medicine, College of Veterinary Medicine, The University of Georgia, Athens, Georgia

Jeanne A. Barsanti, D.V.M. Diplomate, American College of Veterinary Internal Medicine; Professor, Department of Small Animal Medicine, College of Veterinary Medicine, The University of Georgia, Athens, Georgia

Clay A. Calvert, D.V.M. Diplomate, American College of Veterinary Internal Medicine—Internal Medicine; Associate Professor, Department of Small Animal Medicine, College of Veterinary Medicine, The University of Georgia, Athens, Georgia

Jonathan N. Chambers, D.V.M. Diplomate, American College of Veterinary Surgeons; Associate Professor, Department of Small Animal Medicine, College of Veterinary Medicine, The University of Georgia, Athens, Georgia

Laine A. Cowan, D.V.M. Diplomate, American College of Veterinary Internal Medicine; Assistant Professor, Department of Clinical Sciences, College of Veterinary Medicine, Kansas State University, Manhattan, Kansas

Craig E. Greene, D.V.M. Diplomate, American College of Veterinary Internal Medicine; Professor, Department of Small Animal Medicine, College of Veterinary Medicine, The University of Georgia, Athens, Georgia

Michael R. Lappin, D.V.M., Ph.D. Diplomate, American College of Veterinary Internal Medicine—Internal Medicine; Assistant Professor, College of Veterinary Medicine and Biomedical Sciences, Colorado State University, Fort Collins, Colorado

Charles L. Martin, D.V.M. Diplomate, American College of Veterinary Ophthalmologists; Professor and Director, Veterinary Medical Teaching Hospital, College of Veterinary Medicine, The University of Georgia, Athens, Georgia

John E. Oliver, D.V.M., M.S., Ph.D. Diplomate, American College of Veterinary Internal Medicine—Neurology; Professor, Department of Small Animal Medicine, College of Veterinary Medicine, The University of Georgia, Athens, Georgia

James P. Toombs, D.V.M. Diplomate, American College of Veterinary Surgeons; Associate Professor of Small Animal Surgery, Department of Clinical Sciences, School of Veterinary Medicine, Purdue University, West Lafayette, Indiana

PREFACE

Since its introduction in 1987 to the veterinary medical profession, *Small Animal Medical Diagnosis* has enjoyed tremendous success with veterinary students and small animal practitioners. Nearly 15,000 copies have been sold. In large part due to the philosophy and organization of its contents, *Small Animal Medical Diagnosis* has proven its usefulness and versatility as an effective aid in the diagnosis of small animal disease.

Small Animal Medical Diagnosis is organized and written in a problem-oriented format similar to the instructional philosophy of the problem-oriented veterinary medical record. It approaches clinical diagnosis in a logical problem-related manner (identical to the process used by the most skilled diagnosticians). *Small Animal Medical Diagnosis* contains the core information necessary to effectively evaluate the major medical problems in dogs and cats. It relates clinical signs to the pathophysiological mechanisms of disease and describes the appropriate causes (ruleouts) for clinical signs or problems.

Small Animal Medical Diagnosis is an excellent textbook for veterinary students and practitioners who need assistance in the formulation of accurate diagnostic plans for the evaluation of their clinical patients. It is very useful for instructors who utilize a problem-based format for their students.

Small Animal Medical Diagnosis does not attempt to describe the factual information of specific disease processes. There are many excellent textbooks available which take this traditional approach to the organization of medical information. What *Small Animal Medical Diagnosis* has accomplished is to effectively relate disease to clinical signs or problems, a most critical step in the management of clinical patients.

The second edition of *Small Animal Medical Diagnosis* follows the identical format to the first edition. Information has been updated and diagnostic plans have been refined or revised based on new information. Sections dealing with symptomatic therapy have been eliminated.

We are indebted to our colleagues who have perfected the problem-oriented approach as a major instructional philosophy. We extend our appreciation to the staff of J. B. Lippincott Company for their assistance in the development of this Second Edition.

Michael D. Lorenz, B.S., D.V.M.
Larry M. Cornelius, D.V.M., Ph.D.

CONTENTS

PART SIX
Cardiovascular Problems

PART SEVEN
Respiratory Problems

PART EIGHT
Digestive Problems

PART FOURTEEN
Laboratory-Defined Problems

CHAPTER ONE

The Problem-Oriented Approach

Michael D. Lorenz

In the 1960s, the problem-oriented medical record (POMR) was introduced in medical practice.[3,4] The POMR encourages the user to employ sound logic in evaluating patients and provides a convenient system for displaying medical data and actions.[1] In 1971, the Department of Small Animal Medicine at The University of Georgia adopted the POMR for use in the Small Animal Teaching Hospital. Since then, the concepts underlying the POMR have become the basis of a system for identifying and managing an animal's problems. These concepts have also been incorporated into lecture and laboratory courses.[2]

The basic tenet of the problem-oriented approach (POA), and thus the POMR, is that disease alters anatomy and function to cause clinical signs and symptoms. These changes in anatomy and function are called "problems." The focus of the POA is different from that in the classic method of diagnostic impressions and lists of differential diagnoses. Instead, emphasis is placed on critical identification of the patient's problems and a clear understanding of the mechanisms (pathophysiology) that create each problem. When the mechanisms are clearly understood, the diseases that cause each problem are more easily recalled. In the POA, the term *rule out* is used to refer to a potential cause of any problem. The most appropriate diagnostic procedure for documentation of each rule out is listed. Thus, possible causes of problems are always coupled with the most appropriate diagnostic procedures.

The clinical reasoning process utilized in the POA is based on four steps: (1) data base collection, (2) problem identification, (3) plan formulation, and (4) assessment and follow-up.

STEP 1: DATA BASE COLLECTION

The initial data base should contain the information necessary to allow identification of all problems in the patient. The size of the data base for any particular patient should be specified in advance. This is the guaranteed data base, and it is collected for each animal. Although the size of the guaranteed data base is often debated, there is no disagreement that it must include a complete history

1

and a complete physical examination. A strong argument can be made for the inclusion of a complete blood count and urine analysis in the guaranteed data base, since these procedures broadly screen many body systems. These diagnostic procedures can be viewed as an extension of the physical examination. In this book, the problems described are largely those identified through the history and physical examination.

A problem-specific data base is the information necessary for properly evaluating the possible causes or rule outs for that problem. Each chapter of this book has a diagnostic plan that lists the data base for each problem.

History

Next to the physical examination, the history is the most important aspect of correct medical problem solving. One must resist the temptation to substitute diagnostic tests for a thorough history. The history alerts the clinician to the presence of potential problems and increases one's curiosity during physical examination of the patient. First, the chief complaint is determined. This complaint is pursued in depth, noting any additional problems and their chronologic development. All medications must be listed, since treatment often alters the normal progression of many diseases. Each body system is reviewed and the owner questioned about the presence of signs that would indicate organ or system dysfunction.

In taking the history, two different techniques are usually employed. The first technique, called the cross-examination or interrogation style, allows the clinician to ask questions in an organized and chronologic manner. Some owners are inhibited by this style, whereas others may answer questions falsely, particularly when the question is not understood. The second technique is the open-ended story style, in which the owner is asked to describe the pet's problems. This style may be disorganized and lack the chronologic specificity needed in a good history. The author prefers a combination of the two techniques, using just enough cross-examination to clarify problems and add good chronology to the history.

Physical Examination

The physical examination is the most important aspect of the data base. Problems not identified in the physical examination are usually also missed when more invasive or expensive diagnostic tests are performed. In addition, the proper interpretation of laboratory tests involves correlation with the history and physical examination findings. A complete physical examination should not require more than 5 to 8 minutes. Each body system should be examined. Particular attention should be given to those body systems in which dysfunction is suspected from the history. Ocular and neurologic evaluations (frequently slighted during the physical examination) must be included.

PRESENTING COMPLAINT OR REQUEST						
REFERRING VETERINARIAN						
ADDRESS						
PHONE						
ADMISSION HR.	PREVIOUS ADMISSION	DISCHARGE HR.				

(1) GEN	☐ N ☐ ABN ☐ NE	(2) INTEG	☐ N ☐ ABN ☐ NE	(3) M	☐ N ☐ ABN ☐ NE	(4) CIRC	☐ N ☐ ABN ☐ NE	(5) RESP	☐ N ☐ ABN ☐ NE	(6) DIG	☐ N ☐ ABN ☐ NE
(7) GU	☐ N ☐ ABN ☐ NE	(8) EYES	☐ N ☐ ABN ☐ NE	(9) EARS	☐ N ☐ ABN ☐ NE	(10) NS	☐ N ☐ ABN ☐ NE	(11) L	☐ N ☐ ABN ☐ NE	(12) MUCOSA	☐ N ☐ ABN ☐ NE

DESCRIBE ABNORMAL (USE NUMBERS ABOVE)   T _____   P _____   R _____   WT _____

STUDENT SIGNATURE _____   PHYSICAL EXAMINATION   ADM. CLINICIAN SIGNATURE _____

FIGURE 1-1. System-oriented physical examination form.

The author suggests that a physical examination form be followed that stresses a complete review of body systems (Fig. 1-1). Abnormalities are recorded for each system on the form. Special examination forms for the integumentary system, eye, and nervous system are very helpful and reduce writing time (Figs. 1-2, 1-3, and 1-4).

Text continues on p. 7

DATE: _____

GRADE LESIONS:

1 if few or mild
2 if several or moderate
3 if many or severe

Primary Lesions

Papule____ Pustule____ Vesicle____ Bulla____
Plaque____ Nodule____ Tumor____ Cyst____
Macule____ Patch____ Wheal____ Abscess____

Secondary Lesions

Scale____ Epidermal Collarette____ Crust____
Alopecia____ Erythema____
Hyperpigmentation____ Lichenification____
Erosion____ Excoriation____ Ulcer____
Comedone____ Hyperkeratosis____ Callus____
Fissure____ Scar____ Hypopigmentation____

(Circle)

Pruritus: Int. Mod. Mild None
Thickness: Norm. Inc. Dec.
Elasticity: Norm. Inc. Dec.
Easy Epilation: Yes No
Hair Coat: Norm. Dry Dull Brittle Oily

INITIAL WORK-UP (Circle)

Scrape: Sarcoptes Demodex Neg.
         Other _____
Parasites: Fleas Flea Dirt Ticks
           Other_____
Woods Light: – +   DTM submitted
Direct Smear: _____

DISTRIBUTION OF LESIONS

VENTRAL   DORSAL

DIFFERENTIAL DIAGNOSIS

Teaching Hospital
College of Veterinary Medicine
University of Georgia
Athens, Georgia

9/85 (#815/3-N)

Dermatology Exam.

FIGURE 1-2. Dermatologic examination form for the integumentary system.

OPHTHALMIC CONSULTATION REQUEST

DATE REQUESTED	TIME AM ☐ PM ☐	LOCATION OF ANIMAL	SPECIES	ADDRESSOGRAPH
REQUESTING CLINICIAN		STUDENT		
Hx/PROBLEMS				
PRIOR OCULAR AND SYSTEMIC THERAPY				

OD	OPHTHALMIC EXAMINATION	OS

ORBIT/GLOBE

LIDS
Palpebral Reflex

CONJUNCTIVA &
MEMBRANA NICTITANS

NASOLACRIMAL SYSTEM

CORNEA
Sensation

IRIS
Direct Reflex
Consensual Reflex

ANTERIOR CHAMBER,
ANGLE, & IOP

LENS

FUNDUS

VITREOUS

VISUAL ACUITY
Menace Reflex

OCULAR MOTILITY &
VESTIBULAR REFLEXES

PROBLEMS		OS-Left Eye OU-Both Eyes NE-Not OD-Right Eye N-Normal Examined
		DATE AND TIME COMPLETED / / AM ☐ PM ☐
		BY

FIGURE 1-3. Ophthalmic examination form.

I. Subjective

II. Objective (circle or describe)

                                     Alert   Stupor

A. Observation: Mental Status: Depressed Coma _____

    Posture: Normal, Head Tilt, Tremor, Falling L-R _____

               Normal, Post Paresis, Tetraparesis

    Gait: Ataxia, Dysmetria, Circling _____

B. Palpation: Muscle or Skeletal Abnormality

C. Postural Reactions

L	Reaction	R
	Hopping, Front	
	Hopping, Rear	
	Proprioception Front	
	Rear	
	Placing, Tactile Front	
	Rear	
	Placing, Visual Front	
	Rear	

E. Spinal Reflexes

L	Reflex Spinal Segment	R
	Triceps C-7–T-1	
	Ext. Carpi Rad. C-7–T-1	
	Quadriceps L-4–6	
	Flexion, Fore C-6–T-1	
	Flexion, Hind L-5–S-1	
	Perineal S-1–2	

G. Assessment:

    Note significant findings and localize lesion.

D. Cranial Nerves

L	Nerve + Function	R
	II vision menace	
	II + III pupil size	
	Stim. L. eye	
	Stim. R. eye	
	II Fundus	
	III, IV, VI Strabismus	
	Nystagmus	
	V Sensation	
	V Mastication	
	VII Facial Muscles	
	Palpebral	
	IX, X Swallowing	
	XII Tongue	

F. Sensation: Location

    Hyperesthesia _____
    Superficial Pain _____
    Deep Pain _____

H. Plan: Dx

Sig: _____ DVM

FIGURE 1-4. Neurologic examination form.

STEP 2: PROBLEM IDENTIFICATION

The second step in medical problem solving is problem identification. In small animal veterinary medicine, a problem is defined as any abnormality requiring medical or surgical management or one that interferes with the quality of life. It is important for problems to be stated at their current level of understanding. An overstated problem may cause expensive, invasive, and needless diagnostic tests to be performed. Many times problems identified in the history need to be documented, since the owner's observations may be erroneous. Problems are numbered consecutively and dated chronologically on a separate sheet of paper called the master problem list (MPL). As additional problems are identified, they are dated and assigned the next number.

The POMR couples all notations in the medical record to numbered problems on the MPL (Fig. 1-5). The MPL should be placed in the front of the medical record. It serves as a table of contents that directs the medical care of each patient.

Problems are subject to several "fates" (see section on assessment and follow-up). Problems can be redefined at a higher level of understanding, or they may be combined. The clinical reasoning process has problem resolution as its primary goal. Problems may be resolved or combined to a diagnosis or only resolved therapeutically. Problems can be inactivated when no further diagnostic or therapeutic action is warranted but resolution has not occurred.

STEP 3: PLAN FORMULATION

Once the problems are identified and the MPL formulated, attention is given to development of an initial plan (Fig. 1-6). This is a critical step in the clinical reasoning process, since it will dictate medical action for the first 24 to 48 hours. Each plan has three components: (1) a diagnostic section, (2) a therapeutic section, and (3) a client/owner education section. The initial plan emphasizes components 1 and 2. Plans are also a component of the assessment and follow-up step described below.

The Diagnostic Plan

A diagnostic plan is formulated and written for each problem. The plan should be organized with the most important or serious problems listed first. Rule outs (causes) are listed under each problem, with priority given to the most likely causes. Diagnostic procedures are coupled with each rule out. In this manner, logical clinical reasoning can be displayed and audited. The clinician in effect has stated the thought process; that is, "Here are the problems I've identified," "These are the most likely causes in my opinion," and "I will perform these diagnostic procedures to test my hypothesis." When displayed in the POMR, the clinical reasoning process can be evaluated by any knowledgeable individual.

DATE ACTIVE	NO.	MASTER PROBLEM LIST CONTINUED	DATE RESOLVED

FIGURE 1-5. Master problem list form (the "table of contents" or "index" to the medical record) (this page, front; page 9, back).

Feline
Health Record

Minor
Problem
List

Vaccinations	Date/Brand (N or PM) Lot				
FPL					
Respir.					
Rabies					

Diagnostic Testing	Dates				
Fecal					
Felv					
FIP					

Type	Parasites (external, internal)	Dates			

Anthelminthics Administered					

FIGURE 1-5 (*continued*)

Temporary Problem List
Initial Plan

Problem	Dx:	Rule outs, Procedures	Rx:	CE·

Student Signature   Clinician Signature

FIGURE 1-6. Form for construction of the initial plan.

Developing a well-founded diagnostic plan is based on the logic and information contained in each chapter of this book. As stated earlier, the POA emphasizes the management of problems through knowledge of their mechanisms and causes. By listing the problems, interrelationships can be more easily elucidated. Certainly, a disease or condition that appears as a major rule out for more than one problem should be highly suspected as the primary target for clinical diagnostic efforts.

The management of certain problems involves the collection of data beyond that contained in the guaranteed data base. This information constitutes the problem-specific data base. It includes tests or procedures that help establish the cause and the metabolic or biochemical consequences of the problem. Clinical algorithms are sequential steps in clinical reasoning based on the results of the problem-specific data base. Clinical algorithms are used in this book to display a logical progression of problem management. "Perfect" algorithms do not exist. Therefore, understanding the reasons for each decision is important. Algorithms are very useful in medical management, since it is impossible to remember all the causes of many problems.

The Therapeutic Plan

Therapy must be coupled with the problem that it is intended to resolve or help. When this is not done, the logic of therapeutic decisions cannot be audited. During formulation of the initial plan, a clinician must weigh the possible benefits of symptomatic therapy against the alterations that therapy may produce in laboratory test results. In many cases, serum should be saved prior to therapy for future biochemical or immunologic tests. In medicine, as much time is spent diagnosing what was done to an animal as is spent in diagnosing the underlying disease.

A therapeutic plan is also part of the assessment and follow-up step.

Client/Owner Education

This section of the initial plan describes the information given to clients about their animals' problems, general condition, and prognosis.

STEP 4: ASSESSMENT AND FOLLOW-UP

The fourth step in medical problem solving is the assessment of data collected from the initial plan (or the problem-specific data base). These results must be correlated with the history and physical findings. The clinician is actually assessing hypotheses stated in the initial plan. The assessment should be written in the medical record in relationship to each problem and should accurately interpret the results of diagnostic tests or procedures. It reflects the logic for changes in the MPL.

Follow-up represents actions to be taken based on the results of the initial plan or daily plans. In the POMR, follow-up is maintained in the daily progress notes. Progress notes contain three sections and are written in a problem-oriented manner; that is, information is grouped according to the problem it affects. Section 1 is for new or additional data, section 2 is the assessment, and section 3 is the plan (remember that plans always have three components). Orienting follow-up information by problems allows the clinical reasoning process to be displayed so that it can be efficiently and effectively audited.

SUMMARY

The problem-oriented approach to medical management is based on logical concepts. Disease creates clinical signs or problems. When problems are logically examined, the underlying disease(s) can be discovered. When the diagnosis still escapes identification, proper problem management improves the quality of life. The POA is not a new system; it follows the logic that clinicians have used for many years. The POMR is new, and it provides a structured format for display of an old system of medical management. The POA is no panacea for the "ills" of medical management. It will not correct the problems created by superficial data collection. Poor histories, poorly performed physical examinations, poorly understood pathophysiologic processes, and deficiencies in basic concepts of therapy are not corrected by this system. It is a system that functions well when all steps are meticulously followed.

This book is about problems: how they are identified, why they occur, what diseases are ultimately responsible, and how they are logically pursued. Other books are available that describe disease in detail. When the knowledge of disease is coupled with the knowledge of problems, the clinical reasoning process operates at its highest level. The author sincerely believes that the clinical reasoning process is greatly improved when problems are understood first, followed by the knowledge of disease.

The POA is a logical way to think about diagnosis and patient management. A POMR is not necessary for the clinician to think in terms of "problem solving." However, when the POMR is used, it reflects a problem-oriented approach to case management.

REFERENCES

1. Hurst JW: Ten reasons why Lawrence Weed is right. N Engl J Med 284:51, 1971
2. Lorenz MD: Problem directed instruction in small animal clinical endocrinology. J Vet Med Ed 12:6, 1985
3. Weed LL: Medical records, patient care, and medical education. Ir J Med Surg 6:271, 1964
4. Weed LL: Medical records that guide and teach. N Engl J Med 278:593, 1968

PART ONE

General (Polysystemic) Problems

CHAPTER TWO

Pyrexia (Fever)

Michael D. Lorenz

Pyrexia is an elevation of body temperature caused by disease. It is a clinical sign that occurs in a wide variety of pathogenic conditions. Fever is a term synonymous with pyrexia. Hyperpyrexia refers to a fever greater than 105°F. Intermittent fever is one in which the temperature falls to normal and rises again each day. A remittent fever is characterized by marked variation in temperature level each day; however, the low point remains above normal. A relapsing fever has short periods of increased temperature interspersed with periods of 1 or more days of normal temperature. A septic fever has large daily oscillations in body temperature.

To understand the significance of fever, it is necessary to have some background information about the regulation of body temperature and the pathogenesis of fever.

REGULATION OF BODY TEMPERATURE

Mammals are endothermic vertebrates that are capable of regulating their body temperature by altering heat production and heat loss. Temperature regulation is a complicated reflex integrated by a thermoregulatory center in the hypothalamus. Thermal sensors are located throughout the body but are most abundant in the skin, spinal cord, abdomen, and hypothalamus.[1] The *effectors* of the reflex are those structures actually involved in raising or lowering body temperature. Examples of these effectors include skeletal muscle, skin, and the respiratory system.

Body heat is largely generated by the liver's oxidation of nutrients. During physical activity, much heat is also generated by the muscles. The muscular system is important to thermal regulation, since its heat production can be rapidly increased or decreased according to need. Heat can be eliminated from the body in three ways: radiation, vaporization, and convection. In dogs and cats, the primary mechanisms for heat loss are radiation and vaporization. Since small animals are covered with hair and have few sweat glands, heat is not rapidly dissipated through the skin. Panting is their primary means of dissipating excessive heat.

The central thermoregulator is set at 101°F to 102°F. It responds to changes of less than 0.2°C,[2] and heat production is greatly augmented when skin temperatures are below 33°C. As the animal senses falling body temperature, two important effectors are stimulated. Peripheral vasoconstriction helps decrease heat loss, and increased muscular activity (shivering) generates additional heat. If body temperature increases in the normal animal, peripheral vasodilation, panting, and decreased muscular activity are mechanisms that dissipate heat. In general, the mechanisms for raising body temperature are sympathetically controlled, whereas depression of temperature is largely parasympathetically regulated.

In summary, body temperature is controlled by a thermoregulator that receives information from a variety of thermal sensors.[2] Small changes in body temperature elicit marked sympathetic or parasympathetic responses that alter heat production and heat loss.

Pathophysiology of Fever

Diseases or substances that induce fever (pyrogenic) do not affect the effector side of the thermoregulatory reflex. Pyrogenic conditions affect the sensory and/or integrating parts of the reflex.[1] Fever represents the ability of an animal to regulate its body temperature at a higher level; that is, the thermoregulatory set point is raised above normal. The body temperature may or may not be raised to the same level.

Activators of Fever

Fever-inducing substances are called *pyrogens.* Bacterial endotoxin, gram-positive bacteria, viruses, hypersensitivity reactions, and tumors are sources of so-called *exogenous pyrogen.* It is unlikely that these substances directly affect the thermoregulatory center, because the size and molecular complexity of most exogenous pyrogens preclude their entrance into the hypothalamus.[3]

All the activators of fever probably induce the formation of protein mediators called *endogenous pyrogen,* which is the actual fever-inducing compound. It is released from neutrophils, monocytes, and eosinophils. Lymphocytes do not release endogenous pyrogens; however, sensitized lymphocytes reacting with antigen release a soluble lymphokine that stimulates production of endogenous pyrogen in neutrophils and macrophages.[4] Endogenous pyrogen is also released from fixed phagocytes such as Kupffer cells, splenic sinusoidal cells, alveolar macrophages, and peritoneal cells. Endogenous pyrogen does not exist as a preformed compound in the cells. Rather, its synthesis is stimulated when leukocytes or macrophages become activated by an exogenous source.

There is considerable evidence that endogenous pyrogen either directly or indirectly elevates the thermoregulatory set point in the hypothalamus. The exact mechanism is unknown but probably involves monoamines, prostaglandins, and cyclic AMP. Once the temperature set point is elevated, the body temperature is perceived as too low. Heat is conserved (vasoconstriction), and heat production increases (chills, shivering). These processes elevate the body temperature. When the fever stimulus is removed, the hypothalamic thermostat is reset at normal and the body temperature is lowered by peripheral vasodilation, sweating, and panting.

FUNCTION OF FEVER

There is no conclusive proof that fever is either harmful or beneficial. The majority of clinicians consider fever to be a condition that should be suppressed to make the patient feel better. Based on experiments in animals, fever may have several beneficial effects. First, it may directly inhibit the growth of microorganisms, both bacteria and viruses. For instance, neonatal puppies have lower body temperatures than adults and are much more susceptible to herpes viral infection. The suppressive effects of fever on the growth of microorganisms may be coupled with host defense mechanisms. For example, serum iron levels decrease in animals with infection. The reaction, which is most likely due to endogenous pyrogen, makes an essential nutrient (iron) less available for bacterial metabolism. In addition, fever reduces the ability of bacteria to trap, or chelate, iron.

Several immune responses may be affected by fever. Lysosomes are more easily broken down during fever, and proteolytic enzymes that are destructive to viral agents are released. Fever may also increase the production of interferon, which interferes with the growth of viruses. There is some evidence that leukocyte mobility and phagocytic activity are enhanced by fever. In addition, the bactericidal activities of leukocytes may be increased by fever. Lastly, fever may enhance lymphocyte transformation.

The fever that accompanies noninfectious conditions apparently has little useful purpose and may aggravate the other clinical signs. However, fevers below 106°F in dogs and cats are potentially beneficial. Fevers above 106°F are potentially harmful to cellular metabolism. These fevers should be suppressed.

DIAGNOSTIC PLAN

Fever that results from acute inflammatory processes is usually easy to explain, and the cause is often found from the physical examination. Obscure or unexplained fevers are usually caused by chronic inflammatory processes that are difficult to define with routine physical or laboratory procedures. These have been defined as fevers of unknown origin; they have three characteristics: (1) a duration of at least 2 weeks, (2) temperature exceeding normal by 1.5°F on several occasions, and (3) obscure etiology. Four major disease categories should be considered when seeking the etiology of an obscure fever: (1) infectious

Text continues on p. 22

TABLE 2-1. Causes of Obscure Fever in Dogs

Diseases	Suggestive Clinical Signs	Diagnostic Clues	Special Tests
Generalized infections			
Bacterial endocarditis	Shifting leg lameness, joint effusion, heart murmur, cardiac arrhythmia, limb edema, history of recent surgical or medical illness	Changing cardiac murmur, splenomegaly, neutrophilic leukocytosis, microscopic hematuria, suppurative joint effusion, cardiac arrhythmia, hypoalbuminemia	Aerobic and anaerobic blood cultures, urine culture, joint fluid culture, ECG
Systemic mycoses	Chronic cough, chronic diarrhea, lymphadenopathy, suppurative skin nodules, history of endemic exposure, neurologic signs (head tilt, circling, paresis, ataxia)	Evidence of diffuse granulomatous pneumonia on thoracic radiographs; granulomatous skin lesions; chorioretinitis, anterior uveitis, occasional neurologic signs	Demonstration of organism in bronchial secretions, exudate, lymph node aspirates, or tissue biopsies; culture of organisms from tissue or exudates; occasional serology to confirm diagnosis
Ehrlichosis	Epistaxis, petechiation, pallor, chronic weight loss, anorexia, serous ocular and nasal discharges	Thrombocytopenia, leukopenia, anemia (nonregenerative); presence of brown dog ticks on patient or in its environment	Demonstration of intracytoplasmic morula in mononuclear cells from peripheral blood or bone marrow; indirect fluorescent antibody test for *Ehrlicha canis* antibody
Rocky Mountain Spotted Fever (*Rickettsia rickettsii*)	Chronic anorexia, weight loss, peripheral limb and scrotal edema	Thrombocytopenia, mild anemia, possible chronic renal failure; evidence of vasculitis; occasional vestibular signs	Serology for *R. rickettsii;* FA test on skin biopsy

Canine Lyme borreliosis	Anorexia, lethargy, lymphadenopathy, shifting lameness and joint pain	Recurrent, intermittent, non-erosive arthritis; area endemic for the vector (*Ixodes damnini, I. pacificus, I. scapularis*)	Histology, cytology, serologic tests
Toxoplasmosis	Variety of clinical syndromes including diarrhea, icterus, chronic cough, muscle pain and weakness, neurologic signs, chorioretinitis	Myositis, chronic liver failure, chronic pneumonia, chronic CNS signs, and chorioretinitis are suggestive	Serologic examination for toxoplasma antibodies and identification of organisms in affected tissue (muscle, liver, brain)

Localized infections

Pyothorax	Chronic cough, dyspnea, muffled lung sound	Pleural effusion on thoracic radiographs	Thoracentesis for fluid analysis and bacterial and fungal cultures
Chronic hepatic disease	Chronic weight loss, vomiting, anorexia; icterus may or may not be present; vague neurologic signs	Persistent increased concentrations of ALT, hypoalbuminemia, low BUN; radiographic evidence of small liver	Bile acid assay, ammonia tolerance test, hepatic biopsy
Chronic pyelonephritis	Signs absent unless disease progresses to chronic renal failure; few dogs may have anterior abdominal pain	Persistent hematuria, pyuria, and bacteria on cystocentesis urine specimens	Excretory urogram, renal biopsy, ultrasonography
Chronic prostatitis or abscess	Dysuria, hematuria, tenesmus	Enlarged or painful prostate found on rectal palpation	Prostatic ejaculate, prostatic biopsy, double-contrast cystography, ultrasonography

Immune-mediated disorders

Systemic lupus erythematosus	Shifting leg lameness, muscle pain or weakness, joint effusion and pain, anemia	Nonerosive suppurative polyarthritis, autoimmune hemolytic anemia, idiopathic thrombocytopenia, polymyositis, glomerulonephritis	ANA titer, LE prep, Coomb's test, antiplatelet antibody, renal biopsy

(*continued*)

TABLE 2-1. Causes of Obscure Fever in Dogs *(continued)*

Diseases	Suggestive Clinical Signs	Diagnostic Clues	Special Tests
Rheumatoid arthritis	Progressive lameness, joint pain, joint enlargement	Progressive erosive polyarthritis	Arthrocentesis, rheumatoid factor titer
Lymphosarcoma	Signs largely depend upon tissue or organ involved. Enlarged peripheral or abdominal nodes are very suggestive	Nonregenerative anemia, pancytopenia, neutropenia	Lymph node aspiration or biopsy, organ biopsy, bone marrow examination
Leukemia and other myeloproliferative disorders	No specific clinical signs	Evidence of leukemia in blood smear; possible association with anemia and thrombocytopenia	Bone marrow examination
Drug-induced disorders			
Tetracycline	None	Associated with antibiotic therapy	Response to withdrawal of medication

ECG, electrocardiogram; FA, fluorescent antibody; CNS, central nervous system; ALT, alanine aminotransferase; BUN, blood urea nitrogen; ANA, antinuclear antibody; LE, lupus erythematosus

TABLE 2-2. Causes of Obscure Fever in Cats

Diseases	Suggestive Clinical Signs	Diagnostic Clues	Special Tests
Systemic infections			
FeLV-related disease	Chronic infections, abortion, anemia, vomiting, diarrhea, dyspnea, anorexia and weight loss	Nonregenerative anemia, immature blood cells in peripheral circulation; pleural effusion, organ enlargement, abdominal masses	FeLV tests, bone marrow examination, organ biopsy
Feline infectious peritonitis	Dependent on form of disease present; abdominal and pleural effusion with effusive form; possible nonspecific neurologic signs, anterior uveitis, renal and liver failure with noneffusive form	Hyperglobulinemia, nonregenerative anemia, suppurative modified transudate in thorax or abdomen	FIP titer, liver or renal biopsy, examination of body cavity effusion, CSF examination
Toxoplasmosis	Dyspnea, icterus, enlarged abdominal lymph nodes, neurologic signs, iritis, retinitis, abortion	Bilirubinemia, diffuse pneumonia, leukopenia, anemia	Serology, demonstration of organism in tissue
Immune-mediated disorders			
Systemic lupus erythematosus	See Table 2-1	See Table 2-1	See Table 2-1
Polyarthritis	Progressive lameness, pain and enlargement of carpal and tarsal joints	Soft tissue swelling, degenerative joint disease, erosion of carpal or tarsal joints	FeLV test

FeLV, feline leukemia virus; FIP, feline infectious peritonitis; CSF, cerebrospinal fluid (bacterial, viral, fungal, rickettsial), (2) immune-mediated, (3) neoplastic, and (4) drug-induced. The diagnostic plan should be formulated to explore each of these potential causes. In the dog, bacterial endocarditis, systemic lupus erythematosus, and lymphoreticular neoplasia are the most common causes of obscure fever. The data base should include a complete blood count (CBC), biochemical profile, urine analysis, aerobic and anaerobic blood cultures, antinuclear antibody test, and thorough palpation of the abdomen and peripheral lymph nodes. Any abnormality detected in these procedures is followed up, since it may be a clue to the location of the fever-inducing disease.

The most common causes of obscure fever in cats are the systemic viral infections: feline infectious peritonitis and feline leukemia-related disease. The data base for a cat with obscure fever should include a CBC, biochemical profile, urine analysis, feline leukemia test, and feline infectious peritonitis titer. The eye grounds should be carefully examined since these viral infections may produce chorioretinitis. If these procedures are negative, blood cultures, antinuclear antibody (ANA) testing, and toxoplasmosis titers are indicated.

Tables 2-1 and 2-2 list the diagnostic criteria for the major diseases that produce obscure fevers in dogs and cats, respectively. The tables do not list every possible cause of obscure fever. Rather, the most common causes are described. Note that localized organ involvement (*i.e.,* hepatic abscess) may cause obscure fever. The initial data base must be carefully examined in order to identify clues that suggest disease in a particular organ. In addition, chest radiographs are useful for evaluation of the lungs and pleural space.

REFERENCES

1. Kluger MJ: Temperature regulation, fever, and disease. Int Rev Physiol 20:209, 1979
2. Pickering G: Regulation of body temperature in health and disease. Lancet 1(1):59, 1958
3. Dinarello CA, Wolff SM: Pathogenesis of fever in man. N Engl J Med 298:607–612, 1978
4. Chao P, Francis L, Atkins E: The release of an endogenous pyrogen from guinea pig leukocytes in vitro: A new model of investigating the role of lymphocytes in fevers induced by antigen in hosts with delayed hypersensitivity. J Exp Med 145:1288–1298, 1977

CHAPTER THREE

Disturbances of Food Intake: Anorexia and Polyphagia

Michael D. Lorenz

Disturbances of food intake are frequently the first signs observed by owners when an animal is ill. Owners tend to be very observant of their animals at meal time, since most people associate a good appetite with good health. Many systemic and even localized disease processes affect food intake. Unfortunately, a disturbance of food intake is not definitive of a specific disease process; rather, it represents a clinical finding common to many diseases. To meaningfully approach this problem, one should understand how food intake is regulated in the normal animal.

REGULATION OF FOOD INTAKE

Definitions

Hunger. Hunger means a craving or a desire to ingest food. In humans, hunger is often associated with intense rhythmic contractions of the stomach. In animals with the stomach removed, the apparent psychic sensations of hunger still occur and the animal still searches for an adequate food supply.

Appetite. In animals, appetite and hunger are often used as synonymous terms; however, appetite actually implies hunger for specific foods. Thus, appetite reflects the quality of food intake, whereas hunger reflects the quantity of food intake.

Satiety. Satiety is the opposite of hunger and results from a filling meal, particularly when the energy and nutritional requirements of the animal are fulfilled.

Neural Regulatory Mechanisms

Hypothalamic Centers for Hunger and Satiety. The hunger or feeding center is in the lateral hypothalamus. Stimulation of this area directly triggers the psychic drive to search for and ingest food and causes an animal to eat voraciously. Stimulation of the ventromedial nuclei of the hypothalamus causes complete satiety, even in the presence of stimuli that would normally incite hunger. The satiety center is believed to inhibit the feeding (hunger) center. Neuronal lesions that destroy the ventromedial hypothalamic nuclei cause complete disinterest in food and progressive weight loss. The function of the hypothalamic center is to control the quantity of food intake by exciting activity of lower centers.

Other Mechanisms for Neuronal Control of Feeding. Centers higher than the hypothalamus also affect feeding, presumably via their influence on the feeding and satiety centers. These higher centers include the amygdala and the cortical areas of the cortex. They are closely related to the hypothalamus. The amygdala is one of the major parts of the olfactory nervous system and probably couples appealing odors with the desire to eat. Although the amygdala may both stimulate and inhibit feeding, its major function appears to be in food discrimination (appetite). The cortical regions of the limbic system function in much the same manner as the amygdala, except that they play a major role in the animal's drive to search for food when hungry.

Nutritional and Alimentary Regulation of Food Intake

Nutritional Regulation. Nutritional regulation primarily refers to the maintenance of normal quantities of nutrients in the body. The body's nutritional status influences the feeding center in the hypothalamus. In general, inadequate nutritional stores cause feeding, whereas abundant nutritional stores favor satiety.

Effects of Glucose and Amino Acid Concentrations. The concentration of blood glucose has important effects on feeding. A raised blood glucose concentration increases the activity of the satiety center and secondarily decreases the activity of the hunger center. The satiety center concentrates glucose, whereas other areas of the hypothalamus do not. Increased blood amino acid concentrations also reduce feeding, although the effect is less dramatic than that of glucose.

Effects of Fat Metabolites. The amount of adipose tissue in the body inversely affects feeding: as the proportion of adipose tissue increases, the rate of feeding decreases. The quantity of free fatty acids and fat metabolites in the blood is directly proportional to the quantity of adipose stores in the body. It is likely that free fatty acids and other fat metabolites have a negative-feedback regulatory effect on feeding. This lipostatic mechanism may be a major factor in long-term feeding regulation.

Alimentary Regulation. Several short-term physiologic stimuli affect feeding. Although habits related to eating are important, factors related to the alimentary tract also play important roles.

Gastrointestinal Distention. Distention of the stomach and intestinal tract inhibits feeding. Nervous impulses arising from mechanoreceptors in the wall of the distended tract stimulate the satiety center and inhibit the feeding center. The inhibitory effects of stomach distention are not completely removed by denervating the stomach wall; overstretching the abdominal cavity and nutritional signals from the liver may also be involved. This possibility is significant since diseases of the liver, stomach, small intestine, and abdominal cavity are frequently associated with anorexia.

Cephalic Regulation. Various factors related to feeding, such as chewing, salivation, swallowing, and tasting, may also inhibit the feeding center after a certain amount of food has passed through the mouth. These cephalic factors decrease feeding in animals with esophageal fistulas that prevent food from entering the stomach.

ANOREXIA

Anorexia is the lack of, or disinterest in, the ingestion of food. In clinical terms, total anorexia is the pathologic absence of hunger. Its presence is associated with many disease processes that either directly inhibit or suppress activity in the hunger center or stimulate activity in the satiety center. Anorexia may be partial or complete, pathologic, physiologic, or psychologic. The major task confronting the veterinary clinician is to determine whether anorexia is pathologic or physiologic/psychologic in origin.

Pathophysiology

Many diseases or disorders produce anorexia because they disturb the normal neurologic, endocrinologic, and mechanical mechanisms that control hunger and feeding. In certain disorders such as cancer, the underlying mechanisms are not totally understood. The basic causes of anorexia have been identified (see Display, Classification for the Causes of Anorexia). This classification scheme may be somewhat artificial, since most diseases produce a combination of factors leading to anorexia. However, it does provide a logical method for finding the cause of anorexia, particularly when other manifestations of the disease are obscure.

Primary Anorexia. For the purpose of diagnosis, it is convenient to initially think of anorexia in three general categories: primary, secondary, or pseudo. Primary anorexia results from direct disease processes involving the appetite centers of the hypothalamus or from psychologic disorders that directly affect neural control of feeding.

Diseases or disorders that destroy or structurally inhibit the appetite center are listed in the Classification for the Causes of Anorexia. Destruction of the appetite center results in complete anorexia. Other neurologic signs related to hypothalamic dysfunction may be present if the lesion is of sufficient size to

Classification for the Causes of Anorexia

I. Primary anorexia
  A. Neurologic dysfunction
    1. Increased intracranial pressure
      a. Cerebral edema
      b. Hydrocephalus
    2. Intracranial pain
    3. Hypothalamic disorders
      a. Neoplasia
      b. Infection
      c. Trauma
  B. Psychologic disorders
    1. Anorexia nervosa (humans)
    2. Unpalatable diets
    3. Stress
    4. Altered daily routine or environment
  C. Loss of smell
II. Secondary anorexia
  A. Pain
    1. Abdominal
    2. Thoracic
    3. Musculoskeletal
    4. Urogenital
  B. Abdominal organ disorders
    1. Enlargement or serosal distention
    2. Inflammation
    3. Neoplasia
  C. Toxic agents
    1. Exogenous
      a. Drugs
      b. Poisons
    2. Endogenous
      a. From organ failure (*e.g.,* metabolic wastes)
      b. Endotoxin
      c. Pyrogens (fever)?
  D. Endocrine
    1. Adrenal insufficiency
    2. Hypercalcemia
  E. Neoplasia of any site
  F. Infectious disease
  G. Miscellaneous
    1. Cardiac failure
    2. Malnutrition with ketosis
    3. Motion sickness
    4. High environmental temperature
    5. Autoimmune disease

III. Pseudoanorexia
   A. Disorders of the oral cavity
      1. Abscessed or broken teeth
      2. Foreign bodies
      3. Stomatitis, pharyngitis, tonsillitis
   B. Hypoglossal paralysis
   C. Mandibular paralysis
   D. Maxillary or mandibular fractures or dislocations
   E. Retrobulbar disease
      1. Abscess
      2. Inflammation
      3. Neoplasia
   F. Blindness
   G. Esophagitis
   H. Tetanus
   I. Temporomandibular myositis

disrupt other neuronal centers in the brain stem. A thorough neurologic examination may detect these abnormalities. This form of anorexia is relatively uncommon in dogs and cats.

Psychologic disorders, although more easily identified in humans, are extremely difficult to differentiate from other causes of anorexia in animals. The psychologic causes of anorexia listed in this chapter are probably common except for anorexia nervosa, which is not documented in small animals. Conditions that evoke fear, anxiety, and depression may result in anorexia. Changes of environment that disrupt normal daily activities may cause anorexia in animals, especially cats.

Severe pain arising from any part of the body may cause anorexia, since it may inhibit the appetite center. Intracranial pain, that is, headache, is probably most important; however, it is nearly impossible to document in animals. When musculoskeletal diseases are present, the administration of analgesics may greatly improve appetite.

Secondary Anorexia. The diseases that produce secondary anorexia occur in areas outside the brain and affect the neural and endocrine control of hunger. In many diseases, compounds may be produced that inhibit the activity of the appetite center. This category is the major cause of anorexia in animals. It must be recognized that anorexia is commonly associated with nausea or vomiting. This is not surprising, since these centers are probably neuronally interconnected. The type of stimuli for anorexia, nausea, and vomiting may be identical, the only difference being the magnitude of the stimulation.

Pain may cause anorexia by inhibiting neuronal stimulation of the appetite center. Pain also produces psychologic abnormalities that inhibit hunger.

Intra-abdominal disorders such as distention of the serosa or capsule of various abdominal organs cause anorexia via neuronal pathways or mechanisms that also produce vomiting. Distention of the stomach and small intestine (most significantly the duodenum) from obstruction are common causes of anorexia. Splanchnic sympathectomy eliminates vomiting from intestinal obstruction; however, vagotomy is required to eliminate the associated anorexia.[4]

Inflammatory involvement of virtually any abdominal organ, pelvic organ, or visceral peritoneum may produce anorexia via neural pathways to the brain stem that inhibit appetite. Inflammatory diseases of the liver, pancreas, stomach, small intestine, and kidneys are the most commonly encountered causes of anorexia, other than vomiting.[4] Severe uterine enlargement, as occurs in pyometra or late pregnancy, may also cause anorexia through stimulation of neuronal pathways that eventually inhibit the appetite center. In pyometra, toxic compounds from the uterus may also inhibit the appetite center.

Toxic agents, either endogenous or exogenous, are common causes of anorexia and nausea. Toxins produce anorexia by two primary mechanisms: directly by affecting the appetite centers and indirectly through involvement of intraabdominal organs, creating inflammation, necrosis, and organ failure. Many drugs and toxins apparently stimulate the chemoreceptor trigger zone in the medulla, producing vomiting, nausea, and anorexia. Digitalis works through this mechanism, whereas amphetamines directly inhibit the appetite center.

Endogenously produced metabolic wastes that result from organ failure (such as uremia from renal failure, hyperammonemia from liver failure, and ketosis from insulin deficiency) are serious causes of anorexia and its closely related problems of nausea and vomiting. Microgram quantities of bacterial enterotoxin are capable of inducing anorexia and may partially explain the anorexia common to a variety of bacterial infection.[4] One must wonder if endogenous pyrogen also has the property of inhibiting the appetite center, since anorexia is so commonly associated with fever from bacterial, viral, mycotic, and autoimmune diseases.

Endocrine disorders (deficiency of glucocorticoid hormones from adrenal gland failure) commonly result in anorexia. The exact mechanism is unknown. In classic Addison's disease, azotemia and hyperkalemia contribute to the anorexia of glucocorticoid deficiency. Hypercalcemia from any cause produces anorexia by an unknown mechanism.

Neoplastic disease is a serious cause of anorexia in animals. In many patients, anorexia is the primary complaint and may not be associated with other clinical signs. Cancer in animals produces peptides or nucleotides that inhibit feeding regulators.[5] Rats with hyperphagia (produced by destruction of the satiety center) develop anorexia within 2 weeks of neoplastic transformation.[1] Liberation of heat from cancer cells and altered taste sensation also appear to promote anorexia in cancer patients.[3] Cancer of intraabdominal organs may produce anorexia by any of the previously described mechanisms.

Cancer is a prime rule out for all patients with chronic anorexia. Other clinical signs may be lacking, which makes diagnosis extremely difficult in some cases.

Miscellaneous causes, including cardiac failure, prolonged malnutrition with ketosis, motion sickness, and inner ear disease, are causes of anorexia, nausea, and sometimes vomiting. Loss of smell, although rare, should not be overlooked as an obscure cause of anorexia.

Pseudoanorexia. Diseases in this category do not directly suppress the desire to eat. Rather, they result in the inability to pick up, masticate, or swallow food. These conditions are frequently so painful that animals will not eat even though they are hungry. The causes of pseudoanorexia listed in the Classification for Causes of Anorexia are usually identified by a thorough physical examination.

Diagnostic Plan

Since anorexia is a common sign of many diseases, the approach to its diagnosis is the identification of the underlying cause. The physical examination is extremely important, since most causes of pseudoanorexia can be identified by observation of the animal when it is presented with food and by careful examination of the head, mouth, and throat. These animals may try to eat but experience pain or discomfort that prevents normal eating. Examination of the head may reveal pain when the jaws are opened or the masticatory muscles are palpated. Oral examination can reveal foreign bodies, tooth disease, stomatitis, or hypoglossal paralysis. Dysphagia and regurgitation are common problems associated with pharyngeal and esophageal disorders.

When no abnormalities of the head or oral cavity are detected, the next diagnostic step is to uncover causes of secondary anorexia. Thorough abdominal palpation is critical and may reveal abnormalities that dictate future diagnostic plans. When the physical examination is unrevealing, a complete blood count (CBC), biochemical profile, and urine analysis should be performed to rule out a variety of systemic, metabolic, and endocrinologic diseases. Abnormalities detected in these procedures may dictate future courses of action.

When no abnormalities are detected in the laboratory procedures just described, the causes of primary anorexia are considered. A thorough neurologic examination is done, with attention given to subtle abnormalities. If the neurologic examination is normal, one then considers the possibility of a psychologic disorder. The history may provide clues to the cause.

The diagnostic plan for anorexia is schematically represented in Figure 3-1.

POLYPHAGIA

Polyphagia (ravenous appetite) is the consumption of food in excess of normal estimated or calculated intake. It must be differentiated from pica, the craving for abnormal substances (for example, soil or plants). As with anorexia, polyphagia may be physiologic, pathologic, or psychologic in origin. Overfeeding that results in obesity may be a form of psychologically acquired polyphagia.

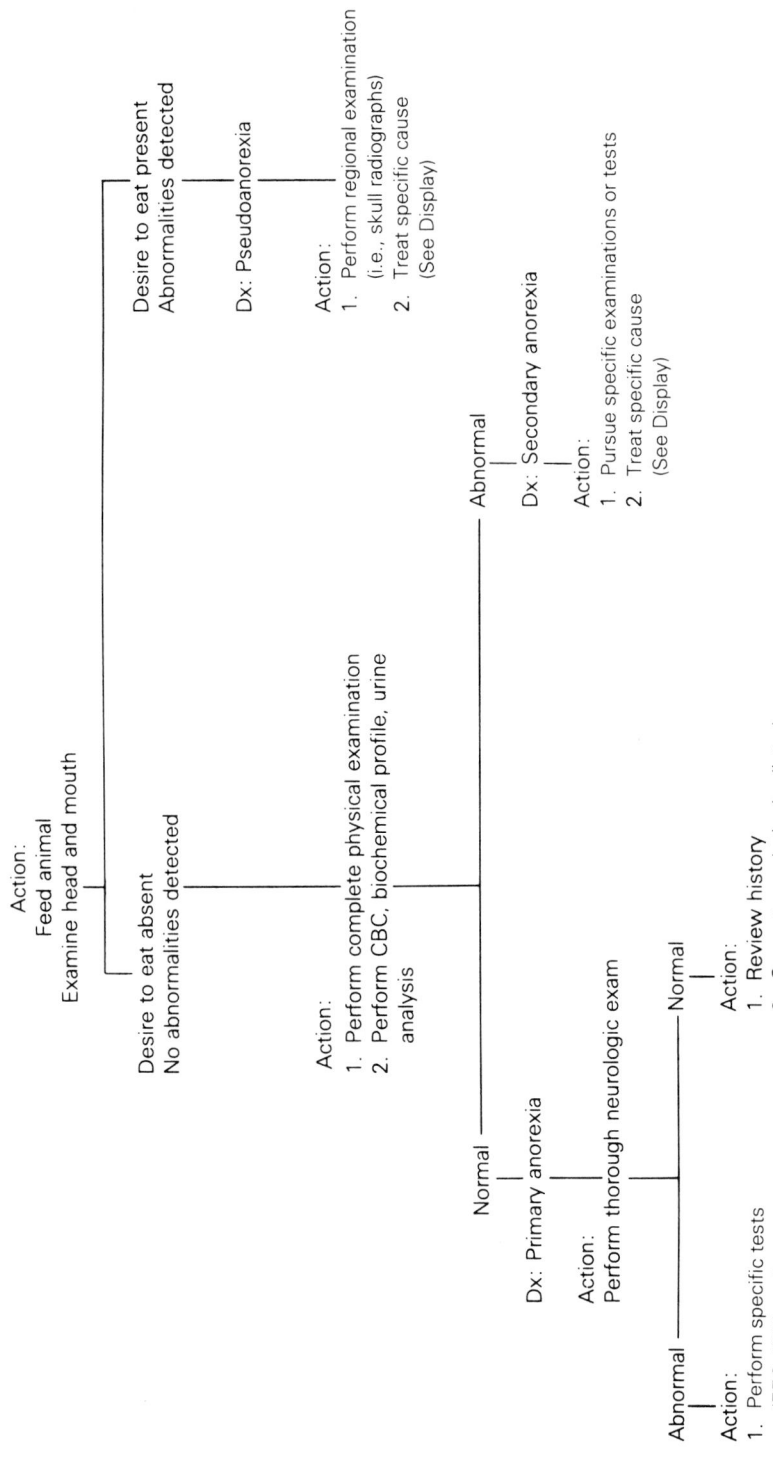

FIGURE 3-1. Algorithm for the diagnosis of anorexia.

Pathophysiology

In small animals, polyphagia usually results secondarily from diseases that create a negative caloric balance or an increased metabolic rate. These diseases cause inhibition of the satiety center and stimulation of the appetite center. Primary examples include hyperadrenocorticism, hyperthyroidism, diabetes mellitus, pancreatic exocrine insufficiency, and primary intestinal malabsorption. These diseases result in muscle wasting as well as polyphagia. Certain drugs such as glucocorticoid hormones and the anticonvulsants phenobarbital, primidone, and phenytoin may directly stimulate the appetite center.

Primary polyphagias are disorders that directly destroy the satiety center in the brain stem and result in severe obesity. These conditions are rarely encountered. Overfeeding that leads to obesity is another form of primary polyphagia. This condition is probably acquired through feeding habits, although a genetic basis may also be responsible in certain breeds. The obese animal appears to lose one part of the feeding regulatory mechanism. In the normal animal, the accumulation of fat stores in the body tends to decrease feeding, whereas in the obese animal, feeding continues despite the obvious accumulation of adipose tissue.

Diagnostic Plan

The causes of polyphagia are classified as primary or secondary (see Display, Classification and Causes of Polyphagia). The secondary causes of polyphagia are most common. All of the causes of polyphagia result in weight gain, except those that develop secondary to an increased metabolic rate or a catabolic disorder. The initial diagnostic step is to determine if the animal's weight has decreased, increased, or remained the same. If weight loss has occurred, the clinician should then search for evidence of caloric deficiency diseases or disorders that result in an increased metabolic rate. The history and physical examination usually provide evidence of associated probems such as polydipsia, polyuria, diarrhea, nervousness, and accelerated heart rate. A CBC, urine analysis, and biochemical profile can confirm a diagnosis of diabetes mellitus and hypoglycemia. Specialized tests such as serum thyroxine determinations and plasma cortisol assay are usually needed to confirm a diagnosis of hyperthyroidism and hyperadrenocorticism, respectively.

Animals with digestive disorders that produce polyphagia usually have diarrhea or bulky, malformed stools. Trypsin-like immunoreactivity, serum folate, and serum cobalamin assays are required to differentiate pancreatic exocrine insufficiency from primary intestinal malabsorption.

If weight has increased, attention should be given to the causes of primary polyphagia or the administration of appetite-stimulating drugs. The most common cause in this category is overeating or overfeeding. The history may be helpful, although most owners deny that they overfeed their pets.

Classification and Causes of Polyphagia

I. Primary polyphagia
   A. Destruction of satiety center (rare)
      1. Neoplasia
      2. Trauma
      3. Infection
   B. Psychologic
      1. Overfeeding
II. Secondary polyphagia
   A. Increased metabolic rate
      1. Hyperthyroidism
      2. Low environmental temperature
   B. Catabolic disorders
      1. Hyperadrenocorticism
      2. Diabetes mellitus
      3. Pancreatic exocrine insufficiency
      4. Malabsorption syndrome
      5. Hypoglycemia
      6. Low calorie diet
   C. Drug-induced polyphagia
      1. Glucocorticoid hormones
      2. Anticonvulsants

REFERENCES

1. Anand B: Nervous regulation of food intake. Physiol Rev 41:667–708, 1961
2. Boyar RM: Endocrine changes in anorexia nervosa. Med Clin North Am 62:297, 1978
3. Crow SE, Oliver J: Cancer cachexia. Comp Cont Ed 3:682, 1981
4. McGuigan JE: Anorexia, nausea, and vomiting. In MacBryde CM, Blacklow RS (eds): Signs and Symptoms, 5th ed. Philadelphia, JB Lippincott, 1970
5. Theologides A: Anorexia-producing intermediary metabolites. Am J Clin Nutr 29: 552–558, 1976

CHAPTER FOUR

Episodic Weakness

Michael D. Lorenz

PROBLEM DEFINITION AND RECOGNITION

Weakness that occurs with exercise and dissipates with rest is termed *episodic.* It is recognized as early fatigue with mild exercise, although in some cases, more vigorous or prolonged exercise may be needed to induce the problem. Signs of weakness include an ataxic or paretic gait, severe panting, reluctance to walk or run, lying down, and collapse. The animal may be alert or depressed. Following rest, muscle strength improves greatly.

PATHOPHYSIOLOGY

The correct approach to diagnosis of this problem is based on knowledge of the normal physiology of muscle function during exercise and at rest. In addition, the function of other organs that support muscle metabolism (*i.e.*, by supplying oxygen, calories) during exercise must be considered. The astute clinician is able to quickly and accurately recall the neuromuscular events that control muscle contraction and relate these to cardiopulmonary support.

Muscle and nerve are tissues that generate electrical activity, called action potentials, along the cell membranes. Action potentials are generated by the movement of sodium and potassium ions through the cell membrane. The movement of these ions is controlled by calcium. Therefore diseases that cause electrolyte imbalances may produce episodic weakness as their primary clinical manifestation. Table 4-1 describes the effects of various electrolyte disturbances on the production of action potentials and the resultant clinical signs or problems.

In the normal animal, skeletal muscle fibers are stimulated to contract by the lower motor neurons. The muscle fibers are connected to the nervous system via neuromuscular junctions (also called motor endplates). The motor endplate transmits electrical activity (action potentials) from the axon to the muscle fiber. Acetylcholine is the neurotransmitting agent released in the motor endplate that initiates action potentials on the muscle fiber membrane. The release of acetylcholine is modulated by calcium ion (see Table 4-1) and is inactivated by acetylcholine esterase enzyme. Thus, disturbances of calcium homeostasis or

TABLE 4-1. Effects of Electrolyte Imbalance on the Production of Action Potentials, Motor Endplate Function, and Muscle Function

Disorder	Effect on Action Potential Production	Effect on Motor Endplate Function	Effect on Muscle Contraction	Primary Clinical Signs or Problems
Hyperkalemia	Decreased intensity due to hypopolarization of membrane Decreased membrane potential	None	1. Decreased strength of contraction 2. Block conduction of cardiac impulse	Muscle weakness, bradycardia, sinoatrial arrest
Hypokalemia	Membrane hyperpolarization	None	Decreased strength of contraction	Muscle weakness
Hypocalcemia	Increased membrane excitability Spontaneous impulses	Decreased release of acetylcholine	Decreased strength of contraction	Tetany
Hypercalcemia	Decreased membrane excitability	Increased release of acetylcholine	Possible spontaneous contractions; possible decrease of muscle strength	Muscle fasciculations and muscle weakness

disorders that affect the activity of acetylcholine may adversely affect neuromuscular transmission and can produce episodic weakness.

Special receptors on the muscle fiber membrane bind the acetylcholine released by the axonal foot process. Although this binding occurs for only a few milliseconds, it creates an action potential on the muscle fiber. Normally, three to four times more electrical activity is generated than needed to stimulate muscle contraction. This is the "safety factor" of the neuromuscular junction; "fatigue" of this synapse almost never occurs under normal exercise conditions. Myasthenia gravis is an autoimmune disease affecting the acetylcholine receptors. In myasthenia gravis, the number of effective acetylcholine receptors is reduced so that normal muscle contractions may occur at rest, but during work or exercise the fibers easily fatigue because effective electrical stimulation cannot be sustained.

An action potential, generated on the surface of muscle fibers, is conducted into the cell, where it stimulates the release of calcium ions stored within the sarcoplasmic reticulum. Calcium ions then stimulate contraction of the myofibrils. A physiologic pump within the muscle cell stores calcium ions in the sarcoplasmic reticulum, and this mechanism keeps the concentration of calcium ions in the myofibrils at an extremely low level except during periods of excitation. Therefore, the concentration of calcium ions within the body is critical for normal muscle contraction. Disturbances of calcium homeostasis at this level may result in episodic weakness.

During muscle contraction, much energy is required. The primary initial source of energy is muscle glycogen, which is utilized by the process of aerobic glycolysis. Muscle glycogen can be rapidly expended during exercise; blood glucose then becomes the primary source of energy. In hypoglycemic conditions, this source of energy is not available; therefore, episodic weakness is a common problem associated with hypoglycemia.

Aerobic glycolysis is the most effective means of generating energy within skeletal muscle. In conditions of reduced oxygen tension (*e.g.*, reduced oxygen in the blood, reduced hemoglobin concentration) or with vigorous exercise, insufficient oxygen is present to maintain aerobic glycolysis. Anaerobic glycolysis, although less effective, generates some energy for muscle function. High levels of lactic acid are produced, which may cause disturbances within the muscle cell. Therefore, conditions of decreased oxygen concentration in the blood may result in episodic weakness, since, during exercise, the increased metabolic demands in muscle tissue cannot be met.

Primary muscle disease such as early degenerative disorders (myopathies) or inflammation (myositis) may cause episodic weakness via damage to any of the steps necessary for normal muscle contraction. These diseases may asymmetrically affect muscle fibers within a muscle or a group of muscles. Thus, sufficient function may be maintained to sustain mild work; however, the increased demands of exercise cannot be sustained because insufficient numbers of healthy fibers are present for recruitment.

TABLE 4-2. Causes of Episodic Weakness

Category	Condition	Documentation	Underlying Disease	Specific Diagnostic Test
Metabolic	Hyperkalemia	Serum K^+	Adrenal insufficiency	Plasma cortisol profile
			Severe acidosis	Blood gases and pH
			Severe renal failure	Blood urea nitrogen
				Urinalysis
				Complete blood count
	Hypokalemia	Serum K^+	Severe vomiting	See Chapter 32
			Diuretic therapy	
	Hypocalcemia	Serum Ca^{++}	Hypoparathyroidism	Urine, calcium, and phosphorus
				Serum phosphorus
				PTH assay
	Hypercalcemia	Serum Ca^{++}	Pseudohyperparathyroidism (Lymphosarcoma)	Complete blood count
				Lymph node aspirate or biopsy
			Primary Hyperparathyroidism (Parathyroid tumor)	Serum PTH assay
				Presence of parathyroid mass
				Urine calcium and phosphorus
				Serum phosphorus

	Hypoglycemia	Fasting blood glucose	Functional beta cell carcinoma	Insulin-glucose ratio Glucagon response test
			Adrenal insufficiency	Plasma cortisol profile Serum electrolytes
			Glycogen storage disease	Glucagon response test Tissue biopsy (liver, muscle)
Cardiovascular	Arrhythmias	ECG		See Chapter 21
	Conduction failure	ECG		See Chapter 21
	Congestive heart failure	Thoracic radiographs Ultrasonography	Dirofilaria immitis	Knott's test Occult heartworm test ECG
Neuromuscular	Myasthenia gravis	Repetitive nerve stimulation	Thymoma Autoimmune disease	Tensilon response test Muscle receptor antibody test
	Polymyositis	Serum muscle enzyme levels Muscle biopsy EMG	Eosinophilic myositis Autoimmune disease (systemic lupus) Toxoplasmosis	Biopsy Antinuclear antibody Direct FA of muscle Biopsy, serology
	Feline hypolalemic polymyopathy	Serum K$^+$ less than 3.5 mEq/l Increased creatine kinase EMG Muscle biopsy	Renal dysfunction	See documentation

PTH, parathyroid hormone; ECG, electrocardiogram; FA, fluorescent antibody; EMG, electromyogram

Minimum Data Base for Episodic Weakness

1. History
2. Physical examination; include neurologic examination
3. Laboratory
   a. Complete blood count
   b. Urine analysis
   c. Complete biochemical profile
   d. Knott's test
4. Electrocardiogram
5. Thoracic radiographs

DIAGNOSTIC PLAN

The diseases or disorders that cause episodic weakness are listed in Table 4-2. The diagnostic plan is based on the mechanisms that cause this problem plus knowledge of their relative frequency of occurrence in dogs and cats.

The history and physical examination may provide clues to the underlying mechanism or disease. In this regard, the history and physical examination usually provide clues of cardiopulmonary disease (*e.g.,* coughing, cyanosis, edema, ascites, pale muscle membranes, abnormal pulse, heart murmurs [see related chapters]). A neurologic examination is valuable, since organic disease of the nervous system usually creates constant signs of weakness (see Chapter 47), and signs may be localizing to a segment or region of the nervous system. Except for depression or, rarely, seizures, the neurologic examination is usually normal with the diseases listed in Table 4-2. Muscle palpation is very important since primary muscle diseases may cause pain (see Chapter 46) and/or atrophy. The presence of polysystemic signs, vomiting, polydipsia-polyuria, anorexia, or weight loss may indicate the presence of a metabolic disorder. A minimum data base (see Display, Minimum Data Base for Episodic Weakness) should be collected to evaluate this problem.

Several diseases that cause episodic weakness may create problems suggestive of other diseases. For instance, polymyositis may cause acquired megaesophagus and thus regurgitation (see Chapter 32). The regurgitation may cause aspiration pneumonia and clinical signs of severe pulmonary disease. The pulmonary disease may be assumed to be the cause of the episodic weakness, and thus the primary disease can be easily overlooked.

CHAPTER FIVE

Polydipsia and Polyuria

Michael D. Lorenz

Polydipsia and polyuria (P&P) are associated clinical signs that commonly occur in small animals as the result of several different polysystemic disorders. In most cases, these signs suggest a disorder in water homeostasis that has disturbed normal plasma and cellular osmolality. Polyuria is the increased production of urine usually of low specific gravity. Polydipsia is increased thirst. In most situations, polydipsia is a compensatory mechanism for polyuria; however, in rare instances, polydipsia is the primary event and polyuria is a compensatory mechanism for excretion of the excess water load. This chapter provides a concise review of P&P and outlines a diagnostic plan for animals with these problems.

Normal regulation of body fluid volume and osmolality depends upon a balance between water loss and water intake. Drinking and urine loss are the most important mechanisms for regulation of body water. If increased drinking is not compensated by increased urine loss, body water must increase, with resulting cellular overhydration. Conversely, if urine loss is not compensated by increased drinking, body water decreases, with resulting cellular dehydration. Water and sodium regulation are closely interrelated, since extracellular fluid osmolality is almost totally determined by sodium concentration. Fluid osmolality and, ultimately, body fluid volume are controlled by neuroendocrinologic and renal mechanisms. To logically pursue the problems of P&P, clinicians should understand these basic mechanisms.

THE THIRST MECHANISM

Thirst is the conscious desire for water. The stimulus to drink is generated in the thirst center in the hypothalamus. The involved neurons lie in close proximity to the antidiuretic hormone (ADH) control centers and are controlled by extracellular fluid osmolality. A 2% increase in osmolality is sufficient to stimulate thirst. The basic stimulus that excites the thirst center is intracellular dehydration; this mechanism has been termed *primary thirst.* A second stimulus for the thirst center arises from volume and pressure receptors located in the left atrium and large vessels. A reduction in blood volume by 8% to 10% can induce thirst by neural stimulation of the thirst center from these pressure receptors. Although the role of these thirst center stimuli is well understood, these are not the primary mechanisms that determine water intake in normal animals. *Secondary thirst* is a poorly understood mechanism that anticipates water needs before actual deficiencies occur. The stimulus for drinking is from oropharyngeal cues or is related to the circadian rhythm of eating. It is well established that in 5 minutes animals will drink nearly the exact amount of water required to relieve anticipated or existing dehydration, even though it may take hours for this fluid load to be distributed within the body. Evidence that supports the concept of secondary thirst includes thirst despite lack of dehydration or maximally concentrated urine.

Other mechanisms may also stimulate the thirst center. For example, both renin and angiotensin stimulate thirst by direct action on neurons in the thirst center. Compounds with this capacity are termed *dipsinogenic.* This mechanism may be important in certain diseases in which these substances accumulate in large amounts.

Pathologic Thirst

Primary polydipsia is increased drinking not explained as a compensatory mechanism for excessive fluid loss. Among the causes of pathologic thirst (see Display, Causes of Pathologic Thirst), compulsive water drinking (pseudopsychogenic polydipsia) is probably most important in animals. Although the cause is not known, psychogenic factors such as anxiety or boredom may be involved. Water intake exceeds body needs, and a compensatory polyuria results. Unlike in humans, osmoregulation remains present in affected animals. When animals are deprived of water, urine is concentrated and thirst decreases when ADH is administered. The condition is treated by controlling water intake and eliminating predisposing factors.

Causes of Pathologic Thirst

- Neuronal irritation (hypothalamic)
    Tumor
    Trauma
    Inflammation
- Compulsive water drinking (pseudopsychogenic polydipsia)
- Increased plasma renin
- Other
    Hypercalcemia
    Thoracic caval constriction

RENAL CONCENTRATING MECHANISMS

The structure of the kidney enables animals to excrete a large solute load and still conserve most of the water that appears in glomerular filtrate. In water excess, urine is diluted and urine volume increases. In water deficit, the opposite process occurs. In a 25-pound (10.5-kg) dog, 68 liters of fluid are filtered by the glomeruli each day; however, less than 500 ml is excreted as urine. Urine volume control is primarily regulated by the ADH and countercurrent systems.

The ADH-Osmoreceptor Control System

Water homeostasis is largely dependent upon extracellular fluid sodium concentration: sodium concentration is inversely related to water content but directly related to fluid osmolality. Osmolality of extracellular fluid is regulated by thirst and the ADH feedback control mechanisms. ADH is produced by specialized neurons in the hypothalamus and is stored in nerve endings in the neurohypophysis. Large amounts of ADH are normally stored in these nerve endings, called *pituicytes*. Increased extracellular fluid osmolality stimulates the osmoreceptors in the hypothalamus to release ADH from the pituicytes. Under the influence of ADH, the permeability of the collecting tubules to water is greatly enhanced. Water is then reabsorbed along concentration gradients established in the renal medulla by the countercurrent system. The increased absorption of water conserves fluid while allowing the excretion of solute waste in the urine. The retention of water in relationship to sodium decreases the osmolality, lowering the output of ADH. When the extracellular fluid becomes hypoosmotic, less ADH is released. Excess water is lost in the urine, increasing the osmolality to normal. A 2% change in osmolality increases or decreases ADH secretion. An 8% decrease in blood pressure or volume also stimulates ADH secretion. Volume receptors in the left atrium and the carotid sinus pressure receptors are responsible for these effects on ADH secretion.

The mechanism of ADH action to increase tubular permeability to water is not known. In addition to increasing water reabsorption, ADH also increases the reabsorption of urea. This is an important step in the renal urea cycle that influences renal medullary hypertonicity.

The Countercurrent System

Water reabsorption from glomerular filtrate is dependent upon a high osmotic gradient in the renal medulla. Two solutes, sodium chloride and urea, are primarily responsible for maintaining this osmotic gradient. Large concentrations of sodium chloride remain in the renal medulla for two reasons: (1) sluggish blood flow in the peritubular capillaries (vasa recta) and (2) a countercurrent multiplier system at work in the loop of Henle (LH) and vasa recta. Urea also becomes highly concentrated in the renal medulla and may contribute nearly half of the hypertonicity of the inner medulla.

Renal Tubular Functions

Glomerular filtrate is *isosthenuric,* meaning it has a specific gravity equal to that of plasma (1.008 to 1.012). Tubular functions (passive and active reabsorption) dilute or concentrate this filtrate depending upon body needs. In most cases, the final product, urine, is more concentrated than glomerular filtrate.

Nearly 75% of glomerular filtrate is reabsorbed in the proximal tubule regardless of need. In a 25-pound (10.5-kg) dog filtering 68 liters a day, 51 liters of fluid are reabsorbed in the proximal tubule and 17 liters pass on to the remainder of the renal tubule. Filtered water is passively reabsorbed in the proximal tubule following osmotic gradients produced by the active transport of solutes such as glucose, sodium, and amino acids. Diseases that affect the proximal tubule (primary renal disease, renal glycosuria, Fanconi syndrome) or those that result in solute loads that overwhelm proximal tubule absorptive capacity (diabetes mellitus) create an osmotic diuresis by overloading absorptive functions in the LH and distal tubules. An obligatory water loss accompanies this increased solute excretion.

Fluid entering the LH has a volume of 17 liters and is nearly isotonic (specific gravity, 1.008 to 1.012). The LH generates a high concentration gradient within the renal medulla, which is necessary for water conservation and urine concentration. The ascending limb of the LH generates solute-free water. Fluid leaving the LH has a volume of 12 liters and a specific gravity of 1.003 (*hyposthenuric*). Thus, the LH dilutes tubular fluid to maintain renal medullary hypertonicity while absorbing approximately 7% of the glomerular filtrate. Urine specific gravities less than 1.008 suggest normal tubular function through the LH, since urine is diluted below isosthenuria at this level. Abnormal LH function results in polyuria because of decreased renal medullary hypertonicity. Disorders that affect LH function include primary renal disease and diuretics such as furosemide.

The final steps in water conservation occur in the distal tubule and collecting ducts. In the distal tubule, sodium and water are reabsorbed while potassium is actively secreted. This process is strongly enhanced by aldosterone. Fluid leaving the distal tubules has a specific gravity of 1.003 to 1.010 and a volume of 8 liters. Approximately 6% of the tubular fluid is reabsorbed in the distal tubule. Epithelial cells in the collecting ducts are relatively impermeable to water unless stimulated by ADH. In the absence of ADH, tubular fluid becomes somewhat more dilute because of sodium and other solute reabsorption. In the presence of ADH, water is reabsorbed; this process is responsible for water homeostasis in normal animals. The collecting ducts in our 25-pound example dog can reabsorb nearly 8 liters of fluid, depending upon body needs.

Table 5-1 illustrates the effects of ADH relative to urine volume and specific gravity. As urine specific gravity doubles, urine volume is halved. Thus, when

TABLE 5-1. Urine Specific Gravity Versus Urine
Volume in ADH Deficiency

Specific Gravity	Volume	Specific Gravity	Volume
1.001	5 liters	1.010	500 ml
1.002	2.5 liters	1.020	250 ml
1.003	1.7 liters	1.040	125 ml
1.004	1.25 liters	1.050	100 ml
1.005	1.0 liters		

urine is hyposthenuric, small changes in specific gravity have profound effects on urine volume. However, as urine becomes hyperosmotic, large changes in specific gravity have smaller effects on urine volume. With ADH deficiency, profound polyuria occurs because the urine has a very low specific gravity.

Several disorders produce P&P by disturbing distal and collecting tubular function. These include primary renal disease, diabetes insipidus, pyometra, hyperadrenocorticism, hypoadrenocorticism, liver failure, and hypercalcemia. Glucocorticoid and spironolactone therapy also has these effects.

Medullary Washout

Certain diseases produce polyuria by decreasing renal medullary osmotic gradients. Failure of the sodium chloride pump in the LH is a primary mechanism for this abnormality. Failure of the urea cycle or urea depletion, as occurs in chronic liver failure, may also decrease renal medullary hypertonicity. Prolonged P&P produces medullary washout by increasing the rate of fluid flow through the LH and vasa recta. This decreases the effectiveness of the countercurrent mechanism and results in the production of isotonic urine. The importance of medullary washout is discussed more thoroughly later in this chapter in regard to its effect on urine concentration tests.

APPLIED PATHOPHYSIOLOGY

As stated previously, many diseases produce polyuria because they affect renal concentrating mechanisms or stimulate primary polydipsia. Table 5-2 lists the various diseases that produce P&P and summarizes the altered physiology that actually produces these signs.

DIAGNOSTIC PLAN

The evaluation of an animal that may have P&P proceeds in four steps: (1) documentation that the problems exist; (2) inspection of the data base for clues to diagnosis; (3) performance of urine concentration tests; and (4) performance

TABLE 5-2. Pathogenesis of Polydipsia and Polyuria in Various Diseases and Iatrogenic Disorders

	Major Abnormality	Mechanism of P&P
Spontaneous disease or abnormality		
Diabetes insipidus		
Neurogenic	Hypothalamic or posterior pituitary injury	Deficiency of ADH
Nephrogenic	Tubular enzyme deficiency or receptor unresponsiveness	Tubule unresponsive to ADH
Diabetes mellitus	Insulin deficiency→hyperglycemia	Glycosuria: excessive absorbable solute in proximal tubule
Hyperadrenocorticism	Excessive endogenous production of glucocorticoids; adrenal cortical hyperplasia or neoplasia	ADH inhibition at collecting duct; may inhibit ADH release
Hypercalcemia (Hypercalcemic nephropathy)	Parathyroid tumor: excessive parathormone Lymphosarcoma: osteoclast stimulating factor	Early: inhibition of ADH Stimulation of thirst Late: mineralization of kidney; chronic renal failure
Hyperthyroidism	Autonomously functioning thyroid tumor→excessive thyroid hormones	Uncertain
Liver failure	Liver insufficiency ↓ Urea synthesis and ↓ renin catabolism	↓ Renal medullary hypertonicity Dipsinogenic activity of renin

44

Medullary washout	Loss of countercurrent multiplier system (various disorders)	↓ Renal medullary hypertonicity
Pyometra	Endometrial hyperplasia Bacterial endotoxins??	Tubule unresponsive to ADH
Pseudopsychogenic polydipsia (compulsive water drinking)	Primary polydipsia	Compensatory polyuria Medullary washout??
Renal disease	Renal tubular dysfunction Renal medullary dysfunction	Alteration of several renal concentrating mechanisms
Iatrogenic disorders (drug therapy)		
Alcohol		Inhibition of ADH release
Glucocorticoids		ADH inhibition
Mannitol	Nonabsorbable solute	Osmotic diuresis
Dextrose	Excessive absorbable solute	Osmotic diuresis
Furosemide	Inhibition of active chloride transport in loop of Henle	Osmotic diuresis Medullary washout
Phenytoin		Inhibition of ADH release
Vitamin D intoxication	Excessive vitamin D absorption→hypercalcemia	Early ↑ ADH inhibition Late ↑ renal mineralization

ADH, antidiuretic hormone

TABLE 5-3.   Water Intake, Urine Output, and Urine
Specific Gravities in Normal Dogs and Cats

Species	Water* Intake	Urine* Output	Urine Specific Gravity Expected Range	Urine Specific Gravity Maximum
Dog	20–90	20–45	1.018–1.045	1.065
Cat	0–45	20–40	1.030–1.050	1.085

*Values in ml/kg/day

of special diagnostic tests or procedures. These procedures also allow the clinician to decide which is the primary versus the compensatory event. In most small animals, polyuria is the primary problem and polydipsia is the compensatory disorder.

Documentation

Many owners may complain that their pets are urinating or drinking excessively. However, it is difficult for owners to quantitate water intake or urine output unless the problem is severe. As related earlier, a 25-pound (10.5-kg) dog with a urine specific gravity of 1.010 produces roughly 500 ml of urine per day. Only very astute owners are able to detect polyuria of this magnitude. The signs of lower urinary tract disease, dysuria and pollakiuria, are often confused by owners with polyuria. Because of false information related by owners, it is important to document the problem of P&P. Initial evaluation includes a complete physical examination, accurate determination of the animal's weight and hydration status, determination of packed cell volume (PCV) and plasma proteins, and assessment of urine specific gravity. Animals with urine specific gravities above 1.035 are probably not polyuric (see Table 5-1). The animal's water consumption should be measured accurately. For many patients, the owner can perform the procedure at home. With hospitalized patients, water consumption, urine output, and urine specific gravities are measured. In marginal P&P, 48- to 72-hour determinations are necessary, whereas in severe P&P, 24-hour determinations usually are sufficient. Normal daily water intake and urine output for dogs and cats are listed in Table 5-3.

Inspection of Data Base

The completed initial data base (history, physical examination, hematology, biochemical profile, and urine analysis) is carefully searched for clues to the cause of P&P. For instance, the presence of glucosuria would imply the possible presence of diabetes mellitus or proximal tubular defects. In this case, further tests to document P&P would be withheld until the glucosuria problem is resolved. Table 5-4 lists the various diseases for which P&P is a major sign and describes the clues most indicative of that disorder.

During the initial evaluation of animals with suspected P&P, approximately 50% are found not to have the problem, suggesting that the owner's observations were probably in error. Many cases have sufficient clues in the data base to suggest a primary cause for the P&P; however, in other documented P&P animals, no cause can be identified. Diabetes insipidus, nonazotemic renal failure, certain cases of hyperadrenocorticism, and psychogenic polydipsia are examples of disorders that are not easily differentiated in the initial data base. At this point, patients with unexplained P&P are evaluated with urine concentration procedures.

Urine Concentration Tests

These tests are indicated for patients with P&P not explained by steps 1 and 2 in the diagnostic plan. In small animals, two procedures are used: the water deprivation test and the ADH (pitressin) response test. In certain cases, the animal may be fluid-deficient (dehydrated) during the evaluation of steps 1 and 2. Obviously, a documented dehydrated patient with low urine specific gravity is not a candidate for water deprivation, since it is already apparent that either renal disease or a deficiency in the action or presence of ADH is likely present. It is more logical and safer to perform an ADH response test in these animals. Therefore, before beginning urine concentration tests, the hydration status of the patient must be accurately assessed. This is done clinically by measuring the PCV, total plasma proteins, and, if possible, plasma osmolality. If little evidence of dehydration is present and no other contraindications exist, one should proceed with water deprivation.

Water Deprivation Test. The abrupt test is indicated when poorly controlled water deprivation results in either negative or equivocal findings. The contraindications for this test are azotemia, dehydration, and hypercalcemia.

The test is conducted as follows:

1. Following a 12-hour fast, obtain a blood sample for serum osmolality.
2. Obtain urine for specific gravity and save a small quantity for osmolality.
3. Store serum and urine in a refrigerator.
4. Allow patient to urinate and defecate before recording accurate body weight.
5. Place animal in metabolism cage and withhold food and water.
6. Evaluate animal every 3 to 4 hours by assessing body weight, urine specific gravity, dehydration, and general well-being.

The water deprivation test is terminated when one of three criteria is achieved: (1) production of concentrated urine, (2) weight loss of 7%, or (3) demonstration of hemoconcentration (increased plasma protein concentration or osmolality). At termination of the test, urine produced during the last half

TABLE 5-4. Differential Diagnosis of Diseases That Produce Primary Polyuria, Polydipsia: Diagnostic Clues and Special Tests

Rule Out	Predominant Clinical Signs (Other Than PePP)	Hematology	Biochemistry	Urine Analysis (Other Than Specific Gravity)	Special Tests
Pseudopsychogenic polydipsia (compulsive water drinking)	No consistent clues; search for predisposing environmental or emotional problems	No consistent clues	No consistent clues	No consistent clues	None Response to control of water intake
Hyperadrenocorticism (also see diabetes mellitus)	Alopecia Thin skin, elasticity ↓ Calcinosis cutis Muscle weakness Polyphagia Hepatomegaly	Lymphopenia Eosinopenia	BUN N or ↓ ALT N or ± ↑ Alk Phos ↑ ↑ Cholesterol ↑ Glucose N or ↑	WBC ↑ or N Bacteria N or ↑ Glucose N or ↑	Plasma cortisol Dexamethasone suppression tests
Hypercalcemia	(Depends on precipitating disease) Weakness, depression Muscle tremors Anorexia	Usually normal unless associated with lymphosarcoma PCV ↓ WBC N	BUN N or ↑ Creatinine B or ↑ Calcium ↑ Phosphorus N, ↓ or ↑ (depends on stage of disease)	Calcium crystals	Lymph node aspirate or biopsy Bone marrow aspirate PTH assay
Hyperthyroidism	Polyphagia Voluminous stools Weight loss Nervousness, hyperactivity	Usually normal	Cholesterol ↓ Glucose N or ↑	Rarely glucosuria	Serum T4 test Thyroid
Diabetes insipidus	Marginal dehydration	PCV N or ↑ TS N or ↑	BUN N or ↑ Na N or ↑ Cl N or ↑		ADH response test Water deprivation test
Diabetes mellitus (also see hyperadrenocorticism)	Weight loss Polyphagia Vomiting Lethargy Hepatomegaly	Lipemia PCV N or ↑ WBC N or ↑ Lymphopenia Eosinopenia	BUN N or ↑ ALT N or ↑ Alk Phos ↑ Glucose ↑ ↑ TCO₂ ↓	Glucosuria Ketonuria	Glycogenated hemoglobin Glucose tolerance Serum amylase, lipase Blood gases

	Clinical signs	Hematology	Chemistry	Urinalysis	Diagnostic tests
Liver failure	Vomiting Diarrhea Weight loss Neurologic signs Icterus	PCV N or ↓ TS ↓	BUN N or ↓ T Prot ↓ Albumin ↓ ALT ↑ Alk Phos ↑	Ammonium biurate crystals	Serum ammonia Bile acids Coagulogram Liver radiographs Biopsy
Early renal failure	No consistent clues	Normal	If not azotemic, no consistent clues	Protein N or ↑	PSP Creatinine clearance Assess renal size: Palpation Radiographically
Renal failure	Weight loss Vomiting Anorexia	Nonregenerative anemia Lymphopenia	↑ BUN ↑ Creatinine ↑ Phosphorus ↓ TCO₂	Protein N or ↑ Casts +	Renal biopsy Renal size Radiographically Ultrasonography
Pyelonephritis	Fever Vomiting Mild abdominal pain Weight loss	WBC N or ↑	Normal unless chronic renal failure develops	WBC ↑ Bacteria + Protein ↑	Urine culture Excretory urogram Ultrasonography
Pyometra	Anorexia Vomiting Depression Enlarged uterus History of estrus Vaginal discharge	WBC ↑ (may be normal if early or cervix is open)	BUN N or ↑	WBC ↑ Protein ↑	Abdominal radiography Ultrasonography Exploratory laparotomy
Hypoadrenocorticism	Anorexia Vomiting Depression Diarrhea Weakness Hypotension	Lymphocytosis Eosinophilia PCV N, ↑, ↓	BUN ↑ Na N or ↓ K N or ↑ Cl N or ↓	No consistent clues	Plasma cortisol profile

BUN, blood urea nitrogen; N, normal; ↓, decreased; ↑, increased; ALT, alanine aminotransferase; Alk Phos, alkaline phosphatase; PCV, packed cell volume; WBC, white blood cells; PTH, parathormone; ADH, antidiuretic hormone; TS, total solids; TCO₂, total carbon dioxide; T Prot, total protein; PSP, phenolsulfonphthalein

TABLE 5-5. Response to Urine Concentration Tests in Certain Diseases That Produce P&P

Disease	Usual Range of Urine Specific Gravity (Nonchallenged)	Response to Water Deprivation	Response to ADH Administration
Diabetes insipidus (neurogenic)	1.001–1.017	Negative	Positive
Diabetes insipidus (nephrogenic)	1.001–1.017	Negative	Negative
Primary renal disease (nonazotemic)	1.008–1.030	Negative	Negative
Hyperadrenocorticism	1.001–1.035	Positive	Positive
Renal medullary washout	1.008–1.012	Negative-abrupt Positive-gradual	Negative
Pseudopsychogenic polydipsia	1.001–1.030	Positive	Positive

hour is collected and the specific gravity is determined. A small amount of urine should be saved for osmolality determination.

Normal dogs, when water-deprived, can maximally concentrate urine to a specific gravity of 1.065. Cats produce even more concentrated urine under similar conditions. It appears that most normal dogs and cats achieve urine specific gravities of 1.045 or greater. Values of 1.035 to 1.045 are considered a "grey" zone, and values below 1.035 are abnormal. Failure to concentrate urine following water deprivation indicates one of the following possibilities: (1) deficiency of ADH, (2) renal unresponsiveness to ADH, (3) primary renal disease, or (4) renal medullary washout. Failure to concentrate urine following this procedure usually eliminates primary polydipsia, unless medullary washout is present.

A gradual water deprivation test is indicated when medullary washout is suspected or for severely polyuric animals that are at increased risk of severe hemoconcentration if suddenly deprived of all water. In this procedure, water intake is measured for 2 days and then gradually decreased over 3 to 4 days. The patient is closely monitored, as for the abrupt procedure. As stated earlier, normal renal medullary hypertonicity is reestablished within 1 to 3 days. Failure to concentrate urine during this procedure eliminates medullary washout as the cause of polyuria. The results of water deprivation tests in various diseases are summarized in Table 5-5.

ADH (Vasopressin) Response Test. This test is indicated for animals that fail to concentrate urine after water deprivation or for animals for which deprivation is viewed as a risky procedure. In most cases, ADH response tests can be performed immediately following water deprivation tests. A urine specific gravity is obtained prior to starting the test. Water and food are withheld. Aqueous vasopressin tannate in oil is given subcutaneously, and urine specific gravities are obtained every 30 minutes for 90 minutes. The dosage of aqueous vasopressin is 3.0 units for dogs weighing more than 6.5 kg and 2.0 units for dogs less than this weight. Adult cats are given 2.0 units. The bladder must be emptied at every 30 minute sampling period. Most animals with normal kidneys achieve urine specific gravities of 1.015 or greater. Failure to respond to vasopressin suggests the presence of primary renal disease, nephrogenic diabetes insipidus, or medullary washout. If questionable results are obtained, the ADH response test should be repeated. The results of urine concentration tests in various diseases are summarized in Table 5-5.

Special Diagnostic Tests

The final step in evaluation of animals with P&P is the selection and performance of specialized tests. These tests vary according to the diseases under investigation. They are listed by the appropriate disease in Table 5-4.

PART TWO

Behavioral Problems

CHAPTER SIX

Misdirected Aggression

John E. Oliver

PROBLEM DEFINITION AND RECOGNITION

Aggression is difficult to define, even by authorities in the field. A comprehensive definition is "an overt act the goal of which is either to eliminate, consume or cause the escape of, an opponent by inflicting organic damage upon the latter, or to induce the opponent to escape by noncontactual means, that is, via a ritualized attack or threat."[10] The meaning of aggression is clearer when the various forms are listed (Table 6-1).[7,9] Many forms of aggression are normal behaviors in a species, and are a problem only when they are misdirected in relation to our environment. Misdirected aggression is the most frequent problem presented to behavioral specialists.[2,7,8,15]

PATHOPHYSIOLOGY

Aggressive behavior may be caused or modified by organic brain lesions, genetic predisposition, learning or conditioning, early socialization, and gender. Although organic brain disease has been considered an infrequent cause of aggression, there is little documentation that it is not important.[2,3,7,9]

The limbic system is considered the anatomic substrate for most behavior. It is a complex interconnection of nuclei in the more primitive parts of the cerebrum with areas in the thalamus, hypothalamus, and midbrain.[4] Stimulation or destruction of some of these structures enhances or reduces aggressive behavior. A summary of some of these findings is included in Table 6-1.[13] Focal lesions of one of these structures could cause aggression in the clinical patient, but few documented cases have been reported. Most of the reported cases of aggression with brain lesions had diffuse or multifocal lesions, generally a nonsuppurative encephalitis.[3,4]

Psychomotor seizures may have an aggressive component.[2,4,7,12] Animals may run blindly, bite at anything in their path, and bite at themselves or inanimate objects; finally they may have a generalized seizure. Some animals exhibit this behavior when fed, attacking themselves or the food dish. The behavior is stereotyped, the animal is not aware of its surroundings, and anticonvulsants may reduce the episodes (see Chapter 50).

TABLE 6-1. Forms of Aggression

| Type | Anatomic Substrate | |
	Activators	Suppressors
Predatory	Lateral hypothalamus	Ventromedial hypothalamus
		Basolateral amygdala
Competitive and	Centromedial amygdala	Olfactory bulbs
intermale	Ventrolateral posterior	Septal nuclei
	thalamus	Head of caudate nucleus
	Central gray matter	
Fear-related	Centromedial amygdala,	Ventromedial hypothalamus
	fimbria of the fornix	Septal nuclei
		Dorsal hippocampus
Territorial	Lateral hypothalamus	Basolateral amygdala
Maternal	Hypothalamus	Septal nuclei
	Ventral hippocampus	Basolateral amygdala
Sex-related	Hypothalamus	Septal nuclei
	Ventral hippocampus	Basolateral amygdala
	Centromedial amygdala	Cingulate gyrus
Irritative	Dorsomedial hypo-	Ventromedial hypothala-
	thalamus	mus, basolateral
	Posterior hypothalamus	amygdala
	Anterior cingulate gyrus	Head of caudate nucleus
		Posterior cingulate gyrus
Learned	Cerebral cortex(?)	Unknown
Pain-related	Unknown	Unknown
Seizures	Limbic system	
Idiopathic	Unknown	Unknown

Early socialization can have a major effect on aggressive tendencies. Most of the information is on dogs, but it probably applies to other species as well. If the dog has little contact with people in early life, especially from 3 to 12 weeks of age, it is likely to be fearful of human contact and may be a fear biter. Removal of the dog from the litter at 3 to 4 weeks of age prevents normal socialization with other dogs, and it may be aggressive toward dogs as an adult. Social dominance in the household is also important. Early obedience training is useful to establish the owner's dominance at an early age. This is especially important in breeds that tend to be aggressive by nature. Hart has rated dogs on reactivity (affection, excitability, excessive barking, snapping, and activity), aggressiveness (territorial defense, watchdog barking, aggression to dogs, and dominance over owner), and trainability (obedience training and housebreaking).[6] The aggressive tendencies are summarized in Table 6-2. It is clear that genetic factors are important in the level of aggression. In addition, a few breeds are reported to have "idiopathic aggression." These include the Saint Bernard,[7] Doberman pinscher,[7] German shepherd,[7] English springer spaniel,[4,15] English cocker spaniel,[11] and Bernese mountain dog.[7,15]

TABLE 6-2. Levels of Aggressive Tendencies in Dogs

Very Low	Low	Medium	High	Very High
Basset hound	Australian	Beagle	Afghan hound	Airedale
Bloodhound	shepherd	Bichon frise	Alaskan mal-	terrier
English	Brittany	Boston terrier	amute	Akita
bulldog	spaniel	Cocker	Boxer	Cairn terrier
Norwegian	Chesapeake	spaniel	Chow Chow	Chihuahua
elkhound	Bay	English	Dalmatian	Dachshund
	retriever	springer	Great Dane	Doberman
	Collie	spaniel	Saint Bernard	pinscher
	German	Irish setter	Samoyed	Fox terrier
	shorthaired	Lhasa apso	Siberian	German
	pointer	Maltese	husky	shepherd
	Golden re-	Pekingese		Rottweiler
	triever	Pomeranian		Schnauzer
	Keeshond	Poodle (all		(miniature)
	Labrador re-	sizes)		Scottish terrier
	triever	Pug		Silky terrier
	Newfoundland	Shetland		West Highland
	Vizsla	sheepdog		white terrier
		Shih Tzu		
		Weimaraner		
		Welsh corgi		
		Yorkshire		
		terrier		

(Data from Hart BL, Hart LA: Selecting pet dogs on the basis of cluster analysis of breed profiles and gender. J Am Vet Med Assoc 186:1181–1185, 1985)

Male animals are more aggressive than females.[7] Prepubertal castration has little effect on this difference, but castration, either prepubertal or postpubertal, reduces intermale aggression in about half of dogs.[7]

Dogs can be taught to be aggressive. Aggressive tendencies can also be shaped by positive feedback (*e.g.,* the fear biter may be reinforced by successfully driving people away). Early training is critical in the development of social behavior, especially in the animals that are normally most aggressive.[7]

DIAGNOSTIC PLAN

Aggressive animals are dangerous, so all procedures should be conducted with the objective of avoiding injury to the examiner, support personnel, and the client. The history is usually the most important part of the evaluation of behavioral disorders. Adequate time should be allowed to extract all of the necessary information. Items to be analyzed include the usual medical information (see Chapter 1), and specific data on the animal's behavior, including early socialization, times of normal and abnormal behavior and events surrounding each, owner-animal interaction, training, and environment. If the behavior is sudden in onset, events occurring at the time should be explored carefully.

The physical, neurologic, and laboratory examination should rule out systemic and neurologic disease in most cases (see Chapter 50). If the animal is normal except for the behavioral problem, then the type of aggression should be determined (see Table 6-1). Factors likely to relate to the type of aggression are also listed in Table 6-1. This information should lead to the source of the problem. The causes of each type of aggression are so numerous that they defy cataloguing. For more details, see one of the references.[1-3,7-9,11,14,15]

REFERENCES

1. Beaver B: Veterinary Aspects of Feline Behavior. St. Louis, CV Mosby, 1980
2. Borchelt PL, Voith VL: Aggressive behavior in dogs and cats. Comp Cont Ed Pract Vet 7:949–960, 1985
3. Caldwell DS, Little PB: Aggression in dogs and associated neuropathology. Can Vet J 21:152–154, 1980
4. De Lahunta A: Veterinary Neuroanatomy and Clinical Neurology, 2nd ed. Philadelphia, WB Saunders, 1983
5. Hart BL: Behavioral indications for phenothiazine and benzodiazepine tranquilizers in dogs. J Am Vet Med Assoc 186:1192–1194, 1985
6. Hart BL, Hart LA: Selecting pet dogs on the basis of cluster analysis of breed profiles and gender. J Am Vet Med Assoc 186:1181–1185, 1985
7. Hart BL, Hart LA: Canine and Feline Behavioral Therapy. Philadelphia, Lea & Febiger, 1985
8. Houpt KA: Aggression in dogs. Comp Cont Ed Pract Vet 1:123–128, 1979
9. Houpt KA, Wolski TR: Domestic Animal Behavior for Veterinarians and Animal Scientists. Ames, Iowa State University Press, 1982
10. Karczmar AG, Richardson DL, Kindel G: Neuropharmacological and related aspects of animal aggression. Prog Neuropsychopharmacol 2:611–631, 1978
11. Mugford RA: Aggressive behavior in the English cocker spaniel. Vet Ann 25:310–314, 1984
12. Oliver JE Jr, Lorenz M: Handbook of Veterinary Neurologic Diagnosis. Philadelphia, WB Saunders, 1983
13. Valzelli L: Human and animal studies on the neurophysiology of aggression. Prog Neuropsychopharmacol 2:591–610, 1978
14. Voith VL: Applied animal behavior for the veterinary practitioner. Proceedings AAHA 47th Annual Meeting, 1980, pp 15–33
15. Voith VL: Diagnosis and treatment of aggressive behavioral problems in dogs. Proceedings AAHA 47th Annual Meeting, 1980, pp 35–38

CHAPTER SEVEN

Self-Mutilation

Michael D. Lorenz

PROBLEM DEFINITION AND RECOGNITION

Self-mutilation is the destruction of any body part through the volitional acts of an animal. It is usually recognized by the injuries induced through biting, chewing, or rubbing of the limbs, feet, tail, or head. Autoamputation of a foot or tail is the result of many severe self-mutilation syndromes. This chapter describes the syndromes that cause self-induced destruction of a body part, other than primary dermatologic conditions (see Chapter 15).

PATHOPHYSIOLOGY

The pathophysiology of self-mutilation syndromes is poorly understood in dogs and cats, since these animals are incapable of expressing their feelings regarding pain, pruritus, or abnormal behavior. In veterinary medicine, the assumption has been that self-mutilation is the animal's response to the perception of altered sensation. More recently, attention has focused on a psychogenic basis for self-mutilation.

Basically, self-mutilation can be classified into the following etiologic categories: (1) primary sensory neuropathy or neuritis, (2) psychogenic causes, (3) psychomotor epilepsy, (4) encephalitis, and (5) intractable severe pruritus or pain secondary to soft tissue or bone inflammation (see Display, Diseases That Cause Self-Mutilation in Dogs and Cats). Category 5 may overlap with category 1.

Primary sensory neuropathies or neuritis may be congenital or acquired. Damage to sensory nerves from trauma, compression, neoplasia (neuroma), or viral infection (herpes virus, pseudorabies virus) may cause pain or paresthesia (morbid or perverted sensation). Paresthesia is described by humans as a burning, searing, or prickling sensation. Causalgia is a burning pain caused by injury or scar tissue in the sympathetic nerves innervating the skin. It is assumed that damage to peripheral nerves or sensory nerve roots in dogs and cats results in similar sensations. The altered sensation may be referred to that area of the skin or limb (tail) innervated by the affected sensory nerve. The animal's re-

Diseases That Cause Self-Mutilation in Dogs and Cats

- Neuropathies
    Traumatic neuropathy
    Neoplasia
        Neuroma
        Neurofibroma
    Compression
        Skeletal fractures
        Skeletal subluxation
        Lumbar spinal stenosis
    Inflammation
        Trigeminal neuritis
        Pseudorabies virus
        Canine distemper virus
    Congenital sensory neuropathy (English pointer, dachshund)
- Behavioral (psychogenic) diseases
    Acral pruritic nodule
    Feline hyperesthesia syndrome/neurodermatitis
- Psychomotor epilepsy
- Encephalitis
    Pseudorabies virus
    Canine distemper virus
- Soft tissue or bone inflammation

sponse to this sensation is severe chewing, biting, and licking. Autoamputation is common.

Psychogenic causes of self-mutilation cannot be conclusively proven in the dog or cat. However, self-mutilation may be worsened or initiated by changes in the environment that could be viewed as "stressful." Certain animals benefit from antianxiety drugs or drugs that block the effects of endorphins. These findings tend to support a psychogenic basis for some of the syndromes recognized in dogs and cats. Acral pruritic nodule, feline hyperesthesia syndrome, and feline lick granuloma are dermatoses commonly attributed to a psychogenic abnormality. Autoamputation is rare, and the neurologic examination is normal.

Psychomotor epilepsy is a seizure disorder characterized by episodes of abnormal behavior such as hysteria, rage, salivation, and hallucinations. During the seizures, especially if rage is a component, self-mutilation of a body part may occur. Frequently when food is the apparent stimulus, dogs will violently attack their pelvic limbs and tail, causing severe lacerations. Autoamputation is rare. Psychomotor seizures are preceded by an aura, and the animal is usually completely unresponsive to commands during the ictus. Loss of consciousness is not a feature of this syndrome. Psychomotor seizures result from functional abnormalities in the limbic system of the brain.

Viral encephalitis may cause self-mutilation through involvement of the brain stem and/or cranial and peripheral nerves (neuritis). Pseudorabies is the outstanding example of those viral diseases that cause intense pruritus and severe self-mutilation. In pseudorabies, self-mutilation is most severe on the head, face, neck, and shoulders. Other signs of viral encephalitis are usually present and include abnormal behavior, fever, hypersalivation, and generalized convulsions. Pets are usually infected by eating contaminated pork.

Viral encephalitis that causes severe behavioral changes from brain stem disease may cause self-mutilation through changes in the function of sensory neurons. Canine distemper encephalitis is one example. In most cases, other clinical signs of neurologic disease are present. There is no evidence that herpes viruses other than pseudorabies virus are associated with self-mutilation syndromes in dogs and cats. Herpes zoster infection in humans frequently causes intense pruritus and burning via inflammation of cranial or peripheral neurons.

Severe inflammation of soft tissue and underlying bone may cause chronic irritation of sensory receptors. This may be perceived as severe pruritus, pain, or burning. Severe excoriations or self-mutilation may result from the animal's intense chewing or licking.

DIAGNOSTIC PLAN

A diagnostic plan for the problem of self-mutilation is presented in Figure 7-1. The initial step is to identify any neurologic signs or deficits that may be present. A thorough neurologic examination is required. If neurologic signs are present, the lesion should be localized to the central or peripheral nervous system (see Chapter 47). The presence of seizures associated with self-mutilation is strong evidence of central nervous system disease. A thorough seizure workup is indicated (see Chapter 50).

Peripheral nerve lesions causing a sensory neuropathy are extremely difficult to diagnose. In some cases, pain perception may be decreased from the affected area; other sensory or motor deficits may be present. In most cases, there are few, if any, signs of neurologic disease. In these animals, one must consider the presence of a sensory neuropathy due to trauma, neoplasia, entrapment, or compression. Radiographs of the affected body part and that region of the vertebral column from which the affected nerves originate should be closely examined for bony or soft tissue changes that might cause a neuropathy. Measurement of sensory nerve conduction times and evoked potentials may be helpful in the identification of a sensory neuropathy. Unfortunately, only a few large referral centers are equipped to perform these electrodiagnostic procedures.

Biopsy of affected skin for histopathology and possible bacterial and fungal

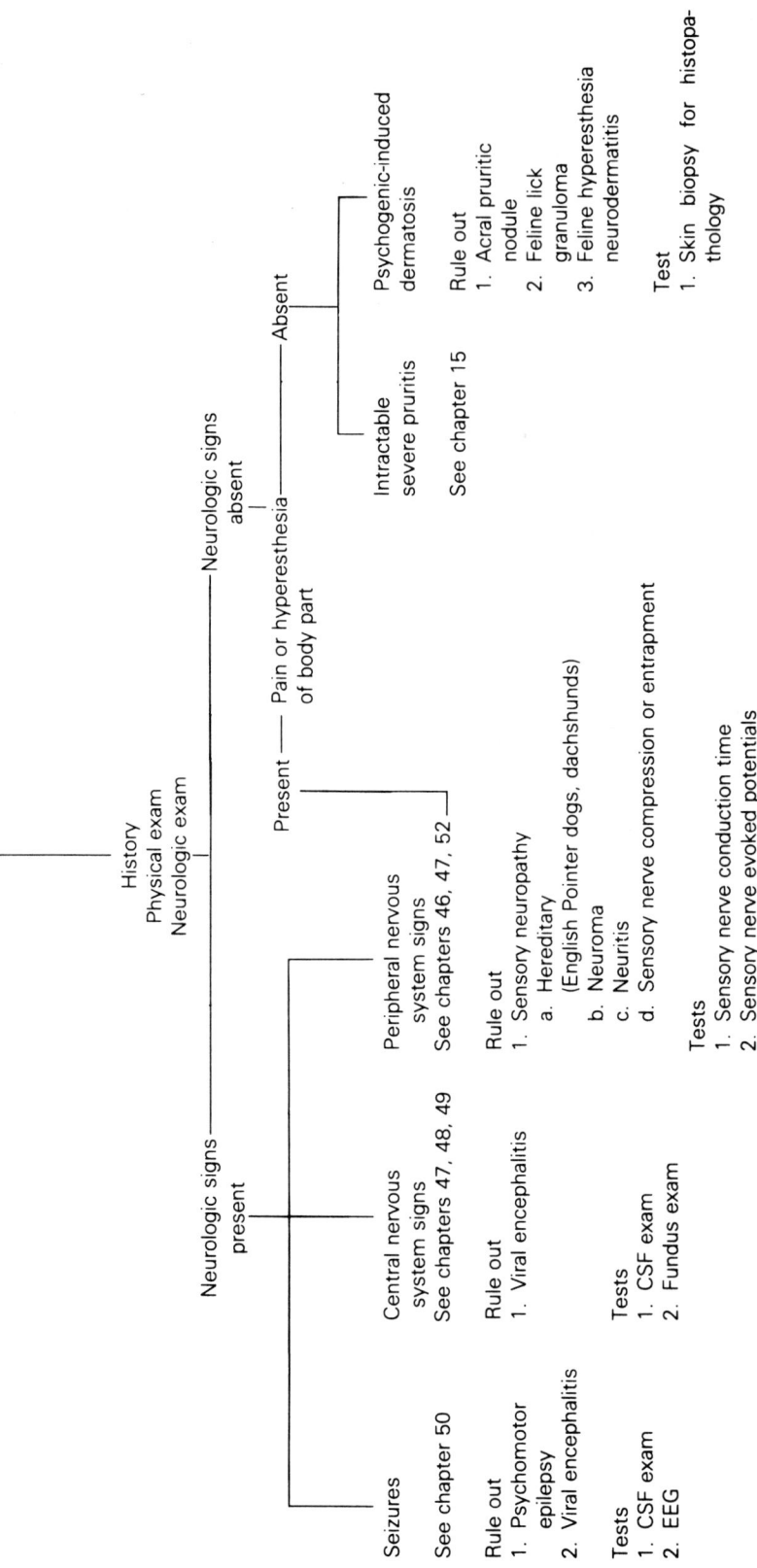

FIGURE 7-1. Diagnostic plan.

culture should be performed, especially when the lesions are swollen, nodular, or infected.

Behavioral studies should be undertaken when there is no evidence of organic disease to explain the self-mutilation. Changes in an animal's "normal" daily routine may be associated with self-mutilation. Introduction of a new animal or person in the environment or moving the animal to new surroundings may initiate excessive chewing and licking. Animals placed under unusual stress such as heavy obedience work from a demanding trainer may also initiate self-mutilation. The response to antianxiety drugs and endorphin antagonists may be useful in establishing a psychogenic basis for the syndrome.

CHAPTER EIGHT

Coprophagy and Pica

Michael D. Lorenz

PROBLEM AND DEFINITION AND RECOGNITION

Coprophagy is the ingestion of feces. It is not uncommon in dogs, but it is rare in cats. Coprophagic dogs usually ingest dog or cat feces although other animal feces may be eaten if available. In certain situations, coprophagy is considered normal animal behavior. For instance, lactating bitches normally ingest the feces of their puppies from birth to 3 weeks of age.

Pica is a craving for and the ingestion of unnatural articles. Dogs may eat dirt (geophagy), rocks, sticks, or cat litter, and may lick concrete. Cats may crave wool yarn. Both dogs and cats may ingest green grass; this is most commonly observed in the spring. Coprophagy is a pica for feces.

PATHOPHYSIOLOGY

Although many causes for pica and coprophagy have been proposed, the underlying cause of these behaviors is unknown. Except for the coprophagy of lactating bitches, most forms of pica should be considered an abnormality of behavior.

Veterinarians and laypeople have assumed that coprophagy results from certain dietary deficiencies. One theory proposes a deficiency of amylase perpetuated by a high-carbohydrate diet.[2] Other theories propose that coprophagy results from a deficiency of proteolytic enzymes.[1] None of these theories has any scientific merit. Coprophagy may occur in well-nourished dogs with no evidence of digestive system disease.

Animals with pancreatic exocrine insufficiency may become severely coprophagic, apparently in an attempt to ingest sufficient calories to prevent starvation. Any disease that causes polyphagia may also cause coprophagy (see Chapter 5). Coprophagy has been associated with hyperadrenocorticism, glucocorticoid therapy, diabetes mellitus, intestinal malabsorption syndromes, intestinal parasitism, hyperthyroidism, and nonspecific dietary deficiencies.

There are usually few deleterious consequences associated with coprophagy. Severe halitosis is a common complaint of owners. Dogs that ingest large quantities of horse manure may develop acute gastroenteritis. The ingestion of dog feces may cause repeated infection with gastrointestinal parasites. The ingestion

65

of foreign matter may cause gastrointestinal obstruction. Some dogs with acquired megacolon may impact the colon with sand, rocks, or garbage material. Geophagic dogs may develop excessive wear of the teeth. In humans, geophagia (ingestion of clay soil) may cause hypokalemia, iron deficiency, and zinc deficiency; this has not been reported in dogs or cats.

DIAGNOSTIC PLAN

Since many animals with coprophagy or pica are thought to have behavioral problems, a thorough history regarding the environment and handling of the pet is indicated. Stressful conditions or abrupt changes in the animal's normal routine should be identified and eliminated. The diet should be carefully analyzed for any deficiencies, especially in the area of trace minerals.

Gastrointestinal disease, pancreatic exocrine insufficiency, hyperthyroidism, hyperadrenocorticism, and diabetes mellitus should be considered as possible etiologies. A urine analysis and biochemical profile should be performed to ascertain the possible presence of these disorders. A complete blood count (CBC) may detect iron deficiency. Fecal flotations are indicated, since chronic intestinal parasitism may be associated with coprophagy.

REFERENCES

1. McCuistion WR: Prevention of Coprophagy. In Kirk RW (ed): Current Veterinary Therapy III. Philadelphia, WB Saunders, 1968
2. Morris ML: Index of Dietetic Management. In Kirk RW (ed): Current Veterinary Therapy VI. Philadelphia, WB Saunders, 1977

CHAPTER NINE

Urine Spraying in Cats

Jeanne A. Barsanti

DEFINITION AND RECOGNITION

Urine spraying in cats is a method of marking territory. The cat typically smells the target area, turns around and forcibly expresses urine while standing with its tail upright. The urine is sprayed horizontally onto a vertical object. Another form of urine marking in cats is voiding a small amount of urine while squatting. Cats may also void outside of litterboxes because of factors related to the litterbox itself as well as because of urinary tract diseases. Spraying becomes a form of inappropriate urination (voluntary urination in the wrong place or at the wrong time) when the target is in the owner's house. Inappropriate urination must always be distinguished from urinary incontinence (see Chapter 40). This chapter addresses inappropriate urination in cats in general as well as spraying in particular, because some clients do not understand the specific terminology and since many identify the problem by finding urine but do not actually observe the act of urination.

PATHOPHYSIOLOGY

Inappropriate urination is the most common behavioral problem in cats, accounting for 56% of all feline behavioral complaints in one survey.[1] The incidence of spraying is highest in intact males, but spraying also occurs in intact females, especially during estrus. Even in cats neutered at less than 10 months of age, 10% of males and 5% of females sprayed urine more than once a month. This high incidence of a "behavioral problem" is related to continuation of a normal feline behavior during indoor confinement with people who obviously find it objectionable. Approximately 26% of cats that urinate inappropriately also defecate inappropriately.[1]

Normal Behavioral Considerations

Cats spray urine or squat to void a small amount of urine to establish their territory and to communicate their presence to other cats. Cats by choice prefer a low population density, where each can establish its own territory. They adhere to regular schedules of movement to avoid confrontations with other cats, except during breeding season. The frequency of spraying is increased by the sight, odor, and sounds of other cats. Androgens also increase the frequency of spraying, while progestogens decrease it. The problem of spraying arises when cats become house pets, particularly when confined with other cats. The incidence of spraying is directly proportional to the number of cats in the household, particularly with male cats. In households of 10 or more cats, a spraying problem is inevitably present in at least one cat. In contrast to popular opinion, one survey found that neutered male cats were more likely to spray in a household including female cats as opposed to a household containing only other males.

Other Considerations

Cats may void urine outside of a litterbox because of aversion to the box. Most cats are easily litter-trained because of their natural tendency to urinate in sand or loose dirt. However, cats possess this tendency to varying degrees. Some cats avoid certain types of litter (especially that containing deodorants such as chlorophyll), dirty litter, litter being used by another cat, and litter in certain types of containers (such as those with lids or with or without high sides). Cats may also learn to avoid a litterbox if it is associated with punishment, injury, or pain either inflicted from without or associated with cystitis or urethritis.

Cats may become attracted to an alternative area for voiding urine, because of house soiling by another pet or because of discovering a surface or material that they prefer to litter.

Environmental changes may also cause a cat to urinate outside the litterbox. These can include moving to a new house, redecorating an existing dwelling, adding a new person or pet to the household, or longer-than-usual absences of the owner.

Urinary tract problems that cause dysuria or polyuria may also result in urination outside of the litterbox (see Chapters 5 and 38).

Once a cat begins to urinate outside a litterbox, it may continue to do so for reasons different from that which initiated the problem. For example, the cat may object to a new litter, but after the litter is changed it continues to urinate outside the box because it has learned to prefer the new location, whether because of odor, material, or the location itself.

DIAGNOSTIC PLAN

Primary rule outs for a cat urinating outside the litterbox are: (1) problems related to disease, such as dysuria (voiding urgency), polyuria (requiring more frequent trips to the litterbox or increased soiling of the box), and musculoskeletal problems (which inhibit access to the litterbox), (2) urine marking, (3) a change in urination area preference (see Display, Rule Outs for Inappropriate Urination in Cats).

Rule Outs for Inappropriate Urination in Cats

Diseases

Those that cause dysuria
    Feline urologic syndrome (idiopathic hematuria)
    Cystic or urethral calculi
    Bacterial cystitis/urethritis
    Lower urinary tract neoplasia
Those that cause polyuria
    Renal failure
    Diabetes mellitus
    Hepatic failure
    Hyperthyroidism
    Others (see Chapter 5)
Musculoskeletal problems inhibiting mobility

Urine Marking

Spraying
Squatting to void small urine volumes without dysuria

Urination Preference

Aversion to litter or litterbox
Preference for a new material or location
Environmental change

History

A thorough history is essential; however, owners seldom know the meaning of terms such as spraying, incontinence, polyuria, and dysuria. Some owners consider any urination outside the litterbox as spraying, while others have never heard the term. An exact description of the cat's position during urination or determining whether the urine is found on a horizontal or vertical surface will help determine if spraying has occurred. The owner should be questioned regarding the presence of dysuria, hematuria, and polyuria (see Chapters 5, 38, and 39), since disease in the urinary tract may cause inappropriate urination. Urinary incontinence must be distinguished from inappropriate urination (see Chapter 40). Any changes in the household or management of the cat are important, as are any other behavioral changes, medical problems, or drug usage. Androgen therapy in cats may induce urine marking.

Sometimes owners of more than one cat do not know which cat is inappropriately urinating. One proposed method of determining the culprit is to inject

0.3 ml of sodium fluorescein subcutaneously (Fluorescite Injectable, 10%, Alcon Laboratories) or to give 0.5 ml orally to the most likely suspect. The urine should fluoresce with a Wood's light for the next 24 hours. Each cat in the household can be checked by evaluating one every other day.

Physical Examination and Diagnostic Tests

A complete physical examination should be performed on the affected cat. A urine analysis should be performed. If abnormalities suggestive of urinary tract infection are present (pyuria, bacteriuria, hematuria), a culture of urine collected by cystocentesis is indicated. Urine analysis and urine culture should be performed on the same day as collection. If the urinalysis is abnormal, survey and contrast radiographs may also be indicated to determine whether urolithiasis or a soft tissue mass (such as a neoplasm) is present. If the urine is marginally concentrated (urine specific gravity less than 1.040), a blood urea nitrogen (BUN) and/or serum creatinine should also be assessed. A blood chemistry profile and complete blood count (CBC) may also be indicated to rule out other causes of polyuria (see Chapter 5).

REFERENCE

1. Beaver BV: Housesoiling by cats: A retrospective study of 120 cases. J Am Anim Hosp Assoc 25:631–637, 1989

SUGGESTED READING

Chastain CB, Graham CL, et al: Adrenocortical suppression in cats given megestrol acetate. Am J Vet Res 42:2029–2035, 1981

Hart BL: Objectionable urine spraying and urine marking in cats: Evaluation of progestin treatment in gonadectomized males and females. J Am Vet Med Assoc 177:529–533, 1980

Hart BL, Barrett RE: Effects of castration on fighting, roaming, and urine spraying in adult male cats. J Am Vet Med Assoc 163:290–292, 1973

Hart BL, Cooper L: Factors relating to urine spraying and fighting in prepubertally gonadectomized cats. JAVMA 10:1255–1258, 1984

Hart BL, Leedy M: Identification of source of urine stains in multi-cat households. J Am Vet Med Assoc 180:77–78, 1982

Henik RA, Olson PN, et al: Progestogen therapy in cats. Comp Cont Ed Pract Vet 7:132–141, 1985

Mansfield PD, Kemppainen RJ, et al: The effects of megestrol acetate treatment on plasma glucose concentration and insulin response to glucose administration in cats. J Am Anim Hosp Assoc 22:515–518, 1986

Voith V: Behavioral disorders. In: Ettinger SJ (ed): Veterinary Internal Medicine, 3rd ed, pp 235–236. Philadelphia: WB Saunders, 1989

PART THREE

Conformational Problems

CHAPTER TEN

Abdominal Distention

Larry M. Cornelius

DEFINITION AND PROBLEM RECOGNITION

Abdominal distention may be defined as a sudden or gradual increase in the size of the abdomen. Distention may be intermittent or persistent and asymptomatic or painful. Abdominal distention may be due to either fluid or nonfluid causes (Fig. 10-1). Ascites is an abnormal accumulation of fluid transudate or modified transudate in the peritoneal cavity. Since exudates must also be ruled out whenever abdominal fluid is present, they will be included in the discussion of ascites. Associated signs such as vomiting, diarrhea, abdominal pain, polydipsia, polyuria, polyphagia, and edema, may be clues to the etiology of abdominal distention and ascites.

PATHOPHYSIOLOGY

Pathophysiologic mechanisms of ascites are similar to those of expansion of extracellular fluid elsewhere in the body (edema). There appear to be two general categories: (1) those in which the primary event is escape of plasma into tissue spaces with resultant hypovolemia and secondary renal retention of electrolytes and water and (2) other types in which the primary disturbance is excessive renal retention of electrolytes and water, leading to extracellular fluid expansion and transudation of fluid from plasma into tissue spaces.[2] General mechanisms of ascites formation include decreased colloid osmotic pressure of plasma (hypoalbuminemia), increased capillary hydrostatic pressure, increased capillary permeability, obstruction of lymph flow, and excessive renal retention of sodium and water. More than one of these causes are often present in clinical cases of ascites.

Hypoalbuminemia, in the absence of other causes of ascites, must be severe (less than 0.8 g/dl) in order to lower plasma oncotic pressure sufficiently to cause ascites; however, lesser magnitudes of hypoalbuminemia facilitate the formation of ascitic fluid whenever other causes, such as increased capillary permeability, are also present. For example, ascites in a patient with a serum albumin concentration of 1.8 g/dl is unlikely to be the result of hypoalbumin-

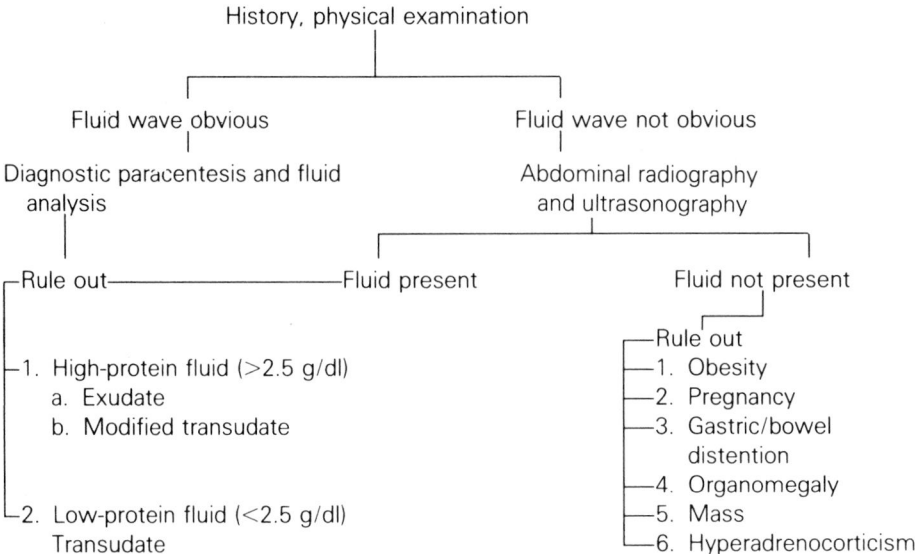

FIGURE 10-1. Initial plan for diagnosing abdominal distention.

emia alone, and the animal should be evaluated for another underlying disorder, such as one of the other general causes listed above.

Thoracic and abdominal venous obstruction results in increased capillary hydrostatic pressure and may cause ascites. Protein content of ascitic fluid varies, depending upon the anatomic site of venous obstruction, and thus may be helpful in localizing and determining the cause of ascites (Table 10-1).[1] Experimentally produced *transient* (duration of a few minutes) portal venous obstruction alone does not cause ascites. Lymph flow from the bowel markedly increases, and it probably compensates for obstructed portal venous drainage. *Sustained* portal hypertension does cause ascites, termed *presinusoidal* obstruction. Persistently increased intestinal capillary hydrostatic pressure causes dilation of intestinal lacteals and increased fluid transudation into the bowel lumen, and from the serosa into the peritoneal cavity. Intestinal lymph is lower in protein than hepatic lymph; therefore, ascites caused by chronic portal stasis is generally *low in protein* (less than 2.5 g/dl).[1] The most common cause of chronic portal stasis in dogs and cats is liver disease characterized by inflammation or fibrosis diffusely affecting portal tracts (see Table 10-1).

Obstruction of blood flow draining hepatic sinusoids, termed *postsinusoidal* obstruction, causes production of high-protein (greater than 2.5 g/dl) ascites derived from hepatic lymph. Protein content is high because hepatic sinusoidal capillaries are much more porous and "leaky" than capillaries elsewhere in the body. With increased hydrostatic pressure in hepatic sinusoids, relatively large albumin molecules readily extravasate into formed lymph. Extrahepatic portal

TABLE 10-1. Causes of Abdominal Effusion

High-Protein (>2.5 g/dl) Ascites		Low-Protein (<2.5 g/dl) Ascites
Exudate	Modified Transudate	Transudate
Protein (g/dl) > 3.5	2.5–6.0	<2.5
Cells/cmm > 30,000	250–20,000	<1000
Inflammatory	Cardiac	Hypoalbuminemia
Bacterial (septic)	Right-sided congestive	(<0.8 g/dl)
Bowel rupture	heart failure	Glomerular disease
Penetrating wounds	Intracardiac tumors	Hepatic insufficiency
Ruptured abscess	Cardiomyopathy (dog)	Gastrointestinal loss
Chemical	Obstruction of hepatic	(diarrhea)
Intraperitoneal drug	vein or thoracic cau-	Chronic starvation
Pancreatitis	dal vena cava	Vasculopathies
Leakage of:	Thrombosis	Immune-mediated
Bile	Stricture	(lupus)
Urine	Vascular anomaly	Infectious (bacterial,
Circulatory com-	Diffuse liver disease with	viral, rickettsial)
promise	post-sinusoidal ob-	Sustained portal hyper-
Thrombosis	struction (rare)	tension
Torsion	Neoplasia in abdomen	Cirrhosis
Intussusception	Chyle	Chronic active hepatitis
Physical injury	Lymphadenitis	Abdominal or hepatic
Postsurgical manipu-	Ruptured lymphatic	neoplasia with sus-
lation	Inflammatory	tained portal hyper-
Trauma	Feline infectious perito-	tension and/or
	nitis	hypoalbuminemia

venous pressure is generally normal or only slightly increased with postsinusoidal obstruction. Examples of postsinusoidal obstruction include right-sided heart failure and lesions of major hepatic veins or thoracic caudal vena cava, such as thrombosis (see Table 10-1).

Abdominal masses (neoplasms, granulomas, "walled-off" abscesses) may cause intraabdominal vascular damage and leakage of blood or plasma, resulting in *high-protein ascites* (see Table 10-1). On the other hand, if the mass restricts portal blood flow (presinusoidal), resulting in sustained portal hypertension, low-protein intestinal lymph contributes to the formation of the ascitic fluid. Low-protein ascites (with normal serum albumin) in the presence of an abdominal mass signifies that portal venous obstruction is present.[1]

The pathophysiologic events of intraabdominal exudate formation vary with the particular exudate. Rapid accumulation of blood in the abdomen, such as may occur following trauma or rupture of a splenic hemangiosarcoma, may be associated with signs of hypovolemic shock. A rent in the urinary system with accumulation of urine in the peritoneal or retroperitoneal spaces will result in signs of uremia. Leakage of bile into the peritoneal cavity causes signs of chemical peritonitis. A ruptured bowel usually leads to septic peritonitis with signs of endotoxemia and septic shock.

For the nonfluid causes of abdominal distention, the pathophysiologic mechanisms also vary, depending on the cause. For example, ileus may be secondary to peritonitis or an obstructed bowel. Lack of normal bowel motility may allow proliferation of pathogenic intestinal bacteria and subsequent absorption of endotoxins. Intraabdominal masses may impinge on normal abdominal organs and cause disruption of function, resulting in signs such as anorexia, vomiting, diarrhea, and icterus. With gastric volvulus, abdominal venous return is severely restricted and signs of hypovolemic shock may occur.

DIAGNOSTIC PLAN

History and Physical Examination

The history may be helpful in narrowing the range of possible causes of abdominal distention. An example would be a history of polydipsia, polyuria, and polyphagia in a dog with a distended, pendulous abdomen suggesting hyperadrenocorticism. The physical examination should be complete. Associated findings such as dyspnea, tachycardia, heart murmurs, and peripheral edema usually help in determining the etiology of abdominal distention and the appropriate diagnostic plan. Ballottement of the abdomen should be done carefully to determine if a fluid wave is present; with experience, false-positive results are infrequent, but small amounts of abdominal fluid usually cannot be detected by this method.

Other Diagnostic Procedures

Whenever an abdominal fluid wave is easily observed, paracentesis and fluid analysis prior to other diagnostic procedures are appropriate. These are accomplished by using a 20- to 22-gauge, 1-inch needle and a 6-ml syringe. If the animal is fractious, it is safer to use a butterfly needle unit. Although the risks of this procedure are minimal, it is probably better to tap the right cranial quadrant to avoid the spleen. Appropriate clipping and skin preparation should be done. Fluid analysis, including protein content (determined using a refractometer), cell count and differential, sediment examination, and culture/sensitivity, if indicated, should be performed. Only a small amount of fluid (less than 1 ml) is required. Removal of large amounts of ascitic fluid causes or worsens hypoalbuminemia and should be avoided unless fluid distention is causing serious respiratory distress.

Abdominal and thoracic radiographs and abdominal sonograms are often needed to evaluate an animal with abdominal distention. Ultrasonography is particularly helpful when large amounts of abdominal fluid obscure radiographic detail. A suggested initial diagnostic plan for abdominal distention is shown in Figure 10-1.

REFERENCES

1. Greene CE: Ascites: Diagnostic and therapeutic considerations. Comp Cont Ed Sm Anim Prac 1:712–719, 1979
2. Schroeder HA: Edema. In MacBryde CM, Blacklow RS (eds): Signs and Symptoms, pp 804–833. Philadelphia, JB Lippincott, 1970

CHAPTER ELEVEN

Edema

Craig E. Greene

PROBLEM DEFINITION

Edema, an accumulation of body fluid in tissues, results from expansion of the interstitial fluid volume. This increase in the extravascular compartment of the extracellular fluid can occur in a localized or generalized distribution, depending on the underlying causes. Determining the reasons for edema formation is usually necessary to its resolution. In many patients, treatment for edema must be instituted immediately and before a diagnosis is established because increased tissue fluid pressure may directly interfere with physiologic functions such as proper tissue nutrition.

PATHOPHYSIOLOGY

The interstitial fluid space is highly structured; it consists of collagen fibers embedded in a gel matrix. Fluid within this network, although relatively immobile, is in dynamic equilibrium with the blood capillary network and enters as a result of hydrostatic pressure on the arteriolar network. Narrow pores in the capillary endothelium normally restrict the migration of large plasma proteins into the interstitial space, while allowing free passage of water and small solute molecules. Since the interstitial fluid protein concentration is normally much lower than that of plasma, the colloidal osmotic pressure from intravascular protein facilitates fluid retention in the vascular space. Under normal circumstances, excess fluid filtered into the interstitial space does not accumulate but is reabsorbed into the venous blood via local lymphatic circulation, so that minimal amounts of extracellular tissue fluid normally exist. The return of fluid via lymphatic circulation is also somewhat influenced by interstitial compartment compliance. Normally, entry of fluid into the interstitial space causes a marked increase in tissue pressure, which further restricts the movement of fluid out of the vascular space.

Disease processes cause edematous fluid formation by disrupting the normal fluid dynamics in the interstitial space. Increased capillary permeability from endothelial damage can result in vascular leakage and interstitial fluid accumulation. Hypoproteinemia will also result in expansion of the interstitial compartment, as will a reduced flow or an obstruction of the lymphatic or venous circulation.

Albumin, the smallest plasma protein, is the primary source of plasma colloidal oncotic pressure and attracts fluid to remain within the vascular space. Edema usually becomes evident when the serum albumin concentration falls below 2.0 g/dl.

Extensive generalized edema is associated with a reduction of plasma volume and a simultaneous increase of extracellular fluid space. This results in decreased renal excretion of sodium by presumed hormonal mechanisms. This solute retention promotes extracellular fluid accumulation and exacerbates edema formation.

An increase in free-fluid volume in tissues accounts for the pitting phenomenon that is seen in edematous states. Pressure applied to an edematous area forces the mobile fluid out of the region, resulting in a permanent indentation. The mobility of fluid also explains the continuous weeping of wounds in edematous tissues and the mobility of edema to the lowest portions of the body. Generalized edema has its greatest effect in the dependent parts of the body because of the increased venous volume and back pressure from the gravitational pooling of blood in these areas.

RULE OUTS AND DIAGNOSTIC PLAN

A thorough history and physical examination can help determine the causes of edema (see Display, Rule Outs for Edema). Any disease process that produces lymph node enlargement can cause secondary lymph stasis and edema. Fever, warm swelling, and enlarged or painful lymph nodes are associated with inflammatory conditions causing lymphadenomegaly. Regional lymph node enlargement may also occur with lymphoreticular neoplasia that produces edema. Arteriovenous fistulas may be detected by the presence of a continuous murmur auscultated in the affected extremity. Generalized edema from cardiovascular disorders may be detected on physical examination on the basis of pulse, respiratory rate, and cardiac auscultation. Suspicious findings can be followed up with electrocardiography, thoracic radiography, and cardiac ultrasonography. Measurement of central venous pressure using a catheter and manometer is useful in determining the presence of venous obstruction or systemic venous hypertension. Venous or lymphatic occlusion can also be detected by contrast radiography.

The presence of concurrent ascites should be ascertained in any edematous patient, since it may help determine the cause of both disorders. Ascitic fluid often forms by itself or prior to subcutaneous edema with cardiac disorders or portal hypertension, but it can also occur in conjunction with edema in hypoproteinemic patients. An analysis of the ascitic fluid to determine cell and

Rule Outs for Edema

- Decreased capillary integrity (increased permeability)
    Inflammation
    Vasculitis
      Infectious
      Immune-mediated
    Allergy
    Trauma
    Burns
    Toxins
- Change in tissue gel
    Myxedema
    Serous atrophy of subcutaneous fat from cachexia
- Noninflammatory increase in tissue fluid
    Decreased plasma oncotic pressure (hypoalbuminemia)
      Increased albumin loss
        Renal
        Gastrointestinal
        Body cavities
        Wounds, burns
        Vasculitis
        Nephrotic syndrome
        Protein-losing enteropathy
      Decreased albumin production
        Protein malabsorption
        Hepatic insufficiency from any cause
    Lymphatic hypertension or obstruction
      Surgical or traumatic injury
      Neoplasia
      Lymphatic or lymph node inflammation
      Congenital lymphedema
    Increased capillary hydrostatic pressure
      Venous hypertension
        Venous obstruction
        Right heart failure or obstruction
        Arteriovenous fistula
        Overhydration
      Arteriolar hypertension
        Hyperaldosteronism
        Inappropriate secretion of antidiuretic hormone
        Acute renal failure

protein composition (see Chapter 10) often distinguishes among causes of edema.

Essential laboratory screening should include a complete blood count with a leukocyte differential and, most importantly, the measurement of plasma and urine protein concentrations. A refractometer can be used for initial screening of plasma protein concentration; albumin and total protein measurements should always be determined. If hypoproteinemia is found, causes of this problem should be considered (see Chapter 63). Electrolyte concentrations in plasma and urine can be examined to determine if the extracellular fluids are being retained in excessive or normal amounts in proportion to the electrolytes; this may help determine whether the process is primary or secondary to renal, adrenal, or caudal pituitary dysfunction. Immune or infectious disorders, suspected on the basis of clinical or laboratory findings, have to be confirmed using additional serologic tests. Enlarged lymph nodes should always be aspirated for cytologic evaluation; when unresolvable, they should be subsequently biopsied for histopathologic study. Edema may originate from a variety of disturbances; therefore, multiple abnormalities in laboratory tests may be apparent.

CHAPTER TWELVE

Retarded Growth

Michael D. Lorenz

PROBLEM DEFINITION AND RECOGNITION

Retarded growth is failure to attain the weight and/or height standards characteristic of a given breed of dog or cat. The problem is more difficult to define in mongrels, since absolute standards are not available to guide one's judgment. Standards for the various breeds of dogs are available from the American Kennel Club. Canine and feline growth charts have been published elsewhere.[7]

Dwarfism is marked underdevelopment of the body. It is one cause of retarded growth; however, not all small animals are true dwarfs.

PATHOPHYSIOLOGY

To understand why growth is retarded, it is necessary to know the mechanisms that control growth in normal animals. Normal growth is a critical balance of proper nutrition, oxygen, hormonal interactions, and genetic influences that control cell division and development.[1]

Genetic Control

The genetic information that ultimately controls cell division and growth is primarily contained in the sex chromosomes, although the autosomes probably contribute to growth regulation. In humans, it is known that the genes that allow normal growth are contained in the X chromosome. In addition, the Y chromosome also contains growth-promoting genes.[1] The greater size of male animals is probably explained by the positive influence of the Y chromosome. If the amount of Y chromosomes is increased, as in XYY individuals, greater-than-normal stature occurs whereas growth is retarded in XO individuals.

Prenatal Growth

Growth of the fetus depends on maternal health and nutrition and the ability of the placenta to transfer necessary nutrients to the developing fetus. Placental size and function may be directly related to the size and weight of newborns.

83

So-called runts may never achieve normal size, since no make-up growth occurs after birth.

Hormonal abnormalities during fetal life appear to exert relatively little influence on somatic growth. Fetal growth is not appreciably impaired by failure of the fetal thyroid, and animals with congenital hormone deficiencies are usually of normal size at birth.

Postnatal Growth

Normal growth is dependent on the secretion and interaction of several key hormones. In addition, adequate nutrition—including calories, protein, essential fatty acids, minerals (especially zinc and calcium), and vitamins (especially vitamin A)—is necessary for maximum growth. Deficiency of growth-promoting hormones, malnutrition, and metabolic diseases are the most common causes of retarded growth.

Hormonal Regulation of Growth. The most commonly recognized hormonal regulator of growth is growth hormone (GH), or somatotropin. This polypeptide hormone of pituitary origin has both catabolic and anabolic effects. The catabolic effects (lipolysis, restricted glucose transport) are directly induced by the hormone, whereas the growth-promoting effects are mediated by insulin-like growth factors (IGFs), or somatomedins.[2]

Studies in German shepherd dwarf dogs have shown that both GH and IGF levels are extremely low compared with those in normal dogs.[5] In addition, the IGF levels in these dogs appear to be controlled by GH.[5] In dogs there is a parallel relationship between body size and plasma IGF levels.[4] Larger dog breeds have the highest IGF levels, which progressively decrease in smaller breeds.[4] Surprisingly, there is little difference in plasma GH levels across the various breeds, regardless of size. In a study of the poodle breed, the small stature of the toy poodle was clearly associated with lower concentrations of IGF and the larger stature of the standard poodle with higher concentrations of IGF, even though GH levels were remarkably similar.[3]

Although GH deficiency results in retarded growth, a deficiency of IGF may also cause this problem. Since IGF is largely made in the liver, any serious liver problem during growth may result in small stature.

Thyroxine is a general stimulator of cellular metabolism and has a strong positive effect on growth. Hypothyroidism that occurs in the neonatal or juvenile animal results in severe growth suppression and slow cerebral development. Congenital hypothyroidism is rare in dogs and cats.

Insulin may be necessary at the cellular level for GH to exert its effects. Small stature (retarded growth) is common in dogs with congenital diabetes mellitus (keeshond, golden retriever).

Malnutrition. Probably the most common cause of retarded growth is malnutrition resulting from dietary deficiency or severe gastrointestinal parasitism.

When these problems are severe or prolonged, reduced growth may never be totally made up during the catch-up growth phase that occurs once normal nutrition is established. Deficiencies of vitamin A almost always cause growth retardation. Initially, deficiency of vitamin D does not slow growth; however, the resulting abnormalities in bone metabolism and bone growth may cause severe growth suppression. The mechanism by which zinc deficiency causes growth suppression is unknown.

Animals with congenital heart defects or chronic progressive lung disease grow slowly and often fail to develop normal size. A deficiency of oxygen in the tissues is the primary mechanism.

Disease of the digestive system that results in maldigestion or malabsorption of nutrients may cause severe growth retardation. Pancreatic insufficiency in dogs may occur prior to puberty and result in severe growth retardation. The syndrome known as *juvenile pancreatic atrophy* occurs in large breeds such as the German shepherd and Great Dane. Congenital megaesophagus may also cause retarded growth.

Metabolic Diseases. The most common metabolic causes of retarded growth are liver disease and kidney failure. Severe liver disease due to portosystemic shunts, copper intoxication (Wilson's syndrome), or infection such as feline infectious peritonitis virus is a common cause of retarded growth. Congenital renal diseases such as polycystic kidneys and progressive renal failure of Lhasa apso and Norwegian elkhound cause severe growth reduction.

Although growth reduction occurs with these diseases, more specific signs are likely to be present.

DIAGNOSTIC PLAN

The classification and causes of retarded growth are listed in the accompanying box. Table 12-1 lists the differentiating features of the most important causes of growth retardation.

The initial step in the diagnosis of growth retardation is to determine the presence or absence of signs suggestive of metabolic or polysystemic disease. The degree of retarded growth and the symmetry of the reduced size should be determined. For example, endocrine disorders usually cause severe but proportional dwarfism. In contrast, chondroplastic dwarfism that occurs in Alaskan malamutes is characterized by bilateral stunting of the forelimbs with carpal enlargement.[6-8] Careful examination of the long bones may provide additional clues. For instance, enlargement of the diaphyseal region of the long bones may suggest vitamin D deficiency and rickets. (See Display, Classification and Causes of Retarded Growth.)

The data base must include radiographs of a long bone, a complete blood count, urine analysis, and biochemical profile. See Table 12-1 for the diagnostic

Text continues on p. 90

TABLE 12-1.   Differential Diagnosis of Retarded Growth

Disease	Major Associated Sign(s)	Suggestive Laboratory Finding(s)	Radiographic Change(s)
Abnormal endocrine regulation			
Growth hormone deficiency	Hyperpigmentation Severe alopecia Absence of primary hair Delay in permanent dentition	Suppression of growth hormone and insulin-like growth factor	Delayed closure of growth plates
Congenital hypo-thyroidism	Sparse hair coat Dull, depressed at-titude	Low serum T4 Inadequate re-sponse to thyroid-stimulating hormone	None
Diabetes mellitus	Polydipsia, polyuria	Glycosuria Elevated blood glucose	None
Genetic disorders of bone and cartilage			
Chondrodysplasia (Alaskan malamutes)	Shortening of the ra-dius and ulna Carpal enlargement Lateral bowing of the forelimbs	Complete blood count (regenera-tive anemia due to hemolysis) Bone marrow (nor-moblastic ery-throid hyper-plasia)	Evidence of chon-drodysplasia at 8–12 weeks of age
Mucopolysaccha-ridosis (*e.g.,* Sia-mese cats)	Dwarfism Severe skeletal de-formities Neurologic deficits Retinal atrophy	Metachromatic in-clusion bodies in circulating leuko-cytes Increased levels of dermatan sulfate in urine	Bony proliferation and fusion of cer-vical vertebrae Entire spine may be involved Broad, irregular epiphyses and an-kylosis of joints
Achondroplasia (collie, basset hound, minia-ture poodle, Scot-tish terrier)	Abnormally short limbs May be associated with muscle weakness	None	Disturbance of epiphyseal, chon-droblastic growth Impaired ossifica-tion of long-bone cartilage
Nutritional deficiencies			
Zinc	Infection Poor wound healing Dry, scaly skin Hyperkeratotic foot pads	None	None

(continued)

TABLE 12-1. Differential Diagnosis of Retarded Growth *(continued)*

Disease	Major Associated Sign(s)	Suggestive Laboratory Finding(s)	Radiographic Change(s)
Calcium	Lameness Bone pain Pathologic fractures Neurologic signs	Serum calcium and phosphorus in low-normal range Alkaline phosphatase may be increased	Generalized skeletal demineralization Evidence of fractures (*e.g.,* healed)
Vitamin A	Thick cranial bones Delayed growth of nervous tissue Xerophthalmia Hydrocephalus Suppurative skin lesions	None	Shortening and thickening of the long bones Thick cranial bones
Vitamin D	Muscle pain Bending and distortion of long bones Nodular enlargements on bones	Low-normal serum calcium	Flattening and mushrooming of the growth plates Bending of the long bones
Oxygen	Cyanosis Rapid breathing Syncope Ascites, etc.	Increased packed cell volume Decreased arterial PO_2	Depends on condition
Congenital (inherited) disorders of cell metabolism			
Lipid storage diseases	Various neurologic signs suggesting cortical, cerebellar, or brain stem disease	None	None
Glycogen storage diseases	Muscle weakness Hepatomegaly Seizures	Blood glucose decreased or normal	Hepatomegaly
Congenital or acquired major organ failure or insufficiency			
Cardiopulmonary failure Congenital heart or great vessel defect Chronic pulmonary disease	Dyspnea Cyanosis Exercise intolerance Syncope Ascites Cough Tachycardia	Packed cell volume may be increased; abdominal transudate Decreased blood PO_2	Depends on cause: cardiomegaly, pulmonary edema, pleural effusion, pulmonary infiltrates, or fibrosis

(continued)

TABLE 12-1. Differential Diagnosis of Retarded Growth *(continued)*

Disease	Major Associated Sign(s)	Suggestive Laboratory Finding(s)	Radiographic Change(s)
Hepatic failure	Seizures Neurologic signs Vomiting Anorexia Hemostatic problems Ascites	Decreased serum albumin Increased serum ammonia	Small liver Angiography may reveal portosystemic shunt
Renal failure	Polyuria Polydipsia Vomiting Anorexia Renal rickets Dehydration	Decreased packed cell volume Increased blood urea nitrogen, creatinine, phosphorus Decreased calcium in some cases Isosthenuria	Small kidneys Bone demineralization
Digestive tract			
Megaesophagus	Regurgitation	None	Decreased esophageal motility and esophageal dilatation Aspiration pneumonia
Pancreatic atrophy	Diarrhea	Decreased trypsin-like immunoreactivity	None

Classification and Causes of Retarded Growth*

Abnormal Endocrine Regulation

- Growth hormone deficiency
     Pituitary dwarfism—German shepherd
- Congenital hypothyroidism
- Diabetes mellitus
     Rottweiler
     Golden retriever
     Keeshond

Genetic Disorders of Bone and Cartilage

- Chondrodysplasia
  Alaskan malamutes—chondrodysplastic dwarfs
- Mucopolysaccharidosis—Siamese cats
- Achondroplasia
  Basset hound
  Collie
  Miniature poodle
  Scottish terrier

Nutritional Deficiencies

- Major nutrients
  Protein (essential amino acids)
  Fats
  Carbohydrates
- Minerals   • Vitamins
  Zinc   A
  Calcium   D
- Oxygen
  Congenital heart disease (development defect)
  Chronic lung disease (as in "swimming puppies")

Congenital (Inherited) Disorders of Cell Metabolism

- Lysosomal storage diseases
- Glycogen storage diseases

Chronic Inflammation, Infection, and Parasitism

- Immunodeficiency diseases
- Intestinal parasitism

Congenital or Acquired Major Organ Failure

- Congenital heart failure due to developmental defects
- Hepatic failure
  Portosystemic shunts
- Renal failure
  Familial progressive renal insufficiency
    Lhasa apso
    Shih tzu
    Norwegian elkhound
  Canine Fanconi syndrome
  Congenital polycystic kidneys
- Digestive tract disease

*Note: The diseases listed above are major examples of the causes of retarded growth. The lists are not inclusive of every breed or disease.

findings associated with the various disorders. Radiographs can be very useful, since various forms of dwarfism have characteristic changes (see Table 12-1).

When endocrinopathies are suspected as the cause of dwarfism, specific hormonal assays are warranted. Thyroxine concentrations measured before and after thyroid-stimulating hormone (TSH) stimulation plus a thyrotropin-releasing hormone (TRH) response test should be performed. If thyroxine levels are normal, GH concentrations before and after intravenous clonidine (10 μg/kg) stimulation should be measured.[2] Blood samples are collected at 0, 15, 30, 45, 60, and 90 minutes after clonidine stimulation. Measurement of insulin-like growth factor I may also be useful.[2] In clinical practice it is difficult to find a reliable laboratory for the assay of GH and IGF.

REFERENCES

1. Daughaday WH: Growth and sex development. In MacBryde CM, Blacklow RS (eds): Signs and Symptoms, 5th ed, p. 32. Philadelphia, JB Lippincott, 1970
2. Eigenmann JE: Growth hormone and insulin-like growth factor in the dog: Clinical and experimental investigations. Dom Anim Endocrinol 2:1–16, 1985
3. Eigenmann JE, Patterson DF, Froesch ER: Body size parallels insulin-like growth factor I levels but not growth hormone secretory capacity. Acta Endocrinol (Copenh) 106:448–453, 1984
4. Eigenmann JE, Patterson DF, Zapf J, Froesch ER: Insulin-like growth factor I in the dog: A study in different dog breeds and in dogs with growth hormone elevation. Acta Endocrinol (Copenh) 105:294–301, 1984
5. Eigenmann JE, Zanesco S, Arnold U, Foresch ER: Growth hormone and insulin-like growth factor I in German shepherd dwarf dogs. Acta Endocrinol (Copenh) 105: 293–298, 1984
6. Fletch SM, Pinkerton PH, Brueckner PJ: The Alaskan malamute chondrodysplasia (dwarfism-anemia) syndrome: In review. J Am Anim Hosp Assoc 11:353–361, 1975
7. Kirk RW, Bistner SI: Normal physiologic data. In Handbook of Veterinary Procedures and Emergency Treatment, 4th ed, pp 885, 888. Philadelphia, WB Saunders, 1985
8. Tarpin T, Roach MR: Chondrodysplasia in the Alaskan malamute: Involvement of arteries, as well as bone and blood. Am J Vet Res 42:1865–1873, 1981

CHAPTER THIRTEEN

Weight Loss

Michael D. Lorenz

PROBLEM DEFINITION AND RECOGNITION

Weight loss is a physical condition that results from a negative caloric balance, such as when metabolic utilization and excretion of essential nutrients exceed the supply. Weight loss does not necessarily imply malnutrition; however, in many disease states it does. When the nutritive deficiency is restricted to calories, stored fats may be lost, which may be desirable (*e.g.,* in obesity). Weight loss may result from the loss of body fluids, as in dehydration, or from the elimination of ascites or edema. In this chapter, only weight loss due to undernutrition (calorie deficiency, protein deficiency, or both) is discussed. The reader is referred to other chapters dealing with the problems of dehydration, edema, and ascites.

Weight loss is considered significant when a 10% decrease in normal body weight occurs unassociated with loss of body fluids. Certainly, undernutrition is present when the small reserves of body protein are gone and body tissue protein is utilized for calories. Growth and weight charts should be consulted when one evaluates the significance of any weight loss. In addition, body conformation, muscle mass, and bone structure characteristics of the various breeds should be considered.

Emaciation is extreme weight loss due to severe undernutrition and is characterized by prominence of the skeleton due to catabolism of body fat and protein. Cachexia is a state of extreme ill health associated with weight loss, anorexia, weakness, and mental depression.

PATHOPHYSIOLOGY

When any of the many etiologic factors discussed in subsequent sections becomes of sufficient magnitude or persists for a sufficient time, the deficient nutrient is withdrawn from body stores or tissues that contain it. The first stage is a negative balance of the nutrient factor, causing abnormalities in growth, repair, or maintenance. Subsequent changes, in approximate order of appearance, are tissue depletion, biochemical changes, functional alterations, and anatomic defects.

In caloric undernutrition (negative caloric balance), balance must be achieved by reducing activity or by utilizing body tissues for energy. During the stage of tissue depletion, body stores of fat and limited stores of protein are used first. As a result, tissue depletion may be advanced before signs develop.

Several biochemical disturbances may occur in the undernourished animal. When tissue protein has been greatly depleted, total serum proteins may decrease, largely because of a decrease in serum albumin. Other biochemical changes likely to occur include an increase in extracellular fluid; vitamin deficiencies; calcium/phosphorus imbalance affecting bone metabolism with an increase in serum alkaline phosphatase activity; low serum iron concentration and microcytic anemia; and decreased concentrations of thyroid hormones.

The functional changes associated with undernutrition occur because of decreased metabolism and tissue depletion. Fatigue, lack of energy, and mental depression are common signs. The body temperature decreases in response to the decreased metabolic rate; decreased thermogenesis obviously saves calories. Bradycardia and hypotension are common. Nonregenerative anemias—in addition to iron deficiency anemia—may occur, since less hemoglobin is required to carry a reduced concentration of oxygen that supports the lower metabolic rate.

Extreme undernutrition results in anatomic lesions that are easily recognized. The fat padding is lost first, and muscles are catabolized later for energy. Pallor; skin hemorrhages; edema; dry, wrinkled skin that is inelastic; dry, brittle hair; reproductive failure or failure to cycle; gonadal atrophy; and periodontal disease are the most common anatomic lesions.

Once all adipose tissue is exhausted, severe depression, hypotension, and death will occur.

CAUSES OF WEIGHT LOSS

In general, there is but a single cause of weight loss: insufficient calories are present to meet the metabolic needs. However, caloric deficiency may be divided into three major categories (see Display, Causes of Weight Loss): (1) inadequate food intake, (2) failure to assimilate calorigenic nutrients, and (3) excessive caloric expenditure. All categories may be in effect, but there is always a negative caloric balance.

The degree of appetite may be an important clue to the diagnosis of certain diseases, since weight loss in the face of a normal or increased appetite suggests an inadequate diet, maldigestion syndrome, or excessive caloric expenditure, as occurs in hyperthyroidism or diabetes mellitus. However, serious undernutrition may cause anorexia in a patient that initially had a normal appetite. Many diseases may cause anorexia late in their courses (see Chapter 3).

Causes of Weight Loss

- Inadequate food intake
    Dietary deficiency
        Inadequate amount
        Poor digestibility
        Protein-calorie imbalance
    Oropharyngeal disease (dysphagia, prehension, and mastication problems)
    Vomiting and regurgitation
    Anorexia (numerous causes; see Chapter 3)
- Malassimilation of calorigenic nutrients
    Maldigestion
        Pancreatic exocrine insufficiency
        Bile salt deficiency
    Malabsorption syndromes
        Villous atrophy
        Infiltrative diseases
            Inflammatory bowel disease
            Lymphosarcoma
            Histoplasmosis
    Diarrhea
- Excessive caloric expenditure
    Increased metabolic rate
        Hyperthyroidism
        Fever
        Infection/sepsis
        Malignancy
        Heart failure
        Trauma
    Loss of caloric nutrients
        Diabetes mellitus (glucosuria)
        Renal disease (proteinuria)
        Burns (serum protein)
        Severe pyoderma (serum protein)
        Protein-losing enteropathy (albumin and globulin)
        Intestinal parasites
        Chronic blood loss
    Physiologic causes
        Pregnancy
        Lactation
        Extreme exercise
        Increased thermogenesis (decreased environmental temperature)

Clinical Manifestations of Undernutrition

- Weight loss
- Failure to grow
- Fatigue, muscle weakness
- Nervous irritability
- Delayed convalescence
- Poor wound healing
- Dehydration
- Anorexia
- Impaired liver function
- Protein deficiency
- Mineral, trace element deficiency
- Vitamin deficiency
- Anemia
- Edema, ascites (hypoalbuminemia)

Effects of Disease on Nutrition and Weight Loss

Various types of illness may affect the absorption, intake, utilization, or excretion of various nutrients. The reader is referred to the Display, Clinical Manifestations of Undernutrition. Two important causes of weight loss will be discussed.

Infection, Pyrexia, and Weight Loss. One of the earliest consequences of infection is anorexia and a tendency to drink only liquids. Antimicrobial therapy may interfere with the intestinal synthesis of certain nutrients such as vitamins. Fever, by increasing metabolic rate, causes catabolism of body tissue.

Infection and fever cause a stress reaction qualitatively similar to that of pain and fear. Cortisol released in response to stress mobilizes amino acids from skeletal muscle for glyconeogenesis in the liver. This process causes a depletion of body protein and a negative nitrogen balance, because the mobilized amino acids are deaminated to make glucose and the nitrogen is excreted as urea in the urine. In certain infections, especially those associated with diarrhea, deficiencies of vitamin A and the B vitamins may develop. This is especially of great concern in cats, in which the gastrointestinal synthesis of B vitamins is limited.

The malnutrition and weight loss associated with infectious disease result in several adverse effects. The outcome of infection is frequently worsened by the malnutrition, since malnutrition may decrease antibody formation, inhibit or delay phagocytic reactions, lower tissue resistance to infection, decrease the rate of wound healing and collagen formation, and delay the destruction of bacterial toxins.

Effects of Neoplastic Disease That Cause Weight Loss

- Anorexia (see Chapter 3)
    Suppression of appetite center
    Pain
    Disease of abdominal organs
- Maldigestion syndromes
    Deficiency of pancreatic enzymes
        Pancreatic cancer
        Diffuse infiltration of duodenum (obstruction of pancreatic ducts)
        Bile salt deficiency
        Obstruction of bile duct (bile duct carcinoma)
- Malabsorption syndromes
    Diffuse small intestinal neoplasia (*e.g.*, lymphosarcoma)
    Gastric hypersecretion (apudomas)
- Protein-losing enteropathies
    Diffuse small intestinal neoplasia with lymphatic obstruction (*e.g.*, lympho-
        sarcoma)
    Carcinoma (gastric, small intestinal, colonic)
- Electrolyte and fluid imbalances
    Vomiting
    Diarrhea
    Hypercalcemia (ectopic production of parathormone-like compounds)
- Increased or altered metabolism
    Induced anaerobic metabolism (lactic acidosis)
    Adrenal cortical neoplasia (*e.g.*, increased gluconeogenesis due to hypercorti-
        solemia)
    Thyroid neoplasia
    Pheochromocytoma
- Cancer therapy
    Surgical resection
        Chewing or swallowing difficulties
        Malabsorption (gastric or intestinal resection)
        Pancreas
            Maldigestion
            Diabetes mellitus
    Radiation treatment
        Anorexia
        Regurgitation
        Diarrhea
        Malabsorption
    Chemotherapy
        Anorexia
        Vomiting
        Diarrhea
        Abdominal pain
        Intestinal ulceration

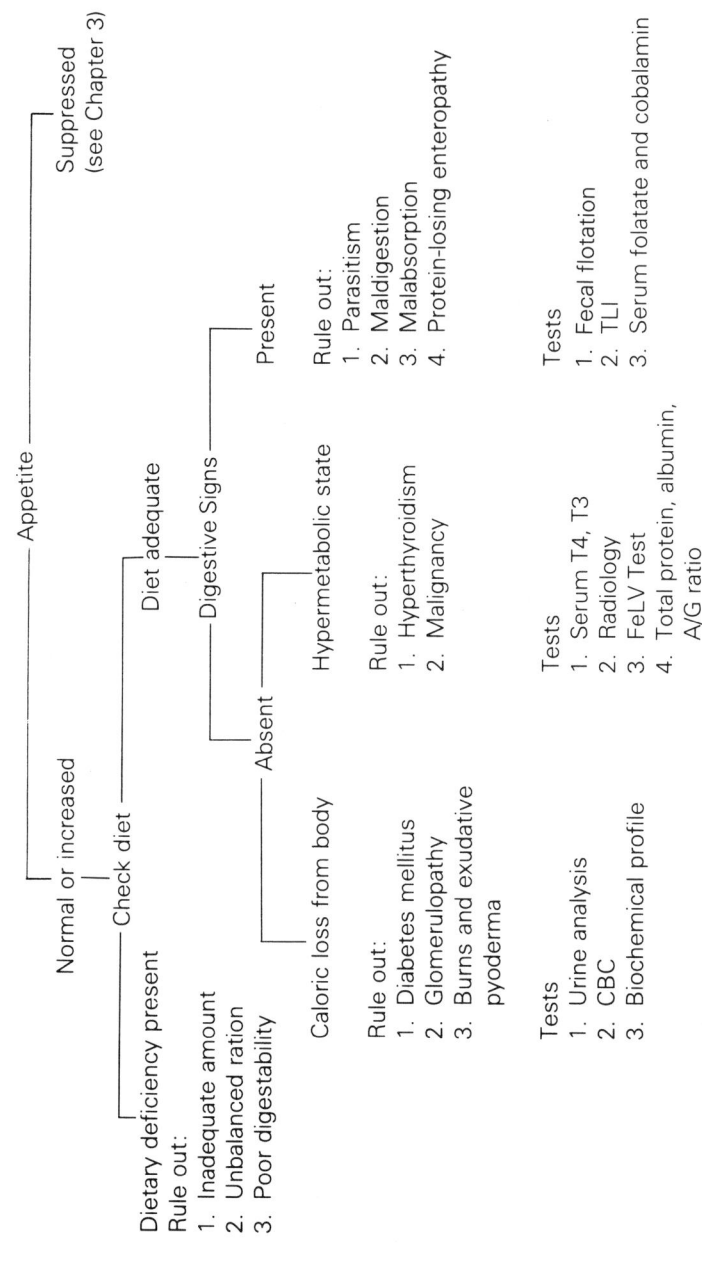

FIGURE 13-1. Diagnostic plan for weight loss.

Appetite
— Normal or increased
— Suppressed (see Chapter 3)

Check diet

Dietary deficiency present
Rule out:
1. Inadequate amount
2. Unbalanced ration
3. Poor digestability

Diet adequate

Digestive Signs
— Absent
— Present

Absent

Caloric loss from body

Rule out:
1. Diabetes mellitus
2. Glomerulopathy
3. Burns and exudative pyoderma

Tests
1. Urine analysis
2. CBC
3. Biochemical profile

Hypermetabolic state

Rule out:
1. Hyperthyroidism
2. Malignancy

Tests
1. Serum T4, T3
2. Radiology
3. FeLV Test
4. Total protein, albumin, A/G ratio

Present

Rule out:
1. Parasitism
2. Maldigestion
3. Malabsorption
4. Protein-losing enteropathy

Tests
1. Fecal flotation
2. TLI
3. Serum folatate and cobalamin

Cancer Cachexia. Malignant disease frequently results in severe weight loss and malnutrition. In fact, weight loss may occur as a very early finding in cancer, even before the development of other clinical signs. Thus, cancer—especially of the liver, pancreas, or intestinal tract—should be considered in the initial diagnostic plan for unexplained weight loss. In the cat, feline-leukemia-virus–associated disease or malignancy should receive priority in the diagnosis of weight loss.

As discussed in Chapter 3, cancer has an unexplained effect in causing anorexia and wasting. This may occur when obvious intestinal obstruction, sepsis, and endocrine disorders are not present.[1] The weight loss observed in animals with cancer is usually associated with anorexia, vomiting, diarrhea, or severe dysfunction of the liver or pancreas (see Display, Effects of Neoplastic Disease That Cause Weight Loss). It is possible that certain types of cancer cause direct suppression of the appetite center through unexplained mechanisms. Human cancer patients may have alterations in taste, although this is usually not the primary factor responsible for anorexia.[1]

A number of metabolic changes that alter energy requirements may occur in cancer patients. Cancer may alter energy metabolism so that requirements are increased beyond those of normal animals.[1] Some cancer patients experience an increased resting metabolic expenditure during a time of decreased caloric intake. Fever, infection, and stress-induced glucocorticoid release are not uncommon, and these cause increased gluconeogenesis and protein catabolism. In addition, the direct metabolic activity of certain tumors may be large enough to cause a significant drain on host tissues. Interestingly, cancer may cause the host to alter its normal aerobic metabolism in favor of a less efficient anaerobic state. This results in lactic acidosis and decreased energy production from carbohydrates such as glucose.

DIAGNOSTIC PLAN

A scheme for the diagnosis of weight loss is presented in Figure 13-1. It is based on the diseases listed under the Display, Causes of Weight Loss. A review of Chapter 3 may also be useful in the diagnosis of weight loss.

REFERENCE

1. Shils ME: Nutritional problems induced by cancer. Med Clin North Am 63:1009, 1979

CHAPTER FOURTEEN

Obesity

Michael D. Lorenz

PROBLEM DEFINITION AND RECOGNITION

Obesity is a condition of excess body fat. It is the most common nutritional disorder in veterinary medicine, with reported prevalence of 25% to 44% in dogs[2,3] and 6% to 12% in cats.[3] It should not be considered synonymous with excess body weight, although the two conditions often occur simultaneously in an animal. The term *common obesity* or *simple obesity* refers to adipose tissue that occurs in a normal body distribution. Dystrophic obesity, with a pathologic alteration in body fat distribution pattern, has not been reported in veterinary medicine. However, canine patients with hypercortisolism often have fatty deposits over the dorsal shoulders and intraabdominally, which may be a form of dystrophic obesity. There are two types of common obesity. *Hyperplastic obesity*, due to excessive numbers of adipocytes, may have a genetic component and is associated with overeating early in life. *Hypertrophic obesity* is due to increased fat cell size; it usually occurs in adult life and is believed to be more prevalent in veterinary medicine.

Variable conformation and body size make it difficult to determine "normal" body weight limit tables in veterinary medicine. Ultrasonography, girth measurements, and water displacement have been utilized to quantitate canine body fat content. Identification of clinically important obesity in veterinary patients is dependent upon a subjective evaluation of body fat stores. This is accomplished by palpation over the rib cage. The outline of the ribs should be readily palpable. Ribs obscured by subcutaneous fat are indicative of obesity; ribs readily visible without palpation suggest the animal is too thin. Excess fat may be deposited over the iliac crests in older, obese dogs. Ventral abdominal subcutaneous fat may be helpful in assessing feline obesity, although fat in this area is frequently confused with mammary gland development. Recognition is subjective, but obesity is often marked and apparent to the veterinarian. Obesity causing a 15% excess in body weight is potentially injurious to the patient and should be treated.[3]

Conditions that may be confused with obesity include generalized subcutaneous edema (anasarca) or abdominal distention due to any cause. Differentiation is generally possible on physical examination. Edematous subcutaneous tissue will generally "pit" upon compression, in contrast to the loose feel of subcutaneous fat. Abdominal distention due to obesity is accompanied by excess subcutaneous fat. Occasional cases of abdominal distention may be difficult to distinguish on physical examination; differentiation may require radiographs and/or abdominocentesis. The radiographic density of fat is intermediate to air and soft tissue (fluid); excess fat offers excellent radiographic contrast.

PATHOPHYSIOLOGY: DEVELOPMENT OF OBESITY

Obesity is always caused by prolonged caloric intake in excess of body needs. It may be due to overeating or reduced physical activity, or both. Genetic, endocrine, and social factors play contributory roles.

Obesity develops in two stages. In the first stage (the dynamic stage), body fat accumulates because of an excess in caloric intake. The pet's diet contains an excessive number of calories during this stage. In the second stage (the static stage), food intake is balanced by energy expenditure. In this stage, the obese sedentary dog may consume relatively few calories. Owners of pets in this stage of obesity are correct when they claim that their dogs eat only small quantities of food daily.

Food intake is under control of the feeding and satiety centers of the hypothalamus, which determine a "set point" for body weight.[3] This set point is not as tightly controlled as that for body temperature (see Chapter 2). It may be affected by psychologic factors (forebrain input), nutrient type, metabolic/endocrine diseases, food availability and palatability, and social factors (competition with other household pets and owner encouragement of food intake).[3] Boredom, idleness, and nervousness increase food intake in humans and may have a similar effect in animals. Highly palatable fatty or sweet foods are likely to be consumed more readily and increase the animal's set point for body weight. The use of predigested animal tissue ("digest") in commercial cat food has contributed to an increased prevalence of obesity in cats.[3] High-fat or high-carbohydrate nutrients are assimilated more efficiently and may lead to the development of obesity.[1,3]

Although an underlying disease condition predisposing the animal to obesity is not usually present, it is important to determine if such a condition exists and institute specific therapy where indicated. Commonly identified predisposing pathologic conditions (Table 14-1) include hypothyroidism and hyperglucocorticoidism (endogenous or exogenous). Other conditions that have been incriminated include cerebral or hypothalamic brain lesions and insulinoma. Even when a predisposing condition is identified, the condition of obesity is still dependent upon caloric intake in excess of needs and can be managed through dietary and exercise regulation.

There appears to be a genetic predisposition to obesity in cocker spaniels; Labrador retrievers; Cairn, West Highland, and Scottish terriers; and collies. Boxers, fox terriers, and Sealyham terriers are reported to have a low incidence of obesity.[2,3] Obesity is more common with advancing age, probably because of

TABLE 14-1. Clinical Diseases Predisposing to the Development of Obesity

Disease	Suggestive Clinical Signs	Laboratory Findings	Special Tests
Hypothyroidism	Lethargy, thick skin, alopecia, bradycardia, thermophilia, somnolence, hypothermia	Nonregenerative anemia	TSH response test
Hypercortisolism	Polyuria/poly-dipsia, pot-belly appearance, thin skin, alo-pecia, hepato-megaly	Stress leukogram, hyperglycemia, elevated alka-line phospha-tase, urinary tract infections	ACTH response test Dexamethasone suppression test ACTH Assay
Cortical/ hypothalamic lesion	Neurologic deficits		Neurologic exami-nation, CSF tap, EEG
Insulinoma	Weakness, sei-zures	Hypoglycemia	Amended glucose-to-insulin ratio

TSH, thyroid-stimulating hormone; ACTH, adrenocorticotropic hormone; CSF, cerebrospinal fluid; EEG, electroencephalogram

a reduction in basal metabolic rate and physical activity. Females are more commonly obese than males. Neutering had been associated with an increase in body weight in both sexes. In males, castration frequently reduces activity levels and also removes the androgenic hormone, testosterone, which normally diverts energy and amino acids into muscle protein production.[1] The result may be increased fat production. In females, ovariohysterectomy does not usually result in marked obesity. However, in occasional cases, spayed female dogs become severely obese. Reduced activity levels and increased food intake are believed to be contributory. Hormonal imbalance[1] (including high follicle-stimulating hormone levels, which stimulate feed intake, and low serum estro-gen levels, which normally inhibit food intake) may also play a role. Prevalence of obesity in pets is higher when the pet is owned by middle-aged, elderly, or overweight individuals.[2] This may be attributable to reduced exercise and/or increased caloric intake due to treats and table scraps.

The prevalence of obesity appears to be on the rise in veterinary medicine. The increased confinement of pets during the work day in suburban and urban environments plays a role by reducing physical activity. The highly palatable energy-dense pet foods on the grocery shelf are a product of a highly competitive industry in which palatability is at a premium. Obesity in veterinary patients is principally attributed to the use of these diets, which are offered in large amounts on a frequent or easily accessible basis. Reduction in energy expendi-ture due to low levels of physical activity, reduced metabolic rate, and genetic and endocrine factors further exacerbate this condition.

TABLE 14-2. Deleterious Effects of Obesity

Organ/System	Effect of Obesity
General	Lethargy, irritability, fatigability, heat intolerance, inactivity, increased risks with anesthesia and surgery, technical difficulty with many diagnostic and therapeutic procedures
Musculoskeletal	Arthropathies, metabolic bone disease
Cardiovascular	Increased cardiac workload, myocardial fatty deposits, myocardial hypoxia, and arrhythmias
Gastrointestinal	Increased risk of pancreatitis and hepatic lipidosis
Endocrine	Glucose intolerance, increased risk of diabetes mellitus
Respiratory	Dyspnea, alveolar hypoventilation ("pickwickian syndrome"), exacerbation of any respiratory disease (especially tracheal collapse)
Immune	Increased susceptibility to infection, delayed healing
Reproductive	Dystocia, infrequent cycling, reduced reproductive efficiency

Data from references 1 through 5

EFFECTS OF OBESITY

A list of health problems linked to obesity in dogs and cats is presented in Table 14.2.[1-5] Obese pets are frequently fed a diet consisting predominantly of table scraps. Such unbalanced, fatty foods cause many health risks beyond obesity and may predispose the animal to nutritional deficiencies, pancreatitis, diabetes mellitus, and other systemic diseases.

DIAGNOSTIC PLAN

Every attempt should be made to diagnose the predisposing pathologic conditions for obesity. A thorough history, physical examination, and basic laboratory tests are very useful in the differential diagnosis of these conditions. Table 14-1 lists the predisposing causes of obesity with their suggestive clinical signs, laboratory findings, and special diagnostic tests.

REFERENCES

1. Anderson GL, Lewis LD: Obesity. In Kirk RW (ed): Current Veterinary Therapy VII. Philadelphia, WB Saunders, 1980
2. Mason E: Obesity in pet dogs. Vet Rec 86:612, 1970
3. Morris ML, Lewis LD: Obesity. In Lewis LD (ed): Small Animal Clinical Nutrition. Topeka, KS, Mark Morris Associates, 1984
4. Sibley KW: Diagnosis and management of the overweight dog. Br Vet J 140:124–131, 1984
5. Ward A: The fat-dog problem: How to solve it. Vet Med 79:781–786, 1984

PART FOUR

Dermatologic Problems

CHAPTER FIFTEEN

Pruritus

Michael D. Lorenz

PROBLEM DEFINITION AND RECOGNITION

Pruritus is defined as an unpleasant sensation that provokes the desire to scratch. In veterinary medicine, this sensation is impossible to differentiate from other stimuli such as burning, since the animal's responses to these stimuli are similar. Self-mutilation (see Chapter 7) is a common sequela to offensive stimuli in the skin of small animals. The presence of excoriations is evidence of a pruritogenic disorder.

PATHOPHYSIOLOGY

Pruritus should be regarded as one of five primary cutaneous sensations; heat, cold, pain, and touch are the other four. Pruritus is an epidermal sensation, whereas pain can also be perceived from denuded skin. The sensory receptors are naked nerve endings located in the epidermis. The axons that carry pruritic sensation are small unmyelinated C fibers. They ascend in the ventrolateral spinothalamic tracts via the thalamus to the cerebral cortex. Certain areas of the skin may have increased numbers of "itch" receptors or are more sensitive to pruritic stimuli. Although fewer nerve endings are present in chronic dermatitic skin, those present have a lower threshold for pruritic sensation.

Mediators of Pruritus

For many years, histamine was believed to be the major pruritogenic substance. It is now believed that proteolytic enzymes are the major mediators of pruritus in dogs and cats. These enzymes may be released from bacteria, fungi, mast cells, epidermal cells (cathepsin), or leukocytes (leukopeptidases), or they may leak from plasma (plasmin) following capillary dilatation. Although pruritus is a common feature of allergic skin disease, many other diseases cause pruritus through the release of proteolytic enzymes (see Display, Factors That May Initiate Pruritus).

Factors That May Initiate Pruritus

- Physical factors
    Heat
    Cold
    Light
    Electrical stimuli
- Vasodilation
- Anoxia
- Proteolytic enzymes
- Histamine
- Serotonin
- Bile acids
- Calcium salts and uremia
- Asteatosis (dry skin)

Factors Affecting Pruritus

Certain conditions may actually potentiate the pruritic sensation. Boredom may increase the cerebral response to physiologic itch stimuli and actually convert the sensation to a pathologic state. This mechanism may play a role in the etiology of acral pruritic nodules, feline lick granuloma, feline hyperesthesia syndrome, and idiopathic acute moist dermatitis ("hot spots"). Chronically diseased skin has limited perception because of decreased pruritic receptors; however, stimuli applied to this skin are perceived as either a burning sensation or an itch. Thus, stimuli not usually considered noxious may be converted to pruritus (conversion itch). In addition, the remaining nerve endings may have a lower threshold for pruritic sensation. Chronic inflammation and secondary bacterial infections potentiate pruritus by increasing the accessibility of proteases to the nerve endings.

Temporary relief from pruritus occurs when other stimuli (heat, cold, touch, pain) suppress the sensation of itch by competing for neuronal circuits within the internuncial sensory neuronal pool in the spinal cord. To be effective, the competing stimulus must be applied to the same dermatome from which the pruritic sensation originated. Scratching is the primary physiologic response for the control or temporary relief of pruritus. However, scratching may actually potentiate pruritus, because the induced epidermal damage causes the release of additional proteolytic enzymes. This potentiates the itch-scratch-itch cycle common in many skin diseases.

Expanded Data Base for the Pruritic Animal

- Microbiologic tests
  Fungal culture
  Bacterial culture
- Immunologic procedures
  Intradermal skin tests
  Direct fluorescent antibody
- Histopathology
- Provocative exposure
  Environment
  Diet
  Drugs

DIAGNOSTIC PLAN

Pruritus is frequently associated with many primary skin lesions. These include papules, pustules, vesicles, and hyperemia. Secondary skin lesions observed with pruritus include excoriations, scales, crusts, lichenification, and hyperpigmentation. The nature of these lesions, their distribution pattern, and the degree of pruritus are very important factors to consider in the differential diagnosis of dermatologic conditions.

The desire to stop pruritus and its associated self-mutilation must be tempered by the desire to establish a correct diagnosis. Unfortunately, glucocorticoid drugs are frequently given to control pruritus with little regard for finding the underlying cause. The dermatologic history and physical examination should answer at least these five basic questions: (1) Is it pruritic? (2) What are the basic skin lesions? (3) What is the distribution pattern? (4) Is it contagious? and (5) Are other body systems involved?

A problem-specific data base should include a complete history, a description of the dermatologic lesions and their patterns, analysis of multiple skin scrapings, and results of Wood's light examination. This data base should be expanded to include a variety of other procedures based on the dermatologic findings (see Display, Expanded Data Base for the Pruritic Animal).

The diseases characterized by pruritus and their differentiating features are listed in Table 15-1.

TABLE 15-1. Classification of Skin Diseases on the Degree of Pruritus Usually Observed

Disease	History	Lesion(s)	Distribution	Special Test(s)
Very pruritic conditions				
Sarcoptic mange	May be contagious Dogs of all ages affected Nonseasonal	Papules, excoriations	Elbows, ear margins, ventral abdomen and chest	Skin scraping, response to therapy
Atopy	Age: 1–5 years Breeds: terriers, golden retrievers, Irish setters Seasonal and nonseasonal	Many cases have only pruritus—later papules, excoriations, erythema, and lichenification occur	Face, ear pinna, axilla, abdomen	Intradermal skin test (IDST)
Flea allergy dermatitis	Dogs and cats usually older than 1 year Seasonal, except in subtropical climates	Papules, excoriations Cat: miliary crusty or papular lesions	Dog: tail, head, inner thighs Cat: neck, back	Response to flea control IDST with flea antigen
Superficial staphylococcal dermatitis	Usually young dogs—more common during warm months Can be chronic Tendency to relapse	Papules, superficial pustules, erythematous collarettes with scales	Abdomen—may generalize	Response to antibiotic therapy
Feline hyperesthesia syndrome	Usually house cats Any age Psychologic episodes	Pulling of hair	Usually back, also limbs	None
Feline miliary dermatitis (see Flea allergy dermatitis)				
Rhabditic dermatitis	Animals on wet straw	Papular	Ventral—abdomen and legs	Skin scraping
Notoedric mange	Cats: contagious	Papules, excoriations, crusts	Head	Skin scraping

108

Subcorneal pustular dermatitis	Recurrent vesiculopapular eruptions Nonresponsive to antibiotics and corticosteroids	Papules—vesicles, erosions, crusts	Body and face (nose and ears)	Histopathology—subcorneal pustules—response to dapsone
Pemphigus (foliaceus and erythematosus)	Dogs and cats of any age Recurrent lesions	Vesiculopustular eruptions—erosions, scales, and crusts	Face, body, and feet Mucocutaneous lesions are rare	Histopathology—subcorneal acantholysis Positive direct FA
Dermatitis herpetiformis	(See Subcorneal pustular dermatitis)	Vesiculopustular eruptions	Body	Histopathology—subcorneal pustules Response to dapsone
Bacterial folliculitis	Younger short-haired dogs	Papules, small pustules	Body	Skin biopsy
Acral pruritic nodule (lick granuloma)	Usually solitary dogs Constant licking of limb	Nodule with eroded surface	Forelimb	Skin biopsy Radiography of limb
Drug eruption	Recent drug therapy	Papulomacular eruption	No specific distribution	Response to drug withdrawal
Food allergy dermatitis	Dogs and cats of any age Nonseasonal occurrence Acute and chronic signs common	Papules, erythematous plaques, excoriations Lesions may be severe Cats: may cause miliary dermatitis	Dogs: no specific distribution Cats: facial, may generalize	Response to hypoallergenic diet Skin biopsy
Allergic contact dermatitis	Nonseasonal occurrence Signs may wax and wane	Papuloeruptive to erythematous plaques	Ventral: feet, legs, abdomen, chest, axilla, neck	Provocative exposure to potential allergens
Mild to moderately pruritic conditions				
Pediculosis	Young animals	Scales—small papules	Generalized	None
Cheyletiella dermatitis	Young animals	Scales—small papules	Generalized	None

(continued)

TABLE 15-1. Classification of Skin Diseases on the Degree of Pruritus Usually Observed *(continued)*

Disease	History	Lesion(s)	Distribution	Special Test(s)
Demodectic mange	Usually dogs less than 3 years of age	Alopecia, scales, erythema, pustules	Localized—face, legs Generalized—face, body, ear canals, feet	Skin scraping
Pyoderma	No significant clues	Pustules Fistulous tracts	Depends on type	Bacterial culture
Dermatophytosis	Young animals	Circular scaling or asymmetric patches of alopecia	Head and legs usually Body in some severe cases	Fungal culture
Seborrhea	Common in spaniels No significant clues	Asymmetric patches of scales	Body, face, ears	None
Nodular panniculitis	Recurrent painful or pruritic nodules	Nodules with necrotic centers	Body	Histopathology—necrosis and inflammation of fat
Sporotrichosis	Often develops following skin injury	Nodules—suppurative lymph nodes Cats—erosive nodules	Limbs—may follow lymphatics Cats—head and face	Cytology Fungal culture Histopathology—PAS and methenamine silver stains

FA, fluorescent antibody; PAS, periodic acid–Schiff

110

CHAPTER SIXTEEN

Diagnostic Significance of Various Skin Lesions

Michael D. Lorenz

The morphology of skin lesions is extremely important in the diagnosis of dermatologic conditions. This chapter describes the morphology and diagnostic significance of the primary and secondary lesions. All lesions must be carefully examined so that the primary lesions are differentiated from the secondary changes.

PRIMARY SKIN LESIONS

Papule

Morphology. Papules are small, solid eruptions in the epidermis and are approximately 1 cm in diameter or smaller. Most papules are erythematous, reddened swellings produced by tissue infiltration of inflammatory cells, epidermal edema, or epidermal hypertrophy. Papules, when present as a group, may form erythematous plaques or rashes. The elevation may not be visible but can usually be felt with the fingertips. The surface epithelium of true papules remains intact unless secondarily traumatized.

Diagnostic Significance. Papules are the basic lesions in many allergic and parasitic skin diseases (*e.g.,* flea allergy dermatitis and sarcoptic mange). Papules are also the earliest stage in pustule formation and may be confused with the initial stages of small vesicular eruptions. Therefore, papules may be observed in pustular diseases such as bacterial folliculitis, pemphigus foliaceus, subcorneal pustular dermatoses, and dermatitis herpetiformis. It is very important to examine the stratum corneum covering the eruption. With pustules and vesicles, the stratum corneum is usually separated from the underlying epidermal layers, and the resulting cleft may be filled with various amounts of fluid or inflammatory exudates. Most diseases with papular eruptions are pruritic. Since scratching may dramatically alter the appearance of the skin, lesions should be characterized in nontraumatized areas.

Pustule

Morphology. Pustules are small circumscribed or larger asymmetric eruptions in the skin. The cavity of the pustule is filled with inflammatory (suppurative) exudate. Pustules may be superficial (just under the stratum corneum, *i.e.,* subcorneal) or deep (extending down to the hypodermis). Pustules may be yellow, erythematous, or hemorrhagic in appearance. Rupture of the pustule may leave a superficial erosion or, with deep pustules, a necrotic fistulating tract.

Diagnostic Significance. Subcorneal pustules are associated with superficial bacterial infection (superficial staphylococcal dermatitis, folliculitis), pemphigus foliaceus, subcorneal pustular dermatoses, and dermatitis herpetiformis. Deep pustules are frequently seen with deep pyodermas and certain fungal diseases such as sporotrichosis. In the differential diagnosis of pustular eruptions, the contents of an intact pustule should be microscopically examined for bacteria and acantholytic epithelial cells, and aseptically cultured for bacteria. Pemphigus foliaceus, subcorneal pustular dermatitis, and dermatitis herpetiformis form pustules that are sterile.

Vesicle

Morphology. Vesicles are circumscribed eruptions in the epidermis filled with clear fluid. Bullae are large vesicular eruptions. The "dome" covering the vesicle or bulla in dog and cat skin is very fragile and easily ruptured. Therefore, vesicular eruptions in dog and cat skin are short-lived and can be easily missed. Ruptured vesicles expose the underlying epithelium, creating erosions. Early vesicles may appear as papules and the term *vesiculopustular eruptions* is used when papules and vesicles coexist in the skin.

Diagnostic Significance. Vesicles may be associated with contact irritants or burns. Bullae are the basic lesions in pemphigus vulgaris and bullous pemphigoid, which are autoimmune skin diseases that produce clefts within the epidermis. Vesiculopustular or vesiculopapular eruptions are also associated with subcorneal pustular dermatoses, dermatitis herpetiformis, pemphigus foliaceus, pemphigus erythematosus, and drug eruptions.

Wheals

Morphology. Wheals are circumscribed, raised lesions, usually with a flat surface. They are usually erythematous and consist of localized edema.

Diagnostic Significance. Wheals may be associated with cutaneous anaphylactoid reactions such as insect bites, drug allergy, food allergy, or contact irritation. The classic wheal in dogs is the positive reaction to intradermal skin test antigens. Wheals are uncommon lesions in most allergic dermatoses of dogs and cats.

Macule

Morphology. Macules are circumscribed to slightly asymmetric spots in the skin, characterized by hyperpigmentation, depigmentation, or erythema.

Diagnostic Significance. Hyperpigmented macules are occasionally associated with endocrine disorders such as hyperadrenocorticism, Sertoli cell tumor, and hypothyroidism. Hyperpigmented macules frequently occur as the final stage in the healing of circumscribed superficial erosions (*e.g.*, superficial staphylococcal dermatitis). Erythematous macules are observed with many acute dermatoses and probably represent erythematous plaques. Depigmented macules are usually large and are called patches. They are associated with vitiligo and, rarely, hypothyroidism. Hyperpigmented macules are characteristic of many dog breeds and may be more apparent in puppies. In some breeds, these juvenile macules disappear near puberty and may reappear in later life.

Nodule

Morphology. Nodules are solid, usually round elevations in the skin that may extend into the deeper layers. The surface may be intact or ulcerated. Nodules are caused by cellular accumulations in the skin.

Diagnostic Significance. Nodules may be granulomatous (inflammatory) or neoplastic. Neoplastic nodules are called tumors. Biopsy of the nodule and histopathologic examination of the tissue are indicated to identify the underlying reaction. Callus, lick granuloma, nodular panniculitis, and histiocytoma are examples of nodular disorders.

SECONDARY SKIN LESIONS

Ulcer

Morphology. Ulcers represent denuded epithelium that exposes the dermis. Hair is usually absent in such lesions.

Diagnostic Significance. Severe necrotizing or inflammatory diseases produce ulcers. Ulcers generally heal with scar formation. Neoplastic conditions such as squamous cell carcinoma, burns, toxic epidermal necrolysis, and severe autoimmune diseases produce ulcers. Ulcerated skin provides a break in the barrier to bacterial infection and must be properly managed to prevent infection.

Erosion

Morphology. Erosions represent denuded epithelium that leaves the basement membrane intact. Hair follicles are usually preserved.

Diagnostic Significance. Erosions are the common lesions that remain when pustules, vesicles, or bullae rupture. Because the basement membrane is intact, erosions heal without scar tissue formation.

Excoriation

Morphology. Excoriations are symmetric or asymmetric superficial erosions caused by scratching, biting, or rubbing. The surface of the lesion is usually moist and contains hair.

Diagnostic Significance. Excoriations reflect the presence of a pruritic skin disease. The term *hot spot* is used by laypeople to describe this lesion.

Scale

Morphology. Scales are loose fragments of keratin debris that accumulate in the coat or on the skin. Most scales in the dog are dry, powdery, or flaky. Occasionally, waxy or greasy scales are found.

Diagnostic Significance. Scales represent a disorder of the keratinization process; they may reflect a lack of hydration in the stratum corneum. Waxy scales or scaly plaques are the basic lesions observed in primary seborrhea. Scales are nonspecific lesions that result from a variety of inflammatory and endocrine disorders.

Crust

Morphology. Crusts are dried blood, serum, pus, scales, or topical medications that cover the surface of ulcers or erosions.

Diagnostic Significance. See above sections on pustules, erosions, and ulcers.

Scar

Morphology. Scars are fibrous tissue that has replaced normal epithelium in the healing of an ulcer. Scars are depigmented and hairless.

Diagnostic Significance. Scars may follow severe burns and deep pyodermas. Irregular scars occur on the face and limbs of dogs and cats with the cutaneous manifestations of systemic lupus erythematosus. Canine solar dermatitis frequently heals with scar tissue formation.

Lichenification

Morphology. Lichenification is thickening of the skin with exaggeration of the superficial skin markings. Histologically, the skin is characterized by marked acanthosis (thickening of the prickle cell layer). Lichenified skin is usually hyperpigmented.

Diagnostic Significance. Lichenification is most commonly observed in chronically inflamed skin and may result from constant scratching or rubbing. It is also observed in acanthosis nigricans and the male feminizing syndrome. In many parts of the United States, the most common cause is chronic flea allergy dermatitis.

Hyperkeratosis

Morphology. Hyperkeratosis is an increased thickness of the stratum corneum. It may occur on the body, planum nasale, and digital pads. Scales are frequently associated with hyperkeratotic reactions.

Diagnostic Significance. See above section on scales. In addition, hyperkeratotic reactions are associated with dermatophyte infections.

CHAPTER SEVENTEEN

Alopecia

Michael D. Lorenz

Alopecia is the loss or lack of hair in any amount or distribution up to complete baldness. Alopecia may be a primary event; however, it most commonly occurs secondary to an acquired disorder.

PATHOPHYSIOLOGY

The basic mechanisms that produce alopecia include (1) abnormalities in follicular structure; (2) abnormalities in follicular function (alteration of hair growth cycle); (3) structural abnormalities of the hair shaft; and (4) traumatic removal of hair.

Abnormalities in Follicular Structure

Primary alopecia is caused by inherited abnormalities of follicular structure. These may range from complete absence of hair follicles to absence of hair follicles that produce hair of a particular color.

Secondary (acquired) alopecia may be caused by diseases that disturb the follicular environment, prompting the disruption of hair growth and the dislodgment of hair from the follicles. Bacterial folliculitis, demodectic mange, severe necrotizing processes, and follicular hyperkeratosis are examples of acquired diseases that adversely affect follicular structure.

Abnormalities in Follicular Function

Diseases in this category do not destroy follicular structure *per se*, but they adversely affect the normal cyclic phases of the hair follicle. The phases of follicular activity are anagen (growth phase) and telogen (resting phase). The normal follicular cycles in the dog and cat have seasonal variations; however, hair growth is not synchronized but follows a mosaic pattern. The majority of follicles are in anagen, yet a few neighboring follicles may be in catagen or telogen. Certain conditions or diseases cause alopecia by prompting the development of telogen follicles. Estrogens, testosterone, and adrenocortical hormones delay the initiation of anagen. Thyroid hormone accelerates follicular activity.

Conditions such as severe illness, fever, pregnancy, and lactation may cause the simultaneous precipitation of many follicles into catagen and telogen. The resulting alopecia is called "telogen effluvium." Certain drugs may also arrest mitotic activity of the follicle, causing alopecia.

The endocrine disorders may also produce follicular hyperkeratosis that results in follicular plugging. Follicular plugging disturbs normal hair growth.

Structural Abnormalities of the Hair Shaft

Certain diseases may weaken the hair shaft so that normal tension on the hair causes it to break. This is a primary mechanism for the alopecia that results from dermatophyte infections. Weakened, brittle hair shafts may be found in certain endocrine disorders, such as hypothyroidism.

Traumatic Removal of Hair

This is a common mechanism for the alopecia associated with pruritic dermatosis. Constant self-mutilation mechanically removes or breaks the hair. The underlying inflammatory process may also delay the initiation of anagen.

CLASSIFICATION

Alopecia may be classified by its onset (primary *versus* secondary) or by its distribution. The distribution pattern of the alopecia may be characteristic of the specific underlying disease. Alopecias may be classified by distribution as diffuse, regional, multifocal, or focal.

Diffuse Alopecia

The generalized or diffuse alopecias are primarily truncal and tend to spare the head and limbs. Endocrine disorders are the most important cause of nonpruritic diffuse alopecia. Their differentiating features are listed in Table 17-1. Occasionally, allergic, bacterial, fungal, or immune-mediated diseases cause generalized alopecia. Telogen effluvium has been previously described as a cause of diffuse alopecia.

Regional Alopecia

Regional alopecias occur in a variety of dermatoses that have a predisposition for certain areas of the body. These distribution patterns are useful in formulating a differential diagnosis. The conditions likely to involve the face, ears, feet, mucocutaneous junctions, and caudal body are given in the accompanying lists. (See Displays: Diseases with Marked Facial Alopecia; Diseases with Ear Alope-

TABLE 17-1. Differential Features of Endocrine Alopecia

Disease	Dermatologic Signs	Major Systemic Sign(s)	Profile Findings	Special Tests
Hypothyroidism	Intense hyperpigmentation Thickened skin Dry, brittle coat	Lethargy Cold intolerance Weight gain Myxedema Anestrus	↑ Serum lipids Rarely, nonregenerative anemia	T4 before and after TSH stimulation
Canine Cushing's syndrome	Thin skin, lack of skin elasticity Calcinosis cutis Pigmented macules	Polyuria/polydipsia Muscle weakness Abdominal enlargement Hepatomegaly Polyphagia Anestrus	Lymphopenia ↑ Alkaline phosphatase ↑ Serum lipids ↑ Glucose ↓ Urine specific gravity	Plasma cortisol before and after ACTH stimulation Dexamethasone suppression tests
Sertoli cell tumor	Gynecomastia Thin skin Pigmented macules	Pendulous prepuce Cryptorchidism	Rarely, anemia and thrombocytopenia	Ultrasonography
Male feminizing syndrome	Hyperpigmentation and lichenification of the caudal abdomen and flanks Gynecomastia	Attraction to male dogs	No consistent clues	None
Adult-onset growth hormone deficiency	Variable degrees of alopecia and hyperpigmentation of rump, flanks, and body	None	No consistent clues	Growth hormone assay before and after xylazine stimulation
Estrogen deficiency	Patchy alopecia of flanks and back Very soft skin Very soft and fine hair	Occasionally urinary incontinence	No consistent clues	Response to estrogen therapy
Feline endocrine alopecia	Alopecia of caudal abdomen, rear legs Occasionally diffuse truncal alopecia	None	No consistent clues	None
Hypotestosteronism	Diffuse truncal alopecia Mild hyperpigmentation	Castrated Testicular atrophy	No consistent clues	Serum testosterone Response to testosterone therapy

↑, increased; TSH, thyroid-stimulating hormone; ACTH, adrenocorticotropic hormone

119

Diseases with Marked Facial Alopecia

- Demodectic mange
- Dermatophytosis
- Canine and feline acne
- Feline food allergy dermatitis
- Systemic lupus erythematosus
- Discoid lupus
- Pemphigus erythematosus
- Pemphigus foliaceus
- Canine solar dermatitis
- Atopy
- Epidermolysis bullosa simplex/dermatomyositis
- Juvenile pyoderma
- Lipfold pyoderma
- Subcorneal pustular dermatosis
- Notoedric mange
- Drug eruption

Diseases with Ear Alopecia

- Dermatophytosis
- Demodectic mange
- Sarcoptic mange
- Pemphigus foliaceus
- Pemphigus erythematosus
- Seborrhea
- Marginal ear pinna alopecia and seborrhea
- Periodic ear pinna alopecia of miniature poodles
- Subcorneal pustular dermatitis
- Solar dermatitis (cats)
- Cold agglutinin disease
- Fly bite dermatitis
- Bacterial otitis externa
- Otodectic otitis externa
- Atopy

Diseases with Alopecia of the Feet

- Atopy
- Contact dermatitis
- Discoid lupus erythematosus
- Demodectic mange
- The pemphigus group
- Bullous pemphigoid
- Interdigital pyoderma
- Thallium poisoning

Diseases with Mucocutaneous Involvement and Alopecia at Mucocutaneous Junctions

- Pemphigus vulgaris
- Bullous pemphigoid
- Candidiasis
- Thallium poisoning
- Drug eruption
- Toxic epidermal necrolysis

---

cia; Diseases with Alopecia of the Feet; Diseases with Mucocutaneous Involvement and Alopecia at Mucocutaneous Junctions; and Diseases with Alopecia of Caudal Trunk and Abdomen.)

Multifocal Alopecia

Multifocal alopecia is probably the most common distribution pattern. It may begin with a focal pattern, but multiple lesions develop as the disease progresses. See Display, Diseases Producing Multifocal Alopecia.

Focal Alopecia

This form of alopecia may initiate a multifocal distribution pattern and is caused by many of the diseases that produce multifocal alopecia. Diseases such as demodectic mange, acral pruritic nodule, dermatophytosis, and solitary neoplasms may remain as a focal pattern throughout the course of the disease.

Diseases with Alopecia of Caudal Trunk and Abdomen

- Flea allergy dermatitis
- Feline endocrine alopecia
- Male feminizing syndrome
- Hypoestrogenism
- Adult-onset growth hormone deficiency

Diseases Producing Multifocal Alopecia

- Demodectic mange
- Dermatophytosis
- Pyoderma
- Superficial staphylococcal dermatitis
- Cutaneous neoplasia
- Autoimmune skin diseases
    The pemphigus group
    Bullous pemphigoid
    Systemic lupus erythematosus
    Discoid lupus erythematosus
- Dermatitis herpetiformis
- Subcorneal pustular dermatosis
- The deep mycoses
- Seborrhea
- Nodular panniculitis
- Cutaneous candidiasis
- Zinc-responsive dermatosis

DIAGNOSTIC PLAN

Although the distribution of alopecia may provide clues to the diagnosis, characterization of the primary and secondary lesions is also very important. The diagnostic significance of the various skin lesions is described in Chapter 16.

In certain cases, direct examination of the hair shaft and root may provide some clues as to the underlying etiology. Club hairs have a tiny white ball at the root end, and root sheaths are absent. Club hairs indicate a telogen hair follicle; however, the removal of club hair may initiate anagen. Anagen hairs plucked from the follicle have a larger expanded root surrounded by a root sheath. Hair can be carefully plucked from the coat so that the anagen-to-telogen ratio can be determined. When telogen hairs predominate, endocrine disorders, normal shedding, and telogen effluvium should be considered. Diseases that attack the hair shaft, such as dermatophytes, cause the hair to break; the root end may appear like a spear. Traumatic alopecias are characterized by hair broken midway up the shaft. These hairs may be more difficult to pluck from the follicle.

PROGNOSIS

The reversibility of alopecia depends on two factors: (1) the presence of viable hair follicles and (2) the correction of the underlying pathology. Alopecia is permanent when hair follicles are congenitally absent or reduced in number (hypotrichosis), or when lesions heal with scar tissue formation. Scar tissue is devoid of hair follicles, since it is derived from connective tissue.

CHAPTER EIGHTEEN

Abnormalities of Skin, Hair, and Mucous Membrane Pigmentation

Michael D. Lorenz

Abnormalities of skin or coat color are of great concern to pet owners, especially when the abnormality is an obvious fault in a show animal. Of greater importance to veterinarians is the realization that these disorders may reflect a serious underlying disease. An understanding of the normal pigmenting process is necessary in order to correctly diagnose these disorders.

NORMAL SKIN AND HAIR PIGMENTATION

Three basic pigments (melanin, hemoglobin, and carotene) and the optical effect called *scattering* are responsible for normal skin color. Scattering is the rearrangement of light as it passes through a turbid medium (*e.g.*, skin, hair, mucosa). The degree of pigment and the density of the medium containing the pigment combine to produce the various colors.

Skin and Hair Pigments

Melanin. Melanin is formed by specialized cells (melanocytes) in the basal cell layer of the epidermis, hair follicle, and mucous membranes. Melanogenesis involves the oxidation of tyrosine to melanin. This reaction is catalyzed by a copper-containing enzyme called *tyrosinase.* Melanin is injected through dendritic processes from the melanocytes into epithelial cells. Some free melanin pigment is engulfed by dermal cells called *melanophages.* Melanogenesis is increased by ultraviolet light, raised temperature, and friction. Sulfhydryl compounds inhibit tyrosinase activity and thus decrease melanin production.

The intensity of melanin pigment is not determined by the number of melanocytes but by the size and number of melanin granules contained in epithelial cells. Dark-skinned animals have larger, more numerous melanin granules in several layers of epithelial cells. Albino individuals have sufficient melanocytes but cannot form melanin because of a defect in tyrosinase activity.

The colors produced by melanin range from brown to yellow, orange, or orange-red. Melanin is a strong pigment and usually obscures the other pigments in dark-skinned animals.

Melanin is the primary black-brown pigment of hair and pheomelanin is the yellow-red pigment. Pigmentation may be uniform throughout the shaft or have alternating bands of varying degrees of pigment. White hair is largely devoid of melanin. Pigment cells within the hair root (bulb) deposit the pigment in or between the cortical and medullary hair cells. The amount of pigment placed in the hair is genetically determined and creates the optical effects characteristic of particular breeds. The distribution of melanocytes within hair follicles is also genetically determined. This accounts for spotting, ticking, and other color patterns.

Hemoglobin. Blood vessels of the mucous membranes, sparsely pigmented skin, and white nails are penetrated by light and thus contribute to the color of these tissues. The primary pigment is hemoglobin. Oxyhemoglobin is more red, and reduced hemoglobin is more blue. Thus, the overall hue is determined by the ratio of oxyhemoglobin to reduced hemoglobin. Rapid changes in skin, mucous membrane, or nail color result from changes in vessel diameter, blood flow, and degree of hemoglobin oxidation. Increased reddening of the skin, mucous membrane, or nails is caused by vasodilation, whereas vasoconstriction or hypotension has the opposite effect. Cyanosis is apparent when reduced hemoglobin is present in concentrations of 5 g or more per deciliter of blood. Extreme cold may also cause increased skin redness, because the lower temperature may decrease oxygen utilization in local tissue; thus, more oxyhemoglobin is present to give the red color.

Carotene. Carotene and its related pigments impart a yellowish color to the skin. It is relatively unimportant in small animals.

INCREASED SKIN PIGMENTATION

This process may involve melanin, hemoglobin, carotene, and pigments of endogenous (bilirubin) or exogenous origin. Melanin and bilirubin are the most clinically important pigments.

Melanosis

Melanosis is hyperpigmentation due to increased amounts of melanin. Several factors may potentiate excessive melanin production. It is more common in canine skin (see Display, Causes of Melanosis in Dogs) and occurs infrequently in cats.

External Causes. Melanosis resulting from ultraviolet light exposure is called tanning. It is of little clinical significance in animals, since the hair coat tends

Causes of Melanosis in Dogs

- Chronic eczematous dermatoses
  - Flea allergy dermatitis
  - Atopy (chronic)
  - Allergic contact dermatitis
  - Food allergy dermatitis
- Focal superficial dermatoses
  - Superficial staphylococcal dermatitis
  - Dermatophytresis
- Hormonal conditions
  - Hypothyroidism
  - Hyperadrenocorticism
  - Sertoli cell tumor
  - Male feminizing syndrome
- Miscellaneous conditions
  - Acanthosis nigricans
  - Friction
  - Tanning (only in areas of alopecia exposed to light)

to prevent light exposure to the skin. The planum nasale and ear tips of white cats may actually suffer sunburn because of insufficient melanin protection.

Heat, radiation therapy, and mechanical irritation (as from a collar or harness) may cause localized melanosis.

Chronic Inflammation. Melanosis is a common finding in chronic inflammatory dermatoses. The pattern may be focal, multifocal, or regional. The underlying mechanism is not completely known but may be related to mechanical irritation (scratching, rubbing). The inflammatory process may also directly stimulate melanin production. Melanosis is most common in lichenified skin that results from chronic allergic conditions (*e.g.,* chronic flea allergy dermatitis).

Hormonal Control. The pituitary gland plays the dominant role in controlling melanin metabolism. Melanocyte-stimulating hormone (MSH) is secreted by the pituitary gland and increases melanin production in the skin. It is structurally similar to adrenocorticotropic hormone (ACTH), which also may stimulate melanosis in humans. Apparently ACTH has little, if any, MSH activity in dogs or cats that is clinically important.

Melatonin is a hormone found in the pineal gland of mammals. It decreases melanin production and may be useful in treating acanthosis nigricans. Melatonin has little effect in humans.

Glucocorticoids have an antimelanin effect. Since ACTH apparently has little MSH activity in dogs, it is difficult to rationalize the diffuse melanosis observed in hypercortisol states such as canine Cushing's syndrome. Unlike the disease in humans, melanosis is not a prominent feature of canine adrenal insufficiency.

Estrogens tend to stimulate melanosis, whereas testosterone has little or no effect. Thus, the melanosis of hyperestrogenism can be explained; however, the hyperpigmentation observed in male feminizing syndrome is difficult to rationalize if the etiology is actually hypoandrogenism.

Thyrotropin (thyroid-stimulating hormone, TSH) has a melatonin-like effect, whereas increased levels of thyroid hormones stimulate melanosis in humans. Hypothyroid dogs frequently develop generalized melanosis. This reaction is difficult to rationalize, since the hormonal changes should reduce melanin production. Obviously, other factors must be operating in hypothyroid dogs.

Melanoplakia. Melanoplakia is focal melanosis of the mucous membranes. It has been observed in certain breeds of dogs and orange tabby cats. Melanoplakia has little clinical significance other than cosmetic. It should be differentiated from malignant melanoma.

Yellow Pigmentation

Jaundice (Icterus). The serum bilirubin must reach 2 to 4 mg/dl before jaundice is clinically detectable. Tissue staining lags plasma staining, whereas the reverse is true when icterus is subsiding. Biliverdin imparts a greenish hue to the yellow color and usually occurs with biliary obstruction. Elastic tissue has a great affinity for bilirubin, which may explain the accentuation of icterus in the sclerae, conjunctivae, and mucous membranes. Icterus cannot be detected in edematous skin.

Medication. Quinacrine hydrochloride (Atabrine) is a drug utilized in the treatment of *Giardia* infection, solar dermatitis, and discoid lupus. It may produce a diffuse yellow color of the skin. Unlike bilirubin, the pigmentation is less intense in the sclerae.

Hemoglobin Pigmentation

Blood diffused through the skin and subcutaneous tissue at first has a purplish-blue or blackish-blue color. As the blood breaks down, bilirubin and biliverdin are formed. These pigments produce localized yellowish or yellowish-green discoloration.

Polycythemia produces an erythematous to purplish-red discoloration of the skin and mucous membranes. The vessels of the mucous membranes are very congested and appear slightly cyanotic. This condition, erythremia, represents the effects of red oxyhemoglobin tinted blue by an increased amount of reduced hemoglobin due to sluggish blood flow through the microcirculation.

Carbon monoxide poisoning produces a cherry-red color of the skin and mucous membranes because of the formation of carboxyhemoglobinemia. Cyanohemoglobinemia due to cyanide poisoning produces a similar effect. If death occurs, the bright red color persists. Methemoglobinemia produces a brownish-blue discoloration.

DECREASED SKIN PIGMENTATION

Abnormal skin, hair, or mucous membrane color may result from the loss of one or more normal pigments or modification of their appearance by some anatomic or physiologic factor.

Anemia

Pallor is the effect of decreased hemoglobin in blood vessels. Hemolytic anemia produces a combination of pallor and icterus. The yellow pallor of intravascular hemolysis may be modified by the presence of hemoglobinemia.

Decreased Melanin Production

Albinism. Albinism is a genetically controlled defect in the conversion of tyrosine to melanin. There is no deficiency of melanocytes or the substrate tyrosine. The entire skin, eyes, and hair are devoid of pigment. All white small animals are not true albinos in that some melanin pigment is present in the eyes and skin. Albino animals are predisposed to sunburn of the ears and nose or the skin when the hair is clipped or lost from disease.

Vitiligo (Leukoderma). Vitiligo is an acquired loss of melanin pigmentation in focal areas of the hair and mucous membranes. It has a patchy distribution of white hair or depigmentation of the gums, mucous membranes, eyelids, and nose. Vitiligo has been recognized in the Belgian truverian, Doberman pinscher, appaloosa horse, and other dark-coated breeds of dogs.

Several potential causes of vitiligo have been recognized. It may result from anatomic destruction of melanocytes (freezing, severe necrosis, scar tissue), inhibition of melanin formation (copper deficiency), nervous influences, and autoimmune antibody formation. The underlying cause in dogs has not been determined. Affected animals are healthy in all other respects, and the disease is usually slowly progressive. In humans, vitiligo may be caused by Addison's disease, hyperthyroidism, diabetes mellitus, and pernicious anemia.

A localized form of vitiligo involving the planum nasale has been observed in dogs eating from rubber food dishes that contain *p*-benzylhydroquinone. Apparently this chemical is absorbed through the skin and inhibits melanin synthesis. The condition is reversible.

Immunologic Dermatoses. Depigmentation of the nose, periocular skin, and/or oral mucosa and lips is a feature of several immunologic disorders including discoid lupus erythematosus, systemic lupus erythematosus, pemphigus foliaceus and erythematosus, and the Vogt-Koyanagi-Harada—like (VKH) syndrome. Ultraviolet light may potentiate the autoimmune response directed at melanocytes or melanin pigment. Severe ulceration of involved skin may result and is aggravated by continual licking or rubbing of the affected areas. VKH syndrome is characterized by loss of pigment in the previously described areas as well as a severe uveitis. The cause of VKH syndrome is unknown, but a hypersensitivity to melanin is suspected. Akitas, Samoyeds, and Siberian huskies are the breeds most frequently affected.

Depigmentation of the nose is the primary feature of canine solar dermatitis. Apparently, sunlight activates a photosensitization resulting in severe ulceration of the planum nasale.

Leukotrichia. Leukotrichia is the loss of pigment from hair causing normally pigmented hair to turn white. In addition to the conditions that cause leukoderma, leukotrichia may be caused by a variety of conditions that disrupt the injection of melanin into the developing hair shaft. Trauma, burns, follicular infections, and ionizing radiation may cause these local effects. In some black-haired animals, hair clipping may cause the growth of white hair. The defect is usually temporary.

PART FIVE

Hematolymphatic Problems

CHAPTER NINETEEN

Prolonged Bleeding

Craig E. Greene

PROBLEM DEFINITION AND RECOGNITION

Bleeding disorders can involve deficiencies in platelets, in the extrinsic or intrinsic coagulation systems, or in vascular integrity, alone or in combination. An outline of extrinsic and intrinsic coagulation sequences is presented in Figure 19-1. The clinical presentation of a bleeding disorder may aid the clinician in arriving at a diagnosis. Purpuric or ecchymotic hemorrhages are usually caused by microscopic lesions in the blood vessel wall, resulting from impaired formation of platelet plugs at sites of microvascular injury. Animals with such defects show multifocal pinpoint petechial or ecchymotic hemorrhages, most commonly on the skin and mucosal surfaces. Epistaxis, melena, and hematemesis may be seen in severe cases of platelet-induced bleeding. In contrast, bleeding associated with abnormalities in the extrinsic and intrinsic clotting systems is usually characterized by large spreading subcutaneous hematomas, body cavity

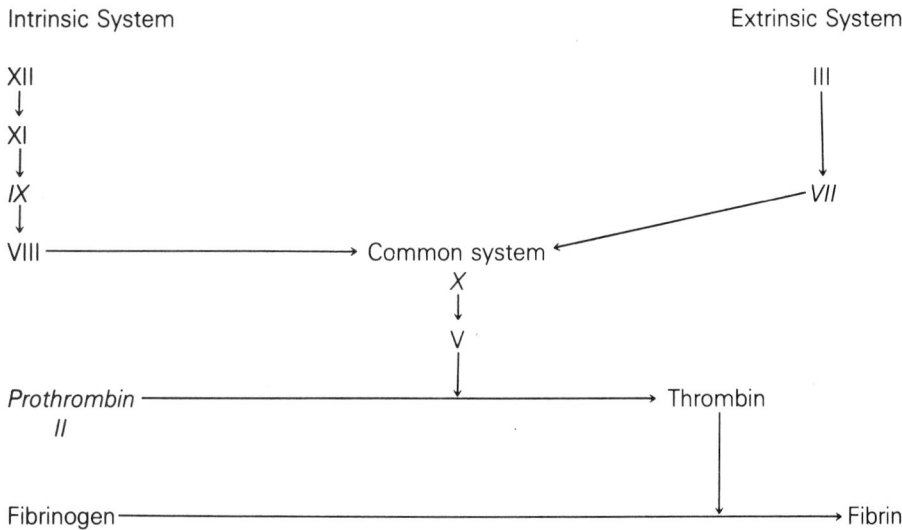

FIGURE 19-1. Coagulation cascade. Vitamin K–dependent factors are in italics.

hemorrhage, and rebleeding following venipuncture and surgical dissection. In general, animals with clotting defects in the latter stages of the intrinsic pathway show greater incoagulability than those with abnormalities in early intrinsic stages or in the extrinsic pathway.

Hemorrhagic disorders, regardless of cause, have also been classified as hereditary or acquired. *Hereditary* clotting disorders are being recognized with increasing frequency in domestic animals, most notably the dog and cat. Frequently, genetically affected animals have a history of recurrent hemorrhagic episodes beginning early in life. The severity of clinical signs depends on several factors, including the type of defect, the degree of the deficiency, and individual variation. Moderately to severely affected animals with hereditary bleeding disorders are commonly young at presentation. Tail-docking, ear-cropping, dew claw removal, and neutering may initiate the problem. However, with the absence of surgical or traumatic insult or of stress, overt clinical signs may not be evident. *Acquired* clotting disorders arise in animals of any age as a pathophysiologic response to preexisting disease. The hemorrhagic diathesis may be the most profound manifestation or, in other cases, only one part of the clinical spectrum associated with the underlying disease.

Hereditary Platelet Disorders

Thrombocytopenia

- Decreased platelet production
    Neonatal virus disease
    X-linked trait (Wiskott-Aldrich syndrome)
    Autosomal traits (various diseases such as Bernard-Soulier syndrome)

Platelet Dysfunction

- Thrombasthenia
    Glanzmann's disease
- Thrombopathia
    Bernard-Soulier syndrome
    Storage pool disease
    Albinism
    Ehlers-Danlos syndrome
    Wiskott-Aldrich syndrome
    Osteogenesis imperfecta
    Others

Susceptible breeds: otterhounds, basset hounds; isolated in other breeds: Simmenthal cattle, cats, fawn hooded rats

TABLE 19-1. Hereditary Clotting Factor Deficiences

Factor	Disease	Species or Breed	Type of Deficit	Clinical Signs
I	Afibrinogenemia Hypofibrinogenemia	Saanen goats	AID	HD; severe
II	Hypoprothrombinemia	Boxers	AID	Neonatal HD; epistaxis, mild
VII	Hypoproconvertinemia	Beagles Alaskan malamutes	AID	Mild; bruising, demodicosis
VIII	Hemophilia A (classic hemophilia)	Most dog breeds, mongrels, cats, horses	X-linked	HD; severe, moderate, or mild
IX	Hemophilia B (Christmas disease)	Cairn terriers, St. Bernards, coonhounds, French bulldogs, particolored cocker spaniels, Alaskan malamutes, British shorthair cats	X-linked	HD; ususally severe
von Willebrand factor + platelets + epithelium	von Willebrand's disease	German shepherds, miniature schnauzers, golden retrievers, Doberman pinschers, Scottish terriers, Pembroke Welsh corgis, Manchester terriers, Chesapeake Bay retrievers, other breeds of less frequency, Poland-China swine, rabbits	AID	HD; usually moderate or mild; severe postsurgical bleeding; otitis externa; panosteitis; epistaxis; melena; stress-induced bleeding; often lethal in homozygotes
X	Stuart factor deficiency	Cocker spaniels, mongrels	AID	Neonatal HD; lethal in homozygotes
XI	Plasma thromboplastin antecedent deficiency	Springer spaniels, Great Pyrenees, Kerry blue terriers, Holstein cattle	AID	HD; mild; hematuria; severe or lethal bleeding 12–14 hr after surgery
XII	Hageman trait Hageman factor deficiency	Cats, marine mammals, reptiles, birds, poodles, sharpei	AR in cats	None

AID, autosomal, incomplete dominance; HD, hemorrhagic diathesis; AR, autosomal recessive

135

Acquired Platelet Disorders

Thrombocytopenia

- Decreased or ineffective thrombopoiesis
  Irradiation, myelophthistic diseases, hypothyroidism, drugs (estrogens, cytotoxic agents)
- Increased destruction, consumption, or sequestration
  Immunologic: idiopathic, isoantibodies, hypersplenism, infectious agents, vaccination, ehrlichiosis, drug-induced disorder, autoimmune disease
  Coagulatory: mechanical (extracorporeal circulation), vascular disease (hemangiosarcoma, vasculitis) disseminated intravascular coagulation
  Sequestration: splenomegaly (splenic neoplasia, portal hypertension)
- Dilutional by transfusion of platelet-free fluids such as stored blood products, crystalloids, or colloids

Thrombocytosis

- Increased production: hemorrhage, hemolysis, iron deficiency, rebound, cirrhosis
- Decreased storage: exercise, stress, epinephrine, vincristine

Platelet Dysfunction

- Disease-associated: hyperfibrinolysis, uremia, hepatic dysfunction, paraproteinemias, scurvy, polycythemia, myeloproliferative diseases
- Drug-induced: aspirin, phenlybutazone, heparin, estrogen, phenothiazines, local anesthetics, plasma expanders, warfarin, sulfonamides, propranolol, many antibiotics, antihistamines

Acquired Clotting Factor Disorders

- Primary hyperfibrinolysis
- Disseminated intravascular coagulation (DIC)
- Vitamin K deficiency
  Rodenticide ingestion
  Complete biliary obstruction
  Prolonged enteric antimicrobial therapy
- Circulating anticoagulants
  Heparin administration
  Plasma expander therapy
  Antifactor antibodies

- Liver disease
  DIC
  Vitamin K deficiency
  Factor dysfunction
  Decreased factor synthesis
  Hyperfibrinolysis

PATHOPHYSIOLOGY

Hereditary coagulation defects (see Display, Hereditary Platelet Disorders and Table 19-1) arise as genetic mutations and have increased in prevalence because of the high degree of inbreeding of domestic dog and cat populations. A defect usually results in a malfunctioning coagulation protein and generally involves one coagulation factor. Undoubtedly, there is some heterogeneity with respect to the severity and underlying cause of the coagulation defect, even within the same disease. Von Willebrand's disease (VWD) is caused by a deficit in a coagulation protein that is responsible for both platelet and coagulation factor dysfunctions. There are a wide variety of quanititative and qualitative deficiencies of the Factor VIII–related proteins with VWD, and affected animals can range from asymptomatic to those with fulminant hemorrhagic episodes.

Although numerous hereditary disorders of coagulation exist, those acquired as a result of another disease process are more frequent. Acquired bleeding disorders can involve abnormalities in platelets or clotting factors, or both (see Displays, Acquired Platelet Disorders and Acquired Clotting Factor Disorders). In contrast to hereditary disorders, clotting disorders that arise as pathophysiologic responses to preexisting disease frequently are associated with a wide variety of hemostatic alterations.

RULE OUTS AND DIAGNOSTIC PLAN

Diagnostic laboratories can screen for coagulation disorders using a number of tests, including the prothrombin time (PT), partial thromboplastin time (PTT),

TABLE 19-2. Summary of Coagulation Screening Test Results in Most Common Hereditary Bleeding Disorders

	Factors XII, XI, IX, and VIII, and von Willebrand	Factors III, VII	Factors I (Fibrinogen), II, V, X	Thrombocytopathy
Screening tests				
Platelet count	N	N	N	N
ACT	P	N	P	N*
Laboratory tests				
PT (extrinsic)	N	P	P	N
PTT (intrinsic)	P	N	P	N
Fibrinogen	N	N	N†	N
FDPs (clot lysis)	–	–	+	–
Decreased factors	As above	As above	As above	–

N, normal; ACT, activated coagulation time; PT, prothrombin time; PTT, partial thromboplastin time; P, prolonged; –, absent; +, present; FDPs, fibrinogen degradation products

*May be slightly prolonged in some cases, only by 20 seconds or less when counts are less than 20,000

†Decreased in Factor I (fibrinogen) deficiency

TABLE 19-3. Summary of Coagulation Screening Test Results in the Most Common Acquired Bleeding Disorders

	Thrombocytopenia	Hepatic Dysfunction	Disseminated Intravascular Coagulation			Vitamin K Deficiency	Hyperfibrinolysis
			Low-Grade	Acute	End-Stage		
Screening tests							
Platelet count	D	N	D	DD	D	N	N
ACT	N*	P	N	P	PP	P	P
Laboratory tests							
PT (extrinsic)	N	P	N	P	PP	P	P
PPT (intrinsic)	N	P	N	P	PP	P	P
Fibrinogen	N	D	N	D	DD	N	D
FDPs (clot lysis)	−	±	−	+	++	−†	+
Decreased factors	−	I, II, V, VII IX, X	I, II, V, VII, VIII, X, XIII			II, VII, IX, X	I, V, VIII

D, decreased; N, normal; DD, very decreased; ACT, activated coagulation time; P, prolonged; PP, very prolonged; PT, prothrombin time; PTT, partial thromboplastin time; FDPs, fibrinogen degradation products; −, absent; ±, variable; +, present

*May be slightly prolonged in some cases but only by 20 seconds or less when counts are less than 20,000

†Increased FDPs are seen in some cases with extensive extravascular hemorrhage.

thrombin time (TT), coagulation factor assays, and fibrin(ogen) degradation products (FDPs) test. Tables 19-2 and 19-3 summarize the tests used to distinguish the most common hereditary and acquired bleeding disorders seen in small animals. Unfortunately, these tests are not routinely available to most practitioners.

In contrast, a platelet count and an activated coagulation time (ACT) can be used as routine screening tests to separate the various bleeding disorders and to aid in the initial decision regarding appropriate therapy. These two tests have the advantages of being simple to perform and readily available to most veterinary practitioners. Enumeration of platelets is performed indirectly by estimating platelet numbers relative to leukocytes on stained blood films or directly by counting with a hemocytometer and a commercially available diluting-lysing solution (Unopette Microcollection System No. 5855, Becton Dickinson Co, Rutherford, NJ). On blood films, there are normally three to five platelets per oil immersion field. Platelet morphology can also be evaluated at this time, since large forms appear in consumptive states. The ACT is a relatively reproducible measure of the intrinsic and common coagulation pathways. Commercially supplied tubes (Activated Coagulation Time Tubes No. 6522, Becton Dickinson Co, Rutherford, NJ) are available for this procedure. Blood taken by clean venipuncture is injected directly into the prewarmed (37.5°C) vacuum tube or transferred by syringe. The time interval from injection of the blood into the ACT tube until the first evidence of a visible clot is determined to be the ACT. In the dog, a normal ACT is less than 120 seconds. In the cat, it is usually less than 75 seconds.

CHAPTER TWENTY

Lymphadenopathy

Craig E. Greene

PROBLEM DEFINITION AND RECOGNITION

There are hundreds of lymph nodes and lymphoid aggregates of varying size in the dog and the cat, but only a few are palpable on routine physical examination. Palpable superficial nodes include the mandibular, superficial cervical, popliteal, and inguinal lymph nodes. Determining what constitutes mild enlargement is somewhat subjective, since the size of lymph nodes varies according to body weight, breed, amount of body weight, and hydration status. Clinical experience is the best judge of the amount of enlargement. If lymph nodes are exceptionally enlarged, thorough clinical and laboratory testing should be performed based on the location and number of lymph nodes involved.

PATHOPHYSIOLOGY

Lymph nodes are the sites of lymphocyte production and formation of antibodies in response to an antigenic stimulus. In certain diseases involving extramedullary hematopoiesis or myeloid metaplasia, the lymph nodes may produce erythrocytes, platelets, and neutrophils. The causes of lymphadenopathy can be classified by cytomorphologic findings (see Display, Causes of Lymphadenopathy). Enlargement of lymph nodes, which can be localized or generalized, usually reflects the extent of the pathologic process. Acute enlargement from inflammatory processes generally is accompanied by warmth, tenderness, and reddening of the overlying skin. The enlargement may be discrete, or—if it extends into surrounding tissues—the node may be adherent and immobile. This latter process is a common finding with severe localized granulomatous conditions. Necrosis and rupture with drainage are common sequelae to chronic lymph node suppuration associated with infection caused by certain bacteria, such as *Pasteurella, Actinomyces, Nocardia,* and *Yersinia.* Marked lymph node enlargement in the absence of signs of local inflammation frequently reflects lymphatic neoplasia. Noninflamed enlarged lymph nodes usually do not cause physical discomfort. An animal with this type of enlargement is not presented for examination unless the owner observes the swelling or unless blood vessels, lymphatics, or airways are sufficiently occluded to cause additional problems such as edema.

Causes of Lymphadenopathy

- Granulomatous
  - Fungus
  - Bacteria
  - Algae
    - Persistent intracellular forms
- Reactive hyperplasia
  - Infectious
    - Protozoa
    - Metazoa
    - Virus
    - Rickettsiae
  - Immune-mediated
    - Allergic
    - Immunologic
    - Autoimmune
- Suppurative
  - Bacteria
    - Extracellular types
    - Streptococci, staphylococci, *Pasteurella*
- Neoplasia
  - Primary or metastatic
    - Lymphosarcoma
    - Plasma cell neoplasia
    - Metastatic neoplasia
  - Cellular proliferation
    - Extramedullary hematopoiesis

Localized infections usually induce lymphadenopathy, which is limited to the area of regional drainage. If the infection becomes systemic or if it spreads, generalized lymph node enlargement occurs.

RULE OUTS AND DIAGNOSTIC PLAN

A summary of diagnostic laboratory testing for lymphadenopathy is listed in the Display, Ordered Diagnostic Plan for Lymphadenopathy. Laboratory testing should always be preceded by a detailed physical examination. The location of lymphadenopathy may suggest the site of origin of the disease causing it. In metastatic neoplasia, the site of primary tumor must be sought carefully, since the secondary lymphadenopathy may be more prominent than the primary lesion. Rectal, deep cervical, and abdominal palpations and thoracic and abdom-

Ordered Diagnostic Plan for Lymphadenopathy

1. Lymph node aspirate
2. Complete blood count, including platelets
3. Biochemistry, including albumin-to-globulin ratio
4. Urine analysis
5. Bone marrow analysis
6. Serum- or immuno-electrophoresis
7. Specific infectious disease testing (serologic or culture)
   a. Persistent bacteria (*e.g., Brucella, Mycobacterium*)
   b. Persistent viruses (*e.g.,* feline leukemia virus, feline infectious peritonitis virus)
   c. Rickettsiae
   d. Fungi
   e. Protozoa (*e.g., Toxoplasma*)
8. Chest or abdominal radiography or ultrasonography to document multisystemic involvement
9. Lymph node biopsy with special staining for microorganisms, if indicated
10. Culture of lymph node or tissue biopsy

inal radiography may be needed when routine physical examination fails to reveal the lesion site. To perform complete oral and nasopharyngeal examinations, sedation and general anesthesia may be necessary.

The most direct and important, but often overlooked, clinical diagnostic procedure for lymphadenopathy is lymph node aspiration. The area over the enlarged node is clipped free of hair and surgically prepared. The operator immobilizes the node securely between the thumb and forefinger of one hand and percutaneously pierces the node using a sterile 20- to 22-gauge needle and 6- to 10-ml syringe held in the other hand. The tissue is aspirated rapidly back and forth, and then the needle is withdrawn while slight negative pressure is placed on the system. Smears of the aspirated tissue are made by gently dispensing the contents of the syringe onto a clean glass slide. The slide can be initially stained with new methylene blue to determine if the collection of cells is satisfactory and to be used for preliminary examination. Subsequently, the smear should be stained with Wright's stain for a permanent slide and a more accurate cytomorphologic assessment. Gram staining for bacteria should be done when suppurative cytologic findings are present. Lymph node aspirates are most helpful in differentiating hyperplastic and neoplastic conditions. Excisional biopsy of an enlarged node should be performed if the findings on needle aspiration are nonspecific. Selection of the site is usually made on the basis of the largest palpable node. Surgical biopsy provides greater amounts of tissue needed for special staining and cultural procedures and gives information about the overall architecture of the diseased lymph node. Impression smears should always be made from the excised nodes prior to fixation. Impression smears of biopsied tissue give more detailed information about the morphology of individual cells than does histologic examination.

The results of cytologic and histologic examination of enlarged lymph nodes can usually be divided into several categories (see Display, Causes of Lymphadenopathy). Neoplasia, either primary or secondary metastatic forms, can be detected on the basis of abnormal cellular morphology. Specific infectious agents such as *Mycobacterium,* some rickettsiae, *Leishmania, Toxoplasma,* and deep mycotic agents may be detected on direct examination of the node. Other bacterial and fungal agents usually produce suppurative or granulomatous reactions, but organisms are seldom seen. Reactive hyperplasia has the cytologic appearance of a normal node in that the small lymphocyte is the predominant cell, while there are lesser numbers of larger, variably sized lymphocytes, macrophages, and plasma cells. Since active lymph nodes can have similar cytologic appearances, the fact that the lymph node is enlarged indicates hyperplasia, which is usually seen as a reaction to viral, rickettsial, or noninfectious antigens. The cytologic appearance of granulomatous lymph node enlargement is similar to that of reactive hyperplasia, with the exception of neutrophils; however, histologic examination may be needed to differentiate between these two syndromes.

Abnormal findings of routine hematologic and biochemical tests and urine analysis done prior to surgical lymph node biopsy may suggest the presence of a systemic disorder. Additional diagnostic testing may be performed on the basis of the cytologic or histologic findings of the node. If an infectious disease is suspected on the basis of lymph node cytomorphology, then specific serologic testing or cultural procedures should be employed. Bone marrow examination may be indicated if lymphoid neoplasia is suspected based on the presence of abnormal cell types.

PART SIX

Cardiovascular Problems

CHAPTER TWENTY-ONE

Disturbances of the Heart: Rate, Rhythm, and Pulse

Clay A. Calvert

PROBLEM DEFINITION AND RECOGNITION

Disturbances of the cardiac rate and rhythm with associated pulse characteristics are among the most common clinical signs of underlying cardiac or extracardiac disorders. The heart rate and rhythm are determined by either cardiac auscultation or palpation of the arterial pulse. Pulse deficits are found when successive contractions occur so rapidly that left-ventricular diastolic filling is insufficient to generate a normal pulse pressure.

CLASSIFICATION

Disturbances of the heart rate can be broadly classified as bradycardias or tachycardias (Table 21-1). Disturbances of the heart rate are termed *arrhythmias* and are abnormalities of the rate, regularity, or site of origin of the cardiac impulse; or of the conduction of the electrical impulse generated by a pacemaker. The mechanism of cardiac arrhythmias involves disturbances of impulse formation or impulse conduction. Arrhythmias arise from abnormalities of automaticity or conduction, or both.

Sinus tachycardia and sinus bradycardia are probably the most common cardiac rhythm disturbances. These arrhythmias are often physiologic in origin and are frequently not associated with organic heart disease.

Ventricular premature contractions, atrial premature contractions, atrial fibrillation, first- and second-degree atrioventricular block, and ventricular tachycardia were the most commonly diagnosed arrhythmias in dogs in one clinical study.[11] In another study, atrial arrhythmias occurred in approximately 10% of 2000 dogs evaluated during routine examinations because of suspected arrhythmias or for the evaluation of antiarrhythmic drug therapy. Ventricular arrhythmias occurred in approximately 6% of the dogs. Atrial premature beats, ventricular premature beats, atrial fibrillation, first- and second-degree atrioventricular block, and ventricular tachycardia were, in that order, the most common arrhythmias.[13]

TABLE 21-1. Classification of Heart Rate Abnormalities and Common Associated Conditions

Classification	Common Association(s)
Tachycardia	
Sinus tachycardia	Physiologic
	Congestive heart failure
	Systemic disorders
	Hypoxemia
	Drug administration
Atrial tachycardia	Atrial enlargement
	Pulmonary disease
	Drug administration
Atrial fibrillation	Cardiomyopathy
	Mitral insufficiency
Ventricular tachycardia	Cardiomyopathy
	Mitral insufficiency
	Myocarditis
	Contusion
	Toxemia
	Bacteremia
	Ischemia
	Drugs
Bradycardia	
Sinus	Physiologic
	Systemic disorders
	Hypoxemia
	Drugs
	Increased vagal tone
Sinoatrial block or arrest	Physiologic
	Drugs
	Sick sinus syndrome
	Increased vagal tone
Sinoventricular conduction	Hyperkalemia
Advanced second-degree and complete atrioventricular heart block	Myocardial fibrosis
	Cardiomyopathy
	Hyperkalemia

PATHOPHYSIOLOGY

The inherent heart rate and rhythm are constantly modified by numerous physiologic mechanisms, primarily chemical and neurologic in nature. Electrocardiographic analysis is required for the definitive diagnosis of disturbances of cardiac rate and rhythm.

Chemical control is exerted by certain ions and endocrine hormones. Sodium and potassium are the predominant electrolytes important in the control of the

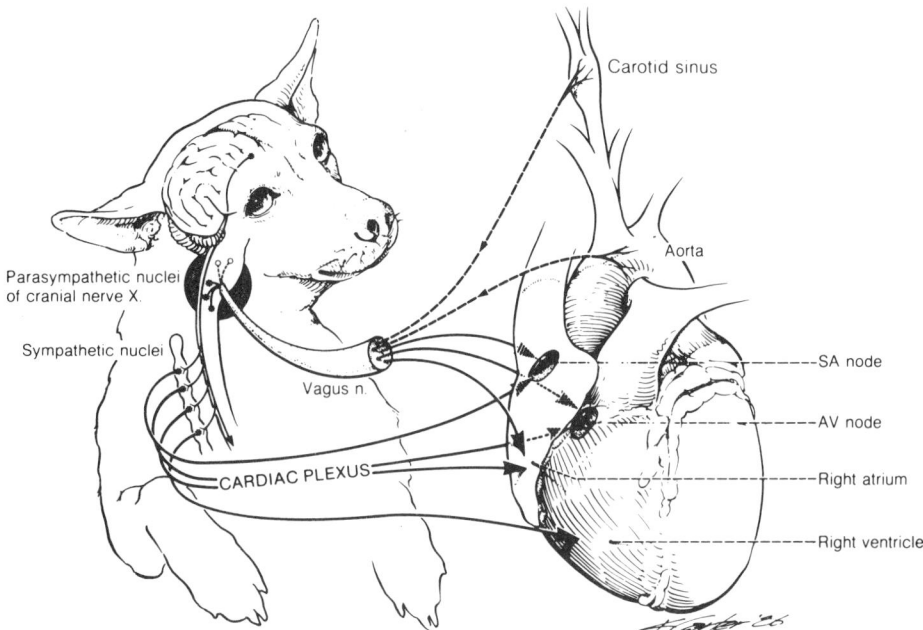

FIGURE 21-1. Schematic representation of the autonomic innervation of the canine heart.

cardiac rate and rhythm. The adrenal gland, when stimulated by its sympathetic nerve supply, secretes a mixture of epinephrine and norepinephrine, hormones that have a profound effect on heart rate and contractility. The autonomic nervous system is responsible for the innervation of the heart (Fig. 21-1). The autonomic nervous system regulates the rate of intrinsic impulse formation, controls the conduction of impulses, and influences the state of myocardial contractility.[1,3,6,9]

The nerve impulses of the autonomic nervous system are transmitted by a chemical mediator. The neurotransmitter of both the sympathetic and parasympathetic preganglionic neurons as well as the postganglionic parasympathetic neurons is acetylcholine. They are cholinergic neurons. The neurotransmitter of the postganglionic sympathetic neurons is norepinephrine.[2] They are adrenergic neurons.

The sympathetic preganglion neurons originate in the first four or five thoracic segments of the spinal cord and extend to the sympathetic chains.[2] The cardiac sympathetic nerves arise from the anterior thoracic sympathetic ganglion. Sympathetic stimulation of the heart increases both the rate and force of myocardial contraction.

The cardiac parasympathetic nerves originate in the medulla oblongata, specifically in the parasympathetic nuclei of the vagus nerve. The efferent fibers terminate primarily in the sinoatrial node, atria, and atrioventricular node.[8]

The right vagus nerve innervates primarily the atrioventricular node.[5] Vagal stimulation results in a slowing of the sinoatrial rate and a decrease in the rate of impulse conduction through the atrioventricular node.[5] The vagus nerve is the efferent limb of a reflex arc with the vagal center in the medulla. Generally speaking, the potential afferent pathways capable of affecting the vagal center include all of the afferent nerves of the body. The more important afferent impulses for controlling the heart arise in portions of the circulatory system, especially those regions from which it receives and into which it discharges the blood: the right atrium and aorta, respectively. On the venous (receiving) end, the Bainbridge reflex causes acceleration of the heart when venous return is excessive to the point of overdistending the right atrium. The sensory endings are in the right atrium and adjacent vena cava and are stimulated by increased tension. The resultant nerve impulses are transmitted by the afferent fibers of the vagus nerve and inhibit the vagal center, thus increasing the heart rate.

On the arterial side is a depressor reflex, whose afferent fibers arise from the left ventricle and the root and the arch of the aorta, and course to the medulla within the vagus nerve. Increased pressure within or contractility of the left ventricle as well as increased tension within the aorta results in vagal stimulation and a slowing of the heart rate. The reverse occurs if the intraaortic pressure becomes subnormal. A similar depressor reflex, dependent on the carotid artery pressure, has its afferent nerve endings in the carotid sinus. The afferent fibers from the carotid sinus reach the medulla via the glossopharyngeal and vagus nerves and the sympathetic trunk. The carotid sinus is a specially innervated part of the arteries and adjacent tissues located at the carotid artery bifurcation. Highly developed nerve endings in the carotid body, in the same location, are chemoreceptors sensitive to hypoxemia and hypercarbia, the response to which is cardiac acceleration.

The higher centers of the brain also may be a source for initiating afferent impulses to the medulla. Increased intracranial pressure is usually associated with slowing of the heart, brought about by overstimulation of the vagal center. This effect may be directly mechanical and due to ischemia resulting from increased pressure upon the blood supply of the medulla. Ischemia stimulates all of the medullary centers, including the vasomotor center, resulting in peripheral vasoconstriction and hypertension. Hypertension, in turn, acts on the aorta and carotid sinus to stimulate depressor reflexes that contribute to bradycardia.

The sympathetic and vagal centers in the medulla form a functional unit referred to as the cardiac center. The quantity and quality of blood reaching this center affect the heart rate. Slight hypoxia of the cardiac center results in an increased heart rate, as does slight hypercarbia. Severe hypoxia results in bradycardia; severe hypercarbia may produce a heart block. Such effects occur by means of efferent impulses coursing along the vagus or sympathetic nerves, or both. Increased temperature of the blood perfusing the cardiac center accelerates the heart rate.

The sympathetic control of the heart is subordinate to vagal control. The afferent pathways of the sympathetic system are identical to those of the vagus nerve. The cardiovascular sensory areas of the right atrium, aortic root, and carotid sinus have an analogously intimate relationship with sympathetic control. Consequently, cardiac acceleration from an overdistended atrium, although predominantly brought about by inhibition of the vagus center, is partially produced by sympathetic nerve stimulation. Slowing of the heart by the vagus in the depressor reflex is enhanced by a concomitant decrease in sympathetic tone.

CONDUCTION SYSTEM ANATOMY

The cardiac conduction system consists of the sinoatrial node, the internodal tracts, the atrioventricular node, the bundle of His, the right and left bundle branches, and the Purkinje fibers (Fig. 21-2).[4,7,10,14,15] The sinoatrial node, situated in the upper right atrium, is the primary pacemaker. The internodal pathways conduct the electrical impulse generated by the sinoatrial node to the atrioventricular node. The atrioventricular node is on the right side of the lower portion of the interatrial septum and is continuous with the bundle of His.

The bundle of His establishes an electrical link between the atria and ventricles as it penetrates the atrioventricular ring. The bundle of His continues along the interventricular septum and bifurcates near the aortic valve. The right bundle branch courses down the right side of the interventricular septum to the anterior papillary muscle. Branching fibers then radiate over the right ventricular free

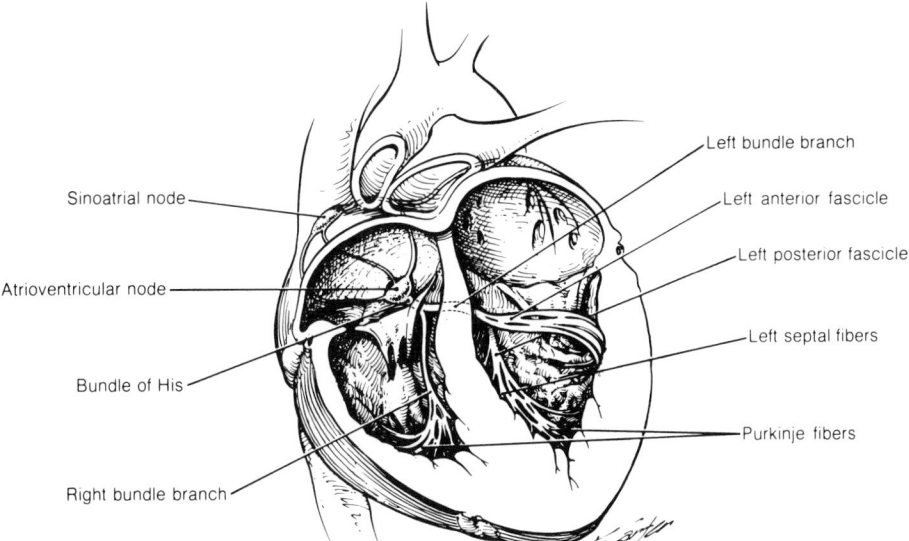

FIGURE 21-2. Schematic representation of the cardiac conduction system of the dog.

wall. The left bundle branch courses along the left side of the interventricular septum and arborizes into two largely interconnected fascicles that course to the two papillary muscles. All diversions of the bundle branches divide into the Purkinje fiber network, which penetrates the ventricular myocardium.

TACHYCARDIA

The most common type of tachycardia is referred to as sinoatrial or, usually, sinus tachycardia. In dogs and cats, the normal sinus rate is between 70 and 120 beats per minute. Most small dogs and cats have a resting sinus rate of 90 to 120 per minute. The causes of sinus tachycardia are numerous (Table 21-2) and are usually the result of extracardiac physiologic or pathologic stimuli. Transient tachycardia is a daily occurrence as a physiologic response to exertion, pain, and heat. Sinus tachycardia is usually the result of altered activity of the autonomic nervous system, rather than a primary disorder in the function of the sinus node. Physiologic sinus tachycardia occurs during and after stimuli resulting in anxiety and is an integral part of the "fight-or-flight" adaptive responses mediated through the sympathetic nervous system.

In congestive failure the heart rate may accelerate to maintain normal tissue perfusion. Extrinsic mechanisms, nervous or chemical, such as the Bainbridge and carotid sinus and aortic reflexes, are involved in the production of compensatory tachycardia in heart failure.

TABLE 21-2. Common Causes of Sinus Tachycardia

Category	Causes
Physiologic	Exercise
	Pain
	Excitement
Pathologic	Fever
	Shock
	Hemorrhage
	Hypotension
	Feline hyperthyroidism
	Anemia
	Hypoxia
	Drugs
	Atropine
	Catecholamines
	Hydralazine
	Congestive heart failure
	Toxicity
	Hexachlorophene
	Endotoxins
	Infections

Sinus tachycardia tends to be persistent as long as its etiology persists. It is usually not paroxysmal unless the stimulus is also short-lived. As a general rule, the rate of sinus tachycardia is usually between 120 and 180 beats per minute, although rates of up to 210 to 220 per minute may occur. In puppies, kittens, and cats, rates may reach 240 to 260 per minute.

Atrial Tachycardia

Unlike sinus tachycardia, atrial tachycardia is usually paroxysmal, that is, it persists for a few beats, to seconds, to minutes but may be sustained in some instances (Fig. 21-3). The rate associated with paroxysmal atrial tachycardia is usually in excess of 200 beats per minute and is typically in the range of 240 to 300 beats per minute. The exceedingly rapid rate and paroxysmal nature of atrial tachycardia are the most useful clues to the differential diagnosis (Table 21-3). An electrocardiogram is necessary for proof of the correct diagnosis. The exact character of the P wave and PR interval during normal sinus rhythm must be recorded to confirm the diagnosis. Since paroxysmal atrial tachycardia is usually of short duration, the P wave configuration and PR interval during normal sinus rhythm can usually be assessed and compared with those associated with the tachycardia.

Atrial tachycardia in dogs and cats may be associated with chronic cardiac disease; if so, severe left atrial enlargement is usually present. In the dog, these changes are most often the result of chronic mitral valve insufficiency (Table 21-4). In the cat, hypertrophic cardiomyopathy is the most common etiology.

TABLE 21-3. Differential Diagnosis of Sinus and Atrial Tachycardia

Tachycardia	Criteria
Sinus	Sustained
	Vagal maneuvers unsuccessful*
	P wave morphology unchanged†
	PR interval unchanged†
	RR interval slightly irregular‡
Atrial	Paroxysmal or sustained
	Vagal maneuvers successful§
	P-wave morphology different†
	RR interval regular‡

*Vagal maneuvers result in deceleration, but tachycardia recurs after vagal maneuvers, unless the etiology had abated.

†Compared with P wave morphology and PR interval during normal sinus rhythm.

‡Inconsistent finding

§Vagal maneuvers break the tachycardia, and normal sinus rhythms persist for minutes, hours, or indefinitely.

TABLE 21-4. Causes of Atrial Tachycardia

Cause	Association(s)
Atrial enlargement	Mitral valve insufficiency (regurgitation) Chronic acquired Congenital Cardiomyopathy Canine dilated congestive Feline hypertrophic
Hypoxemia	Congestive heart failure* Pulmonary disease*
Neoplasia	Hemangiosarcoma of the right auricle
Drugs	Digitalis glycosides Anesthesia
Hypokalemia	Diuretics
Idiopathic	May have early cardiomyopathy

*Often coexistent

Chronic pulmonary disease in middle-aged and old, small-breed dogs is often coexistent with mitral valve disease and may contribute to the genesis of the arrhythmia. The "sick sinus syndrome" of middle-aged and old female miniature schnauzers is sometimes associated with paroxysmal atrial tachycardia; periods of prolonged sinus arrest follow the tachycardia, interspersed with junctional or, less frequently, ventricular escape beats and sinus arrhythmia (see Fig. 21-3). Prolonged sinus arrest results in varying degrees of episodic weakness and syncope. Not all dogs manifesting the sick sinus syndrome experience paroxysmal atrial tachycardia.

Some degree of myocardial fibrosis, myocytolysis, edema, and inflammation are associated with most instances of atrial enlargement severe enough to result in paroxysmal atrial tachycardia. Atrial tachycardia may result from automaticity or reentry mechanisms. Most instances associated with severe left atrial dis-

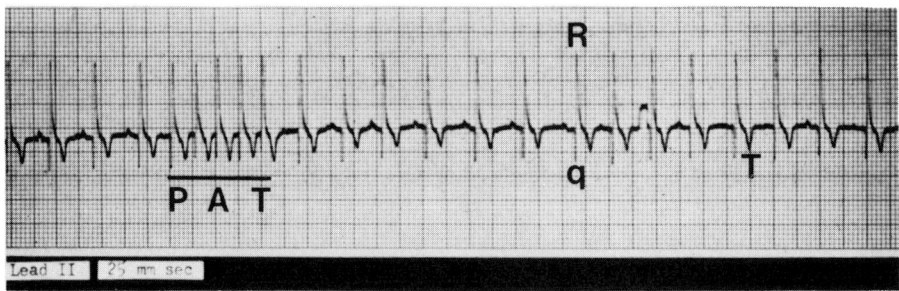

FIGURE 21-3. Paroxysmal atrial tachycardia (*PAT*) in a 12-year-old miniature poodle with mitral valve insufficiency and radiographic evidence of left atrial enlargement.

ease probably result from reentry. Digitalis glycosides can produce abnormal impulse formation, that is, ectopic atrial tachycardia. Paroxysmal atrial tachycardia with concomitant atrioventricular block (first-degree or second-degree, or both) or junctional tachycardia is usually the result of digoxin intoxication. Multifocal atrial tachycardia (also called "chaotic" atrial tachycardia) is also of ectopic origin and, although it may complicate severe cardiac disease, is usually the result of chronic lung disease.[12]

Although atrial tachycardia is unlikely to result in heart failure in younger animals and in those lacking severe cardiac disease, patients with cardiomyopathy or advanced mitral valve disease may experience a significant decrease in cardiac output. Congestive heart failure (pulmonary edema) or shock may occur unless the tachycardia is short-lived.

Sustained or persistent atrial tachycardia is sometimes encountered in young to middle-aged medium- and large-breed dogs that have no history of—or overt evidence of—organic heart disease. Affected dogs may be asymptomatic, may exhibit exercise intolerance and tachypnea, or may occasionally experience syncope. The atrial tachycardia rate in these dogs is typically 260 to 320 beats per minute.

Atrial Flutter

Atrial flutter is an unusual tachycardia in dogs and cats, and it results from a circus movement and reentry. In most cases, the ventricular rate is considerably less than the atrial rate because of a variable and often high degree of atrioventricular block. The atrial flutter rate, although usually exceeding 180 beats per minute, is variable. In dogs, this arrhythmia is most often associated with atrial neoplasia or cardiac catheterization. It may occur with severe left atrial enlargement due to chronic mitral valve insufficiency or cardiomyopathy.

Atrial Fibrillation

Atrial fibrillation is a common arrhythmia in dogs but is uncommon in cats (Fig. 21-4). It is usually associated with severe organic heart disease (Table 21-5). Cardiomyopathies are the most common group of disorders associated with atrial fibrillation in the dog (dilated) and the cat (hypertrophic). Atrial fibrillation occurs occasionally in small dogs with acquired mitral valve insufficiency and severe left atrial enlargement. Since mitral valve disease is very common in small-breed dogs, atrial fibrillation, although uncommon on a percentage basis, is relatively common on an absolute basis.

Atrial fibrillation exacts two hemodynamic penalties: the ineffective writhing of atrial muscle deprives the heart of its atrial transport function, and the incessant and irregular bombardment of the atrioventricular junction (with the latter's variable physiologic block) excites a rapid but irregular ventricular response. These hemodynamic consequences may precipitate congestive heart

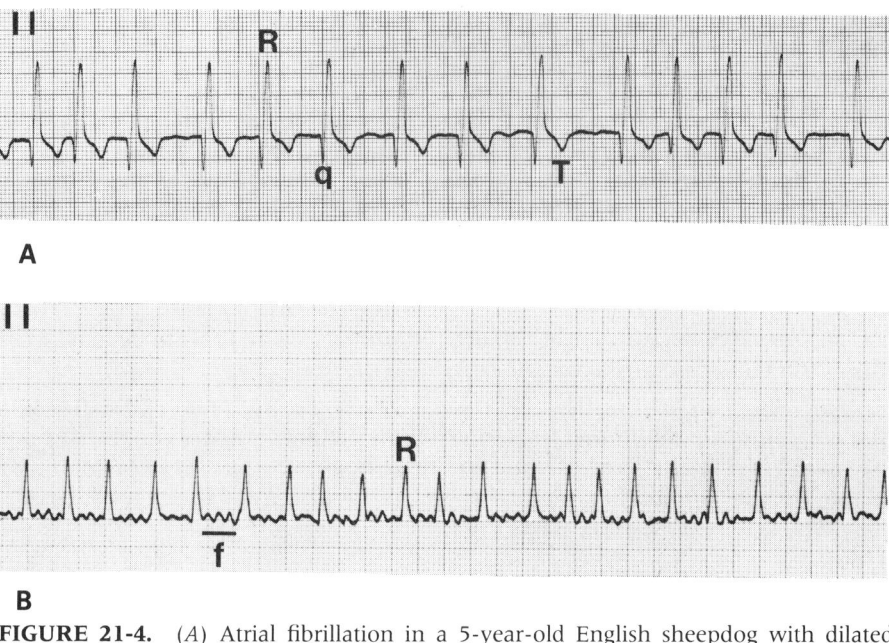

FIGURE 21-4. (*A*) Atrial fibrillation in a 5-year-old English sheepdog with dilated congestive cardiomyopathy and bilateral congestive heart failure. The heart rhythm is rapid (200 to 200/min) and irregular. No P waves are visible. (*B*) Atrial fibrillation in a 7-year-old male Persian cat with radiographically confirmed severe left atrial enlargement and pulmonary edema. P waves are absent, and f waves dominate the baseline.

failure in dogs with advanced mitral valve disease or in dogs and cats with cardiomyopathy.

Atrial fibrillation may be paroxysmal at the onset, converting spontaneously to sinus rhythm. However, in association with organic heart disease, paroxysmal atrial fibrillation portends subsequent sustained atrial fibrillation. Initially, digoxin or digoxin plus propranolol therapy may result in conversion to sinus rhythm, but relapse usually occurs. Atrial fibrillation is occasionally found in overtly normal Irish wolfhounds, a condition analogous to ''lone fibrillation'' in humans, but the arrhythmia should be treated if the rate exceeds 170 beats per minute.

The diagnosis of atrial fibrillation should be suspected on the basis of the physical examination. The heart rhythm is rapid and chaotic (irregularly irregular), and pulse deficits are frequent. Clincial signs consistent with advanced cardiac disease and heart failure are usually present. Auscultation of this chaotic-sounding tachycardia in a giant-breed dog exhibiting weight loss, dyspnea, ascites, pale mucous membranes, and exercise intolerance should leave little doubt as to the clinical and electrocardiographic diagnosis.

The physiologic mechanism of atrial fibrillation has not been conclusively

TABLE 21-5.   Causes of Atrial Fibrillation

Cause	Association(s)
Left atrial enlargement	Canine dilated cardiomyopathy
	Feline hypertrophic cardiomyopathy
	Mitral insufficiency
Hyperkalemia	Hypoadrenocorticism*
Hypothermia*	

*Usually associated with ventricular rates of less than 180 beats per minute

established. Experimental evidence suggests that reentry phenomena are the basis for sustaining this arrhythmia.

Ventricular Tachycardia

Ventricular tachycardia is a life-threatening arrhythmia and is strongly indicative of a diseased heart (Fig. 21-5; Table 21-6). In general, older, small-breed dogs that experience ventricular tachyarrhythmias often have advanced mitral valve disease or chronic obstructive pulmonary disease, or both. Middle-aged, large-breed dogs exhibiting ventricular tachyarrhythmias may have dilated cardiomyopathy; the differential diagnosis depends on associated clinical signs, laboratory findings, and echocardiographic and radiographic abnormalities. Ventricular tachycardia occurring in middle-aged and especially old cats is usually the result of cardiomyopathy, particularly dilated cardiomyopathy. The rapid and accurate diagnosis of this arrhythmia is essential and vital to the survival of the patient.

The mechanisms of ventricular tachycardia are numerous and include micro-reentry circuits in the ventricle, and macro-reentry circuits confined to the specialized conduction system, automaticity, and triggered activity. Even in the same disease, the mechanism of the arrhythmia may vary.

BRADYCARDIAS

Bradyarrhythmias may result from disturbances of impulse formation or impulse conduction (see Display, Classification of Bradyarrhythmias and Their Common Associations). The mechanism of such disturbances is often physiologic but may be pathologic.

Sinus Bradycardia

Sinus bradycardia is probably the most common bradyarrhythmia and is most often the result of increased vagal tone in brachiocephalic breeds (with concomi-

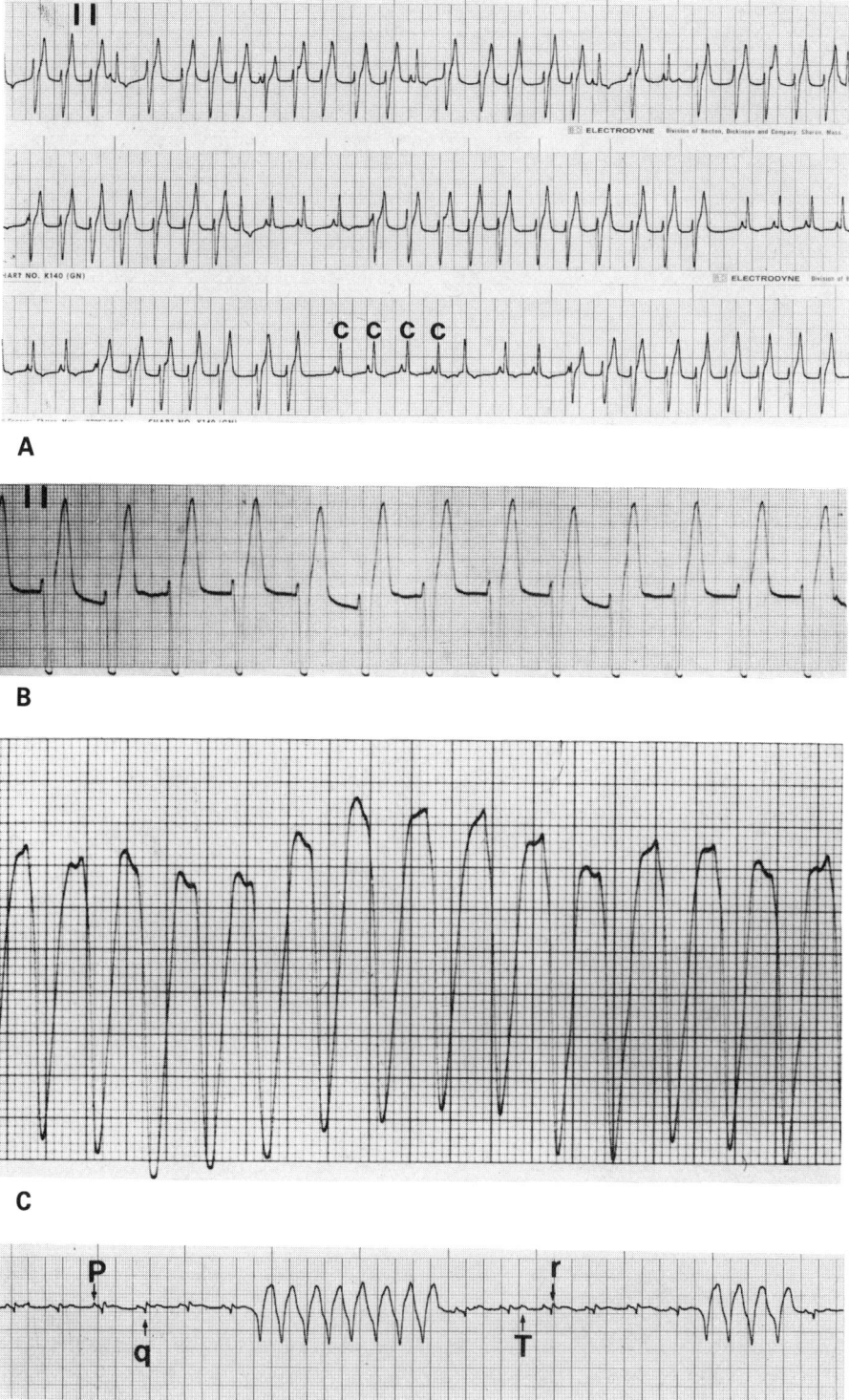

A

B

C

D

TABLE 21-6. Common Diseases and Disorders Associated with Ventricular Tachycardia

General Etiology	Specific Disorders
Myocardial disease or disorder	Cardiomyopathy Contusion Myocarditis Neoplasia (infiltrative cardiomyopathy)
Myocarditis	Parvovirus infection Bacteremia
Idiopathic cardiomyopathy	Doberman pinscher cardiomyopathy Boxer cardiomyopathy Canine dilated Feline cardiomyopathies
Congestive heart failure	Cardiomyopathies Mitral valve disease (advanced)
Toxemia	Postgastric torsion Bacteremia Pancreatitis Peritonitis
Hypoxemia	Congestive heart failure Anemia Pulmonary disease
Drug treatment	Digitalis glycoside Doxorubicin Anesthetic agents Ketamine Antiarrhythmic drugs
Metabolic disturbances	Uremia Hypokalemia Feline hyperthyroidism

FIGURE 21-5. (*A*) Paroxysmal ventricular tachycardia in a 12-year-old Yorkshire terrier with chronic mitral valve insufficiency and pulmonary edema. Capture beats (*c*) represent normal sinus beats that interrupt the tachycardia (25 mm/sec, ½ sensitivity). (*B*) Ventricular tachycardia (180/min) in a 7-year-old male Doberman Pinscher with dilated cardiomyopathy and severe pulmonary edema. (*C*) Ventricular tachycardia (440/min) in a 5-year-old overtly healthy Doberman Pinscher that collapsed suddenly. Ventricular fibrillation and death occurred shortly after this electrocardiogram was obtained. (*D*) Paroxysmal ventricular tachycardia (480/min) in a 12-year-old Siamese cat with dilated cardiomyopathy. Severe weakness, hypothermia, and pleural effusion was present.

Classification of Bradyarrhythmias and Their Common Associations

Disturbances of Impulse Formation

- Sinus bradycardia
  Physiologic
    Increased vagal tone
      Endogenous
      Exogenous
        Vagal maneuvers
        Surgery
        Drugs
      Normal variant in large dogs
  Pathologic
    Systemic disease
      Uremia
      Toxemia
      Peritonitis
    Cardiac arrest
    Hypoxemia
    Hypothermia
    Increase cerebrospinal fluid
      pressure
    Hyperkalemia
  Drug-induced
    Narcotics
    Tranquilizers
    Anesthetics
    Antiarrhythmics
    Beta-adrenergic blocking drugs

Disturbances of Impulse Conduction

- Sinoventricular conduction
  Hyperkalemia
    Hypoadrenocorticism
    Oliguric renal failure
- Advanced atrioventricular heart blocks
  Acquired
    Idiopathic myocardial fibrosis
    Cardiomyopathy
      Feline dilated congestive
      Feline hypertrophic
      Canine hypertrophic
    Infiltrative cardiomyopathy
      (neoplasia)
    Hereditary stenosis of bundle of His
    Bacterial endocarditis
    Hyperkalemia
  Drug-induced
    Digoxin
    Xylazine
    Beta-adrenergic blocking drugs
    Narcotics
    Tranquilizers
    Doxorubicin
    Antiarrhythmic drugs

tant sinus arrhythmia) and a normal variant in large-breed dogs. Sinus bradycardia is usually the result of a disturbance of impulse formation. It is common in large-breed dogs, at rest and during sleep periods. Sinus bradycardia is a part of the normal reaction to vagal stimuli. Pharmacologic sinus bradycardia may result from digitalis glycosides, narcotics, beta-adrenergic blocking agents (propranolol), quinidine, quinidine-like antiarrhythmic drugs, xylazine, and anesthetics.

Pathologic sinus bradycardia may accompany the vagal stimulation produced by vomiting. It is also seen in association with obstructive jaundice, increased intracranial pressure, severe hypoxemia, and depressed mental status. Sinus bradycardia may portend cardiac arrest. Intrathoracic masses may produce a reflex sinus bradycardia due to irritation of the vagus nerve. Cervical masses such as thyroid gland neoplasia and carotid body tumors may produce sinus bradycardia through autonomic reflex arcs.

Vagal tone may be increased during surgical manipulation of abdominal organs, producing a marked sinus bradycardia. Hypothermia is associated with a number of cardiac rhythm disturbances, including sinus bradycardia.

Sinoventricular Conduction

Sinoventricular conduction is pathognomonic for hyperkalemia, most often resulting from hypoadrenocorticism. In this condition, the response of the sinoatrial node is slowed, but conduction via the specialized internodal pathways continues. However, because of the atrial myocardium's increased susceptibility to the resting membrane potential effects of hyperkalemia, an exit block occurs at the sinoatrial junction (junction between the sinoatrial node and perinodal-myocardial tissue). Thus, as the serum potassium concentration increases, a gradual decrease in the sinoatrial rates occurs (associated with gradual prolongation of the PR interval and decreasing P wave amptitude). The P wave eventually disappears (atrial standstill). Tall, spiked, T waves are typically present when this bradycardia develops. The ventricle is activated by the antegrade sinoatrial impulse being conducted via the specialized conducting fibers (internodal pathways, atrioventricular node, bundle of His), which are somewhat resistant to the depressant effect of hyperkalemia.

Sick Sinus Syndrome

The sick sinus syndrome causes episodic weakness and is characterized by sinus node depression, including sinus bradycardia and prolonged sinus (sinoatrial) arrest (Fig. 21-6). Prolonged sinus arrest is followed by delayed junctional and ventricular escape beats and rhythms, alternating with sinus arrhythmia, sinus bradycardia, and prolonged sinus arrest. In some dogs, paroxysmal atrial tachycardia alternates with prolonged periods of sinus nodal inertia and often atrioventricular junctional inertia as well. This syndrome is common in middle-aged and older miniature schnauzers (particularly females), but a similar pattern may be seen in the dachshund, cocker spaniel, and other small-breed dogs. Mitral valve disease and chronic pulmonary disease are often coexistent. Congestive heart failure due to mitral valve insufficiency eventually complicates the management of this syndrome.

Persistent Atrial Standstill

Persistent atrial standstill is a rare condition seen mostly in English springer spaniels.[1] Atrial hypoplasia is present to varying degrees, and sinoatrial node impulse conduction is absent. A junctional or ventricular escape rhythm maintains the ventricular rate at 40 to 60 beats per minute. P waves are persistently

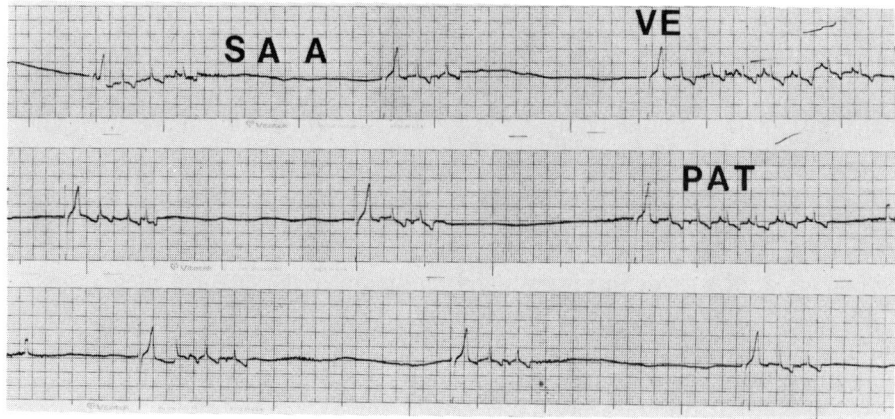

FIGURE 21-6. Sinoatrial arrests (*SA A*) followed by ventricular escape beats (*VE*) and paroxysmal atrial tachycardia (*PAT*) in a 7-year-old female miniature schnauzer that was suffering from synocopal episodes.

absent from the electrocardiogram. Dilated cardiomyopathy often develops within months to a few years after diagnosis of the bradycardia.

HEART BLOCK

A variety of factors may affect propagation of cardiac impulses, particularly in depressed tissues. Thus, decremental conduction is likely to develop in the presence of a lower level of membrane potential and a slower rate of rise of phase 0 depolarization. These conditions can occur in any fibers showing incomplete repolarization or partial depolarization caused by various pathophysiologic factors. Fibers of the atrioventricular node (and possibly of the bundle of His) show the above characteristics even under physiologic conditions; therefore, decremental conduction is common in these tissues. Cardiac glycosides, hypokalemia, and ischemia enhance the degree of decremental conduction and thus may impair atrioventricular conduction, leading to heart block.

Advanced Heart Blocks

Advanced second-degree (Fig. 21-7) and complete (third-degree) (Fig. 21-8) atrioventricular heart block results in bradycardia. The ventricular rate of advanced second-degree heart block depends on the severity of the block (*i.e.,* 2:1, 3:1, 4:1, *etc.*) and the inherent sinoatrial rate. Thus, a 2:1 second-degree block associated with a sinus rate of 120 beats per minute results in a ventricular rate of 60 beats per minute. A 3:1 block with a sinus rate of 180 beats per minute also produces a ventricular rate of 60 beats per minute.

Advanced (high-degree) second-degree atrioventricular heart blocks in dogs

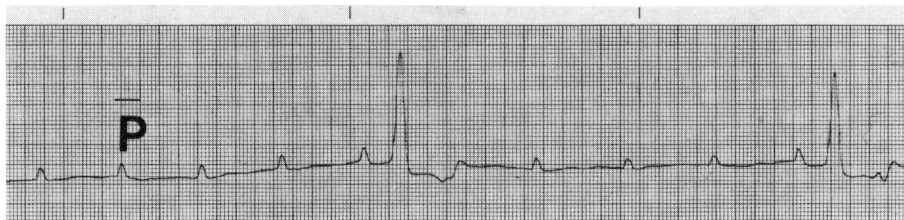

FIGURE 21-7. Advanced second-degree atrioventricular (AV) heart block in a 10-year-old male cocker spaniel that was weak and lethargic. The sinus rate is 160/min, while that of the ventricles is 40/min. Notice that there is a consistent and normal PR interval preceding each R wave. Thus, the diagnosis of second-degree AV block is made. The R wave is of excessive duration, indicating that the block is below the AV node (type B block). This specific type of second-degree AV block often does not respond to atropine and may progress to complete heart block, as was the case in this dog.

are most often associated with idiopathic myocardial fibrosis and mitral valve insufficiency in older, small-breed and brachycephalic breeds. Such conduction disturbances are often precipitated or complicated by digoxin therapy. In the cat, advanced second-degree heart block is usually associated with hypertrophic cardiomyopathy. Electrolyte disturbances (hyperkalemia), hypoxemia, and hypercarbia from any cause can produce heart blocks.

Complete heart block results in a ventricular rate of 30 to 65 beats per minute. Complete heart block is often associated with idiopathic myocardial fibrosis and mitral valve insufficiency in brachycephalic dog breeds and cocker spaniels. In

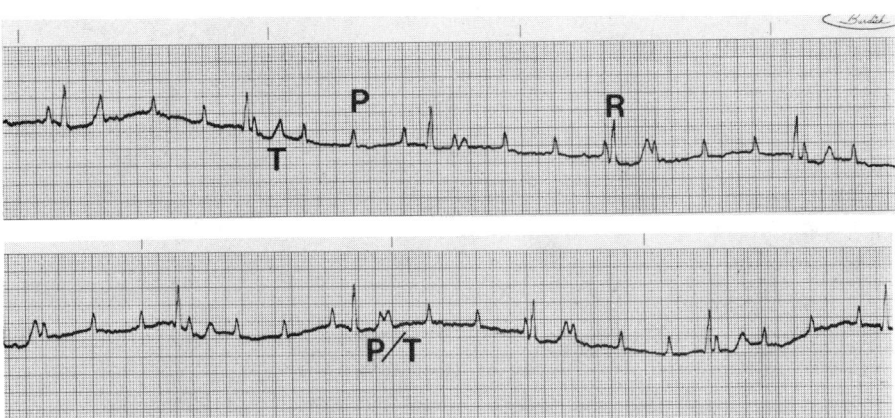

FIGURE 21-8. Complete (third-degree) AV block in a 7-year-old English bulldog that was lethargic. Mitral and tricuspid valve endocardiosis and extensive ventricular fibrosis were present. There are no PR relationships; thus, the diagnosis of complete heart block was made. The sinus rate is 200/min, while the ventricular rate is 60/min.

cats, complete heart block is usually the result of hypertrophic cardiomyopathy. Hyperkalemia may result in complete heart block.

ARRHYTHMIAS NOT PRODUCING ABNORMAL RATES

Some cardiac arrhythmias can result in rhythm disturbances without producing either a tachycardia or a bradycardia (Table 21-7). The physiologic, pathologic, and drug associations of these arrrhythmias parallel those of more advanced arrhythmias of similar etiologies. Pulse deficits are common with premature contractions, while pauses are associated with sinoatrial arrest (or block), and simple second-degree heart block (one block of the antegrade sinoatrial impulse at the atrioventricular node and bundle of His occurs sporadically).

ABNORMALITIES OF THE PULSE

The arterial pressure pulse is produced by ejection of blood from the left ventricle into the great arteries at a rate faster than its run-off into the peripheral circulation. Although the peak rate of ejection of blood occurs prior to the peak pressure in the left ventricle or aorta, the pressure continues to rise in the aorta as long as blood is ejected into the aorta faster than it runs off into the peripheral arteries.

TABLE 21-7. Cardiac Rhythm Disturbances, Which May or May Not Be Associated with Tachycardia or Bradycardia, and Common Associations

Arrhythmia	Association(s)

Sinus arrhythmia	Normal variation
	  Inherent vagal tone
	  Bradycardia possible
	  Brachycephalic breeds

Supraventricular premature contractions	See Tables 21-1, 21-4, and 21-5
Ventricular premature contractions	See Tables 21-1 and 21-6

Sinoatrial block or arrest	Normal variation
	  Exaggerated vagal tone; bradycardia possible
	  See Table 21-1 and Display, Classification of Bradyarrhythmias and Their Common Associations

Simple second-degree AV block	See Table 21-1 and Display, Classification of Bradyarrhythmias and Their Common Associations

AV, atrioventricular

The form of the venous pressure pulse is determined by the rate of the blood return from the peripheral tissues into the venous segment, the pressure-volume characteristics of the segment of vein, the nature of the resistance to flow, the distensibility of the right atrium and ventricle, and the tissue overlying the veins at the point of observation. Although the venous pressure pulse wave travels peripherally away from the heart, there is at the same time a venous blood flow in the opposite direction toward the heart.

Arterial Pulse

The arterial pulse wave at any site is influenced by many factors, including the left ventricular stroke volume, the rate of ejection, the compliance of the aorta and large arteries, the peripheral vascular resistance, the heart rate, the systolic and diastolic blood pressures, the distance from the heart, the blood viscosity, and the size and pressure-volume characteristics of the artery.

The arterial pressure pulse enters the proximal aorta and travels distally at a velocity many times faster than maximum blood flow. The pressure wave is accompanied by a traveling wave distending the arterial wall; the pulse wave velocity increases as arterial wall distensibility diminishes. This increased velocity normally occurs distally as the arteries branch into smaller channels and their walls become stiffer.

The usual technique for palpating the arterial pulse is to press with the examining finger until the maximum pulse is sensed. The pulse is felt as changing displacement superimposed on the "baseline" displacement produced by compressing the artery.

The arterial pressure is divided into two phases: systole and diastole. Arterial pressure begins with the opening of the aortic valve and rapid ejection of blood into the aorta. This is followed by run-off of blood from the proximal aorta to the peripheral arteries. The arterial pressure waveform is characterized by a sharp rise in pressure followed by a decline in pressure. Diastole follows closure of the aortic valve and continues to the next systole. During this time, run-off to the peripheral arteries occurs without further flow from the left ventricle. The lowest point of diastole (end-diastole) is referred to as the arterial diastolic pressure. The systolic arterial pressure rises immediately after ventricular depolarization, that is, after the QRS complex of the electrocardiogram (Fig. 21-9).

Hyperkinetic Pulse. Large, bounding (hyperkinetic) arterial pulses usually indicate the rapid ejection of an increased volume of blood from the left ventricle. Commonly, the arterial pulse pressure is increased, and the peripheral arterial resistance is diminished. The hyperdynamic arterial pulse is sometimes referred to in terms that describe a particular component of the pulse wave. Thus, the "water-hammer pulse," named after a Victorian toy, refers to an extremely rapid, forceful ascending limb of the arterial pulse wave. By contrast, "collapsing pulse" refers to a quick, marked decrease in the arterial pulse wave following its peak.

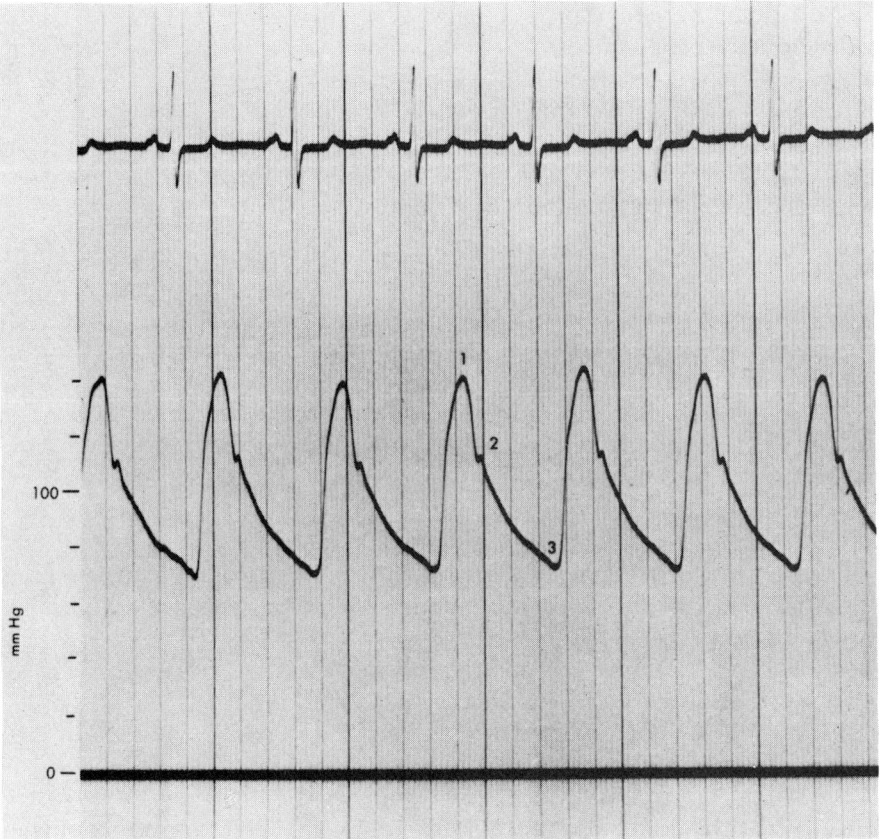

FIGURE 21-9. Normal arterial pressure waveform. 1, arterial systolic pressure (140 mm Hg); 2, dicrotic notch; 3, arterial end-diastolic pressure (72 mm Hg). The dicrotic notch coincides with aortic valve closure as the blood flow in the aorta temporarily reverses direction and blood pressure decreases.

Hyperkinetic arterial pulses occur during exercise, fever, cardiac diseases associated with increased stroke volume, and marked bradycardia with increased stroke volume. A hyperdynamic pulse also occurs when abnormally rapid run-off of blood from the arterial system occurs (Table 21-8). The most striking examples of hyperdynamic pulses are the result of bacterial endocarditis of the aortic valve. The resultant aortic regurgitation results in volume overload, increases stroke volume, and "collapsing postsystolic pulse" due to rapid aortic diastolic run-off back into the left ventricle.

A hypokinetic (small, weak) arterial pulse may be present in patients with diminished left ventricular stroke volume (Table 21-9). Hypokinetic pulses are commonly associated with advanced mitral valve disease and left-sided congestive heart failure in the dog and dilated cardiomyopathy in the dog and cat.

TABLE 21-8. Causes and Associations of Hyperdynamic (Hyperkinetic) Pulses

Cause	Association(s)
Physiologic	Exercise Fever
Increased stroke volume	Hyperthyroidism Aortic regurgitation (insufficiency)
Bradycardia	Sinus bradycardia Advanced and complete heart blocks
Rapid run-off	Patent ductus arteriosus Peripheral arteriovenous fistulas Aortic regurgitation (insufficiency)

Pulsus Alternans. Pulsus alternans is a characteristic pulse pattern in which the beats occur at regular intervals but in which there is a regular attenuation of the pulse pressure. Pulsus alternans is seen in association with ventricular bigeminy and myocardial failure. In dilated cardiomyopathy, it is postulated that alteration of the contractile state of at least part of the myocardium, which may be caused by the failure of electrochemical coupling in some cells during weaker contractions, can produce sustained pulsus alternans. Echocardiographic examination reveals alternating greater and lesser left ventricular shortening fractions. Pulsus alternans may be better appreciated on a peripheral rather than a carotid artery. The patient's respirations should be held, since changes in arterial pressure may be produced by respiration.

Pulse Deficit. Pulse deficits can occur with various types of cardiac rhythm disturbances. Supraventricular or ventricular premature contractions (extrasys-

TABLE 21-9. Pulse Abnormalities and Associated Conditions

Pulse Type	Association(s)
Pulsus bisferiens	Aortic regurgitation (insufficiency) Aortic valve bacterial endocarditis Aortic stenosis with aortic regurgitation Patent ductus arteriosus Feline hypertrophic obstructed cardiomyopathy
Hypokinetic	Dilated cardiomyopathy Mitral valve insufficiency Aortic valve stenosis Hypovolemia Shock
Pulsus alternans	Ventricular bigeminy Dilated cardiomyopathy
Pulsus paradoxus	Pericardial tamponade

toles) may be associated with no pulse, a small-amplitude pulse, or a normal pulse, depending upon the timing and whether the left-ventricular pressure generated is able to open the aortic valve. The arterial pulse following a ventricular premature contraction may be enhanced because of decreased aortic impedance, increased left ventricular filling (compensatory pause), and augmented contractility (postextrasystolic augmentation). Pulse deficits are commonly associated with ventricular tachycardia and atrial fibrillation.

Venous Pulse

The evaluation of the venous pulse is an integral part of the physical examination, since the venous pulse reflects both the right atrial pressure and the hemodynamic events in the right atrium. Factors influencing the right atrial and central venous pressure include the total blood volume, the distribution of blood volume, and right atrial contraction. The two main objectives of examining the jugular veins are the estimation of the central venous pressure and the inspection of the waveform. Clipping of the hair, wetting the jugular furrow, and shining a light across the skin overlying the jugular vein enhance the detection

TABLE 21-10. Causes of Elevation of Jugular Vein Pressure
and Jugular Pulses

Cause	Associations
Right-sided congestive heart failure	Pulmonic stenosis (congenital)
	Tricuspid insufficiency
	Congenital
	Acquired
	Cardiomyopathies
	Cor pulmonale
	Chronic pulmonary disease
	Pulmonary hypertension
	Heartworm disease
	Chronic mitral insufficiency
Right ventricular inflow obstruction	Pericardial effusion
	Idiopathic
	Pericarditis
	Idiopathic
	Infectious
	Neoplastic
	Pericardial constriction
	Neoplastic
	Heart base tumor
	Intracardiac tumor
	Right atrial myxoma
	Sarcoma

of the jugular pulse. The patient should be relaxed and placed in recumbency, with the trunk inclined to various degrees.

The difference between venous distention and venous pressure must be considered. Veins may be markedly dilated with minimal increase in pressure or may not be visibly distended despite a very high venous pressure. Increased venous pressure may be detected with the patient in lateral recumbency. The saphenous vein is visualized, and the extremity is slowly and passively elevated from a dependent position. The vein should collapse at a level nearly parallel to the thoracic inlet (approximate level of the right atrium).

Distention of the jugular veins, the presence of a jugular pulse, and elevation of the jugular venous pressure are most often produced by right-sided congestive heart failure (Table 21-10). Right ventricular inflow obstruction may also produce elevation of the jugular venous pulse.

Cannon "a" waves are jugular pulses that occur when the right atrium contracts while the tricuspid valve is closed during right ventricular systole. They are associated with cardiac rhythm disturbances such as ventricular premature contractions, ventricular tachycardia, and complete heart block. Cannon "a" waves may occur in the presence or absence of right-sided congestive heart failure.

REFERENCES

1. Agostini E: Functional and histologic studies of the vagus nerve and its branches of the heart, lungs and abdominal viscera in the cat. J Physiol 135:182–185, 1957
2. Anderson MI, Castillo J: Cardiac innervation and synaptic transmission in the heart. In DeMellow WC (ed): Electrical Phenomena in the Heart. New York, Academic Press, 1972
3. Armous JA, Randall WC: Functional anatomy of canine cardiac nerves. Acta Anat 9:510–528, 1975
4. Baird JA, Robb JS: Study, reconstruction and dissection of the atrioventricular conducting system of the dog heart. Anat Sec 108:747–751, 1950
5. Berne RM, Levy MN: Cardiovascular Physiology. St. Louis, CV Mosby, 1977
6. Kaye MP, Geesbrecht JM, Randall WC: Distribution of autonomic fibers to the canine heart. Am J Physiol 218:1025–1029, 1970
7. Liu SK, Tilly LP, Tushajian RJ: Lesions of the conduction system in the cat with cardiomyopathy. Recent Adv Stud Cardiac Struct Metab 10:681–693, 1975
8. Mizeres NJ: The anatomy of the autonomic nervous system in the dog. Am J Anat 96:290–296, 1966
9. Muir WW: Effects of atropine on cardiac rate and rhythm in dogs. J Am Vet Med Assoc 172:917–921, 1978
10. Myerberg RJ, Nillsson K, Celband H: Physiology of canine intraventricular conduction and endocardial excitation. Circ Res 30:217–243, 1972
11. Patterson DF, Detweiler DK, Hubben K, et al: Spontaneous abnormal cardiac arrhythmias and conduction disturbances in the dog. Am J Vet Res 22:355–369, 1961

12. Tilley LP: Essentials of Canine and Feline Electrocardiography, pp 164, 165, 371. Philadelphia, Lea & Febiger, 1985
13. Tilley LP: Transtelephonic analysis of cardiac arrhythmias in the dog. Vet Clin North Am 13:395–408, 1983
14. Truex RC, Smythe MQ: Comparative morphology of the cardiac conduction tissue in animals. Ann NY Acad Sci 127:19–33, 1965
15. Uhley HN, Rivkin L: Peripheral distribution of the canine A-V conduction system: Observations on gross morphology. Am J Cardiol 5:688–698, 1960

CHAPTER TWENTY-TWO

Heart Murmurs

Clay A. Calvert

PROBLEM DEFINITION AND RECOGNITION

Murmurs are audible successive sounds with distinct duration, as opposed to normal heart sounds, which are short transitory events. Cardiac murmurs result from turbulence created in laminar blood flow.[16] When the flow velocity of fluid within a pipe exceeds a certain value, turbulence develops and energy is dissipated, which generates audible vibrations. Turbulence may also arise when fluid passes through a small hole in a plate that partially occludes a pipe, when the pipe diameter changes abruptly, or when a jet of fluid strikes a surface. A critical level of turbulence must be achieved to produce a sound that is clinically evident. The characteristics of the murmur depend upon the velocity of blood flow and the surrounding structures that are caused to vibrate. Blood velocity and blood density variations can also produce turbulence within the heart and arteries.

CLASSIFICATION

Heart murmurs may be classified as (1) innocent, (2) functional, or (3) pathologic (Table 22-1). It is useful to describe murmurs on the basis of five auscultatory criteria (Table 22-2). First, they may be categorized according to their timing in the cardiac cycle (Table 22-3); accordingly, murmurs are identified as being systolic, diastolic, or continuous. A second aspect of the description of a heart murmur is its intensity (Table 22-4).[6] Unfortunately, murmur intensity does not necessarily indicate flow volume. Thus, although a very small jet does not usually generate a loud murmur, torrential flow through a large hole, as in a large ventricular septal defect, occasionally produces no murmur. The ear perceives higher-frequency noises as being louder than those of the same amplitude but of lower frequency. Third, the frequency, or pitch, of the murmur over each of the heart valves and at the thoracic inlet should be characterized. The fourth aspect of the characterization of a murmur is the modulation or shape of the murmur (Fig. 22-1). Although the holosystolic plateau murmur of mitral insufficiency (regurgitation) is relatively easy to recognize, not all plateau or

TABLE 22-1. Classification of Heart Murmurs and Examples

		Characteristic	
Classification	*Intensity*	*Frequency*	*Association*
Innocent	I/VI–II/VI	Medium	Systolic ejection Puppies, kittens Thin-chested dogs
Functional	I/VI–III/VI	Medium to high	Systolic ejection Anemia Tachycardia Fever Hyperthyroidism High cardiac output
Pathologic	I/VI–VI/VI	Low to high	Congenital heart defects Acquired valvular disease Aortic outflow tract obstruction Systolic anterior mitral valve motion AV valve annulus dilation, dilated cardiomyopathy
Continuous		Crescendo- decrescendo	PDA

AV, atrioventricular

ejection (crescendo-decrescendo, also called diamond-shaped) murmurs are easily discerned. A phonocardiogram is necessary to confirm the modulation of many murmurs. Last, the location of the murmur where the intensity is loudest and the area of radiation should be succinctly described. The classification of systolic murmurs[10] into systolic ejection murmurs and holosystolic (regurgitant systolic) murmurs is of clinical value.

TABLE 22-2. Description of Cardiac Murmurs Based on Auscultatory Criteria

Criteria	*Characterization*
Timing (see Table 22-3)	Systolic Diastolic Continuous
Intensity	I/VI–VI/VI
Frequency (pitch)	Low Medium High Mixed
Modulation (shape)	Plateau Crescendo-decrescendo (diamond-shaped) Decrescendo
Location	Variable

TABLE 22-3. Cardiac Murmurs Based on Location Within the Cardiac Cycle (Timing) and Character (Modulation)

Timing	Modulation	Associations
Systolic	Crescendo-decrescendo (diamond-shaped ejection murmur)	Congenital pulmonic stenosis Congenital aortic stenosis Innocent murmurs
	Plateau holosystolic	Mitral regurgitation (insufficiency) Tricuspid regurgitation (insufficiency) Ventricular septal defect
Diastolic	Decrescendo	Aortic regurgitation (insufficiency) Aortic valve bacterial endocarditis Secondary to chronic aortic stenosis Secondary to a high ventricular septal defect
Continuous		Patent ductus arteriosis

TABLE 22-4. Classification of Cardiac Murmurs by Degree of Intensity

Intensity (Grade)	Description
I/VI	Barely audible
II/VI	Audible after a few seconds of auscultation, low intensity
III/VI	Immediately audible, moderate intensity
IV/VI	Loud intensity without a precordial thrill
V/VI	Loud intensity with a precordial thrill
VI/VI	Loudest intensity, precordial thrill, audible with stethoscope slightly away from thoracic wall

PATHOPHYSIOLOGY

Systolic ejection murmurs imply turbulent blood flow at the time of right or left ventricular ejection into its corresponding great artery. They are typical of the murmurs produced by congenital aortic and pulmonic stenosis. The origin of such murmurs is likely to be along the ventricular outflow at the semilunar valve level or at the immediate artery (pulmonary or aorta). Since actual blood flow is an essential ingredient in the genesis of turbulence responsible for the murmurs, the murmur begins after semilunar valve opening and ends upon cessation of flow with the closure of the same semilunar valve. Such murmurs are known as crescendo-decrescendo, or diamond-shaped (see Fig. 22-1, *B*).

Holosystolic or regurgitant systolic murmurs, that is, those associated with mitral or tricuspid valve regurgitation (insufficiency), begin as soon as the atrioventricular valve closes and continue beyond semilunar valve closure. Because the pressure difference (gradient) between ventricle and recipient chamber

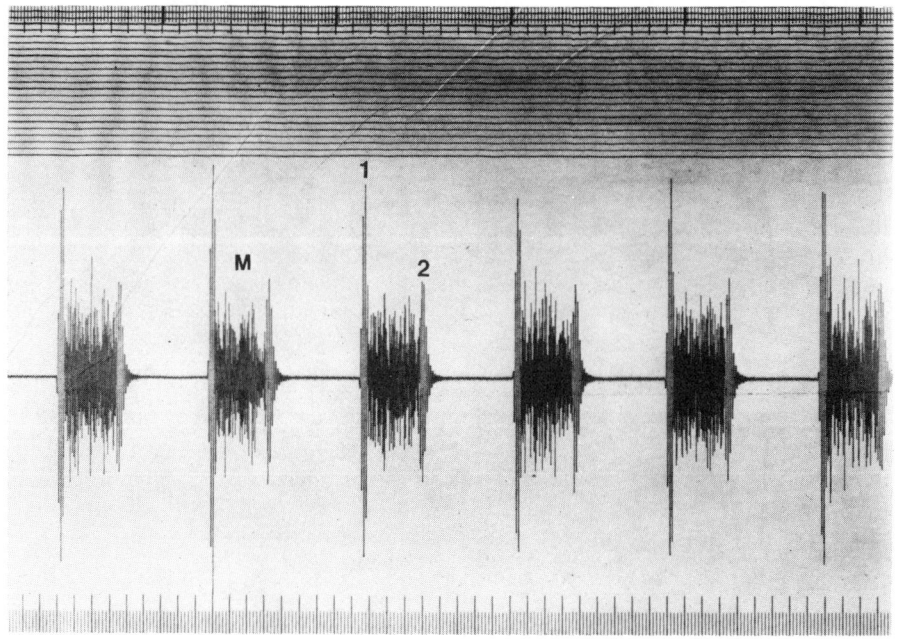

A

B

(atrium) is considerable throughout systole, the murmur tends to have an even or plateau configuration (see Fig. 22-1, A). A holosystolic murmur is also typical of a ventricular septal defect.

Innocent systolic ejection murmurs are produced by normal turbulent flow through the proximal great arteries at the time of ventricular ejection.[11] The intensity of the murmur, as influenced by stroke volume or velocity of ejection, and proximity of the great arteries to the chest wall determine whether the murmur is audible with the stethoscope. Such murmurs are typically heard when a tachycardia exists, and in puppies, kittens, and young lean dogs; these animals tend to have a brisk circulation and a smaller thoracic cage with a narrow transverse diameter. The murmur tends to be of medium frequency, peaks in early to midsystole, usually ends before the second heart sound, and is best heard on the left side over the mitral or aortic valve or at the thoracic inlet. The murmur may be the result of turbulent flow into the pulmonary artery[3] or aorta,[17] or both.

Functional systolic murmurs are produced by increased velocity of blood within the cardiovascular system and by extracardiac factors.[6] Pleural or pericardial effusion, anemia, fever, hyperthyroidism, and tachycardia of any cause may produce functional murmurs. Such murmurs are often detected during anesthesia when a sinus tachycardia exists due to atropine administration.

Decreased blood viscosity and increased velocity of blood flow produce turbulence if the blood hemoglobin level falls below 6 mg/dl (packed cell volume is usually less than 15% to 20%). The functional murmur of anemia is usually of low intensity and high frequency and occurs during early systole to midsystole. Anemic murmurs are best heard over the mitral valve or aortic valve area.[4-6]

Functional murmurs may be audible when states of high cardiac output exist. Chronic anemia can lead to increased cardiac output, although the exact pathophysiology is not completely understood. The increased cardiac output is produced by both tachycardia and increased stroke volume. Reduction of blood viscosity is an important aspect of the increased cardiac output of anemia,[7] as is decreased peripheral resistance.[5] Thyrotoxicosis is characterized by an increased cardiac output. There is probably a direct effect of thyroid hormone on the heart, producing a tachycardia. In addition, there is an increased sensitivity to

FIGURE 22-1. (A) Phonocardiogram of a holosystolic plateau murmur (M). The intensity of the murmur is constant between the first (1) and second (2) heart sounds. Holosystolic plateau murmurs are associated with atrioventricular valvular insufficiencies and ventricular septal defects. (B) Phonocardiogram of a crescendo-decrescendo (diamond-shaped) or ejection murmur (M). Such murmurs are associated with semilunar valve stenosis, usually congenital pulmonic or aortic valve stenosis. 1, first heart sound; 2, second heart sound.

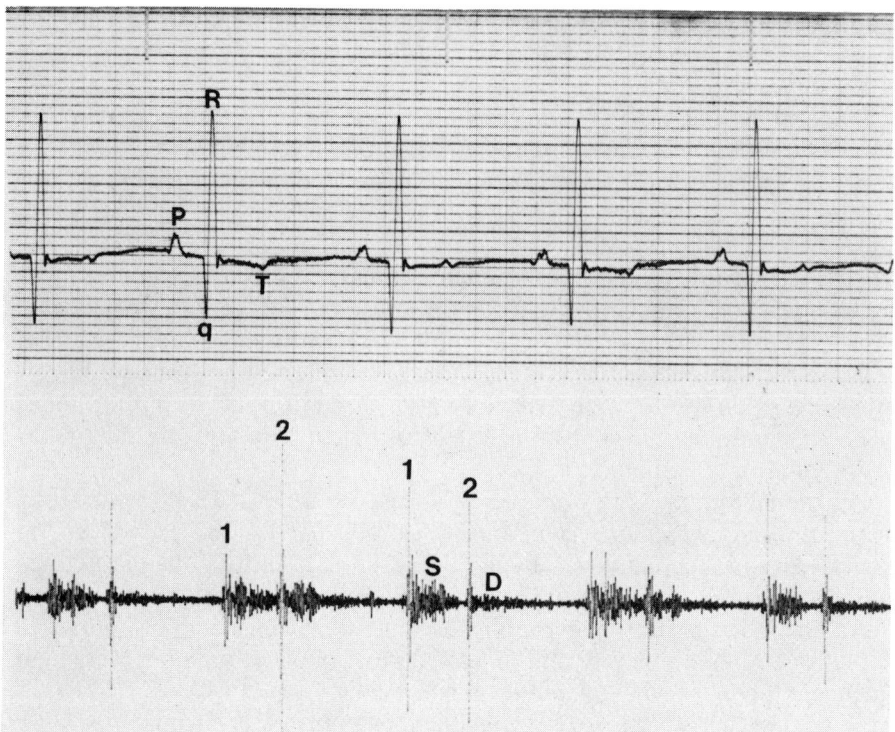

FIGURE 22-2. Decrescendo murmur (*D*) resulting from aortic valvular regurgitation (insufficiency) in a 5-year-old male German shepherd with bacterial endocarditis. A systolic murmur (*S*) is also present and is the result of blood turbulence created by vegetations on the aortic valve. *1,* first heart sound; *2,* second heart sound.

circulating catecholamines, and there may also be a decreased peripheral vascular resistance.[9,12,18]

Murmurs in diastole are unusual and occur in dogs and cats, most often across the aortic valve. The murmur of aortic regurgitation (insufficiency) strongly implies the presence of aortic valvular bacterial endocarditis. The murmur begins immediately after aortic valve closure (second heart sound) and is usually of high frequency, with a decrescendo configuration (Fig. 22-2).

A continuous murmur extends from systole into diastole. Such a murmur results from blood flow continuing from a high-pressure to a lower-pressure area, despite semilunar valve closure. Patent ductus arteriosus is the prototype, and only common example in dogs and cats, of a continuous murmur that peaks in intensity at the second heart sound (Fig. 22-3).

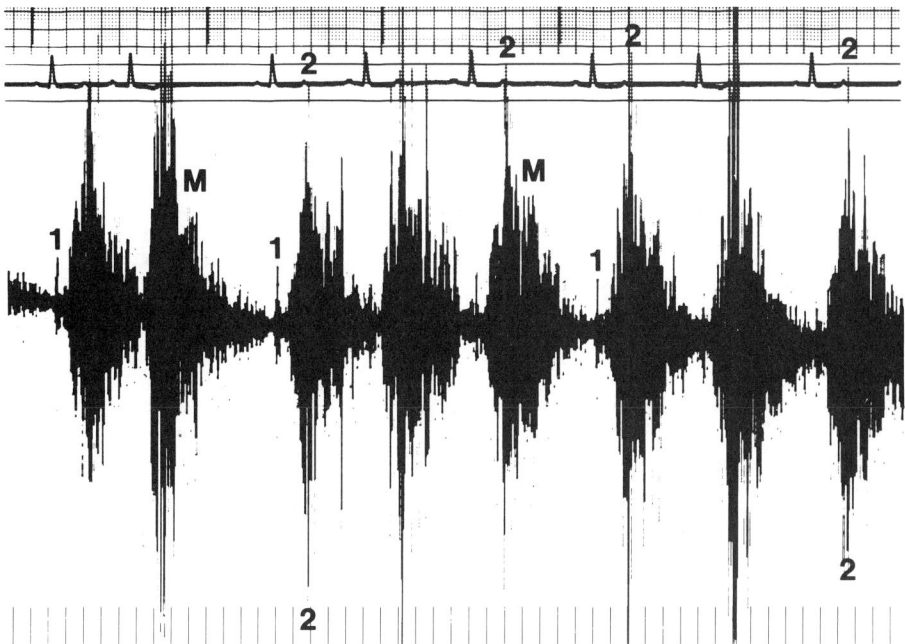

FIGURE 22-3. Continuous murmur (*M*) associated with congenital patent ductus arteriosus. *1*, first heart sound; *2*, second heart sound.

CLINICAL ASSOCIATIONS

Mitral Insufficiency

The murmur of mitral insufficiency (regurgitation) is of mixed frequency and is usually harsh in character (Table 22-5). It is best auscultated from the mitral valve area to the left, caudal sternal border. Loud murmurs (IV/VI to VI/VI) are audible on the right thoracic wall and are difficult to distinguish in that location from concomitant tricuspid insufficiency. Occasionally these murmurs have a whooping or a musical, high-frequency quality. The louder intensity mitral insufficiencies (IV/VI to VI/VI) do not necessarily correlate to the severity of valvular dysfunction. The first heart sound is often accentuated[8] and the second heart sound may be difficult to detect (Fig. 22-4). Mitral insufficiency produces a sequential volume overload, dilatation and eccentric hypertrophy of the left ventricle, left atrial enlargement, pulmonary venous hypertension, and pulmonary edema (left-sided congestive heart failure). By far, the most common clinical cause of mitral insufficiency is endocardiosis (fibrosis, polysaccharidosis) of the mitral valve of unknown etiology in middle-aged to older miniature, toy,

TABLE 22-5. Characteristics of Cardiac Murmurs and Their Associations

Murmur	Timing	Frequency	Intensity	Modulation	Associations*
Mitral insufficiency	Systolic	Mixed	Variable	Plateau (holosystolic)	Acquired in small-breed dogs, spaniels, beagles, and chondrodysplastic breeds Congenital in large-breed dogs, especially great Danes Mitral valvular bacterial endocarditis Dilated cardiomyopathy in cats and dogs Hypertrophic cardiomyopathy in cats Dysplasia (congenital) in cats
Pulmonic stenosis	Systolic	High	Variable	Crescendo-decrescendo	Congenital
Aortic stenosis	Systolic	High	IV/VI–VI/VI	Crescendo-decrescendo	Congenital
Patent ductus arteriosus	Continuous	Mixed	IV/VI–VI/VI	Crescendo-decrescendo	Congenital

Tricuspid insufficiency	Systolic	Mixed	Variable	Plateau (holosystolic)	Acquired in small breeds, especially dachshunds, and brachycephalic breeds, and usually coexists with mitral insufficiency Acquired in Doberman pinschers Congenital in large-breed dogs Congenital (dysplasia) in cats
Ventricular septal defect	Systolic	Mixed	Variable	Plateau (holosystolic)	Usually asymptomatic Common in dogs and cats Frequently associated with atrioventricular valvular defects in cats
Aortic insufficiency	Diastolic	High	I/VI–III/VI	Decrescendo	Aortic valve bacterial endocarditis Secondary to aortic stenosis and ventricular septal defects

*Most common associated conditions

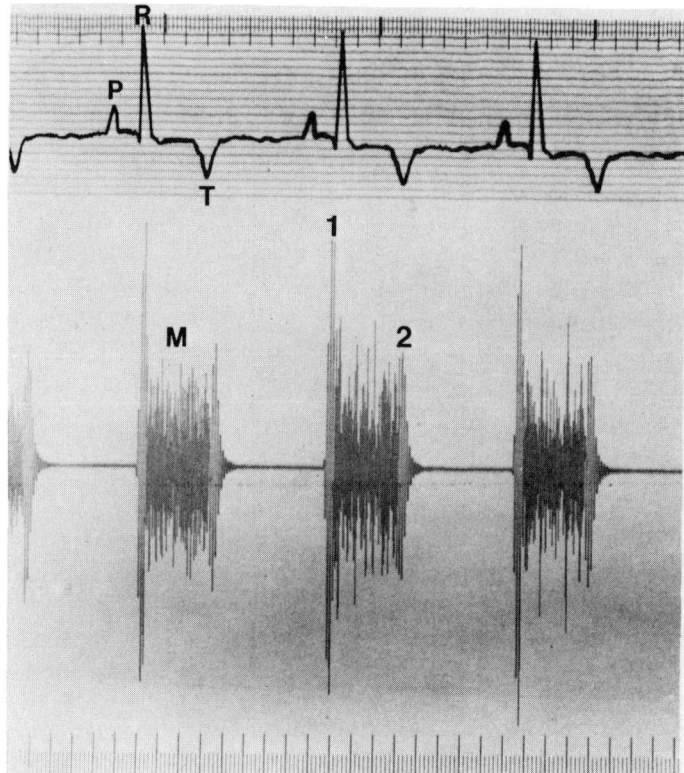

FIGURE 22-4. Holosystolic (plateau) murmur *(M)* of mitral valvular insufficiency (regurgitation). Such murmurs are most often associated with valvular endocardiosis (fibrosis) in middle- and old-aged toy, miniature, and chondrodysplastic breeds, as well as beagles and spaniels. The valvular pathology is progressive, and left-sided congestive heart failure often occurs after several years. Tricuspid valvular insufficiency often occurs concomitantly.

small, and chondrodysplastic breeds; beagles; and spaniels. Doberman pinschers, great Danes, and other giant-breed dogs often develop low-grade mitral valve murmurs due to endocardiosis by middle age or later, but these lesions do not lead to heart failure.

Pulmonic Stenosis

The systolic ejection murmur of congenital pulmonic stenosis is best ausculted over the pulmonic valve area. The murmur is of high frequency, and its intensity correlates with the degree of stenosis. The intensity of this crescendo-decrescendo murmur tends to peak early with mild stenosis and late with more severe stenosis. A palpable thrill is often detected over the left anterioventral precardium. The second heart sound is often split, but a phonocardiogram may be required for detection, since the murmur may obscure the second heart sound.[14] Congenital pulmonic stenosis occurs most often in English bulldogs, terriers, chihuahuas, miniature schnauzers, and bradycephalic breeds. Pulmonic stenosis is uncommon in cats. Clinically significant pulmonic stenosis is associated with electrocardiographic evidence of right ventricular hypertrophy. Radiographic evidence of a poststenotic dilation of the main pulmonary artery segment may be present. Decreased exercise tolerance, syncope, and right-sided congestive heart failure are the consequences of severe pulmonic stenosis. Heart failure, when it occurs, usually does so between the ages of 1 and 3 years.

Aortic Stenosis

The systolic ejection murmur of aortic stenosis is most audible over the aortic valve, although the murmur radiates along the aorta and is audible over the right cranioventral thoracic wall. A thrill is often palpable over the left cranial precordium. The murmur is usually detectable at the thoracic inlet and may be traced along the course of the carotid arteries to the angle of the mandible and, in some cases, to the top of the cranium. This congenital cardiac defect occurs most commonly in large-breed dogs such as the golden retriever, Newfoundland, boxer, and German shepherd. It is also a relatively common defect in cats. Affected animals may remain asymptomatic, but many develop left-sided congestive heart failure between the ages of 3 and 6 years. Episodic weakness and sudden death are common in golden retrievers, rottweilers, and the Newfoundland.[13,15] Atrial fibrillation may occur in middle-aged dogs as a result of secondary mitral insufficiency and left atrial enlargement. Electrocardiographic evidence of chamber enlargement is commonly associated with severe lesions. A poststenotic dilatation of the aorta may be seen radiographically.

A murmur of subaortic stenosis may be produced by left ventricular systolic outflow obstruction in some cats with hypertrophic cardiomyopathy.

Patent Ductus Arteriosus

The murmur of congenital patent ductus arteriosus (machinery-like murmur) is most audible over the aortic valve area, although this murmur is often audible over the entire thoracic wall. Often only a systolic murmur is detected over the left caudoventral thorax; the diastolic humming portion of the murmur may be detected only over the heart base on the left side. This murmur is usually audible at the thoracic inlet and frequently radiates up the carotid arteries. Breeds of dogs most often affected are the miniature and toy poodle, collie, Shetland sheepdog, Pomeranian, and German shepherd. Females are more commonly affected. This congenital defect is also relatively common in cats.

Patent ductus arteriosus produces a volume overload and subsequent enlargement of the left atrium and left ventricle. Evidence of myocardial failure (decreased contractibility) is often detected by echocardiography in advanced cases. The electrocardiogram may be normal or reflect left atrial or ventricular enlargement. Lateral thoracic radiographs are characterized by enlargement of the cardiac silhouette, elevation of the trachea, and the left atrial enlargement. The right ventricle is often enlarged, and the cranial waist may be absent because of the widened aortic arch. Since the defect produces left-to-right shunting of blood, the cranial lobar pulmonary arteries are often larger than the corresponding veins. Severe pulmonary overcirculation is sometimes indicated by increased linear caudal lung lobe densities produced by enlarged arteries and veins. The dorsoventral radiograph typically reveals an elongated cardiac silhouette, partly due to the enlarged aortic arch. The left cranial border of the cardiac silhouette is characterized by enlargements of the descending aortic arch, main pulmonary artery segment, and left atrium.

Patent ductus arteriosus, if not surgically corrected, almost always produces left-sided congestive heart failure (coughing, exercise intolerance, dyspnea, pulmonary edema) before 3 years of age, and often before 1 year of age.

Tricuspid Insufficiency

Tricuspid insufficiency (regurgitation) is usually detected in association with mitral insufficiency in middle-aged to old small-breed and chondrodysplastic breeds. The dachshund may develop tricuspid insufficiency without an audible mitral valve murmur. Although right-sided congestive heart failure may develop, left-sided congestive heart failure is more commonly associated with this disorder because of concomitant mitral valve disease. Congenital tricuspid valve insufficiency, which is most common in large-breed dogs such as Doberman pinschers, setters, and retrievers, often results in right-sided congestive heart failure.

Large-breed dogs such as Doberman pinschers and great Danes often develop tricuspid insufficiency due to endocardiosis by 5 to 7 years of age, but this lesion does not result in heart failure.

Radiographic abnormalities associated with tricuspid valve insufficiency are right atrial and right ventricular enlargement. The electrocardiogram is often normal but may reveal high-voltage P waves (greater than 0.4 mV in leads II and aVF) or, occasionally, evidence of right-ventricular enlargement. In large-breed dogs with congenital tricuspid insufficiency, large Q waves are common and may produce a right axis deviation.

Aortic Insufficiency

The murmur of aortic insufficiency occurs during early diastole and is difficult to hear in most instances. This murmur is seldom loud and is most difficult to detect in the presence of a tachycardia. A phonocardiogram is often useful in confirming the presence of this murmur. Aortic insufficiency is most often de-

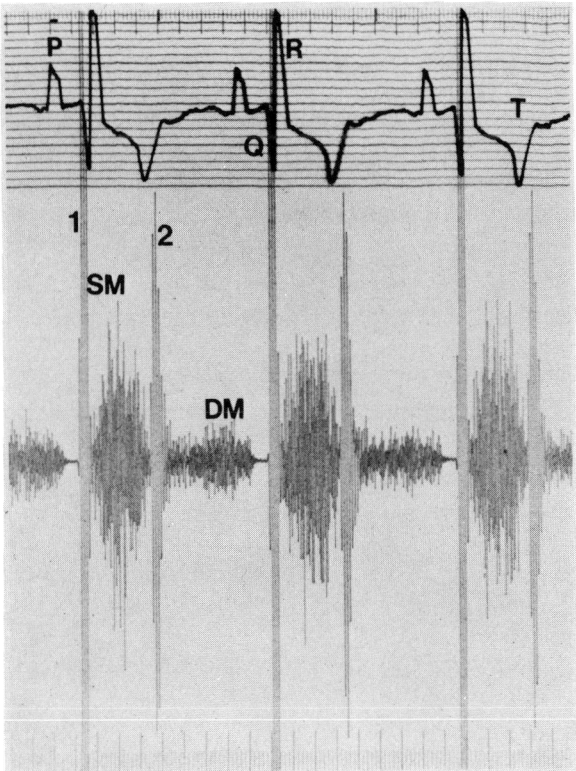

FIGURE 22-5. Diastolic murmur (*DM*) associated with aortic valvular insufficiency (regurgitation). A systolic murmur (*SM*) is also present and may be due to blood flow turbulence caused by vegetations on the aortic and/or mitral valve leaflets. *1*, first heart sound; *2*, second heart sound.

tected in association with bacterial endocarditis affecting at least the aortic valve (Fig. 22-5). Congenital aortic stenosis is often associated with a mild aortic insufficiency, and the latter may be progressive as chronic blood flow turbulence produces abnormalities of the valve cusp margins. A high ventricular septal defect (most common type) may also result in a mild aortic insufficiency due to a loss of septal support of the septal leaflet of the aortic valve, resulting in a sagging effect.

Aortic insufficiency associated with bacterial endocarditis usually produces severe, intractable left-sided congestive heart failure. Aortic insufficiency secondary to aortic stenosis or ventricular septal defect usually does not result in clinical deterioration.

DIAGNOSTIC PLAN

The minimum data base for patients with cardiac murmurs is a complete physical examination and characterization of the murmur (timing, intensity, frequency, location, and modulation). If the murmur is considered to be due to anemia or pathologic conditions, then the data base is extended (Table 22-6). The possibility of a cardiac murmur being due to a high cardiac output state (anemia, hyperthyroidism) depends on the history and physical examination findings.

If the cardiac murmur is thought to be pathologic, then the first steps that are indicated to generate a rank-ordered ruleout list are to consider the epizootiologic factors pertaining to the patient and to characterize the murmur. The age, breed (or type of dog), and historic evidence of a preexisting murmur should be assessed (Tables 22-7 and 22-8). Most puppies, kittens, and young dogs with loud murmurs (IV/VI to VI/VI) have a congenital heart defect. Most middle-aged to old, small, or miniature dog breeds, chondrodysplastic breeds, and beagles with heart murmurs have acquired mitral valvular insufficiency, often with concomitant tricuspid valvular insufficiency. However, even middle-aged dogs of any breed or type may have a congenital defect, and the client may or may not be aware of its presence; therefore, such a history should be ascertained. Unfortunately, because of incomplete physical examinations or poor skill on the part of the veterinarian, the absence of a history of a heart murmur in animals of any age does not rule out the possibility of a congenital defect.

Spaniels may develop heart murmurs due to either AV valvular fibrosis (endocardiosis), dilated cardiomyopathy, or both. Giant- and large-breed dogs, 4

TABLE 22-6. Minimum Data Base for Patients with Cardiac Murmurs

Murmur Intensity	Suspected Etiology	Data Base
I/VI–III/VI	Innocent	Sequential physical examination
	Functional	Sequential physical examination
		CBC, serum chemistry profile, UA if indicated by physical or historic findings
II/VI–VI/VI	Pathologic	CBC, serum chemistry profile, UA
		Thoracic radiographs
		Electrocardiogram
		Special tests*

*Phonocardiogram, echocardiogram, nonselective angiogram, selective cardiac catheterization

CBC, complete blood count; UA, urine analysis

TABLE 22-7. Common Rule Outs for Pathologic Heart Murmurs

Age and Type	Most Common Rule Outs
Puppies, kittens, young animals	Congenital
Adult	
Giant- and large-breed dogs	Cardiomyopathy (dilated)
	Mitral insufficiency
	Tricuspid insufficiency
	Bacterial endocarditis
Small-breed dogs	Mitral insufficiency
	Tricuspid insufficiency
	Bacterial endocarditis
Cats	Cardiomyopathy
	Hyperthyroidism

years of age or older, may develop murmurs of mitral insufficiency secondary to dilated cardiomyopathy. Frequently, such dogs already manifest clinical signs of heart failure.

Most commonly, heart murmurs associated with bacterial endocarditis are aortic in origin, but systolic murmurs of mitral insufficiency are also common. The presence of a diastolic murmur should alert the clinician to the probability of bacterial endocarditis, especially when clinical and laboratory evidence is consistent with bacteremia. Fever, leukocytosis, monocytosis, lameness, hypoalbuminemia, increased serum alkaline phosphatase activity, hypoglycemia, and bacteriuria are variably present in dogs with bacteremia.[1,2] The incidence of bacterial endocarditis in cats is unknown but is probably much lower than that in dogs.

Heart murmurs in middle-aged to older cats are most likely the result of cardiomyopathy, as are new murmurs in young adult cats. A careful history is necessary to rule out the possibility of the murmur having been present since birth (*i.e.*, congenital heart defect).

The most likely disorders associated with many cardiac murmurs can be quickly rank-ordered based on epizootiologic factors. The characteristics of the heart murmur are then determined during the physical examination. The character of the murmur associated with a patent ductus arteriosus in young animals is pathognomonic, and the diagnosis can usually be supported by thoracic radiographic findings. Young dogs, especially those of a breed or type known to have an increased incidence of pulmonic stenosis, with cardiac murmurs that are clearly or suspected to be of pulmonic valve origin will usually have evidence of right ventricular hypertrophy and a right axis deviation on the electrocardiogram.

It is imperative that the patent ductus arteriosus and pulmonic stenosis be correctly diagnosed, since surgical correction or valvuloplasty is feasible. For

TABLE 22-8. Differential Diagnosis of Common Disorders Associated with Pathologic Heart Murmurs

Rule Out	Murmur	Typical Breed or Type	Age (Usual)	Possible Associated Signs	Radiographic Abnormalities	ECG Abnormalities
Aquired mitral valve endocardiosis	Holosystolic plateau	Toy, miniature, small, chondrodysplastic; spaniel; beagle	>7 years	Asymptomatic Cough Exercise intolerance Dyspnea Crackles Syncope Ascites	↑LA ↑RCLPV Pulmonary edema Generalized cardiomegaly Chronic interstitial lung disease Collapsing trachea	None P > 0.04 second ↑LV SVPC VPC
Dilated cardiomyopathy	Holosystolic plateau	Giant, Doberman pinscher, boxer, standard poodle, German shepherd, large dogs	>4 years	Exercise intolerance Cough Dyspnea Crackles Syncope Pale mucous membranes Gallop heart rhythm Muffled heart, lung sounds Ascites Pulse deficits	Generalized cardiomegaly ↑LA ↑RCLPV Pulmonary edema Pleural effusion	P > 0.04 second ↑LV Atrial fibrillation VPC
Patent ductus arteriosus	Continuous (machinery)	Poodle, Shetland sheepdog, collie, German shepherd, many others	Puppy, kitten, young	None Exercise intolerance Cough Dyspnea Crackles	↑LA ↑RCLPA/V Pulmonary edema Elongated cardiac silhouette Aortic, pulmonic, La bulges	None P > 0.04 second ↑LV

Disease	Murmur	Breed	Age	Clinical signs	Radiographs	ECG
Pulmonic stenosis	Ejection (crescendo-decrescendo)	Terrier, brachycephalic, miniature schnauzer, many others	Puppy, young	None	↑RV, ↓Pulmonary artery segment	RVH
Bacterial endocarditis	Holosystolic or diastolic	Middle to large breeds	2–7 years	Exercise intolerance, Syncope, Ascites, Fever, ↑WBC, Monocytosis, Lameness, ↓Albumin, ↑SAP, Hypoglycemia / Fever, ↑WBC, Monocytosis, Lameness, ↓Albumin, ↑SAP, Hypoglycemia	None, Pulmonary edema, Pneumonia	None, VPC
Feline cardiomyopathy Hypertrophic	Systolic	Any	4–12 years	Dyspnea, Gallop heart rhythm, Crackles, Rear limb monoparesis or paraparesis/paralysis	↑LA-RA, Pulmonary edema, Pleural effusion (mild to moderate)	↑Atrial, ↑LV, Atrial fibrillation, SVPC
Dilated congestive	Systolic	Any, Siamese	6–15 years	Dyspnea, Muffled heart, lung sounds, Rear limb monoparesis or paraparesis/paralysis	Generalized cardiomegaly, Pleural effusion	↑Atrial, ↑LV, VPC

ECG, electrocardiogram; LA, left atrium; RCLPV, right cranial lobar pulmonary vein; SVPC, supraventricular premature contractions; VPC, ventricular premature contractions; RV, right ventricle; RVH, right ventricular hypertrophy; WBC, white blood cells; SAP, serum alkaline phosphatase; RA, right atrium most practical purposes, the mere diagnosis of a congenital defect of other types is adequate. Special tests are usually required for a specific diagnosis, and surgical intervention is seldom feasible.

The character of the acquired mitral insufficiency in older, small-breed dogs usually allows for the clinical diagnosis. Thoracic radiographs are indicated to assess the severity of cardiac enlargement and the therapeutic indications. The historic findings are also important in assessing the indications for treatments.

The historic and physical findings in dogs with dilated cardiomyopathy usually overshadow the significance of a cardiac murmur. The diagnosis is usually suspected during the physical examination and supported in most instances by radiographic and electrocardiographic abnormalities. Echocardiography is the safest and easiest method of confirming the diagnosis.

Feline cardiomyopathy and hyperthyroidism account for virtually all heart disease in the adult. The diagnosis is supported by abnormalities of thoracic radiographs or the electrocardiogram, or both. The diagnosis is confirmed by echocardiography and/or thyroid hormone assay.

Cyanosis in association with a heart murmur in a young animal is usually the result of a right-to-left shunt or severe left-sided congestive heart failure. In older dogs, cyanosis is associated with severe left-sided congestive heart failure.

REFERENCES

1. Calvert CA: Valvular bacterial endocarditis in dogs. J Am Vet Med Assoc 180:1080–1084, 1982
2. Calvert CA, Greene CE, Hardie E: Aerobic cardiovascular infections in dogs. J Am Vet Med Assoc 187:612–616, 1985
3. de Leon AC, Perloff JK, Twigg H, et al: The straight back syndrome. Circulation 32:193–203, 1965
4. Detweiler DK, Patterson DF: A phonograph record of heart sounds and murmur of the dog. Ann NY Acad Sci 127:322, 1965
5. Duke M, Abelmann WH: The hemodynamic response to chronic anemia. Circulation 39:503–515, 1969
6. Ettinger SJ, Suter PF: Heart sounds and phonocardiography. In Canine Cardiology, pp 29, 38. Philadelphia, WB Saunders, 1970
7. Fowler NO, Holmes JC: Blood viscosity and cardiac output in acute experimental anemia. J Appl Physiol 39:453–456, 1975
8. Gould L, Ettinger SO, Lyon AF: Intensity of the first heart sound and arterial pulse in mitral insufficiency. Dis Chest 53:545–549, 1964
9. Graettinger J, Muenster JJ, Silverstone LA, et al: A correlation of clinical and hemodynamic studies of patients with hyperthyroidism with and without congestive heart failure. J Clin Invest 38:1316–1321, 1959
10. Leatham A: A classification of systolic murmurs. Br Heart J 17:574–576, 1955
11. Lewis DH: Phonocardiology. In Handbook of Physiology. Bethesda, American Physiological Society, 1962
12. Lewis BS, Ehrenfeld EN, Lewis N: Echocardiographic LV function in thyrotoxicosis. Am Heart J 97:460–468, 1979

13. Patterson DF: Epidemiologic and genetic studies of congenital heart disease in the dog. Circ Res 23:171–202, 1968

14. Patterson DF, Detweiler DK: The diagnostic significance of splitting of the second heart sound in the dog. Zentralbl Veterinarmed 10:121–124, 1963

15. Patterson DF, Flickinger GL: Clinico-pathological conference. J Am Vet Med Assoc 180:1080–1084, 1982

16. Sabbah HN, Stein PD: Turbulent flow in humans: Its primary role in the production of ejection murmurs. Circ Res 38:513–525, 1976

17. Stein PD, Sabbah HN: Aortic origin of innocent murmurs. Am J Cardiol 39:665–671, 1977

18. Theilen EO, Wilson WR: Hemodynamic effects of peripheral vasoconstriction in normal and thyrotoxic subjects. J Appl Physiol 22:207–210, 1967

CHAPTER TWENTY-THREE

Pale Mucous Membranes

Clay A. Calvert

PROBLEM DEFINITION AND RECOGNITION

Pale mucous membranes (pallor) are a common clinical sign of a variety of disorders or diseases. Although pallor may be found by examining the skin, it is best evaluated by examination of the mucous membranes, primarily of the oral cavity. Physiologic vasoconstriction may result in visible pallor in normal cats and many nervous or apprehensive dogs. Other factors such as excitement and physical exertion can produce the appearance of a "healthier" color, particularly of the oral mucous membranes.

CLASSIFICATION

Pale mucous membranes are a manifestation of either decreased red blood cell mass (anemia) or decreased peripheral perfusion (see Display, Classification of Disorders Producing Pale Mucous Membranes). Although moderate to severe anemia produces pale mucous membranes, many conditions result in pallor without a reduction of red blood cell mass. Decreased peripheral perfusion may result from severe dehydration, loss of plasma protein resulting from severe thermal burn, or shock.

PATHOPHYSIOLOGY

The pathophysiology of anemia is discussed in Chapter 60. Anemia results from blood loss, blood destruction, or decreased erythrocyte production. The former two types result in a bone marrow response (regenerative anemia), while the latter, by definition, results from atrophy of some component of the erythroid series of cells.

Pale mucous membranes resulting from dehydration or selective loss of plasma protein are produced by peripheral vasoconstriction in an attempt to maintain sufficient blood pressure and blood perfusion of vital tissues and organs.

Shock is a complex group of acute cardiovascular syndromes that defy precise definition because of their varied origins. It is practical, however, to consider

Classification of Disorders Producing Pale Mucous Membranes

- Anemia
- Decreased peripheral perfusion
    Hypovolemic shock
        Exogenous loss of fluid
            Dehydration
            Selective loss of plasma
            Loss of whole blood
        Endogenous loss of fluid
            Exudative (peritonitis)
            Modified transudative (heart failure)
            Transudative (hypoalbuminemia)
        Hypoadrenocortism
    Cardiogenic shock
        Myocardial failure
            Dilated cardiomyopathy
            End-stage volume overload
                Mitral insufficiency
                Aortic insufficiency
                Congenital defects (some)
        Tachyarrhythmias
        Cardiac tamponade
        Pulmonary thromboembolism
    Vasomotor shock
        Septic
        Neurogenic
        Trauma
        Pain
        Anaphylaxis

shock as a disturbance of circulation, resulting in ineffective or critical reduction of perfusion of vital tissues with associated hypoxia and a wide range of systemic effects. The clinical signs associated with shock are paleness of the mucous membranes, arterial hypotension, rapid and weak pulse, oliguria, and a tendency toward a progressive, refractory irreversible phase.

Pale mucous membranes in shock conditions result from hypovolemia, cardiac insufficiency (myocardial failure), and vasoconstriction. When a patient is in shock, several hemodynamic mechanisms are at work simultaneously, so continuous monitoring of multiple parameters of cardiovascular function is required. Hypovolemia and altered peripheral resistance may be significant factors

TABLE 23-1. Diagnostic Plan for Pale Mucous Membranes

Rule Out	Diagnostic Plan
Anemia	Packed cell volume Reticulocyte count
Dehydration	Total solids BUN Urine specific gravity
Plasma loss	Total solids Total protein Albumin
Whole blood loss	Packed cell volume Total solids
Endogenous fluid loss	CBC Serum chemistry profile Urine analysis Cytology of effusion Radiographs Electrocardiogram
Cardiogenic shock	Thoracic radiographs Electrocardiogram Blood pressure Toe-web rectal temperature differential
Vasomotor shock	CBC Serum chemistry profile Urine analysis Blood pressure Toe-web rectal temperature differential Blood culture (if indicated) Urine culture (if indicated)

BUN, blood urea nitrogen; CBC, complete blood count

in cardiogenic shock. Pump failure (myocardial failure) may be an important feature of severe hypovolemia.

Hypovolemic shock results from oligemia, hemorrhage, traumatic loss of fluids, or burns. There is a true diminution of blood volume due to loss of whole blood or constituents thereof from the intravascular compartment. Compensatory vasoconstriction temporarily reduces the intravascular fluid compartment, and thereby maintains adequate blood pressure. Peripheral vasoconstriction results in pallor.

Cardiogenic shock results from an inability of the left ventricle to perform effectively as a pump in maintaining adequate cardiac output. Pale mucous membranes result from poor peripheral perfusion and vasoconstriction.

Vasomotor shock may begin by expansion of the intravascular fluid compartment, resulting from vasodilation. This produces a relative inadequacy of blood volume. The increase in capacitance results from widespread dilatation of the arteries and arterioles or from venous pooling. This so-called warm shock is not characterized by pale mucous membranes, even though the arterial blood pressure is reduced and peripheral or splanchnic pooling of blood is occurring.

The most common form of vasomotor shock is septic shock. As septic shock proceeds, the typical clinical signs of shock (*e.g.,* tachycardia and pallor) develop as peripheral vasoconstriction occurs in an attempt to restore blood pressure and perfusion of vital tissues and organs.

Neurogenic factors elicited by trauma or pain may result in a type of vasomotor shock. Initially, epinephrine release results in tachycardia and vasoconstriction, which produce pallor. A reflex autonomic stimulation follows and produces splanchnic pooling of blood due to venous dilatation. A relative inadequacy of blood volume then exists. In the absence of hemorrhage or lung trauma, this type of vasomotor shock is self-limiting.

Vascular shock may also result from anaphylaxis, histamine response, and arteriolar dilator drug therapy. All of these factors result in hypotension and pale mucous membranes.

DIAGNOSTIC PLAN

The diagnostic plan for pale mucous membranes varies with the severity of the patient's overall condition, history, and specific clinical findings (Table 23-1). The primary differential diagnosis is anemia versus shock. In most instances, the history and physical examination findings are consistent with one or the other of these problems. When anemia is not suspected to be the primary problem, then the differentiation of hypovolemic, septic, and cardiogenic shock is necessary.

CHAPTER TWENTY-FOUR

Cyanosis

Clay A. Calvert

PROBLEM DEFINITION AND RECOGNITION

Cyanosis refers to a bluish color of the skin or mucous membranes, resulting from an increased amount of reduced hemoglobin, or hemoglobin derivatives, in the small blood vessels of those areas. The most superficial cutaneous capillaries contribute little to the color of the skin in most areas of the body.[8] The subpapillary venous plexus makes the largest vascular contribution to skin color.[8,10] Cyanosis is not synonymous with hypoxemia or hypoxia. The presence of cyanosis implies hypoxemia, but the absence of cyanosis does not preclude severe hypoxia. The degree of cyanosis is modified by the quality of cutaneous or mucosal pigments and the color of the blood plasma as well as by the state of the surface capillaries.

PATHOPHYSIOLOGY

Under normal conditions, during passage through the pulmonary capillaries, blood is exposed to an alveolar oxygen tension of approximately 100 mm Hg and leaves the capillaries in almost complete equilibrium with the alveolar gas. Normal blood leaves the lungs with an oxygen content of approximately 20 ml/dl. The arteriovenous blood oxygen difference under resting conditions is approximately 4 ml/dl.[5] Thus, the mixed venous blood in the pulmonary artery contains approximately 15 ml of oxygen per deciliter, which represents an oxyhemoglobin saturation of 75% and an oxygen tension of 40 mm Hg. Oxygen saturation of arterial blood is normally 95% to 97% and is associated with an arterial partial pressure of oxygen (PaO_2) of 85 to 100 mm Hg. As long as the PaO_2 is at least 60 mm Hg, cyanosis is uncommon. Thus, hypoxemia can exist without cyanosis.

The increase in the amount of reduced hemoglobin in subpapillary venous plexuses, which produces cyanosis, may be brought about either by an increase in the quantity of venous blood in the cutaneous tissue, as the result of dilatation of the vessels and venous ends of the capillaries, or by a decrease in the oxygen saturation in the capillary blood. In general, cyanosis becomes apparent when the mean capillary concentration of reduced hemoglobin exceeds 5%.[6] The absolute, rather than the relative, amount of reduced hemoglobin is important in producing cyanosis. Thus, in severe anemia, the relative amount of reduced hemoglobin in the venous blood may be very large in relation to the total amount of hemoglobin. However, since the latter is severely lowered, the absolute amount of reduced hemoglobin may be small; therefore, patients with severe anemia and marked arterial desaturation do not display cyanosis. Conversely, patients with marked polycythemia, such as with polycythemia vera, tend to be cyanotic at higher levels of arterial oxygen saturation than patients with normal hematocrit values. Local passive congestion, which causes an increase in the total amount of reduced hemoglobin in the vessels of a given area, may cause cyanosis, even though the average percentage arterial saturation is not altered. Cyanosis is also observed when nonfunctioning hemoglobin is present in the blood; as little as 1.5 g/dl of methemoglobin or 0.5 g/dl of sulfhemoglobin is sufficient to produce cyanosis.

Cyanosis may result from a number of different mechanisms. Increased deoxygenated (reduced) hemoglobin can result from arterial hypoxemia, increased extraction of oxygen from capillary blood, dilatation or congestion of the venous system leading to an increased volume of oxygen-poor blood, and the presence of abnormal hemoglobins.

CLASSIFICATION

True cyanosis may be divided into two categories: central and peripheral (Table 24-1). In the central type, there is arterial blood unsaturation or an abnormal hemoglobin derivative, and the warm mucous membranes and skin both are affected (generalized cyanosis). Central or generalized cyanosis is due to arterial hypoxemia or abnormal hemoglobins. Peripheral cyanosis is due to a slowing of blood flow to an area and an abnormally great extraction of oxygen from normally saturated arterial blood. The most common type of peripheral cyanosis is the result of decreased blood flow through the peripheral capillary bed. This may result from cooling of the extremities, vasoconstriction of superficial vessels, polycythemia, thrombophlebitis with thrombosis, and low cardiac output. In low cardiac output states, the arteriovenous oxygen differential is increased. During exercise, this differential increases because cardiac output does not increase appropriately. Consequently, cyanosis is more apparent during exertion. Peripheral cyanosis occurs usually on cool portions of the body, such as digits, nose, and ears. In conditions such as cardiogenic shock with pulmonary edema, there may be a mixture of both central and peripheral types.

Hypoxemia, and therefore cyanosis, may occur when the normal state of gas exchange between alveolar air and pulmonary capillary blood is disturbed. Decreased arterial oxygen saturation results from a marked reduction in the oxygen tension of the arterial blood (PaO_2). Hypoxemia can result from reduced

TABLE 24-1. Causes of Cyanosis and Common Associations

Cause	Association(s)
Central	
Decreases arterial oxygen saturation	Impaired pulmonary function
	Alveolar hypoventilation
	Ventilation-perfusion mismatch
	Impaired oxygen diffusion from alveoli to capillaries
	Anatomic shunts
	Congenital heart defects
	Pulmonary arteriovenous shunting
Hemoglobin abnormalities	Methemoglobinemia
	Sulfhemoglobinemia
Peripheral	
Reduced cardiac output	Myocardial failure
Vasoconstriction	Cold exposure
Venous obstruction	Thrombophlebitis
Arterial obstruction	

inspired oxygen concentration, alveolar hypoventilation, diffusion impairment, ventilation-perfusion mismatch, and right-to-left shunts.

Reduction of inspired oxygen can occur at high altitudes or when insufficient oxygen is delivered during anesthesia. Seriously impaired pulmonary function, through alveolar hypoventilation, ventilation-perfusion mismatch (perfusion of poorly ventilated areas of the lung), or impaired oxygen diffusion is the most common cause of central cyanosis. Pneumonia, pulmonary edema, or chronic obstructive lung disorders, if severe, may produce cyanosis by these means.

Central Cyanosis

Hypoxemia can result from alveolar hypoventilation, ventilation-perfusion mismatch, impaired diffusion, anatomic right-to-left cardiac shunts, and abnormal hemoglobins.

Alveolar hypoventilation is associated with hypercarbia (increased partial pressure of CO_2) of arterial blood ($PaCO_2$). Although alveolar hypoventilation produces hypoxemia, the increase in $PaCO_2$ is most important, and hypoxemia is seldom severe unless hypoventilation is severe. In such cases, the signs of respiratory acidosis dominate. Alveolar hypoventilation can result from depression of the respiratory control center due to drug administration (narcotics, barbiturates, other anesthetics) or organic disorders (trauma, hemorrhage, inflammation); cervical spinal cord damage interfering with efferent nerve traffic to the muscles of respiration; poor respiratory muscle function due to massive chest wall trauma or neuromuscular diseases; and severe upper airway destruction. The latter is most commonly associated with recurrent laryngeal nerve palsy in old dogs, but has been seen as a hereditary disorder in young large-breed dogs, especially the Bouvier des Flanders. Cyanosis occurs only when upper airway obstruction is nearly complete.

Ventilation-perfusion mismatch means that either poor alveolar ventilation is occurring in areas where blood flow is adequate or that blood flow is severely impaired in areas where alveolar ventilation is continuing. Ventilation-perfusion mismatch occurs in association with pulmonary edema, pulmonary thromboembolism, pneumonia, pulmonary contusion, and atelectasis.

Diffusion impairment is often associated with disorders causing ventilation-perfusion mismatch. Diffusion of oxygen across the alveolar epithelium, interstitium, capillary basement membrane, and endothelium is associated with considerable functional reserve. Thus, even when the contact time with pulmonary capillaries is reduced, oxygen diffusion is still adequate under most circumstances. Diffusion impairment may contribute to hypoxemia when patients with lung disease undergo exertion. Decreased diffusion capacity of the alveolar-capillary membrane can result from alveolar destruction, pulmonary edema, severe pulmonary fibrosis, or infiltrative inflammatory or neoplastic diseases. Cyanosis is often absent in association with chronic lung disease with perfusion of underventilated areas.

Another cause of decreased arterial oxygen saturation is shunting of venous blood into the arterial circuit. Certain types of congenital heart defects, such as tetralogy of Fallot and Eisenmenger's complex, are associated with cyanosis. Since blood normally flows from a high-pressure to a low-pressure region, in order for a cardiac defect to result in a right-to-left shunt, it must ordinarily be combined with an obstructive lesion distal to the defect or with elevated pulmonary vascular resistance (Table 24-2). In patients with cardiac right-to-left shunts, the presence and severity of cyanosis depend on the size of the shunt relative to the systemic flow as well as on the oxyhemoglobin saturation of the venous blood. If the systemic blood flow is less than normal in a patient with cyanotic congenital heart disease, the arteriovenous oxygen difference is increased, and the mixed venous blood shunted into the arterial circuit is less saturated with oxygen. Under such circumstances, a small shunt may produce a significant degree of hypoxemia. The oxyhemoglobin saturation of mixed venous blood normally decreases during exercise. This decrease is exacerbated in patients with congenital cyanotic heart disease, since the cardiac output cannot be increased appropriately; thus, some patients may not be cyanotic except during exercise. A useful means of differentiating cyanosis caused by a shunt in the heart or lungs from that caused by primary lung disease is to administer 100% oxygen. Cyanosis caused by a right-to-left shunt will be unaffected, whereas that due to parenchymal lung diseases will decrease.

Intrapulmonary shunting can occur with severe lung lobe consolidation, wherein ventilation is absent while blood continues to flow through the lobe.

TABLE 24-2. Congenital Heart Defects with Associated Right-to-Left Shunting

Obstruction	Defect(s)
Pulmonic valve stenosis	Tetralogy of Fallot
	Pulmonic stenosis and ventricular septal defect
Pulmonary hypertension	Pulmonary hypertension associated with chronic left-to-right shunting occasionally results in reversal of shunting (right-to-left).
	Patent ductus arteriosus
	Ventricular septal defect

This is also an example of severe ventilation-perfusion mismatch. However, in this example breathing 100% oxygen does not improve cyanosis, whereas most other examples of mismatching are favorably influenced by breathing 100% oxygen.

The syndrome known as shock lung (adult respiratory distress syndrome) can occur in association with a number of clinical problems. Classically, shock lung is associated with hypovolemic or septic shock, but an identical syndrome is also seen with head trauma, respiratory assisted ventilation, aspiration pneumonia, pancreatitis, electric cord bite, and seizures.

The onset of shock lung is characterized by an increase in tracheobronchial secretions, tachypnea, and cyanosis. The arterial partial pressure of oxygen (PaO_2) gradually decreases; the arterial partial pressure of carbon dioxide ($PaCO_2$) is initially low but may increase as the patient's condition deteriorates. Metabolic acidosis followed by combined metabolic and respiratory acidosis is common. The tidal volume decreases as does the pulmonary compliance; increased inspiratory pressure is required in order to maintain a given tidal volume.

No single cause of shock lung has been identified. The disorder is probably the result of several insults, including excessive fluid administration, oxygen toxicity, central nervous system injury, aspiration, disseminated intravascular coagulation, microembolization, and infection.

The incidence of pulmonary embolism in dogs is unknown but is surely underdiagnosed. Pulmonary embolism is most often identified in association with advanced heartworm disease and hyperadrenocorticism in dogs, but it is also seen with protein-losing glomerulopathies, sepsis, and neoplasia. In some cases a cause cannot be identified. Pulmonary embolism, when massive, is associated with a high mortality, but when it is diagnosed quickly by lung scanning or pulmonary angiography, appropriate therapy may reduce the risk of mortality.

No clinical sign is pathognomonic for pulmonary embolism. Dyspnea, cough, and hemoptysis are commonly seen in association with severe heartworm disease. Tachypnea, crackles, and tachycardia are nonspecific signs that may be detected. When massive embolism is present, syncope, cyanosis, a gallop heart rhythm, or a splitting of the second heart sound may be detected. Echocardiographic evidence of right ventricular dilatation with reduced shortening fraction is a common finding.

Cyanosis is produced by small amounts of circulating methemoglobin[3] and by even smaller amounts of sulfhemoglobin, although such conditions are uncommon. Methemoglobin contains iron oxidized to the ferric state, which is unable to bind oxygen. Methemoglobinemia may be hereditary (methemoglobin reductase deficiency) but is usually acquired via drug or chemical ingestion or contact. These agents preferentially oxidize hemoglobin and may overcome the normal reducing mechanism of the erythrocytes. Nitrates, after ingestion, may be converted to nitrites by intestinal bacteria. Certain sulfonamides, such as sulfanilamide, sulfathiazole, and sulfapyridine, may produce methemoglobinemia. Acetanilid and phenacetin readily cause methemoglobinemia and sulfhemoglobinemia in cats.[4] Local anesthetics containing benzocaine, when sprayed onto the larynx of cats prior to intubation, are capable of producing methemoglobinemia and sometimes cyanosis.[2] Cats treated with urinary antiseptics containing methylene blue often develop Heinz body (erythrocyte refractile body) anemia of variable severity with associated methemoglobinemia. Urinary tract compounds containing phenazopyridine (analgesic) can produce Heinz body anemia and methemoglobinemia when administered at high dosages.[1] In the dog, onion ingestion can produce methemoglobinemia via the major component of onion oil (alylpropyl disulfide).[7,9]

Peripheral Cyanosis

Peripheral cyanosis is uncommon in dogs and cats but may be caused by generalized vasoconstriction from cold exposure. Cutaneous vasoconstriction may occur in shock or congestive heart failure as a compensatory mechanism, so that blood is diverted to vital areas (kidneys, brain, heart). Even though the arterial blood may be normally saturated, cyanosis can result from the reduced peripheral blood flow through the surface vessels and the reduced oxygen tension at the venous end of the capillaries. Increased oxygen extraction from capillaries because of sluggish blood flow (as in right-sided congestive heart failure) may result in peripheral cyanosis. Peripheral cyanosis alone is not associated with cyanosis of warm mucous membranes, such as the insides of the lips, cheeks, tongue, and conjunctiva.

Venous obstruction associated with thrombophlebitis produces stagnation of blood flow and increased oxygen extraction. Massage or warming of the cyanotic extremity will increase peripheral blood flow and abolish peripheral but not central cyanosis. Other causes of thrombosis are feline cardiomyopathy, bacterial endocarditis, hypercoagulability (nephrotic syndrome), and cold agglutinin disease.

DIAGNOSTIC PLAN

The diagnostic plan indicated for the differential diagnosis of the cyanotic patient is dependent on the associated clinical signs (Tables 24-3 and 24-4). In most instances, the diagnosis of central cyanosis is assumed to result from the presence of severe respiratory distress. Such dyspnea may result from severe pulmonary disease, congestive heart failure with associated severe pulmonary edema, or upper airway obstruction.

The auscultation of pulmonary crackles indicates parenchymal lung disease. Rule outs should include pulmonary interstitial fibrosis, especially in small terriers and miniature and toy breeds; pulmonary edema of cardiogenic or neurogenic origin; pulmonary contusion; pneumonia of various causes; heartworm disease with associated embolism; and shock lung. The presence of congestive heart failure is often suspected on the basis of the age, breed, history, and presence of a heart murmur or gallop heart rhythm.

Central cyanosis in a young dog or cat without evidence of parenchymal lung disease raises the possibility of a right-to-left cardiac shunt. A cardiac murmur may or may not be present. Radiographic assessment may reveal evidence of pulmonary vascular overcirculation and hypertension. Hemoconcentration is often present, depending on the age of the patient and severity of the shunt. The degree of cyanosis is exacerbated with exercise. Arterial oxygen saturation (PaO_2) measurements will reveal hypoxemia.

Upper airway destruction is characterized by inspiratory dyspnea (stridor). These sounds are harsh, high-pitched, and exacerbated by exercise. Stridor may be palpated in the laryngeal region.

Peripheral cyanosis alone is not associated with cyanosis of warm mucous membranes, and the arterial oxygen saturation (PaO_2) is normal. Massaging or

TABLE 24-3. Diagnostic Tests Often Indicated in the Cyanotic Patient

Test	Finding(s)	Association(s)
Arterial blood gas analysis	Reduced PaO_2	Central cyanosis
Thoracic radiographs	Enlarged arteries	Heartworm disease Right-to-left shunt
	Parenchymal disease	Pulmonary edema Pneumonia Contusion Shock lung Pulmonary embolism associated with severe heartworm disease
Electrocardiogram	Right ventricular hypertrophy	Severe heartworm disease Right-to-left shunt
Hematocrit	Elevated	Chronic hypoxemia Right-to-left shunt

TABLE 24-4. Diagnostic Plan and Differential Diagnosis of Cyanosis

Diagnostic Test	Findings	Assessment
Physical examination	Cyanosis of warm mucous membranes	Central cyanosis
	Cool extremities	Peripheral cyanosis
		Mixed cyanosis
	Crackles (severe)	Central or mixed
	Respiratory distress	Central or mixed
Thoracic radiographs	Severe disease	Central or mixed
	Pulmonary arterial	Heartworm disease
		Pulmonary embolism
	Parenchymal	Pulmonary edema
		Pulmonary contusion
		Pneumonia
		Bacterial
		Fungal
		Aspiration
		Neoplasia
		Shock lung
		Heartworm disease
Blood analysis	Hemoconcentration	Central or mixed
		Right-to-left shunt
		Polycythemia vera
	Decreased $PaCO_2$	Central
	Brown color	Central (methemoglobinemia)

warming the affected tissues may abolish the cyanosis by increasing regional blood flow.

Since most causes of cyanosis are the result of thoracic, pulmonary, or cardiac disease, thoracic radiographs are often the single most useful diagnostic test. However, caution is advised when attempting to restrain cyanotic patients for radiographs—death may result. The lateral projection is taken first. The ventrodorsal position is not recommended, and the dorsoventral position is less stressful to the patient. In some instances the cause of the cyanosis is strongly suspected, in which case radiographs are not taken immediately but possibly after the patient's condition has been stabilized.

The hematocrit should be determined. Polycythemia implies chronic hypoxemia and in young dogs is usually associated with cardiac right-to-left shunts. Chocolate brown or brownish dark blood indicates methemoglobinemia. A drop of blood placed on white filter paper enhances the brown color. Placing a sample of such blood in a test tube and shaking it in room air, or bubbling oxygen into the blood, does not produce the bright red blood that normal venous blood produces.

Electrocardiographic evidence of right ventricular hypertrophy is often found with chronic, severe lung disease causing pulmonary hypertension (cor pulmonale) and is usually present with right-to-left cardiac shunts. The latter are usually associated with pulmonary hypertension or pulmonary outflow obstruction.

Blood gas analysis is often helpful. Hypoxemia (decreased PaO_2) is associated with central cyanosis but is usually absent with peripheral cyanosis. Hypercarbia (increased $PaCO_2$) indicates alveolar hypoventilation, and respiratory acidosis usually coexists. Hypercarbia is absent with other lung disorders except severe ventilation-perfusion mismatch. Most patients with mismatching have increased ventilation in response to hypercarbia, which usually normalizes the $PaCO_2$ by the time the patient is evaluated. Likewise, right-to-left shunts, although producing increased CO_2 in the arterial blood, are associated with normal $PaCO_2$ because of a centrally mediated hyperventilation response to the CO_2.

Breathing 100% oxygen usually eliminates cyanosis, unless it is due to a right-to-left shunt. Shunted blood bypasses the ventilated alveoli and is thus never exposed to the high alveolar oxygen concentration.

REFERENCES

1. Harvey JW, Kormick HP: Phenazopyridine toxicosis in the cat. J Am Vet Med Assoc 169:327–331, 1976
2. Harvey JW, Sameck JH, Bargard FJ: Benzocaine-induced methemoglobinemia in dogs. J Am Vet Med Assoc 175:1171–1175, 1979
3. Letchworth GJ, Bentinck-Smith J, Bolton GR, et al: Cyanosis and methemoglobinemia in two dogs due to NADH methemoglobin reductase deficiency. J Am Anim Hosp Assoc 13:75–79, 1977
4. Leyland A: Probable paracetamol toxicity in a cat. Vet Rec 94:104–105, 1974
5. Lukas DA: Cyanosis. In MacBryde CM, Backlow RS (eds): Signs and Symptoms, Philadelphia, JB Lippincott, 1970
6. Lundsgaard C, Van Slyke DD: Cyanosis. Medicine 1:1–5, 1923
7. Rebar AH, Lewis HB: Blood cells in disease. In Catcott EJ (ed): Canine Medicine. Santa Barbara, CA, American Veterinary Publications, 1979
8. Rothman S: Physiology and Biochemistry of the Skin. Chicago, University of Chicago Press, 1954
9. St Omer UV, McKnight EB: Acetylcysteine for treatment of acetaminophen toxicosis in the cat. J Am Vet Med Assoc 197:911–915, 1980
10. Winklemann RK, Scheen SR, Pyka RA, et al: Cutaneous vascular patterns in studies with injections preparation and alkaline phosphatase reaction. In Montagna W, Ellis RA (eds): Advances in Biology of Skin. New York, Pergamon Press, 1961

PART SEVEN

Respiratory Problems

CHAPTER TWENTY-FIVE

Coughing

Larry M. Cornelius

PROBLEM DEFINITION AND RECOGNITION

Coughing is defined as a sudden noisy expulsion of air from the lungs.

PATHOPHYSIOLOGY

The function of coughing, a normal protective reflex, is to remove undesired material from the respiratory tract. It is regarded as a backup defense mechanism to the mucociliary transport apparatus of the respiratory mucosa, which normally clears particles from the respiratory tract.[2] Cough receptors in the respiratory system are most numerous in the large airways; none is present beyond the respiratory bronchioles. Afferent pathways for the cough reflex—located in the vagus, trigeminal, glossopharyngeal, and phrenic nerves—carry impulses to the coughing center in the medulla oblongata. Efferent conduction is carried out in the vagus, phrenic, and other spinal nerves, which supply the larynx, tracheobronchial tree, diaphragm, and other respiratory muscles. A few cough receptors are also present in other locations, such as the nose, paranasal sinuses, and pharynx. Cough receptors respond to both chemical and mechanical stimuli.

The beneficial effect of coughing is the clearing of the air passages, especially the trachea and large bronchi. Severe, persistent coughing, especially when dry and unproductive, may be harmful because it may (1) cause dissemination of infection, (2) further exacerbate inflammation and irritation of the respiratory mucosa, (3) cause overdistention of alveoli resulting in emphysema, (4) induce pneumothorax by causing rupture of bullae or airways, and (5) increase weakness and exhaustion in the patient.[3]

Causes of coughing can be grouped into three general classes by the location of the cause: (1) upper airway, (2) lower airway, and (3) cardiovascular (Table 25-1).

TABLE 25-1. Causes of Coughing in Dogs and Cats

Upper Airway	Lower Airway	Cardiovascular
Pharyngitis	Acute or chronic bronchitis	Left-sided heart failure
Tonsillitis	Bronchiectasis	Left atrial enlargement
Tracheitis	Pneumonia (including aspiration)	Heartworm disease
Collapsed trachea	Immotile cilia syndrome	Pulmonary thrombosis
(dogs)	Pulmonary fibrosis or abscess	Pulmonary edema
Neoplasia or trauma of	Hilar lymph node enlargement	
pharynx, tonsils, or	Neoplasia	
trachea	Fungal infections	
	Allergic bronchitis; PIE	
	Nodular eosinophilic granulomatosis	
	Fungal infections	
	Histoplasmosis	
	Blastomycosis	
	Parasites (lungworms)	
	Trauma or physical	
	Bronchial foreign body	
	Irritating gases or smoke	
	Collapsing bronchi	
	Neoplasia of mediastinum, bronchi,	
	or lungs	

PIE, pulmonary infiltrates with eosinophils

DIAGNOSTIC PLAN

History and Physical Examination

Other signs may be confused with coughing by owners. Gagging and expectoration of phlelgm, dysphagia, regurgitation, and vomiting are sometimes mistakenly reported as coughing. In many cases, an animal with a coughing problem can be induced to cough by vigorously manipulating the trachea. This should be done in the owner's presence to confirm that this is the sign they have observed.

The signalment (age, breed, sex) may help in the assessment of likelihood of particular disorders causing cough. For example, toy-breed dogs have a higher incidence of collapsing trachea. Young animals are more likely to be affected with infectious diseases.

It is important to ask about the pet's environment. If the animal has recently been in contact with groups of other dogs or cats, the likelihood of an infectious disease is increased. Environmental air pollutants, such as cigarette smoke and urban smog, may cause chronic coughing in dogs and cats. Indoor pets are less likely to have heartworm disease and other parasites, such as lungworms, than are outside animals.[1] Asking if the animal has shown other abnormal signs, such as depression, lethargy, anorexia, dyspnea, and exercise intolerance, often

TABLE 25-2. Differentiation of General Causes of Coughing

	Causes of Coughing		
	Upper Airway	Lower Airway	Cardiovascular
Depression/lethargy	Absent or mild	Mild to severe	Moderate to severe
Fever	Absent or mild	Mild to marked	None to marked
Dehydration	Absent or mild	Mild to marked	Mild to marked
Inducible cough	Usually	Occasionally	Occasionally
Dyspnea	Absent to severe	Mild to severe	Mild to severe
Exercise intolerance	Absent to marked	Mild to marked	Moderate to marked
Lung sounds	Normal	Abnormal	Abnormal
Heart sounds	Normal	Normal	Abnormal
White blood cell count	Normal	Normal or increased	Normal or increased
Thoracic radiographs	Normal	Abnormal	Abnormal

helps one decide which groups of rule outs should be considered first (Table 25-2).

Although insufficient for definitive diagnosis and treatment, certain characteristics of a cough may be of diagnostic value. A loud, harsh, dry cough is often a sign of irritation or inflammation in the larynx, trachea, or mainstem bronchi and is a common observation in dogs with infectious tracheobronchitis (kennel cough) and cats with viral rhinotracheitis. A characteristic "goose-honk" cough is heard in many toy-breed dogs with collapsing tracheas (Table 25-3).

Thoracic auscultation should be done carefully in the coughing animal. Both the heart and lungs should be carefully ausculted (see Chapters 21 and 28). It is often helpful to induce coughing by tracheal manipulation and then reauscult the thorax. Abnormal lung sounds are often heard for the first time or intensified, after the animal has a series of coughs. Crackles, wheezes, and increased normal breath sounds are commonly heard in coughing patients. Cardiac murmurs and an abnorml heart rhythm may be ausculted in animals with a cough caused by cardiac disease.

Laboratory Evaluation

A laboratory workup should be done in most patients with signs of illness, such as fever, depression, anorexia, and dyspnea accompanying coughing, or if the coughing is chronic (more than 1 week in duration). A complete blood count and differential, serum biochemical profile, fecal examination for parasites, urine analysis, heartworm check, and feline leukemia virus test (in cats) are usually indicated.

Radiography

Radiographic examination of the thorax is an extension of the physical examination in the coughing patient. Normal anatomy and disease conditions of the

Text continues on p. 212

TABLE 25-3. Common Causes of Coughing in Dogs and Cats and Characteristic Findings

	History/Physical Examination	Laboratory Studies	Radiographs
Dogs			
Acute			
Pharyngitis/ laryngitis	Hacking cough followed by gagging and swallowing of phlegm Hoarse voice Reddened pharynx and tonsils No systemic signs	Normal	Normal
Tracheitis	History of being in contact with a group of dogs Dry, hacking cough No systemic signs	Normal	Normal
Aspiration pneumonia	History of general anesthesia, regurgitation, vomiting, or megaesophagus Deep, moist cough Worsening dyspnea Fever	↑ WBC Neutrophilia and left shift *or* Stress leukogram	Consolidated alveolar pattern with cranioventral distribution
Chronic			
Infectious tracheobronchitis	History of exposure to a group of dogs Deep, dry, persistent cough No systemic signs	Normal	Normal
Tracheal collapse	Toy breed Obese "Goose-honk" cough Dyspnea May palpate collapsing trachea at thoracic inlet	Normal	Tracheal collapse, either intrathoracic or extrathoracic Best seen with bronchoscopy or fluoroscopy Bronchial collapse
Allergic bronchitis/ PIE	Deep cough, dry or productive Mild to severe dyspnea Crackles and wheezes on ausculation No systemic signs	Peripheral eosinophilia Eosinophilic inflammation on transtracheal or bronchial wash	Prominent bronchial or bronchointerstitial pattern
Heartworm disease	Weight loss Persistent coughing Mild to severe dyspnea Exercise intolerance	Peripheral eosinophilia Hyperglobulinemia Microfilaria positive *or* Occult heartworm positive	Right-sided heart enlargement Pulmonary arterial enlargement, pruning, and tortuosity Focal consolidations in lungs, especially diaphragmatic lobes

(continued)

TABLE 25-3. Common Causes of Coughing in Dogs and Cats and Characteristic Findings *(continued)*

	History/Physical Examination	Laboratory Studies	Radiographs
Dogs *(cont.)*			
Chronic *(cont.)*			
Deep mycotic infections Histoplasmosis Blastomycosis	Weight loss Persistent coughing Fever Mild to severe dyspnea Multisystem involvement	↑ WBC Neutrophilia and left shift	Diffuse nodular interstitial densities Thoracic lymph node enlargement
Left-sided heart failure	Old, small-breed dogs Cough most prominent at night Dyspnea and exercise intolerance	ECG variable, LVH pattern, PVCs	Left atrial enlargement Enlarged pulmonary veins Pulmonary edema around base of heart
Cats			
Acute			
Viral rhinotracheitis	Exposure to a group of cats Sneezing and red, watery eyes Oral ulcers	Normal or ↑ WBC with neutrophilia and left shift	Normal
Chronic			
Feline asthma	Deep, productive, paroxysmal cough with neck extended Severe dyspnea and cyanosis	Peripheral eosinophilia Eosinophilic inflammation on tracheal wash	Bronchial or bronchointerstitial lung pattern Hyperinflated lungs
Lungworms	Deep, productive, paroxysmal cough with neck extended Dyspnea Fever Positive FeLV test	Peripheral eosinophilia Ova or larvae in tracheal wash or in the feces (Baermann technique)	Bronchial or bronchointerstitial lung pattern
Heartworms	Outside cat from endemic area Listless, decreased appetite Sporadic vomiting Occasional cough	Peripheral eosinophilia Hyperglobulinemia Microfilaria negative Occult heartworm positive	Enlarged caudal lobar pulmonary arteries Mildly enlarged right ventricle

↑ Increased; WBC, white blood cell; PIE, pulmonary infiltrates with eosinophils; ECG, electrocardiogram; LVH, left ventricular hypertrophy; PVCs, premature ventricular contractions; FeLV, feline leukemia virus thorax are ideally suited for radiographic examination because of the natural contrast between the solid organs, such as the heart and large vessels, and the air-containing lung parenchyma. Proper radiographic technique, including two views, should be strictly followed. Fluoroscopy, available at some referral centers, is helpful in the diagnosis of airway collapse.

Electrophysiologic Testing

If cardiac disease is suspected to be the cause of coughing, an electrocardiogram should be done. Other specialized tests, such as echocardiography, may need to be performed but are generally available only at referral centers.

Transtracheal Wash

In moderate- to large-sized dogs, an evaluation of the lining of the respiratory mucosa from the trachea to the alveoli can usually be obtained from a proper transtracheal wash. This can be accomplished by using a tranquilizer (e.g., acepromazine) and a local anesthetic and penetrating the cricothyroid membrane with a commercial flexible polyethylene intravenous catheter placement device. Because of the risk of tracheal damage in small dogs and cats, tracheal aspiration should be done in these animals by lightly anesthetizing the patient with intravenous ketamine and diazepam and doing the transtracheal wash through a sterile endotracheal tube. Sterile, isotonic fluid such as Ringer's lactate or 0.9% saline solution should be used to do the wash (10 to 30 ml for a moderate- to large-sized dog and 5 to 10 ml for a small dog or cat). The wash will usually be productive if the animal coughs vigorously during the procedure. Samples should be submitted for cytologic evaluation and culture/sensitivity.

Bronchoscopy

A bronchoscopic examination is an excellent means of evaluating airway integrity in dogs and cats. It is especially useful in the workup of a patient with chronic cough. Flexible fiberoptic bronchoscopic equipment for dogs and cats is available but is relatively expensive. Another disadvantage is that general anesthesia is required. Most bronchoscopes permit through-the-scope infusions for bronchial washing and fluid collection by suction for cytologic examination and culture. Cells and tissue for examination can be obtained by using flexible brushes (bronchial brush biopsy) and biopsy instruments (transbronchial biopsy) passed through the bronchoscope.

Fine-Needle Lung Aspiration

When diffuse pulmonary parenchymal disease is visualized radiographically in a chronically coughing (or dyspneic) patient, and procedures described above fail to provide a diagnosis, consideration should be given to fine-needle aspiration of lung tissue. Risk of serious hemorrhage or pneumothorax is relatively low when the following rules are adhered to: (1) do not aspirate from a patient with a bleeding or clotting disorder; (2) restrain the patient well (sedate if necessary); (3) avoid the heart and major vessels (locate the preferred site for aspiration on the thoracic radiographs); (4) do not use a needle larger than 20-gauge (22 gauge or 1- or 1.5-inch needle is preferred); (5) use good technique by advancing the needle straight in, aspirating, and withdrawing straight out (do not allow the needle point to pass to and fro in a shearing motion).

Some of the material aspirated should be saved for culture and the remainder smeared out on a glass slide for cytologic examination.

Lung Biopsy

If the less invasive diagnostic procedures fail to yield a diagnosis in a coughing (or dyspneic) patient with radiographic evidence of focal or diffuse lung disease, thoracotomy and lung biopsy may be necessary. Surgical excision of discrete focal lesions or lobectomy may be curative in some cases.

REFERENCES

1. Ettinger SJ: Differential diagnosis of coughing. In Ettinger SJ (ed): Textbook of Veterinary Internal Medicine, 2nd ed, pp 95–97. Philadelphia, WB Saunders, 1983
2. Ford RB, Roudebush P: Chronic cough. In Ford RB (ed): Clinical Signs and Diagnosis in Small Animal Practice, pp 203–219. New York, Churchill Livingstone, 1988
3. Head JR, Suter PF: Approach to the patient with respiratory disease. In Ettinger SJ (ed): Textbook of Veterinary Internal Medicine, pp 544–564. Philadelphia, WB Saunders, 1975

CHAPTER TWENTY-SIX

Dyspnea

Larry M. Cornelius

DEFINITION AND PROBLEM RECOGNITION

Dyspnea is a condition of a difficult or labored breathing that is recognized as being uncomfortable for the animal. Tachypnea (polypnea) refers to an increased rate of breathing and may accompany dyspnea.[1] In many cases tachypnea may be a normal or adaptive secondary response (physiologic) associated with hyperthermia, exercise, excitement, or stress, and may not be an indication of pathologic respiratory distress. The differentiation between dyspnea and tachypnea, although quite important, may not be obvious, especially to owners and inexperienced clinicians. Orthopnea is difficult breathing in a recumbent position.

PATHOPHYSIOLOGY

Dyspnea may occur for the following basic reasons: (1) need for additional oxygen (most common), (2) compensation for metabolic acidosis, (3) excessive environmental heat (heatstroke), (4) damaged or diseased central nervous system (CNS) respiratory centers, (5) weakness of the respiratory muscles or dysfunction of the motor nerves of respiration, and (6) pain from structures involved in breathing (*e.g.,* pleura, spinal nerves, respiratory muscles, ribs).[1]

Lack of adequate tissue oxygenation can be caused by either diminished oxygen in the environment, disorders interrupting the transfer of oxygen from the environment to the blood (diseases of the upper or lower airway or restrictive diseases), decreased oxygen-carrying capacity in the blood (anemia, methemoglobinemia), excessive need for oxygen (such as with strenuous aerobic exercise), or cardiac insufficiency. Compensation for metabolic acidosis involves the "blowing off" of CO_2 through the lungs and may cause an increase in both the rate and the depth of respiration. Dogs and cats dissipate heat through the respiratory system by panting (tachypnea). An excessively hot environment may cause dyspnea and result in heatstroke. Any disorder causing damage to the CNS respiratory centers in the medulla (*e.g.,* head trauma, inflammation, mass) may disrupt the control of breathing and cause dyspnea. Decreased ventilation and labored breathing may result from disorders causing the dysfunction of motor nerves and muscles involved in breathing, such as polyradiculoneuritis or diaphragmatic paralysis. Dyspnea may also be caused by painful processes of respiratory sensory nerves and muscles and other structures such as the pleura and ribs, which can be the result of trauma, pleuritis, or other factors. Causes of dyspnea in dogs and cats are shown in Table 26-1.

DIAGNOSTIC PLAN

History and Physical Examination

Consideration of the signalment can be helpful. Certain breeds are more prone to various disorders causing dyspnea. For example, brachycephalic dogs often have upper airway problems, and hunting dogs are more likely to have dyspnea caused by the deep mycoses. Large- and giant-breed dogs are more commonly affected with laryngeal paralysis associated with hypothyroidism. Age is also an important consideration; neoplastic disorders are more likely to occur in older animals. The history should include questions about whether the dyspnea was sudden in onset or slowly progressive. Also, a complete history includes questions about other signs the owner has noticed. Asking if the animal is always confined or under the direct supervision of someone helps to assess the possibility of trauma. Considering where the animal lives and what areas it has visited may be revealing. Examples of regional problems often associated with dyspnea include heartworm disease and deep mycoses such as blastomycosis.

A thorough physical examination including all systems may provide important diagnostic clues in a dyspneic patient. A good example would be the presence of a draining skin lesion in a dyspneic dog with blastomycosis; however, care must be taken not to stress a severely dyspneic animal unduly, or death may occur. Allowing the animal to sit quietly in a high-oxygen environment and providing other symptomatic treatment prior to diagnostic procedures may be necessary.[2,3]

Careful observation of the pattern of respiration, usually while the patient is resting, may be of great help in localizing the cause of dyspnea. Upper airway disorders are associated with inspiratory dyspnea characterized by a prolonged, often noisy, labored inspiratory effort and a quick, relatively easy expiratory phase. Lower airway diseases and restrictive disorders generally cause labored breathing characterized by both inspiratory and expiratory dyspnea with a rapid respiratory rate (Table 26-2).

Sometimes it is necessary to exercise the animal in order to incite the dyspnea and characterize it. This is particularly true with certain upper airway disorders, such as laryngeal paresis or paralysis. However, *caution should be used when exercising these patients,* especially in a hot, humid environment. Potentially fatal hyperthermia and hypoxemia can occur rapidly (in a few minutes) in such patients under these circumstances.

Text continues on p. 223

TABLE 26-1. Causes of Dyspnea in Dogs and Cats

Upper Airway	Lower Airway or Pulmonary Parenchyma	Restrictive	Miscellaneous
Stenotic nares	Bronchial diseases	Pneumothorax	Anemia
Rhinitis/sinusitis	Chronic bronchitis	Pleural effusion	Methemoglobinemia
Elongated soft palate	Allergic bronchitis (asthma,	Right heart failure	Compensation for metabolic ac-
Laryngeal diseases	PIE)	Neoplasia	idosis
Laryngitis	Lungworms	Hypoalbuminemia	Heatstroke
Edema	Pneumonia	Hemothorax	Damage to respiratory center
Paralysis	Pulmonary edema	Chylothorax	Head trauma
Spasm	Left heart failure	Pyothorax	Encephalitis
Traumatic rupture of airway	Hypoalbuminemia	Feline infectious peritonitis	Neoplasia
Collapse	Others	Pericardial effusion	Neuromuscular weakness
Intraluminal tracheal or bron-	Pulmonary thromboembolism	Diaphragmatic hernia	Polyradiculoneuritis (coon-
chial foreign body or mass	Heartworm disease	Neoplasia of the mediastinum	hound paralysis)
Extraluminal tracheal or bron-	Hyperadrenocorticism	or thoracic wall	Diaphragmatic paralysis
chial obstruction	Others	Thoracic wall trauma	Others
Mediastinal mass	Pulmonary contusions	Flail chest	Pain
Tracheal or bronchial col-	(trauma)	Extreme obesity	Fractured ribs or vertebrae
lapse	Pulmonary fibrosis	Severe hepatomegaly	Pleuritis
Hilar lymphadenopathy	Pulmonary granulomatosis	Marked ascites	Others
	Deep mycosis	Large intraabdominal mass	Paraquat poisoning
	Pulmonary neoplasia	Severe gastric distention (gas-	Electric cord bite
		tric volvulus)	

PIE, pulmonary infiltrates with eosinophils

TABLE 26-2. Differentiation of General Causes of Dyspnea

	Cause of Dyspnea			
	Upper Airway	*Lower Airway*	*Restrictive*	*Miscellaneous**
Type of dyspnea	Inspiratory	Expiratory	Rapid, shallow	Rapid, shallow or deep
Fever	Absent	Variable	Variable	Variable
Dehydration	Absent	Present	Present	Present
Lung sounds	Referred from upper airway	Abnormal	Abnormal, often muffled	Increased normal breath sounds
Heart sounds	Normal	Variable	Variable	Usually normal
White blood count	Normal	Increased or normal	Increased or normal	Increased or normal
Thoracic radiographs	Normal	Abnormal	Abnormal	Usually normal

*See Table 26-1.

TABLE 26-3. Common Causes of Dyspnea in Dogs and Cats and Characteristic Findings

	History/Physical Examination	Laboratory Studies	Radiographs
Dogs			
Acute			
Aspiration pneumonia	Chronic vomiting or regurgitation Recent anesthesia	↑ WBC Neutrophilia and left shift, or stress leukogram	Consolidated areas in lungs (alveolar and interstitial patterns), especially in ventral areas
Pulmonary thromboembolism	Recent heartworm treatment Rapid, shallow breathing Coughing Hemoptysis Fever Lethargy/depression	↑ WBC Neutrophilia and left shift, or stress leukogram Biochemical panel variable	Evidence of heartworm disease (enlarged right ventricle and pulmonary arteries) Consolidated areas in lungs (alveolar and interstitial patterns), especially caudal lobes
Pulmonary contusions	Recent trauma Expiratory dyspnea or rapid, shallow breathing Muffled lung sounds in certain lung fields Other signs of trauma	↑ WBC Neutrophilia and stress leukogram Anemia ↓ Plasma protein	Patchy consolidation of lung lobes (alveolar and interstitial patterns) Pleural effusion
Pneumothorax	See pulmonary contusions	↑ WBC Neutrophilia and stress leukogram	Evidence of air in the pleural space with the heart apparently elevated off the sternum
Diaphragmatic hernia	See diaphragmatic hernia listed under common causes of chronic dyspnea in dogs in this table.		
Severe anemia	Recent blood loss ± Lethargy, weakness Deep, labored breathing Dyspnea worsened by exercise Tachycardia	Severe anemia, regenerative or nonregenerative WBC variable Biochemical panel variable	Usually normal (depends on cause of anemia)

(continued)

219

TABLE 26-3. Common Causes of Dyspnea in Dogs and Cats and Characteristic Findings *(continued)*

	History/Physical Examination	Laboratory Studies	Radiographs
Dogs *(cont.)*			
Acute *(cont.)*			
Heatstroke	Exposure to hot environment Marked hyperthermia (temperature > 107) Deep, rapid, labored breathing Signs of shock	↑ WBC Neutrophilia and stress leukogram Evidence of DIC (prolonged clotting time and abnormal coagulogram	Normal
Chronic			
Stenotic nares/elongated soft palate/laryngeal malformation or paralysis	Snoring/snorting type breathing Inspiratory dyspnea Brachycephalic breed	Usually normal → Baseline T4 → Response to TSH ±	Normal
Mediastinal mass	Regurgitation Gagging Rapid, shallow breathing Decreased compressibility of thoracic inlet Muffled lung sounds	Hematology variable Cytology of fluid or tissue obtained by thoracentesis variable	Evidence of consolidation (mass) in anterior mediastinum Pleural fluid
Megaesophagus	Regurgitation Coughing Rapid, shallow breathing Lethargy and depression Crackles and wheezing	↑ WBC Neutrophilia and left shift Acetylcholine receptor antibodies in serum ±	Dilated esophagus Consolidated areas in lungs (alveolar and interstitial patterns), especially in ventral areas
Tracheal collapse Allergic bronchitis/PIE Heartworm disease Left-sided heart failure	See Table 25-3. See Table 25-3. See Table 25-3. See Table 25-3.		
Deep mycosis	Hunting dog Labored breathing and tachypnea Fever Mucopurulent nasal discharge Lethargy and depression Crackles and wheezes	↑ WBC Neutrophilia and left shift Mild to moderate nonregenerative anemia Biochemical panel variable	Nodular interstitial pattern diffusely throughout the lungs

Diaphragmatic hernia	Outside dog or history of trauma Rapid, shallow breathing Areas of reduced lung sounds on auscultation and areas of dullness on percussion	WBC usually normal Biochemical panel variable Increased SAP Hyperbilirubinemia	Indistinct diaphragmatic shadow Pleural effusion Intestinal loops, stomach, or liver in thoracic cavity
Cats			
Acute			
Pulmonary contusions	See Pulmonary contusions under Dogs.		
Pneumothorax	See Pneumothorax under Dogs.		
Cardiomyopathy	Expiratory dyspnea or rapid shallow breathing Muffled lung sounds or crackles Gallop rhythm Heart murmur Tachycardia Weak pulse Depression, weakness, lethargy	Hemogram variable Azotemia (prerenal) Arrhythmias and conduction disturbances on ECG Echocardiographic abnormalities	Pleural effusion or pulmonary edema Enlarged heart, valentine-shaped
Feline asthma	See Table 25-3.		
Acetaminophen intoxication	History of acetaminophen administration Tachypnea and labored breathing Cyanosis Pale mucous membranes Mild icterus Facial edema Severe depression	Anemia (nonregenerative if acute) Methemoglobinemia ↑ WBC Stress leukogram ↑ SAP and S-ALT	Normal
Severe anemia	See Severe anemia under Dogs.		
Diaphragmatic hernia	See Diaphragmatic hernia under Dogs.		

(continued)

221

TABLE 26-3. Common Causes of Dyspnea in Dogs and Cats and Characteristic Findings (*continued*)

	History/Physical Examination	Laboratory Studies	Radiographs
Cats (*cont.*)			
Chronic			
Rhinitis and sinusitis	Snoring noises Sneezing Nasoocular discharge Nasal swelling Conjunctivitis	Hemogram and biochemical panel variable Cytology of nasal exudate variable FeLV test often positive	Increased fluid density in nasal passages and sinuses Variable bony lysis and proliferation of nasal and frontal bones
Mediastinal mass	See Mediastinal mass under Dogs.		
Feline asthma	See Table 25-3.		
Lungworms	See Table 25-3.		
Diaphragmatic hernia	See Diaphragmatic hernia under Dogs.		
Pyothorax	Depression and lethargy Fever or hypothermia Tachypnea and labored breathing Muffled lung sounds Dull sounds on percussion of thorax	WBC variable Neutrophilia and left shift, or neutropenia and degenerative shift with toxic neutrophils Nonregenerative anemia FeLV test often positive Biochemical panel variable Cytology of pleural fluid—septic, purulent exudate	Pleural effusion
Feline infectious peritonitis	Depression and anorexia Rapid, shallow breathing Fever Weight loss Abdominal effusion Uveitis CNS signs (*e.g.*, ataxia, paresis)	WBC variable Moderate nonregenerative anemia Hyperglobulinemia FIP titer variable Pleural and abdominal fluid Protein > 3.5 g/dl Cell count < 5000/cm^3	Pleural effusion Abdominal effusion

↑, increased; WBC, white blood cell; ↓, decreased; ±, variably present; DIC, disseminated intravascular coagulation; PIE, pulmonary infiltrates with eosinophils; SAP, serum alkaline phosphatase; S-ALT, serum alanine transaminase; FeLV, feline leukemia virus; CNS, central nervous system; TSH, thyroid stimulating hormone; FIP, feline infectious peritonitus

Careful auscultation of heart and lung sounds is an important part of the physical examination. See Chapters 21, 22, and 28 for further information.

Laboratory Evaluation

A complete blood count, serum biochemical panel, and urine analysis are usually indicated, but they may be delayed until after thoracic radiographs are complete and essential symptomatic therapy[2,3] has been given in some severely dyspneic animals. Other procedures, such as testing for heartworms and feline leukemia virus and determination of feline infectious peritonitis titers, should be done if appropriate (Table 26-3).

Radiography

Thoracic, and sometimes cervical and skull, radiographs should be taken (see Chapter 25).

Cytology

If pleural effusion is observed on thoracic radiographs, a thoracocentesis should be done using aseptic technique, and the fluid should be examined. The protein content can be measured by refractometry; a cell count and differential should be recorded. A portion of the fluid should be saved for bacterial and (sometimes) fungal culture, if indicated.

Fine-Needle Lung Aspiration

If either a mass or diffuse pulmonary parenchymal disease is observed radiographically, a percutaneous, fine-needle aspirate should be considered. For aspirating a mass, ultrasound guidance is helpful. Otherwise, careful estimation of the location of the mass from radiographs should be done to aid in selection of the site for aspiration (see Chapter 25).

Lung Biopsy

Thoracotomy and lung biopsy are sometimes necessary to establish a diagnosis. See Chapter 25 for additional information.

Electrophysiologic Testing

If cardiac disease is suspected, electrocardiography and sometimes echocardiography are indicated (see Chapter 21).

REFERENCES

1. Ettinger SJ: Dyspnea and tachypnea. In Ettinger SJ (ed): Textbook of Veterinary Internal Medicine, 3rd ed, pp 88–90. Philadelphia, WB Saunders, 1989
2. Otto C: Medical emergencies. In Lorenz MD, Cornelius LM, Ferguson DC (eds): Small Animal Medical Therapeutics, pp 503–562. Philadelphia, JB Lippincott, 1992
3. Smallwood L: Respiratory diseases. In Lorenz MD, Cornelius LM, Ferguson DC (eds): Small Animal Medical Therapeutics, pp 219–237. Philadelphia, JB Lippincott, 1992

CHAPTER TWENTY-SEVEN

Hemoptysis

Larry M. Cornelius

DEFINITION AND PROBLEM RECOGNITION

The coughing up of blood is termed *hemoptysis,* and by definition includes only hemorrhage originating from the lower respiratory tract. In the clinical situation, however, it may be difficult to differentiate true hemoptysis from blood that has been regurgitated or vomited, or that has originated from the nasopharynx or oral cavity. Also, when blood from the lower respiratory tract is cleared to the pharynx by coughing or mucociliary transport, it may be swallowed. Hematemesis or melena may be reported instead of hemoptysis. If blood remains in the pharynx, epistaxis or oral bleeding may occur.[1]

PATHOPHYSIOLOGY

Hemoptysis is the result of one of more of the following basic abnormalities: (1) damage to blood vessels in either the bronchial (rare) or pulmonary circulation, (2) severe hypertension in either the bronchial (rare) or pulmonary circulation, or (3) a clotting or bleeding problem.[2] Vascular damage can be the result of inflammation (infectious or noninfectious), necrosis, neoplasia, or trauma. Pulmonary hypertension can be due to precapillary, postcapillary, or combined pre- and postcapillary hypertension.[1] Congenital heart defects characterized by left-to-right shunt and dirofilariasis are examples of precapillary pulmonary hypertension. Postcapillary pulmonary hypertension, and frequently pulmonary edema, occur with passive congestion of pulmonary veins associated with left ventricular failure. Chronic passive congestion of pulmonary veins can cause changes within the pulmonary arterial circulation resulting in both pre- and postcapillary pulmonary hypertension.[1] Clotting or bleeding disorders are caused by abnormalities of clotting factors or platelets (see Chapter 19 and Display, Causes of Hemoptysis in Dogs and Cats).

Although hemoptysis usually results in minimal blood loss, most conditions causing hemoptysis are potentially life-threatening. Occasionally, massive hemoptysis occurs and may cause death due to asphyxiation or hypovolemia. A history of coughing up blood always warrants a thorough evaluation of the patient.

Causes of Hemoptysis in Dogs and Cats

- Cardiovascular
  - Pulmonary thromboembolism
    - Heartworm disease
    - Hyperadrenocorticism
    - Glomerulonephropathies
    - Acute pancreatitis
    - Neoplasia
    - Sepsis
    - Disseminated intravascular coagulation
  - Pulmonary edema
    - Left heart failure
    - Congenital heart defects
- Inflammatory
  - Bronchitis
  - Bacterial bronchopneumonia
  - Fungal pneumonia
    - Blastomycosis
    - Histoplasmosis
  - Lung abscess
- Neoplastic
  - Bronchogenic carcinoma
  - Metastatic carcinoma
- Miscellaneous
  - Trauma
  - Clotting or bleeding disorder
  - Foreign body in airway
  - Transtracheal wash or bronchoscopy
  - Needle biopsy of lung
  - Cavitary lung lesion

DIAGNOSTIC PLAN

History and Physical Examination

The signalment of the patient should be considered in assessing the problem of hemoptysis. For example, dirofilariasis should be a strong consideration in an intact male dog, especially a hunting breed from 1 to 7 years of age that is not on heartworm-preventive medication and is living in a heartworm-endemic area. Older male small-breed dogs, such as toy and miniature poodles, Chihuahuas, and miniature schnauzers, have a higher incidence of mitral insufficiency leading to left heart failure and pulmonary edema.

Before proceeding with an extensive diagnostic workup of hemoptysis, it is important to localize the source of bleeding. Careful questioning of the client may help localize the site of bleeding. Severe persistent sneezing with a bloody nasal discharge prior to the onset of hemoptysis usually indicates that the source of bleeding is the nasal cavity. A history of severe coughing or dyspnea preceding hemoptysis suggests that the blood is coming from the respiratory tract. Animals with a history of serious gastrointestinal disease (*e.g.*, vomiting, diarrhea, weight loss) may vomit blood and aspirate the vomitus, leading to hemoptysis. A history of abnormal bleeding from other sites or easy bruising suggests a clotting or bleeding disorder. Any history or possibility of trauma should be determined.

The owner should be asked to describe the expectorated blood. Blood-streaked sputum is more likely to be caused by a necrotic condition in the lungs, such as purulent bronchopneumonia or neoplasia, than by trauma, which is more likely to result in more profuse bleeding. Expectoration of pink-tinged froth is characteristic of acute pulmonary edema.[1]

A thorough physical examination should be done to evaluate all systems. A complete knowledge of the various clinical manifestations of diseases resulting in hemoptysis makes it less likely that the examiner will overlook important physical findings or fail to appreciate their significance. For example, finding a small skin lesion draining purulent material and mild to moderate peripheral lymphadenopathy in a dog with hemoptysis should alert the clinician to consider blastomycosis. The lips, oral cavity, and nasopharynx should be carefully observed for signs of recent bleeding (due to inflammation, masses, foreign bodies, or other factors) as well as for the presence of petechiae. Blood in the oral cavity may be the result of hemorrhage from the structures of the mouth or nasopharynx, or from the respiratory or gastrointestinal tract. Aspiration of blood from the nasopharynx, or of regurgitated or vomited blood from the gastrointestinal tract, may lead to hemoptysis. Thoracic auscultation is important in determining the possible involvement of the cardiopulmonary system.

Laboratory Evaluation

If hemoptysis is not massive and life-threatening, thoracic radiographs should be obtained after the history and physical examination are completed. Depending on the results, other tests to consider are a complete blood count, platelet count, serum biochemical panel, urine analysis, heartworm testing, clotting panel, blood gas analysis, electrocardiogram, transtracheal wash, bronchoscopy, and fine-needle aspiration biopsy of the lung (see Chapters 21, 25, and 26). Additional special tests (*e.g.*, serology, echocardiography, ultrasonography, angiography, pulmonary scintigraphy), some of which may necessitate referral to a specialty center, may need to be done.

For massive, life-threatening hemoptysis, diagnostic procedures should be delayed until the patient's condition is stabilized.[3] After stabilization, thoracic radiographs should be taken and other tests considered as previously outlined.

REFERENCES

1. Armstrong PJ: Hemoptysis. In Ford RB (ed): Clinical Signs and Diagnosis in Small Animal Practice, pp 239–256. New York, Churchill Livingston, 1988
2. Howard WJ: Hemoptysis—causes and a practical management approach. Postgrad Med 77:53–57, 1985
3. Otto CM: Medical emergencies. In Lorenz MD, Cornelius LM, Ferguson DC (eds): Small Animal Medical Therapeutics, pp 503–562. Philadelphia, JB Lippincott, 1992

CHAPTER TWENTY-EIGHT

Abnormal Lung Sounds

Larry M. Cornelius

DEFINITION AND PROBLEM RECOGNITION

Abnormal lung sounds are heard upon auscultation of the thorax in many patients with diseases of the airway.

PATHOPHYSIOLOGY

Lung sounds can be divided into normal breath sounds and adventitious sounds.[2,4] Normal breath sounds are produced by air movement through the tracheobronchial tree, whereas adventitious sounds are abnormal sounds (crackles and wheezes) superimposed upon breath sounds.[2]

Normal breath sounds are produced by turbulent flow in the central airways (trachea, segmental and lobar bronchi). The sounds are filtered and dampened as they travel within the lung outward through the thoracic wall. It is a common misconception that normal lung sounds are generated in the alveoli. Flow at the acinar and alveolar levels is laminar with low velocity; neither turbulence nor sound is produced. Breath sounds heard at the chest wall probably are the result of filtration and attenuation by the lung and chest wall of the sounds produced in the mouth and central airways. Abnormally loud or soft breath sounds can be the result of either changes in sound production in central airways or altered transmission of sound through the various tissues to the chest wall.[2]

Normal breath sounds differ according to the age of the animal, respiratory pattern, thickness of the thoracic wall, site of auscultation, and pattern of respiration. Breath sounds in young or thin animals are louder, apparently because of less attenuation by fewer intervening alveoli and thinner thoracic walls. In older or obese animals, normal breath sounds may be barely detectable. Loudness or intensity of breath sounds also varies with airflow velocity—the faster the velocity, the louder the breath sounds. Variation in normal breath sounds may be caused by changes in the respiratory pattern, such as panting (increased intensity) and neuromuscular weakness (decreased intensity).

Changes in intensity or loudness of breath sounds may be heard in a variety of other conditions associated with changes in either airflow velocity or transmission of respiratory sounds (increased ventilation, lung consolidation or mass, obstructive respiratory disease, hyperinflation of the lungs, emphysema, pleural effusion, pneumothorax, diaphragmatic hernia).[3] An animal with increased ventilation has abnormally loud breath sounds, which can be ausculted over both the trachea and thoracic wall (unless other factors have changed the sound transmission properties of the respiratory system—see following paragraph). Narrowing of airways, such as occurs with obstructive lung diseases (*e.g.*, airway mass or foreign body or chronic bronchitis), is often accompanied by loud breath sounds (both on inspiration and expiration), because the narrowness increases the velocity of the air. Extrathoracic airway obstruction—for example, laryngeal paralysis or extrathoracic tracheal collapse—results in louder inspiratory breath sounds, because extrathoracic airways narrow during inspiration.

Abnormally loud breath sounds can also be the result of changes in the transmission of respiratory sounds. Areas of pulmonary consolidation or atelectasis transmit breath sounds more efficiently. Thus, louder breath sounds may be heard over consolidated areas. Whether breath sounds are actually louder or quieter over a consolidated area depends on the balance between the competing processes of (1) less sound production due to decreased ventilation in the consolidated area and (2) enhanced transmission of breath sounds through the consolidated area.[3]

Decreased intensity of breath sounds, or silent lung, can be a result of disorders of the pleural space such as pleural effusion and pneumothorax, or other disorders such as diaphragmatic hernia (Table 28-1).

Abnormal sounds produced by pathologic processes within the tracheobronchial tree and lungs are termed *adventitious sounds*. The point of maximal intensity is usually near the diseased area. Adventitious sounds may be either discontinuous (crackles) or continuous (wheezes).

Crackles are intermittent, nonmusical, explosive sounds that have been characterized as fine or coarse. Fine crackles are the most common type and have been described as "Velcro" or "cellophane-type" sounds. Coarse crackles are lower-pitched, louder bubbling and gurgling sounds. Results from experiments show that fine crackles are usually produced by the explosive equalization of pressure following the reopening of airways associated with interstitial lung disease (fibrosis, inflammation, edema).[1] Loud, coarse crackles are caused by conditions in which excessive sputum or fluid is in the airways (inflammation, severe pulmonary edema) (see Table 28-1).

Noting the timing of crackles during the respiratory cycle may help differentiate their causes. Early inspiratory or early expiratory crackles are often caused by obstructive pulmonary diseases, bronchopneumonia, and tracheobronchial fluid accumulation. Late inspiratory crackles are frequently associated with restrictive lung diseases (pulmonary edema, interstitial pneumonia/infiltrates, diffuse interstitial diseases) and lung, pleural, or thoracic wall tumors.[3]

Wheezes are continuous musical or whistling sounds generated by air passing through a narrowed airway and causing a regular vibration or oscillation of the

TABLE 28-1. Causes of Abnormal Lung Sounds in Dogs and Cats

Breath Sounds		Adventitious Sounds	
Loud	*Silent Lung*	*Crackles*	*Wheezes*
Increased ventilation	Pneumothorax	Course	Inspiratory
Exercise	Pleural effusion	Severe pulmonary edema	Laryngeal obstruction
Excitement	Right heart failure	Left heart failure	Necrotic laryngitis
Metabolic acidemia	Neoplasia	Hypoalbuminemia	Laryngeal paralysis
Severe anemia	Hypoalbuminemia	Others	Laryngeal edema
Lung disease	Hemothorax	Bronchopneumonia	Laryngeal collapse
Increased sound	Chylothorax	Pulmonary contusions	Tracheal stenosis
transmission	Pyothorax	(trauma)	Tracheal foreign
Atelectatic lung lobe	Feline infectious peritonitis	Fine	body
Lung mass	Diaphragmatic hernia	Interstitial pulmonary	Extrathoracic tracheal col-
	Intrathoracic neoplastic mass	edema	lapse
	Consolidated lung lobe	Chronic interstitial pneu-	Extraluminal tracheal com-
	Abscess	monia	pression
	Granuloma	Chronic interstitial fibrosis	Neoplastic mass
	Neoplasm		Lymphadenopathy
	Lung lobe torsion		Expiratory
	Extreme obesity		Bronchitis
	Neuromuscular		Allergic (asthma, PIE)
	weakness		Infectious
	Polyradiculoneuritis (coon-		Bronchopneumonia
	hound paralysis)		COPD
	Diaphragmatic paralysis		Pulmonary contusions
	Others		Lungworms
			Pulmonary granulomatosis
			Deep mycosis
			Heartworm disease

PIE, pulmonary infiltrates with eosinophils; COPD, chronic obstructive pulmonary disease airway wall. Wheezing noises occur when an airway lumen is narrowed. If conditions are right, the airway wall flutters between open and nearly closed to produce a continuous sound. The amplitude, pitch, and duration of the wheeze depend on the velocity of airflow and mechanical properties of the airway involved. Pitch may be constant (monophonic) or variable (polyphonic). A common misconception is that the pitch of the wheeze depends on the size of the diseased airway. The pitch is actually determined by the mass and elasticity of the solid structures set into oscillation, as well as the linear velocity of the airflow through the stenosed airway.[3]

Wheezes may be present throughout the respiratory cycle or may be predominantly inspiratory or expiratory. In the majority of pulmonary diseases, wheezing is more common during expiration than during inspiration. Causes of expiratory wheezes include bronchospasm (especially with allergic bronchitis or asthma), mucosal edema, mucous plugging, foreign bodies, tumors, and hilar lymphadenopathy (see Table 28-1). Lower-pitched wheezes are often caused by secretions in the airways, such as occur with bronchopneumonia, and change markedly after a deep cough. Inspiratory wheezing, sometimes termed stridor, is associated with a rigid stenosis of the upper airway, trachea, or mainstem bronchi. Examples include laryngeal edema or inflammation, tracheal foreign body, or segmental tracheal stenosis (see Table 28-1).

Other abnormal sounds that may be heard upon thoracic auscultation include pleural friction rub. A pleural friction rub is characterized by a loud, coarse sound resembling creaking or rubbing of new leather and is not commonly heard in dogs and cats.

DIAGNOSTIC PLAN

History and Physical Examination

Signs most often reported by owners of animals with abnormal lung sounds are coughing, difficult breathing, and wheezing (see Chapters 25 and 26). The wheezing described by clients is often due to abnormal sounds originating from the nasal passages and upper airway. Careful questioning should be done to avoid confusion.

A thorough physical examination should be performed in a quiet area so that accurate thoracic auscultation can be accomplished. Heart and lung sounds should be evaluated while the patient is standing. If the animal is panting, an assistant should intermittently close the animal's mouth while auscultation is done. Purring in a cat can usually be stopped for a short period of time by either exerting moderate pressure on the animal's larynx or distracting the cat by turning on the water flow in a sink. Skin and hair noises can be minimized by first wetting the hair over the area to be ausculted and holding the head of the stethoscope firmly against the thoracic wall. Both sides of the thorax should be ausculted in several areas to evaluate each lung field. Referred sounds from the nasal passages and pharyngeal/laryngeal areas can be differentiated by alternating the site of auscultation from the thorax to the laryngeal area back and forth and comparing the quality and intensity of sounds. If referred sounds from these areas are being heard during thoracic auscultation, the sounds will be similar except less intense over the thorax. It may be helpful to compare the intensity of inspiratory and expiratory sounds. Also, special attention should be given to noting areas of inhomogeneity of lung sounds. After listening to each lung field, it is often useful to induce coughing with digital pressure on the trachea and then reevaluate lung sounds.

Laboratory Evaluation

Diagnostic procedures for evaluation of a patient with abnormal lung sounds are similar to those used for animals with coughing and dyspnea (see Chapters 25 and 26).

REFERENCES

1. Forgacs P: The functional basis of pulmonary sounds. Chest 73:399–405, 1978
2. Kotlikoff MI, Gillespie JR: Lung sounds in veterinary medicine. Part I: terminology and mechanisms of sound production. Comp Cont Ed Pract Vet 5:634–639, 1983
3. Kotlikoff MI, Gillespie JR: Lung sounds in veterinary medicine. Part II: deriving clinical information from lung sounds. Comp Cont Ed Pract Vet 6:462–467, 1984
4. Roudebush P: Lung sounds. J Am Vet Med Assoc 181:122–126, 1982

CHAPTER TWENTY-NINE

Sneezing and Nasal Discharge

Michael R. Lappin

PROBLEM DEFINITION

Sneezing is a superficial reflex that originates in the mucous membranes lining the nasal cavity and is easily induced by chemical or mechanical stimuli. The sneeze results in forceful expulsion of air that passes through the airways with great velocity.[3] This airstream helps clear the respiratory passages, which is the primary function of the sneeze.

Nasal discharge is any material that escapes the respiratory passageways via the external nares. Discharges are classified by their physical characteristics as serous, mucoid, purulent, or hemorrhagic, or a combination of these types. Food or fluid that had been previously ingested may occasionally be passed secondary to conditions affecting the oronasal cavities. The nasal discharge may be unilateral or bilateral, continuous or intermittent, or present only associated with sneezing.

PATHOPHYSIOLOGY

The afferent impulses generated by stimulation of the nasal mucous membranes are carried via the trigeminal nerve to the medulla of the brain, where a complex automatic sequence of events is initiated. After rapid inspiration, the vocal folds and epiglottis close; this is followed by a forceful contraction of the abdominal, external intercostal, and other respiratory muscles, which greatly elevates the air pressure within the respiratory passageways. The epiglottis and vocal folds then open rapidly, allowing air to pass, which results in the sneeze.

Sneezing and nasal discharge occur primarily with conditions directly affecting the nasal cavity and secondarily to pharyngeal or more distal respiratory passageway disease. The nasal cavity function includes olfaction and the filtration, warming, humidification, and conduction of air. The nasal cavity is composed of cartilagenous turbinates covered by a ciliated pseudocolumnar epithelium. This epithelium is primarily respiratory peripherally and olfactory caudomedially and caudodorsally. The lamina propria of the respiratory portion contains serous, mucous, and mixed tubuloalveolar glands. Goblet cells are also present throughout the nasal cavity. The lateral nasal gland is a serous gland in the lateral mucosa that functions primarily in heat exchange. Paranasal sinuses, including the maxillary recess, the frontal sinus, and the sphenoidal sinuses, are connected with the respiratory passageways and occasionally are primarily or secondarily involved with diseases resulting in nasal discharge and sneeze.[5]

The nasal cavity can respond to insult only in a limited number of ways. Most conditions leading to inflammation of the nasal mucosa result in glandular secretions that generally progress from a serous discharge early in the course of disease to a mucoid or mucopurulent discharge as chronicity and secondary bacterial infection develop. Hemorrhage can occur with trauma, coagulopathies, systemic hypertension, and acute deep insult to the richly vascularized nasal mucosa; chronic erosive or invasive disease; or acute multiple sneezing induced by any etiology. Food or water draining from the external nares may result from a communication of the oral and nasal cavities or by passage of ingesta from the nasopharynx into the nasal cavity.

RULE OUTS AND DIAGNOSTIC PLAN

The common causes of sneeze and nasal discharge in the dog and cat are listed in Table 29-1. The signalment, history, physical examination, and physical characteristics of the nasal discharge, if present, will help direct the veterinary clinician to appropriate diagnostic procedures and subsequent therapy.

Signalment

Animal signalment occasionally suggests likely etiologies. Young, very old, and immunosuppressed animals tend to be more susceptible than others to infectious agents. Clinical signs associated with congenital diseases often appear in the very young. Brachycephalic breeds often have nasal discharge directly related to stenotic nares, or they may have nasal discharge secondary to poor handling of ingesta or respiratory secretions in the pharyngeal region caused by an elongated soft palate. Nasal neoplasia and dental disease are more common in older dogs and cats. Diseases leading to systemic hypertension are more common in older animals. Medium- to large-breed dogs with long noses may have higher frequencies of nasal neoplasia. Nasal foreign bodies and fungal disease are more likely to occur in free-roaming animals. Sneezing is much more common with acute disease than in chronic disorders.

History

Acute sneezing or nasal discharge accompanied by ocular discharge is suggestive of viral disease. Animals with acute viral infection commonly have elevated body temperature, and their clinical signs of disease are often more severe than animals with local nasal disease only or chronic viral infection. Animals with viral diseases often have histories of exposure to other animals, particularly in animal shelters and boarding kennels. Vaccination series may or may not have been completed. Congenital abnormalities or pharyngeal disorders cause clinical signs soon after the animal eats or drinks. Gagging is commonly reported by the owners of animals with pharyngeal disease. Foreign bodies, nasopharyngeal polyps in cats, neoplasia (including tonsilar), cricopharyngeal dysphagia, and inflammation of any etiology may be present with a history of gagging and nasal discharge. Recurrent sneezing and nasal discharge that respond to antibiotic therapy are suggestive of bacterial rhinitis secondary to any etiology, including trauma, allergic disease, nasal foreign body, fungal infection, and neoplasia. Seasonal bilateral serous to mucoid nasal discharge accompanied by sneezing and ocular discharge is consistent with allergic rhinitis. Nasal foreign bodies often lead to acute violent sneezing accompanied by pawing or rubbing of the face. Animals with neoplasia and fungal infection often present with a history of nasal discharge that slowly changed in character from serous to mucopurulent to hemorrhagic. Animals with a history of chronic otitis externa or media occasionally present with nasal discharge and sneezing due to communication of the middle ear with the nasopharynx via the eustachian tube. Immunosuppressive diseases such as feline leukemia virus infection or feline immunodeficiency virus infection that predispose an animal to secondary bacterial infection may present with a history of concurrent polysystemic disease such as weight loss, diarrhea, skin disease, cystitis, and general malaise. Animals with diseases leading to systemic hypertension and resultant epistaxis often have a history of polysystemic clinical signs such as polyuria/polydipsia (renal disease, hyperadrenocorticism), weight gain, and lethargy (hypothyroidism).

Physical Examination

A thorough examination of the entire animal, with emphasis on the respiratory system, eyes, and oropharyngeal cavity, is indicated in any animal with sneezing and nasal discharge. Stenotic nares, cleft palate, traumatic oronasal fistula, otitis externa or media, dental disease, and elongated soft palate may be detected on examination of the head and mouth. Redness of the oropharynx or red and enlarged tonsils can occur with many diseases leading to sneezing and nasal discharge. Facial or palate deformity is most consistent with severe fungal disease or neoplasia. Exophthalmos suggests retrobulbar disease and is most consistent with neoplasia. Fractures of the bones overlying the nasal cavity often can be palpated. *Pneumonyssus caninum* is occasionally seen crawling from the external nares.

Many upper respiratory disorders (*e.g.,* infectious disease, allergy, and facial deformities) also cause ocular discharge. Feline viral rhinotracheitis may cause dendritic corneal ulceration, anorexia, and ptyalism secondary to oral ulceration. Both canine distemper and cryptococcosis can cause chorioretinitis; cryp-

Text continues on p. 242

TABLE 29-1. Common Causes of Sneezing and Nasal Discharge in the Dog and Cat

Cause	Signalment	History	PE*	Discharge	Dx†‡	Comments
Congenital						
Stenotic nares	Brachycephalic dogs	Snoring	Stenotic nares	Serous to mucoid	Physical examination	Often without respiratory signs
Cleft palate	Young, all breeds	Poor suckling Milk from nares Chronic discharge postweaning	Cleft palate Abnormal lung sounds with aspiration pneumonia	Food or fluid Mucopurulent with secondary infection Usually bilateral	Physical examination	Less common in cats
Elongated soft palate	Brachycephalic dogs	Gagging, snorting ± association with eating	Elongated soft palate Reddened pharynx Inflamed tonsils	Food or fluid Serous to mucopurulent Usually bilateral	Physical examination	Diagnosis may require sedation; often without respiratory signs
Dysphagia	All breeds Congenital—young Acquired—older	Coughing, gagging Multiple swallowing attempts	Reddened pharynx Inflamed tonsils Abnormal lung sounds with aspiration pneumonia	Food or fluid Serous to mucopurulent Usually bilateral	Physical examination Fluoroscopy Metabolic workup Electromyogram	Many acquired etiologies, often without respiratory signs
Infectious‡						
Viral						
Feline viral rhinotracheitis (FVR)	All breeds All ages; more common in young	Animal contact Poor vaccination history Anorexia common Pytalism	± Oral ulcers ± Conjunctivitis ± Dendritic ulcer ± Abnormal lung sounds Fever common	Mucopurulent	Direct fluorescent antibody staining of conjunctival scraping Serology	Often severe clinical disease; abortion and bronchopneumonia can occur
Feline calcivirus	All breeds All ages (more common than FVR)	Animal contact Poor vaccination history Anorexia common Pytalism	Oral/nasal ulcers ± Conjunctivitis ± Abnormal lung sounds Fever common	Mucopurulent	Diagnosis by clinical signs and exclusion	Ulcers and bronchopneumonia more common than FVR Oculonasal discharge less common than FVR
Reovirus	Cats—all breeds, all ages	Mild symptoms	Fever rare Often ocular signs alone	Rare	Diagnosis by exclusion	Generally mild respiratory signs

238

Etiology	Signalment	History / Clinical findings	Clinical signs	Discharge	Diagnosis	Comments
Canine distemper virus	All breeds, all ages	Poor vaccination history / Animal contact / Multiple system involvement (CNS, gastrointestinal)	Fever / ± Vomiting/diarrhea / ± Abnormal lung sounds / ± CNS disease / ± Ophthalmologic changes / ± Foot pad hyperkeratosis	Mucopurulent	Clinical signs / Complete blood cell count (lymphopenia) / Direct fluorescent antibody staining of conjunctival scraping / Serology / Characteristic cerebrospinal fluid	Immunosuppressive disease with multiple system involvement
Bacterial Many species	Dogs—all breeds / Common in cats / All ages	Chronic sneezing / Snuffling respiration / Often secondary to a primary inflammation	Decreased air flow / Dull percussion / Signs of primary etiology / ± Anorexia and dehydration	Mucopurulent / Usually bilateral	Clinical signs / History of primary etiology / Culture occasionally valuable	Generally a secondary disease / Often secondary to virus, trauma, fungus, congenital, and neoplasia
Chlamydia	Cats / All breeds, all ages / More frequently in young	Animal contact / Usually no polysystemic illness	Mild conjunctivitis	Serous to mucopurulent / Usually bilateral	Cytology / Exclusion / History	Frequently recurrent / Mildest feline infectious upper respiratory disease
Mycoplasma	All breeds, all ages	Usually no polysystemic illness	Mild conjunctivitis	Rare / Serous, if it occurs	Cytology / Culture	Primarily conjunctivitis
Fungal *Aspergillus* and *Penicillium*	Brachycephalic less common / All ages	Progressive / Secondary to trauma (15%)	Fever—rare / Facial or palatal deformity rare / Decreased air flow / Dull percussion / ± Lymphadenopathy or anorexia	Mucoid, mucopurulent, or hemorrhagic / 1/3 unilateral / 2/3 bilateral	Cytology / Culture / Serology / Radiographic changes	Difficult to distinguish from neoplasia / Not recognized in cats

(continued)

TABLE 29-1. Common Causes of Sneezing and Nasal Discharge in the Dog and Cat *(continued)*

Cause	Signalment	History	PE*	Discharge	Dxp†	Comments
Cryptococcus neoformans	Dogs and cats All ages	Upper respiratory signs Polysystemic progression	± Fever ± CNS signs ± Abnormal lung sounds due to dissemination ± Ophthalmologic changes	Mucoid to mucopurulent	Cytology Serology Culture	Most common mycotic infection in cats
Trichosporon sp			Nasal polyp or granuloma			Rare
Rhinosporidium seeberi			Nasal polyp or granuloma			Rare
Parasitic						
Linguatula serrata	Dogs—all ages	Mild sneezing	None	Serous to none	Cytology (isolation)	Often subclinical
Pneumonyssus caninum	Dogs—all ages	Mild sneezing	None	Serous to none	Cytology (isolation)	Often subclinical
Eucoleus boehmi	Dogs—all ages	Mild signs	None	Serous to none	Biopsy Fecal examination	Rare
Neoplastic	Dogs—common Cats—rare Older animals	Progressive	Decreased air flow Dull percussion ± Exophthalmos ± Facial or palatal deformity	Progressive from mucopurulent to hemorrhagic	Cytology Radiographic changes Biopsy	Facial deformity, exophthalmos, unilateral more common than fungal
Allergic	Dogs and cats Usually young	Acute, mild signs Seasonal	± Conjunctivitis ± Dermatologic change	Serous to mucoid	History	May predispose to secondary bacterial infection
Inflammatory polyps	Cats—young	Gagging Dysphagia ± Respiratory signs	± Reddened pharynx ± Reddened tonsils	Serous to mucopurulent	Caudal pharyngeal examination	Likely congenital and arise from the middle ear

240

Disease	Signalment	History	Physical Examination Findings	Nasal Discharge	Diagnostic Plan	Comments
Systemic hypertension	Generally older	Dependent on primary etiology	Retinal vasculature tortuous, retinal hemorrhage; Abnormalities associated with primary etiology	Hemorrhagic	Blood pressure determination	Epistaxis is rare
Dental disease	All animals; More common in old animals	Halitosis; Paroxysms of sneezing; Pawing face	Fistula; Gingival recession; Dental calculi; Facial abscess; Halitosis	Unilateral; Mucopurulent; Occasionally blood-tinged	Physical examination; Skull radiographs	
Otitis media	All animals	Mild signs; Otitis externa	Keratoconjunctivitis sicca; Otic lesions	Dry, crusty	Otoscopic examination; Aspirate and culture	Damage to chorda tympani or facial nerves leads to decreased nasal mucosal gland secretion
Trauma	All animals	Acute; History of trauma	Fractures often palpable	Hemorrhagic; Unilateral or bilateral	History; Radiographs	Secondary bacterial osteomyelitis common
Foreign body	All animals; Cats less likely	Acute paroxysms of sneezing; Head-banging; Free-roaming	Nonspecific	Serous to mucopurulent, depending on chronicity; Occasionally hemorrhagic	Sedation and nasal and caudopharyngeal examination	Secondary bacterial infection common; Commonly secondary to plant materials
Coagulation abnormalities	All animals; Dogs more frequently	Hemorrhage without trauma; Hemorrhage in other areas	Pale mucous membranes; ± Hemothorax; ± Hemoperitoneum; ± Petechiae/ecchymoses; Dependent on etiology	Hemorrhagic	Platelet count; Activated coagulation time; Bleeding time; Factor VIII–related antigen	Multiple etiologies—can occur with thrombocytopenia, platelet dysfunction, or factor deficiency

*Physical examination

†Diagnostic plan

‡Feline leukemia virus and feline immunodeficiency virus immunosuppression may be involved with recurrent upper respiratory infections.

tococcosis may cause anterior uveitis.[6] Chorioretinitis may also be seen with neoplastic diseases. Enlargement of the mandibular lymph nodes is common with many causes of rhinitis including neoplastic disease, diseases with secondary bacterial infection, and viral disease. Immunosuppressive diseases such as feline leukemia virus infection or feline immunodeficiency virus infection that predispose animals to secondary bacterial infection may present with concurrent polysystemic physical examination findings such as weight loss and chronic skin changes.

Unilateral nasal discharge is most consistent with neoplasia, fungal disease, foreign bodies, tooth root abscess, trauma, and oronasal fistulas. Aggressive neoplasia or severe chronic fungal infection may invade both sides of the nasal cavity, leading to bilateral discharge. Bilateral nasal discharge occurs with infectious diseases, congenital deformities, pharyngeal diseases, and allergic rhinitis. Dullness on percussion of the nasal cavity and paranasal sinuses is often present with many diseases but is most consistent with fungal granulomas and neoplasia. Diminished airflow through one or both external nares occurs with most nasal diseases.

Pulmonary parenchymal sounds may be abnormal in disseminated fungal disease or neoplasia, in primary pulmonary disease resulting in secondary nasal discharge, or in diseases affecting both upper and lower respiratory systems (canine distemper virus). Coagulopathies may induce clinical evidence of bleeding in other areas, including petechiation or ecchymoses of the skin and mucous membranes, abdominal distention due to hemoperitoneum, dull heart and lung sounds due to hemothorax, or joint swelling due to hemarthrosis. Animals with diseases leading to systemic hypertension and resultant epistaxis often have other evidence of cardiovascular disease or polysystemic changes evident on physical examination.

Physical Characteristics of the Nasal Discharge

Serous nasal discharge is present in the initial stage of most diseases affecting the nasal cavity. Continuous or long-term serous discharges are most consistent with mild irritative disease such as allergy or nasal parasitism. Mucoid discharge is most consistent with allergic disease, fungal disease, or neoplasia. Viral infection or any long-term inflammatory disease process with secondary bacterial overgrowth produces a mucopurulent discharge. Hemorrhage is present most often with neoplasia, trauma, coagulopathies, systemic hypertension, vasculitis, and fungal infection.

Diagnostic Plan

Diagnostic procedures with the greatest potential yield include detection of airflow through the nasal cavity, cytology, serology, culture and sensitivity, oral and nasal examination under sedation, thoracic and nasal radiographs, direct fluorescent antibody techniques, coagulation profiles, platelet counts, caudal nasal cavity examination with a dental mirror, endoscopy, indirect measurement of blood pressure, fecal examination, lymph node aspiration, and nasal biopsy.

Detection of airflow through the nasal cavities to determine evidence of unilateral or bilateral involvement can be performed using several techniques. Holding a cotton ball over the external nares and observing it for movement during expiration is a relatively insensitive way to detect airflow. Holding a refrigerated microscope slide over the external nares and comparing the amounts of vapor that form under each nostril can be helpful in evaluating airflow.

Cytology characterizes the type of nasal discharge present and occasionally detects fungal elements, neoplastic cells, or parasites. Direct swabs can be evaluated; if deep disease is suspected, nasal flushing with sterile saline may be indicated. It is difficult to assess the importance of bacteria when present, since the nasal cavities contain a rich normal flora and secondary bacterial infection can occur with most causes of nasal discharge. The detection of a homogenous population of bacteria may be significant. Direct fluorescent antibody staining of cells obtained by conjunctival scrapings can be used to detect viral elements of canine distemper virus and feline viral rhinotracheitis. False-positive and false-negative results occur.[2] *Chlamydia* and *Mycoplasma* inclusion bodies may be detected on cytologic evaluation of conjunctival scraping.

Bacterial and fungal cultures are usually of low yield in that the nasal cavity has a large population of normal bacterial flora, and *Aspergillus* and *Penicillium* may be isolated from normal animals. Occasionally, chronic bacterial sinusitis and rhinitis in cats yield a pure bacterial culture that may be useful in determining appropriate antibiotic therapy.

Serologic assays to detect circulating antibodies to *Aspergillus, Penicillium,* and *Cryptococcus* are available.[4,7] A positive titer for *Aspergillus* or *Penicillium* may reflect previous exposure and may not be indicative of ongoing or active disease. The presence of serum antigens of *Cryptococcus* suggests that the organism is currently in the body, although it may not be the cause of the sneeze and nasal discharge. A diagnosis of nasal *Aspergillus* or *Penicillium* infection should be made on the basis of a combination of positive serology, cytologic demonstration of fungal elements, positive fungal cultures, characteristic radiographic findings, and characteristic rhinoscopic findings. Cats with chronic nasal discharge or recurrent sneezing should be assessed for feline leukemia virus infection and feline immunodeficiency virus infection.

Radiographs of the head and thoracic cavity are often indicated in animals with chronic nasal discharge or signs of polysystemic involvement. Thoracic radiographs are best performed in an awake animal, but anesthesia is desirable when evaluating the nasal cavities and paranasal sinuses, because observing fine detail is imperative. Destruction of the nasal turbinates or nasal bones can be detected radiographically; its presence is most consistent with neoplasia and fungal disease. Destruction of the lamina dura is indicative of dental disease. Fractures are often detected in cases of traumatic rhinitis.

Neoplastic cells may be noted on cytologic evaluation of mandibular lymph node aspirations. However, not all nasal neoplasms have metastases to local lymph nodes at the time of diagnosis. If destructive disease is present radiographically, biopsy is indicated. Biopsy of nasal masses has been described utilizing endoscopy, open surgical exploration, and techniques utilizing various biopsy punches.[2,8] Endoscopically obtained biopsies can lead to false-negative results because of the small size of the tissue sample obtained and the tendency for nasal neoplastic or inflammatory diseases to have a fibrinous reaction covering the lesion site. Surgery may be required to make a definitive diagnosis.

If a hemorrhagic discharge is present with or without signs of polysystemic disease, coagulation should be evaluated. This is best done in a practice situation by performing a platelet count, an activated coagulation time; if they are normal, a bleeding time is obtained. In certain breeds, primarily the Doberman pinscher, a von Willebrand's factor antigen assay should be performed in animals with spontaneous idiopathic hemorrhagic nasal discharge to help rule out von Willebrand's disease.[1] Direct or indirect blood pressure determination may help document that systemic hypertension is present. If hypertension is detected, diagnostic procedures for the detection of the primary etiology are indicated. Fecal examination may detect ova of *Eucoleus boehmi*.

REFERENCES

1. Dodds WJ: von Willebrand's disease in dogs. Mod Vet Pract 65:681–686, 1984
2. Hawkins EC: Chronic viral upper respiratory disease in cats: differential diagnosis and management. Comp Cont Ed Pract Vet 10:1003–1012, 1988
3. Jenson D: The Principles of Physiology, pp 227, 739. New York, Appleton-Century-Crofts, 1976
4. Medleau L, Marks MA, Brown J, Borges WL: Clinical evaluation of a cryptococcal antigen latex agglutination test for diagnosis of cryptococcosis in cats. J Am Vet Med Assoc 196:1470–1473, 1990
5. Miller ME: Anatomy of the Dog, pp 716–719. Philadelphia, WB Saunders, 1964
6. Slatter DH: Fundamentals of Veterinary Ophthalmology, pp 228, 701–703. Philadelphia, WB Saunders, 1981
7. Sharp NJH: Aspergillosis and penicilliosis. In Greene CE (ed): Infectious Diseases of the Dog and Cat, pp 714–721. Philadelphia, WB Saunders, 1990
8. Withrow SJ, Jusanek SJ, Macy DW, et al: Aspiration and punch biopsy techniques for nasal tumors. J Am Anim Hosp Assoc 21:551–554, 1985

PART EIGHT

Digestive Problems

CHAPTER THIRTY

Ptyalism

Larry M. Cornelius

PROBLEM DEFINITION AND RECOGNITION

Ptyalism is excessive secretion of saliva. This condition is also called sialosis. Drooling may be the result of either excessive production of saliva or reduced or abnormal swallowing (See Chapter 31). It may be difficult to distinguish between true ptyalism and inadequate swallowing of normal quantities of saliva (pseudosialosis). In this discussion, ptyalism will be used to describe any condition characterized by an excessive loss of saliva from the mouth.

PATHOPHYSIOLOGY

Saliva is normally produced by four major paired salivary glands: the parotids, mandibulars, sublinguals, and zygomatics. Both sympathetic (inhibitory) and parasympathetic (stimulatory) nerves supply the salivary glands, the latter through cranial nerves V, VII, and IX. Salivation is stimulated by both taste and tactile stimuli from the tongue and other areas of the mouth. Salivation also occurs in response to reflexes originating in the gastrointestinal tract when certain gastrointestinal diseases are present.[1] Salivation can be stimulated by impulses originating in higher centers of the brain as a result of conditioned reflexes (pavlovian response).

The saliva of dogs and cats has no significant enzyme content; its function is to soften and lubricate food in preparation for its passage through the pharynx and esophagus into the stomach. Evaporation of saliva from the oral mucosa is also important for heat loss in dogs. Ptyalism may be caused by several disorders that can be categorized as (1) conformational disorders of the lips and mouth; (2) morphologic disorders of the gastrointestinal system; (3) metabolic disorders; (4) neurologic disorders; and (5) drugs or toxins.[1]

Conformational disorders of the lips and mouth causing drooling are often seen in giant-breed dogs. Morphologic disorders of the gastrointestinal system may cause ptyalism by causing pain and nausea. Drooling is most often caused by a reluctance to swallow due to painful lesions such as stomatitis, pharyngitis, and esophagitis. Less commonly, ptyalism is caused by neuromuscular disorders affecting the oral, pharyngeal, or esophageal stages of swallowing and is associated with dysphagia (see Chapter 31). Inflammatory, infiltrative, and obstructive lesions of the gastrointestinal tract stimulate receptors, which may cause nausea and drooling. Diseases of the salivary glands are usually characterized by swelling of the glands rather than by ptyalism.

Metabolic disorders such as hepatic encephalopathy and uremia often cause excessive salivation, but the mechanism is not defined. Increases in the blood levels of ammonia, urea, and other nitrogenous wastes may cause nausea, which in turn causes ptyalism.

As previously mentioned, salivation aids in heat loss in dogs. Overheating due to a hot, humid environment or nervousness and excitement cause ptyalism.

Neurologic disorders causing ptyalism include neuromuscular swallowing disorders (see Chapter 31), nausea caused by excessive stimulation of the vestibular apparatus (motion sickness), and conditioned reflexes (pavlovian response). The neurologic effects of the rabies virus cause drooling due to interruption of swallowing.

Several drugs and toxins may cause ptyalism by different mechanisms. Oral drugs or toxins may have a bitter or noxious taste or be caustic. Other agents, such as apomorphine, cause nausea by stimulating the chemoreceptor trigger zone or the vomiting center in the midbrain. Organophosphates result in parasympathetic stimulation of salivary secretion.

Prolonged, severe ptyalism, especially when accompanied by decreased appetite and water intake, may cause dehydration. Electrolyte and acid-base balance is minimally affected.

DIAGNOSTIC PLAN

History and Physical Examination

Morphologic lesions of the lips, mouth, or pharynx account for most cases of ptyalism. The diagnosis can often be established by history and physical examination (Table 30-1). Access to drugs, toxins, or caustic agents should be established. Associated signs such as nausea, retching, and vomiting are indications for a workup for either a gastrointestinal or metabolic cause of vomiting (see Chapter 32). A history of "staring into space," depression, head-pressing, and intermittent blindness is typical of hepatoencephalopathy. Weight loss, coughing, and difficulty in eating often are reported in animals with swallowing disorders (see Chapter 31). Rabies vaccination history and possible exposure to unvaccinated animals should always be established prior to physical examination. *Protective gloves should be worn and caution used whenever rabies is a possible cause of drooling.*

Sedation or general anesthesia may be required to adequately examine the oral and pharyngeal cavities, but this should be delayed until laboratory results are obtained if a systemic or metabolic cause is likely. Thorough palpation

Text continues on p. 252

TABLE 30-1. Characteristic Findings of Common Disorders Causing Ptyalism

Disorder	Clinical Signs Other Than Ptyalism	Hematology	Biochemistry	Special Tests
Conformational disorders of the lips (giant breeds)	Secondary cheilitis	Normal	Normal	None
Lesions or disorders of the mouth and pharynx				
Gingivitis/stomatitis Pemphigus vulgaris	Anorexia Fever ± Mucocutaneous ulcerative lesions Painful mouth	Normal *or* Leukocytosis with neutrophilia and left shift	Normal *or* ↑ globulin	Biopsy of mucocutaneous lesions for histopathology and immunofluorescence testing
Secondary infection due to FeLV or FIV in cats	Anorexia Depression Weight loss Pale mucous membranes Sneezing and nasoocular discharge Oral ulcers Painful mouth Chronic diarrhea	Nonregenerative anemia Leukopenia with inappropriate left shift ±	Variable	FeLV and FIV tests on blood
Viral upper respiratory infection	Anorexia Depression Fever Sneezing Nasoocular discharge Oral ulcers Painful mouth	Normal *or* Mild nonregenerative anemia Mild leukocytosis with mature neutrophilia	Normal	None
Uremia	Anorexia Depression Vomiting Oral ulcers Polydipsia/polyuria ±	Variable	Variable ↑ BUN ↓ TCO$_2$	Variable Urine culture Abdominal radiographs and sonograms Excretory urogram Renal biopsy

(continued)

249

TABLE 30-1. Characteristic Findings of Common Disorders Causing Ptyalism *(continued)*

Disorder	Clinical Signs Other Than Ptyalism	Hematology	Biochemistry	Special Tests
Ingestion of caustic agent	Anorexia Vomiting Diarrhea Oral ulcers Painful mouth Ptyalism	Normal *or* stress leukogram	Normal	None
Foreign body	Anorexia Pawing at mouth Painful mouth	Normal	Normal	Radiograph mouth and neck
Neoplasm	Anorexia Oropharyngeal mass	Variable	Normal *or* ↑ globulin	Radiograph mouth and thorax
Functional disorder of the pharynx or cricopharynx	Dysphagia (see Chapter 31)			
Esophageal disorders	Regurgitation (see Chapter 32)			
Other gastrointestinal disorders				
Gastroenteritis	Nausea Vomiting Diarrhea Depression	See Chapters 32 and 33.		
Metabolic disorders				
Hyperthermia	Hot, humid environment Marked panting Polydipsia	Normal *or* ↑ PCV and plasma protein Stress leukogram	Normal *or* ↑ albumin and globulin	None

250

	Clinical Signs			Diagnostic Tests
Hepatoencephalopathy	Head-pressing Apparent blindness Stupor/coma	See Chapter 51.	Variable	↑ Plasma ammonia or abnormal ammonia tolerance ↑ Serum bile acids, pre- and post-prandial Portal venography Radionuclide scan of liver and portal system
Congenital portosystemic shunt Acquired portosystemic shunt (primary liver disease) Hepatic failure				
Uremia	See above			
Drugs or toxins				
Bitter or disagreeable taste	Anorexia Excessive licking and swallowing Shaking head	Normal	Normal	None
Organophosphates	Vomiting Diarrhea Muscle trembling Miosis Seizures Other CNS signs	Normal *or* Stress leukogram	↑ Creatine phosphokinase (CPK) ±	↓ Serum cholinesterase level
Neurologic disorders				
Rabies	Depression Paresis/paralysis Aggressiveness Others	Normal	Normal	None before death Fluorescent antibody evaluation of brain after death
Disorders causing dysphagia	See Chapter 31.			
Conditioned reflex (pavlovian response)	None	Normal	Normal	Normal

±, present or absent; ↑, increased; FeLV, feline leukemia virus; FIV, feline immunodeficiency virus; BUN, blood urea nitrogen; TCO$_2$, total carbon dioxide; PCV, packed cell volume; CNS, central nervous system; ↓, decreased should include the salivary glands and the abdomen. Neurologic examination is indicated if a neurologic disorder is suspected.

Laboratory Evaluation

Laboratory tests needed depend upon the suspected cause of ptyalism (see Table 30-1). For some oropharyngeal lesions, such as a foreign body or stomatitis caused by a caustic substance, further evaluation may not be needed. Biopsy of oral ulcers for histopathology and immunofluorescence testing is sometimes indicated. Other causes, such as suspected hepatoencephalopathy, require a complete blood count, urine analysis, biochemical profile, and special tests such as blood ammonia, an ammonia tolerance test, and serum bile acids (pre- and postprandial). Radiographic studies of the oral and pharyngeal cavities or other parts of the gastrointestinal tract may be needed (see Chapters 31 and 32).

REFERENCE

1. Harvey CE, O'Brien JA, Rossman LE: Oral, dental, pharyngeal, and salivary gland disorders. In Ettinger SJ (ed): Textbook of Veterinary Internal Medicine, 2nd ed, pp 1126–1191. Philadelphia, WB Saunders, 1983

CHAPTER THIRTY-ONE

Dysphagia

Larry M. Cornelius

DEFINITION AND PROBLEM RECOGNITION

Dysphagia is difficulty in swallowing and is usually noticed by the owner while the animal is eating. Gagging, drooling, and dropping food from the mouth are commonly reported.

PATHOPHYSIOLOGY

Swallowing is a complex reflex action coordinating many muscular functions, including those of the tongue, hard and soft palates, pharynx, esophagus, and gastroesophageal junction. It is coordinated by cranial nerves V, VII, IX, X, and XI and their nuclei in the brain stem, which in turn are controlled by the swallowing center in the reticular formation of the brain.[1]

The normal swallowing sequence has been divided into three phases for detailed study: (1) oropharyngeal, (2) esophageal, and (3) gastroesophageal. The oropharyngeal phase is subdivided into oral, pharyngeal, and cricopharyngeal phases.[1] The oral stage includes uptake of food or liquid by the tongue, teeth, and/or lips. During the oral stage, the bolus is accumulated at the base of the tongue. Rostral to caudal pharyngeal contractions then propel the bolus from the base of the tongue to the cricopharyngeal passage (pharyngeal stage). The cricopharyngeal stage consists of the relaxation of the cricopharyngeal sphincter, passage of the bolus into the cranial esophagus, closure of the upper esophageal sphincter, and relaxation of the pharyngeal muscles.

As the esophagus receives the bolus, the esophageal phase starts. Both primary and secondary peristaltic waves have been observed in the esophagus.[4] The final phase of swallowing is the gastroesophageal phase, during which the lower esophageal sphincter relaxes and the bolus passes into the stomach. This phase overlaps prior phases.

Dysphagia results from partial or complete interruption of one or more of the above phases of swallowing. Swallowing disorders can result from morphologic lesions or functional disorders of any of the structures involved at any time during the passage of a bolus from the mouth to the stomach (Table 31-1).[2]

Text continues on p. 258

TABLE 31-1. Characteristic Findings of Selected Disorders Causing Dysphagia

Disorder	Clinical Signs Other Than Dysphagia	Hematology	Special Tests
Oral			
Morphologic			
Gingivitis, stomatitis	Decreased appetite Weight loss Drooling Halitosis	Normal	Consider biopsy for histopathologic and immunofluorescent studies.
Foreign body	Evidence of oral pain (*e.g.*, pawing at mouth) Drooling Gagging	Normal	Radiographs of head may show foreign body.
Temporamandibular lesion	See Foreign body.		
Fracture			Radiographs of head show fracture or luxation.
Luxation			
Neoplasia	Decreased appetite Weight loss Halitosis Gagging Enlarged submandibular lymph nodes	Variable	Radiographs of thorax may show metastasis. Biopsy of mass by needle aspiration or wedge
Functional			
Myopathies			
Eosinophilic myositis	Anorexia Depression Difficulty in opening mouth Late atrophy of masticatory muscles	Usually normal	Biopsy of masticatory muscles may show eosinophilic inflammatory response.

Neuromuscular junction—myasthenia gravis	Weakness worsened with exercise Coughing Dyspnea Weight loss Voice change or loss of voice Regurgitation	Normal or leukocytosis with neutrophilia and left shift	Transient regaining of strength after 0.1–0.5 mg Tensilon* IV EMG and repetitive nerve stimulation show decremental response, which disappears after Tensilon. Serum acetylcholine receptor antibody test positive ±.
Neuropathies (cranial nerves V, IX, XII) Idiopathic bilateral trigeminal palsy	Dropped jaw, unable to close mouth Signs usually transient for 1–2 weeks	Normal	EMG of masseter and temporalis muscles
Hydrocephalus	Brachycephalic and toy breeds Open fontanelle Mild depression to severe seizures Visual deficits and motor dysfunction	Normal	Skull radiography including pneumoventriculography EEG
Pharyngeal Morphologic Pharyngitis/tonsillitis	Depression Anorexia Fever ± Weight loss	Variable—leukocytosis with neutrophilia and left shift	None
Retropharyngeal abscess	See pharyngitis/tonsillitis. Swelling in pharynx	Leukocytosis with neutrophilia and left shift	Fine-needle aspirate of pharyngeal swelling shows septic, purulent exudate.
Foreign body Neoplasia	See Foreign body under Oral. See Neoplasia under Oral.		

(continued)

255

TABLE 31-1. Characteristic Findings of Selected Disorders Causing Dysphagia *(continued)*

Disorder	Clinical Signs Other Than Dysphagia	Hematology	Special Tests
Pharyngeal (cont.) Functional Myopathies—polymyositis	Variable ↓ Exercise tolerance Lameness Stiff gait Painful muscles Weakness Loss of muscle mass Regurgitation with signs of aspiration pneumonia (cough, dyspnea)	Normal or leukocytosis with neutrophilia and left shift (due to aspiration pneumonia)	Contrast radiographs of pharynx following barium swallow show retention of barium in pharynx and cranial esophagus. ↑ CPK ± EMG may show positive waves, fibrillation potentials and bizarre high-frequency discharges. Muscle biopsy may show muscle necrosis and lymphocytic inflammation. Immunofluorescence may show staining along muscle sarcolemma.
Neuromuscular junction— see Myasthenia gravis under Oral.			

Esophageal See Chapter 32.
Morphologic
  Esophagitis
  Stenosis
  Perforation
  Diverticulum
  Neoplasia
  Parasitic (*Spirocerca lupi*)
  Foreign body
  Vascular ring anomaly

Functional—megaesophagus
  Congenital and acquired

Gastroesophageal See Chapter 32.
Morphologic
  Esophagitis
  Sliding hiatal hernia
  Intussusception
  Neoplasia
  Pharyngostomy tube

Functional—neuromuscular disorders
  Megaesophagus
  Myasthenia gravis

---

*Trade name for edrophonium chloride
IV, intravenously; EMG, electromyogram; EEG, electroencephalogram; ±, present or absent; CPK, creatine phosphokinase

Structural changes that interfere with swallowing include foreign bodies, traumatic lesions, strictures, or mass lesions, either inflammatory or neoplastic. Gingivitis and stomatitis associated with poor dental care are especially common causes of dysphagia. Functional or motility disorders affecting swallowing include failure, spasticity, or incoordination of muscular contractions and are due to neurologic, neuromuscular junction, or muscular diseases. They may be either congenital or acquired (see Table 31-1).[4]

Disorders affecting the oropharyngeal phase of swallowing usually cause more clinically pronounced dysphagia, whereas abnormalities of the esophageal and gastroesophageal stages are typified by regurgitation (see Chapter 32). Discussion in this chapter will be limited to oropharyngeal dysphagia.

DIAGNOSTIC PLAN

Because treatment and prognosis are different, careful differentiation between oral, pharyngeal, and cricopharyngeal dysphagias has been stressed.[1] Swallowing disorders are complex and therefore should be approached systematically.

History and Physical Examination

The chief complaints and presenting clinical signs of swallowing disorders in dogs and cats often are more directly related to the secondary effects of dysphagia than to the swallowing problem itself. Gagging, drooling, "vomiting," coughing, dyspnea, excessive mandibular or head motion while eating, dropping food from the mouth while eating, reluctance to eat, and weight loss or failure to grow may be the main signs reported by the owner. It is very important to consider a swallowing disorder in an animal with any of these signs, so that appropriate diagnostic procedures can be done to document the exact cause.

A thorough physical examination should include both neurologic and careful oral examinations. The gag reflex should be evaluated by placing a finger in the pharynx. Sedation or general anesthesia is often required to thoroughly examine the oropharyngeal regions for morphologic lesions such as foreign bodies and masses.

Laboratory Evaluation

A complete minimum data base (complete blood count, biochemical profile, urine analysis, and fecal parasite examination) should be done to rule out associated problems. An increased serum creatine phosphokinase (CPK) may be present in some animals with polymyositis. An antinuclear antibody (ANA) titer and lupus erythematosus cell test (LE prep) should be performed if an immune-mediated disorder is suspected. Evaluation of serum for the presence of acetylcholine receptor antibodies is indicated if myasthenia gravis is suspected. Neuropathy due to primary hypothyroidism can be ruled out by doing a thyroid-stimulating hormone stimulation test with pre- and post-serum T4 levels.

Special Studies

Survey radiographs of the mouth and upper cervical area are usually helpful for recognizing gross morphologic abnormalities causing oropharyngeal dysphagia. For functional (motility) disorders of the pharynx, cricopharyngeal sphincter, and esophagus, special studies (cinefluorography or videofluorography) are needed. The barium swallow must be done using both liquids and solids. Manometry, electromyography, and biopsy are required in some cases to establish a diagnosis.

REFERENCES

1. Suter PF, Watrous BJ: Oropharyngeal dysphagia in the dog: A cinefluorographic analysis of experimentally induced and spontaneously occurring swallowing disorders. I. Oral stage and pharyngeal stage dysphagias. Vet Radiol 21:24–39, 1980
2. Watrous BJ: Dysphagia and regurgitation. In Ford RG (ed): Clinical Signs and Diagnosis in Small Animal Practice, pp 389–423. New York, Churchill Livingstone, 1988
3. Watrous BJ: Esophageal disease. In Ettinger SJ (ed): Textbook of Veterinary Internal Medicine, 2nd ed, pp 1191–1233. Philadelphia, WB Saunders, 1983
4. Watrous BJ, Suter PF: Oropharyngeal dysphagias in the dog: A cinefluorographic analysis of experimentally induced and spontaneously occurring swallowing disorders. II. Cricopharyngeal stage and mixed oropharyngeal dysphagias. Vet Radiol 24: 11–24, 1983

CHAPTER THIRTY-TWO

Vomiting and Regurgitation

Larry M. Cornelius

DEFINITION AND PROBLEM RECOGNITION

Vomiting is the forceful ejection of food or fluid through the mouth from the stomach and, sometimes, the proximal duodenum. Regurgitation is more passive and results in expulsion of food or fluid from the oral or pharyngeal cavity or the esophagus.

PATHOPHYSIOLOGY

The Vomiting Reflex

Vomiting is a reflex act that requires a coordinated effort of the gastrointestinal, musculoskeletal, and nervous systems. Stimulation of the vomiting center in the medulla causes vomiting. The neurons of the vomiting center can be activated directly by certain blood-borne drugs or toxins or indirectly through afferent nerves or the chemoreceptor trigger zone (CTZ) located on the floor of the fourth ventricle. Stimulation of receptors in abdominal viscera as well as many other sites throughout the body may result in vomiting. Impulses travel along afferent nerve fibers located in the vagus and sympathetic nerves and synapse in the vomiting center. Receptor activation can occur as a result of inflammation, irritation, distention, or hypertonicity, among other factors. The CTZ can be thought of as a receptor, because the vomiting center must be functional for the animal to vomit when the CTZ is stimulated. The CTZ is stimulated by blood-borne drugs or toxins, such as apomorphine and uremic toxins, and by impulses from the inner ear during motion sickness.

Electrolyte and Acid-Base Changes

Vomiting may result in dehydration because of water lost in secretions of the gastrointestinal tract and lack of dietary intake. Potassium depletion, which is a frequent complication of profuse vomiting (see following discussion), may impair renal tubular concentrating ability and worsen dehydration. Prerenal azotemia may develop if dehydration is severe. In patients with preexisting borderline renal insufficiency, dehydration caused by vomiting may cause decompensation and renal failure.

Electrolyte and acid-base changes caused by vomiting are variable and difficult to predict in both magnitude and type. Deficits of body sodium, potassium, and chloride are likely, but the plasma concentrations depend upon the amount of ion lost relative to the quantity of plasma water lost.

Hyponatremia is commonly associated with persistent vomiting despite the lower concentration of sodium in gastric juice than in plasma. Hyponatremia probably occurs as a result of the dilution of extracellular fluid caused by the patient's consumption of water. Clinical signs attributable to hyponatremia generally are not obvious. Dehydration associated with hyponatremia is termed *hypotonic dehydration.* Extracellular fluid is hypotonic, and water is transferred from the extracellular space into the cellular compartment by osmotic attraction. This type of dehydration markedly reduces the volume of extracellular fluid because this compartment has lost volume to the external environment and to the cells. Therefore, such patients are more prone to vascular collapse (shock) and warrant prompt and aggressive fluid therapy.

Deficit of body potassium and hypokalemia are frequent during profuse vomiting. Clinical signs due to a potassium deficit include weakness, ileus, and impaired renal concentrating ability. Potassium losses during vomiting are primarily the result of excretion of potassium in urine caused by alkalemia and loss of potassium in vomitus. Lack of dietary intake may contribute to this depletion. Alkalemia also causes transfer of potassium from extracellular to intracellular fluid in exchange for hydrogen ions, thus worsening hypokalemia.

Serum chloride levels and acid-base status of blood during profuse vomiting depend upon the source of most of the fluid lost and are difficult to predict without laboratory data. Loss of mostly gastric secretions, as occurs with functional or structural causes of pyloric outlet or high duodenal obstruction, results in loss of mostly hydrochloric acid. Pancreatic and biliary secretions contain large quantities of bicarbonate. Obstruction of pancreatic and biliary flow, as may occur during pancreatitis and cholestatic disorders, can significantly reduce the amount of bicarbonate entering the duodenum. Vomitus produced as a result of obstructive disorders of the pancreas and biliary system is more acidic. Acute pancreatitis may also impede pyloric outflow (as a result of pressure caused by swelling), resulting in loss of mostly hydrochloric acid in vomitus. The usual outcome is hypochloridemia, high serum bicarbonate concentration (metabolic alkalosis), and sometimes metabolic alkalemia (see Display, Causes of Vomiting Usually Associated with Increased Plasma Bicarbonate [TCO_2] and Decreased Plasma Chloride). Paradoxic aciduria (urine pH less than 7.0) may be observed as the kidneys preferentially reabsorb bicarbonate ions to defend against anion (chloride) deficit. Thus, the body's defense against metabolic alkalemia caused by vomiting is inadequate.

Plasma bicarbonate concentration may be increased, normal, or decreased, and blood pH may be increased, normal, or low during vomiting. As mentioned

Causes of Vomiting Usually Associated with Increased Plasma Bicarbonate (TCO₂) and Decreased Plasma Chloride

- Gastric atony with sequestration of fluid in stomach
- Pyloric outlet obstruction
    Pyloric stenosis
    Pylorospasm
    Gastric foreign body
    Neoplasm (intramural or extramural)
- High duodenal obstruction
    Foreign body
    Neoplasm
    Others
- Acute pancreatitis
- Biliary obstructive disorders

above, the location of the lesion causing vomiting and the acidity of vomitus affect the plasma bicarbonate concentration. Other concurrent abnormalities may affect acid-base balance (see Display, Causes of Vomiting Usually Associated with Normal or Decreased Plasma Bicarbonate [TCO₂] and Normal or Increased Plasma Chloride). For example, dehydration may cause poor renal perfusion and the retention of metabolic acids. Lactic acidosis can also result from poor tissue perfusion caused by dehydration or any condition causing hypoxia (such as aspiration pneumonia secondary to vomiting). Net plasma bicarbonate is determined by the process that is quantitatively more severe.

Regurgitation usually does not cause severe changes in electrolyte or acid-base status. Dehydration and weight loss may result primarily from lack of dietary intake. Aspiration pneumonia, sometimes severe, is a common complication of chronic regurgitation.

Causes of Vomiting Usually Associated with Normal or Decreased Plasma Bicarbonate (TCO₂) and Normal or Increased Plasma Chloride

- Gastroenteritis
- Uremia
- Toxins or drugs
- Hypoadrenocorticism
- Others

DIAGNOSTIC PLAN

History and Physical Examination

Signs of vomiting are often confused with those of regurgitation, dysphagia, gagging, and coughing (Fig. 32-1). In none of these disorders, except for vomiting, are hypersalivation, retching, and forceful contractions of the abdominal muscles and diaphragm present. Regurgitation is the effortless expulsion of fluid or food from the pharyngeal cavity or esophagus. Gagging may be followed by either regurgitation or vomiting. Dysphagia means difficulty in swallowing and is most commonly observed during eating or drinking. Drooling of saliva often accompanies dysphagia (see Chapter 31). Coughing is often misinterpreted as vomiting, especially when it is characterized by expectoration of excessive phlegm. Paroxysmal coughing may also be followed by regurgitation or vomiting, making the situation even more confusing for the client and sometimes the veterinarian. Coughing can often be elicited by firm palpation of the trachea. This should be done while the client is present so that the animal's problem can be confirmed or denied.

A carefully taken history is well worth the time it requires. If doubt still exists about which sign is present, it is very important to hospitalize the animal to observe the abnormal signs. If possible, to save time and money, this should be done prior to initiating a laboratory workup.

Since it is not feasible to hospitalize and work up every vomiting animal, initial efforts should be directed at distinguishing patients requiring only symptomatic care from those with more serious disorders. For this purpose, it is helpful to consider the duration (acute versus chronic) and frequency of vomiting and the presence or absence of associated signs. Whenever vomiting has been of short duration (less than 3 or 4 days) and infrequent (once or twice daily) and there are no associated signs, the workup may consist of a minimum data base, including only history and physical examination (emphasis on thorough abdominal palpation) followed by symptomatic therapy. Chronic vomiting (more than 3 or 4 days), increased frequency of vomiting (more than one or two times daily), and vomiting of blood, as well as associated signs such as depression, fever, dehydration, abdominal pain, and signs of shock, often indicate a potentially serious or life-threatening disorder and require an immediate, in-depth laboratory workup.

Laboratory Evaluation

The initial diagnostic consideration for patients hospitalized because of vomiting is to distinguish primary gastrointestinal causes from metabolic or nongastrointestinal causes (see Fig. 32-1; Table 32-1). History may or may not be helpful. Careful abdominal palpation, abdominal radiography, and abdominal ultrasonography are the diagnostic methods of choice to rule out gastrointestinal causes

Text continues on p. 272

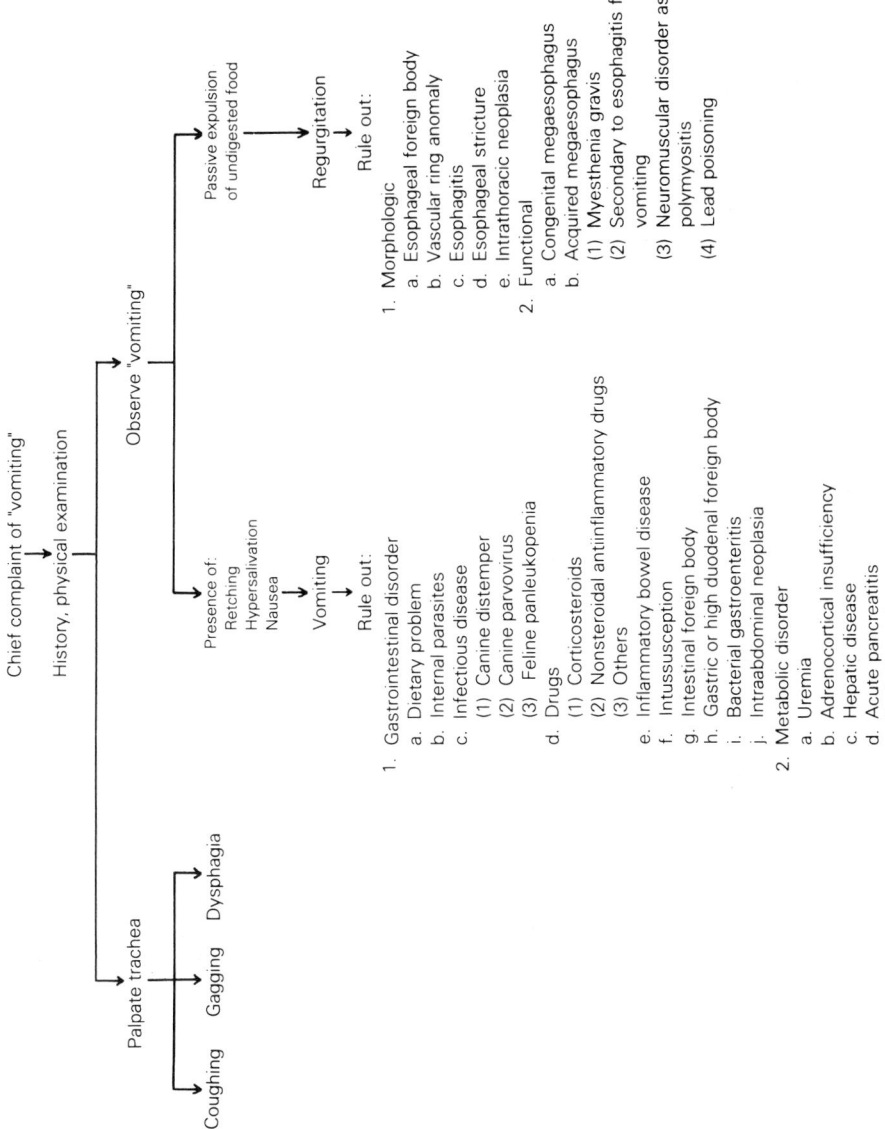

FIGURE 32-1. Initial plan for evaluating vomiting.

265

TABLE 32-1. Characteristic Findings of Common Disorders Causing Vomiting

Disease	Clinical Signs Other Than Vomiting	Hematology	Urine Analysis	Biochemistry	Special Tests
Gastrointestinal tract disorders					
Dietary problem	Few systemic signs Diarrhea and flatulence are sometimes present.	Normal	Normal	Normal	None
Internal parasites	Weight loss and poor hair coat Diarrhea	May have regenerative anemia Eosinophilia	Normal	Normal	Fecal flotation or sedimentation ×3
Drugs Corticosteroids	Polyuria Polydipsia Melena Dermatologic changes (alopecia, thin skin)	Regenerative anemia ± (blood loss) Stress leukogram	Specific gravity 1.010–1.030	↓ Albumin and globulin (blood loss) ↑ SAP and ALT	None
NSAIDS	Melena	Regenerative anemia	Normal	↓ Albumin and globulin (blood loss)	None
Others					
Lymphocytic-plasmacytic enteritis	See Table 33-2.				
Eosinophilic enteritis	See Table 33-2.				
Infectious disease Canine distemper Canine parvovirus Feline panleukopenia	See Table 33-1.				

	Clinical signs	CBC	Urinalysis	Serum chemistry	Radiography/Other
Intussusception	Anorexia, Depression, Dehydration, Abdominal pain, Palpable abdominal mass	↑PCV and plasma protein, Stress or inflammatory leukogram, Toxic granulation of neutrophils ±		Normal albumin and globulin, Electrolytes and acid-base variable, ↓BUN (prerenal)	Abdominal radiographs show gas-distended intestinal loops, indicative of intestinal obstruction.
Intestinal foreign body	Same as intussusception				Abdominal radiographs show gas-distended bowel loops, indicative of intestinal obstruction.
Gastric or high duodenal foreign body	Chronic intermittent vomiting with few other signs or acute, profuse vomiting, Dehydration, Anorexia, Depression	Normal or ↑PCV and plasma protein, Stress leukogram	Variable specific gravity, Paradoxic aciduria ±	Normal or ↑albumin and globulin, ↑BUN (prerenal), ↓Na$^+$, ↓K$^+$, ↓Cl$^-$, ↑TCO$_2$	Abdominal radiographs may show fluid- and gas-distended stomach and gastric or high duodenal foreign body. Upper gastrointestinal study may show delayed gastric emptying.
Bacterial gastroenteritis	Anorexia, Depression, Dehydration, Fever, Diarrhea	↑PVC and plasma protein, Variable WBC, Stress or inflammatory leukogram and toxic granulation of neutrophils	Normal	↑Albumin and globulin, ↓BUN (prerenal), Electrolytes and acid-base variable	Fecal cultures positive for *Salmonella* or *Campylobacter* in some cases

267

(continued)

TABLE 32-1. Characteristic Findings of Common Disorders Causing Vomiting *(continued)*

Disease	Clinical Signs Other Than Vomiting	Hematology	Urine Analysis	Biochemistry	Special Tests
Intraabdominal neoplasia	Decreased appetite Lethargy Weight loss Palpable abdominal mass Vomiting Diarrhea	Mild nonregenerative anemia Variable WBC	Normal	Variable	Abdominal radiographs and sonograms may show evidence of a mass. Thoracic radiographs may show metastatic disease.
Metabolic disorders Uremia	Anorexia Depression Dehydration Weight loss Polyuria/polydipsia Oliguria/anuria	PCV variable ↑ Plasma protein ± WBC variable—stress leukogram	Variable depending on cause	↑ Albumin and globulin ↑ BUN Electrolytes variable ↓ TCO$_2$	Depends on cause
Adrenocortical insufficiency	Lethargy Weakness Intermittent diarrhea Bradycardia Collapse and shock	↑ PCV and plasma protein Eosinophilia and lymphocytosis ±	↓ Specific gravity ±	↑ Albumin and globulin ↑ BUN ↓ Na$^+$ ↑ K$^+$ Na$^+$:K$^+$ ratio < 23:1	↓ Baseline plasma cortisol and no response to ACTH stimulation

Disease	Clinical signs	Hematology	Urinalysis	Chemistry	Other tests
Hepatic disease	Depression, anorexia Head pressing, stupor, coma ± Polyuria, polydipsia ± Icterus Ascites Diarrhea, melena ±	Variable Stomatocytosis	Variable ↓ Specific gravity ± Bilirubinuria Ammonium biurate crystals	Variable ↓ Albumin and globulin ↑ ± BUN ± ↑ Bilirubin ± ↑ ALT and SAP ± ↓ Glucose ±	↑ Serum bile acids, pre- and postprandial ↑ Plasma NH_3 ↓ NH_3 tolerance
Acute pancreatitis	Depression, anorexia, dehydration Obesity Vomiting Abdominal pain upon palpation ± Diarrhea, melena ± Icterus ± Dyspnea ±	↑ PCV and plasma protein ↑ WBC with either inflammatory or stress leukogram Toxic granulation of neutrophils ±	Usually normal Bilirubinuria ± Proteinuria ± Casts ±	↑ Albumin and globulin ↑ BUN ± ↑ SAP ± ↑ ALT ± ↓ K^+ ± ↓ Cl^- ± ↓ Ca^+ ± ↑ TCO_2 ±	↑ Serum lipase Abdominal radiographs may show lack of contrast in pancreatic area and displacement of cranial duodenum. Abdominal sonograms may show mixed echogenic pattern in pancreatic area.
Toxin ingestion	Variable depending upon the toxin ingested				

±, present or absent; ↑, increased; ↓, decreased; SAP, serum alkaline phosphatase; ALT, alanine transaminase; NSAIDs, nonsteroidal antiinflammatory drugs; PCV, packed cell volume; BUN, blood urea nitrogen; WBC, white blood cell; TCO_2, total CO_2; ACTH, adrenocorticotropic hormone

TABLE 32-2. Characteristic Findings of Common Disorders Causing Regurgitation

Disease	Clinical Signs Other Than Regurgitation	Hematology	Urine Analysis	Biochemistry	Special Tests
Morphologic Esophageal foreign body	See Megaesophagus.				Esophagoscopy for visualization and removal of foreign body
Vascular ring anomaly	Young animal Failure to gain weight See Megaesophagus.	See Megaesophagus.			
Esophagitis	History of persistent vomiting Coughing Dyspnea Dehydration Weight loss	Variable ↑PCV and plasma protein ↑WBC with inflammatory leukogram	Normal	↑Albumin and globulin ± Electrolytes and acid-base variable	Esophagoscopy for visualization of esophageal mucosa
Esophageal stricture	See Megaesophagus.				

Intrathoracic neoplasia	Coughing Dyspnea Weight loss Anorexia Depression Dehydration	Mild to moderate nonregenerative anemia ± WBC and leukogram variable	Normal	↑ Albumin and globulin ±	Thoracic radiographs may show mass. Barium swallow for esophageal study
Functional Megaesophagus, congenital and acquired	Coughing Dyspnea Drooling ± Weight loss Fever ± Episodic weakness ±	WBC and leukogram variable	Normal	Normal	Esophagoscopy Barium swallow for esophageal study ↓T4 values pre– and post–TSH stimulation ± Serum acetylcholine receptor antibody test positive ± Transient regaining of strength after 0.1–0.5 mg Tensilon* IV

* Trade name for edrophonium chloride
↑, increased; PCV, packed cell volume; ±, present or absent; WBC, white blood cell

of vomiting. Metabolic causes are best ruled out by an initial data base consisting of a complete blood count, serum biochemical profile, and urine analysis. Ideally, complete arterial blood gas and/or pH analysis is needed for thorough evaluation of a vomiting animal. Because of difficulties in obtaining these data, measurement of plasma bicarbonate is an acceptable alternative. Plasma total CO_2 (TCO_2) consists mostly of bicarbonate and, for clinical purposes, can be substituted for plasma bicarbonate. Automated methods for measuring TCO_2 are routinely available, and TCO_2 should always be included whenever a plasma biochemical profile is requested for a vomiting patient. Special laboratory tests, such as determination of serum lipase activity, serum bile acids, and plasma ammonia level, may be needed in some cases. Common causes of regurgitation and associated clinical signs are shown in Table 32-2.

CHAPTER THIRTY-THREE

Diarrhea

Larry M. Cornelius and Michael D. Lorenz

PROBLEM DEFINITION AND RECOGNITION

Diarrhea is a change in one or more of the characteristics of the bowel movement: increased frequency, increased fluidity, or increased volume. Disease involving the small or large intestine or both may result in diarrhea. Many diseases involving other organs produce similar pathophysiologic changes that culminate in diarrhea. The management of diarrhea is often based on these altered physiologic mechanisms.

PATHOPHYSIOLOGY

A common abnormality found in diarrhea is increased fecal water. Most diseases that produce diarrhea cause an increased concentration of fecal water. Several pathophysiologic mechanisms, including hypersecretion, altered permeability, altered motility, and malabsorption, result in increased fecal water.[1,2] Diarrhea of small bowel origin usually results from fluid being delivered to the colon at a rate or volume that overwhelms normal colonic absorptive capacity (colon overload). Diarrhea of large bowel origin usually occurs because fluid normally delivered to the colon is not absorbed as a result of decreased absorptive capacity of the colon.

Hypersecretion

Hypersecretion occurs with several enteric bacterial diseases of domestic animals. In the normal small intestine, fluid and electrolytes are secreted by immature cells in the base of the intestinal villi. These fluid and electrolytes are promptly absorbed by the mature epithelial cells lining the tips of the villi. This process is called "bidirectional flux," and in the normal animal absorptive flux always exceeds the secretory flux so that a net absorption of fluid and electrolytes occurs. In certain diseases, secretion of fluids is stimulated to such a degree that the absorptive capacity of the small and large intestine is overwhelmed, allowing a marked increase in fecal water. Enterotoxigenic bacteria, such as *Escherichia coli*, produce substances that stimulate hypersecretion and watery diarrhea, even though the gut appears intact structurally. In small animals, hypersecretion is of less importance than in large animals; however, in certain diseases, hypersecretion is partially responsible for increased fecal water.

Altered Permeability

Many enteric diseases dramatically alter gut permeability. Small changes in permeability result in the secretion of electrolyte-rich, protein-poor fluid. Greater permeability changes produce the exudation of fluid containing considerable quantities of plasma proteins. An example of this process is lymphangiectasia, a protein-losing enteropathy. Characteristically, both albumin and globulin are lost in equal amounts, resulting in both hypoalbuminemia and hypoglobulinemia. Structural damage to mucosal integrity produces tremendous permeability changes. A 10,000-fold increase in gut permeability produces hemorrhagic exudates and suggests that the gut defense barriers have been greatly compromised.

Altered Motility

Unfortunately, many veterinarians were taught that diarrhea resulted from hypermotility of the gut. Certainly, in diarrhea luminal contents are transported aborally at an accelerated rate. However, hypermotility is not the primary cause; rather, hypomotility is the usual intestinal response to disease. Two major intestinal movements are normally present: rhythmic contractions, or segmentations, and peristalsis. *Rhythmic segmentations* retard the passage of ingesta through the intestine, thereby aiding digestion and absorption. In diarrheal states, the strength of these contractions is greatly reduced, resulting in decreased resistance to the flow of ingesta. Anticholinergic drugs tend to further decrease the strength and rate of segmental contractions, further complicating the hypomotile condition of the diseased gut. *Peristaltic waves* move ingesta in the aboral direction. There is little evidence to support the widely held concept that peristaltic activity is exaggerated in diarrheal states. In fact, when resistance to flow is decreased by lack of rhythmic contractions, very little peristaltic activity is required to move luminal contents a great distance. In summary, one should view the diseased gut as a hypomotile tube with decreased resistance to the aboral movement of luminal contents. Therapy regarding alteration of motility should be predicated on this assumption.

Malabsorption

Both structural and biochemical mechanisms may produce malabsorption. Diseases that destroy the villous integrity result in malabsorption of fluid, electrolytes, and basic nutrients; infections with the enteric coronaviruses and paroviruses are examples. Altered permeability, hypomotility, and even hypersecretion (which occurs in the recovery phase of these diseases) are also encountered. Gluten enteropathy is another example of a disease that decreases the absorptive surface of the intestine via villous atrophy. Infiltrative disease of the gut wall (inflammatory or neoplastic) may also cause malabsorption. Forms of malabsorption have been recognized in dogs that have little structural abnormality in their gut. In these cases, biochemical malabsorption has been suspected (deficiency of brush border enzyme systems, lymphatic obstruction or malfunction, failure of active transport systems). On a clinical basis, biochemical malabsorption is difficult to prove.

There are several sequelae to intestinal malabsorption. Volume overload of the colon is a common mechanism; however, several other mechanisms come together to increase the volume of fecal water. Malabsorbed basic nutrients (*e.g.*, carbohydrates, fatty acids) create significant osmotic effects in the gut lumen. These osmotically active substances tend to hold water in the gut lumen and may even stimulate the secretion of fluid into the lumen. Bacterial action on carbohydrate and fats in the gut lumen may produce substances (*e.g.*, lactic acid, hydroxy fatty acids) that are osmotically active but also irritative to the intestinal mucosa. These substances aggravate the diarrheal state by enhancing gut secretion of fluid and electrolytes. Bacterial deconjugation of primary bile acids may result in accumulation of secondary bile acids, which are toxic to the intestinal mucosa and liver and thereby worsen diarrhea. Malabsorption of primary bile acids may contribute to hypersecretion and decreased fat digestion, because the bile acid pool may become depleted.

Intestinal Resistance to Pathogens

Immunologic Mechanisms. Both antibody-mediated and cell-mediated immune mechanisms are important. IgA is a secretory antibody produced by plasma cells in the gut wall. It contains a unique protein, called *secretory component,* that promotes transport through epithelial cells to the mucosal barrier and protects the antibody from enzymatic digestion. Although IgA has little opsonic, complement-fixing, or bactericidal activity, it functions by preventing adherence of organisms to the intestinal mucosa. Other immunoglobulins (IgM, IgG, IgE) are present in low concentrations in the gut lumen unless inflammation of the bowel wall allows their exudation.

The role of cell-mediated immunity in intestinal defense against pathogens is not well defined. It is known that animals with T-cell dysfunction are susceptible to gastrointestinal disease.

Nonimmunologic Mechanisms. Gastric acidity may render inactive a number of organisms and their toxins before they reach the lower portions of the intestine. Mucins in the mucous coat of the gastrointestinal mucosa act as receptors for organisms or their toxins, thus protecting the epithelium by competitive binding. Lysozymes and bile salts have been shown to inhibit bacterial growth *in vitro.*

Peristalsis helps prevent bacterial overgrowth in the gut. The role of altered intestinal motility in the pathophysiology of diarrhea has been discussed. The intestinal microflora is a very important host defense mechanism against bacterial pathogens. It is normally quite stable; after disruption, it rapidly returns to its previous state. Many diarrheal conditions are treated symptomatically with antimicrobial drugs, even though a primary bacterial pathogen is not suspected. The normal gut flora serves as a primary defense barrier for the host. Bacterial pathogens must attach to the target cell before they can produce disease, either by invasion or secretion of enterotoxins. Normal gut bacteria inhibit this attachment by occupying spaces available to pathogenic bacteria. Reduction of the normal gut flora with antimicrobial agents decreases this beneficial competition, allowing pathogenic bacteria to attach to target cells, proliferate, and potentially invade the gut mucosa. Proliferation of enteric pathogens such as *Salmonella* is enhanced when antibiotics are given. In certain situations, such as intestinal ileus and exocrine pancreatic insufficiency (EPI), overgrowth of bacteria may contribute to diarrheal states. The use of antimicrobial drugs should be limited to conditions in which gut permeability has been greatly increased or to circumstances involving suspected bacterial overgrowth. Parenteral antibiotics should then be used, rather than poorly absorbed luminal antibiotics that adversely affect normal intestinal microflora.

DIAGNOSTIC PLAN

The initial step in the diagnosis of diarrhea is to localize the problem to either the small or large intestine. This is accomplished by history, physical examination, and gross fecal examination (Table 33-1).[3] Small bowel diarrhea is characterized by increased fecal volume (either watery or bulky). The frequency of defecation is increased; however, tenesmus is absent. Mucus and fresh blood are not prominent, except in young puppies or kittens. In adults, blood is usually digested, resulting in melena. Associated clinical signs include vomiting, rapid weight loss, and dehydration. Gross steatorrhea is pathognomonic of small

TABLE 33-1. Localization of Diarrhea from History and Physical Examination

	Small Bowel	Large Bowel
Fecal volume	Increased	Decreased or normal
Frequency of defecation	Increased	Markedly increased
Tenesmus	Absent	Present
Blood in feces	Melena	Hematochezia
Mucus in feces	Absent or small amount	Large amount
Steatorrhea	Present in some	Absent
Associated signs	Vomiting	Less severe weight loss
	Marked weight loss	Dehydration
	Dehydration	

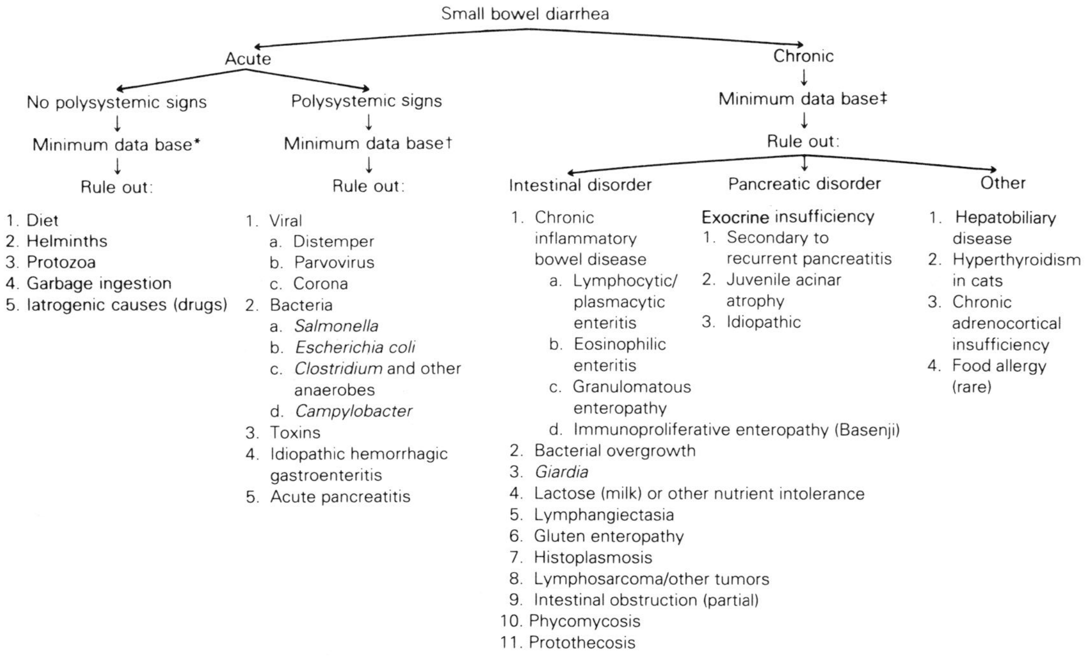

Small bowel diarrhea

Acute → Chronic

Acute:

No polysystemic signs → Minimum data base*

Rule out:
1. Diet
2. Helminths
3. Protozoa
4. Garbage ingestion
5. Iatrogenic causes (drugs)

Polysystemic signs → Minimum data base†

Rule out:
1. Viral
   a. Distemper
   b. Parvovirus
   c. Corona
2. Bacteria
   a. Salmonella
   b. Escherichia coli
   c. Clostridium and other anaerobes
   d. Campylobacter
3. Toxins
4. Idiopathic hemorrhagic gastroenteritis
5. Acute pancreatitis

Chronic: → Minimum data base‡

Rule out:

Intestinal disorder
1. Chronic inflammatory bowel disease
   a. Lymphocytic/plasmacytic enteritis
   b. Eosinophilic enteritis
   c. Granulomatous enteropathy
   d. Immunoproliferative enteropathy (Basenji)
2. Bacterial overgrowth
3. Giardia
4. Lactose (milk) or other nutrient intolerance
5. Lymphangiectasia
6. Gluten enteropathy
7. Histoplasmosis
8. Lymphosarcoma/other tumors
9. Intestinal obstruction (partial)
10. Phycomycosis
11. Protothecosis

Pancreatic disorder

Exocrine insufficiency
1. Secondary to recurrent pancreatitis
2. Juvenile acinar atrophy
3. Idiopathic

Other
1. Hepatobiliary disease
2. Hyperthyroidism in cats
3. Chronic adrenocortical insufficiency
4. Food allergy (rare)

* History, physical examination (thorough abdominal palpation), fecal flotation ×3, protozoal exam ×3
† As above plus CBC, urine analysis, biochemical profile, electrolytes, lipase, fecal culture ±
‡ As for acute small bowel diarrhea with polysystemic signs plus microscopic examination of feces for fat and starch, fecal trypsin, fat absorption (plasma turbidity) test, D-xylose absorption test, serum trypsin-like immunoreactivity, intestinal biopsies (endoscopy or celiotomy)

FIGURE 33-1. Initial diagnostic plan for small bowel diarrhea.

277

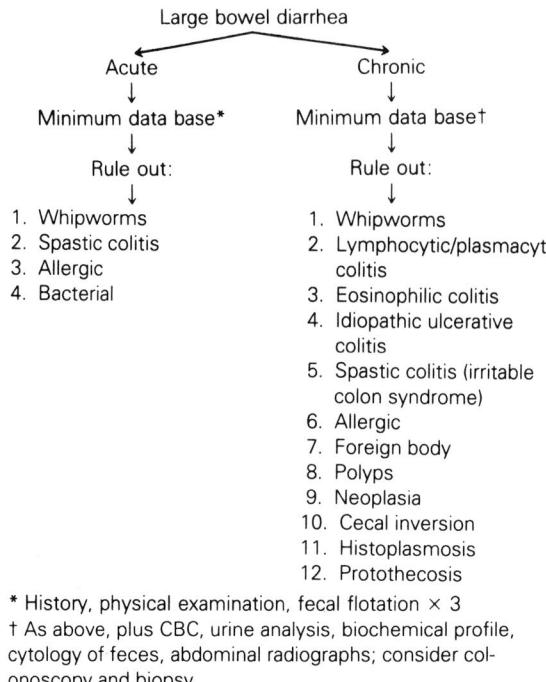

Large bowel diarrhea

Acute → Chronic

Acute
↓
Minimum data base*
↓
Rule out:
↓
1. Whipworms
2. Spastic colitis
3. Allergic
4. Bacterial

Chronic
↓
Minimum data base†
↓
Rule out:
↓
1. Whipworms
2. Lymphocytic/plasmacytic colitis
3. Eosinophilic colitis
4. Idiopathic ulcerative colitis
5. Spastic colitis (irritable colon syndrome)
6. Allergic
7. Foreign body
8. Polyps
9. Neoplasia
10. Cecal inversion
11. Histoplasmosis
12. Protothecosis

* History, physical examination, fecal flotation × 3
† As above, plus CBC, urine analysis, biochemical profile, cytology of feces, abdominal radiographs; consider colonoscopy and biopsy

FIGURE 33-2. Initial diagnostic plan for large bowel diarrhea.

bowel disease or EPI. Large bowel diseases produce stools that are soft, semiformed, occasionally watery, and even excessively firm. The hallmark of large bowel disease is tenesmus, with fresh blood and mucus in the feces. In clinical disease states, signs of either small bowel or large bowel diarrhea may predominate, despite the fact that both segments are affected. The follow-up diagnostic plan depends on whether diarrhea is acute or chronic and on the particular diseases being considered (Figs. 33-1 and 33-2; Table 33-2).

REFERENCES

1. Moon HJ: Mechanisms in the pathogenesis of diarrhea: A review. J Am Vet Med Assoc 172:443–448, 1978
2. Pidgeon GL: Acute onset diarrhea. In Ford RB (ed): Clinical Signs and Diagnosis in Small Animal Practice, pp 437–451. New York, Churchill Livingstone, 1988
3. Sherding RG: Chronic diarrhea. In Ford RB (ed): Clinical Signs and Diagnosis in Small Animal Practice, pp 453–489. New York, Churchill Livingstone, 1988

TABLE 33-2. Characteristic Findings of Common Disorders Causing Diarrhea

Disease	Clinical Signs Other Than Diarrhea	Hematology	Biochemistry	Special Tests
Acute small bowel diarrhea				
Diet change or lactose intolerance	Few polysystemic signs Flatulence often present	Normal	Normal	None
Intestinal parasites	Melena Hematochezia Weight loss Dry hair coat "Unthrifty" appearance	May have regenerative anemia (hookworms, coccidia) Eosinophilia	May have ↓ plasma protein	Fecal flotation or sedimentation ×3
Garbage ingestion	Vomiting ± Few polysystemic signs	Normal	Normal	None
Bacterial enteritis *Salmonella*	Anorexia Depression progressing to signs of shock Fever progressing to subnormal temperature Dehydration Vomiting Melena Hematochezia Abdominal pain	↑ PCV and plasma protein Leukopenia with inappropriate left shift Toxic neutrophils Thrombocytopenia	↓ Albumin ± ↑ Globulin ↑ SAP ± ↓ Glucose ±	Fecal and blood cultures for *Salmonella*
Escherichia coli, Clostridium and other anaerobes	Anorexia Depression Fever Dehydration Vomiting Abdominal pain	Neutrophilic leukocytosis with left shift ↑ PCV and plasma protein	See *Salmonella.*	None

(continued)

279

TABLE 33-2. Characteristic Findings of Common Disorders Causing Diarrhea *(continued)*

Disease	Clinical Signs Other Than Diarrhea	Hematology	Biochemistry	Special Tests
Campylobacter	Those of *E. coli* and *Clostridium* + hematochezia and mucus in feces	See *E. coli.*	↑ Albumin and globulin	Fecal culture for *Campylobacter*
Viral enteritis Parvovirus in dogs	Anorexia Depression Vomiting Dehydration Abdominal pain Fever	Leukopenia (neutropenia with left shift)	Electrolytes variable	ELISA test on feces Electron-microscopy of feces
Panleukopenia in cats	See Parvovirus.	Leukopenia (neutropenia)	See Parvovirus.	None
Distemper	See Parvovirus. Nasoocular discharge Chorea Seizures Paresis Chorioretinitis	Neutrophilic leukocytosis with left shift ↑ PCV and plasma protein	↑ Albumin and globulin	Fluorescent antibody test on conjunctival smear
Toxin (*e.g.*, arsenic, thallium)	Anorexia Depression Vomiting Dehydration Abdominal pain Others depending on toxin	Leukocytosis (stress leukogram)	↑ Albumin and globulin ↑ BUN ↓ TCO$_2$	Analysis of vomitus, feces, urine for toxin
Idiopathic hemorrhagic gastroenteritis	Melena Vomiting Anorexia Depression progressing to signs of shock	Markedly ↑ PCV (60–80%) and plasma protein Leukocytosis (stress leukogram)	↑ BUN ↑ Albumin and globulin	None

Chronic small bowel diarrhea

Lymphocytic/plasmacytic enteritis	Vomiting Weight loss Variable appetite	Mild nonregenerative anemia ↓ Plasma protein	↓ Albumin and globulin ↓ Ca++	D-xylose absorption decreased Small bowel biopsies—infiltration with lymphocytes/plasma cells
Eosinophilic enteritis	Mild weight loss Sporadic vomiting Melena Hematochezia	Regenerative anemia ± Eosinophilia	↓ Albumin and globulin (blood loss) ±	Fecals negative for parasites Small bowel biopsies—infiltration with eosinophils Rapid response to glucocorticoids
Bacterial overgrowth	Weight loss Variable appetite Vomiting ±	Normal	Normal	Normal serum trypsin-like immunoreactivity (TLI) ↑ Serum folate ± ↓ Serum cobalamin ±
Lymphangiectasia	See lymphocytic/plasmacytic enteritis	As for lymphocytic/plasmacytic enteritis	↓ Albumin and globulin	Small bowel biopsies—dilated lymphatics
Small intestinal neoplasia (*e.g.*, lymphosarcoma)	Severe weight loss Variable appetite Sporadic vomiting	As for lymphocytic/plasmacytic enteritis	↓ Albumin and globulin Ca++ variable	Abdominal radiographs show thickened bowel loops Small bowel biopsies
Intestinal parasites (*e.g.*, giardiasis)	Light colored "cowflop" stools Mild weight loss	Normal	Normal	Direct smears of fresh diarrheal feces for motile trophozoites Fecal sedimentation ×3 for cysts Duodenal aspirates Therapeutic trial with metronidazole for 5–7 days

(continued)

281

TABLE 33-2. Characteristic Findings of Common Disorders Causing Diarrhea (*continued*)

Disease	Clinical Signs Other Than Diarrhea	Hematology	Biochemistry	Special Tests
Histoplasma enteritis	Severe weight loss Variable appetite Fever	Neutrophilic leukocytosis Eosinophilia ± Basophilia ± ↓ Plasma protein *Histoplasma* organisms in monocytes or bone marrow ±	↓ Albumin Globulin variable	Complement fixation titer Small bowel and mesenteric lymph node biopsies
Exocrine pancreatic insufficiency	Severe weight loss Ravenous appetite "Unthrifty" appearance Bulky, light, greasy feces	Mild nonregenerative anemia	Normal	Plasma turbidity test Negative 1–4 hours after fatty meal Positive 1–4 hours after fatty meal + pancreatic enzyme supplement ↓ Serum TLI ↑ Serum folate ± (bacterial overgrowth) ↓ Serum cobalamin ± (bacterial overgrowth)
Iatrogenic (antibiotic and antimotility drug abuse)	Mild weight loss Variable appetite	Normal	Normal	Stop all drug administration and feed bland diet for 1 week.

Acute large bowel diarrhea

Chronic large bowel diarrhea

Spastic (nervous colitis, irritable bowel syndrome)	Tenesmus Hematochezia Mucus in feces Nervous animal	Normal	Normal	Fecal negative for parasites Colonoscopy and colon biopsies normal
Whipworms	Hematochezia Mucus in feces Intermittent depression and abdominal pain	Eosinophilia ±	Normal	Fecal flotation ×3 (commonly negative) Response to anthelmintic therapy
Lymphocytic/plasmacytic colitis	Mucus in feces Hematochezia ± Tenesmus Mild weight loss Variable appetite	As for lymphocytic/plasmacytic enteritis	Usually normal	Colonoscopy and colon biopsies—infiltration with lymphocytes and plasma cells
Eosinophilic ulcerative colitis	Mild weight loss Sporadic vomiting Tenesmus Hematochezia Mucus in feces	Eosinophilia	Normal	Fecals negative for parasites Proctoscopy and colonic biopsies—infiltration with eosinophils
Histiocytic ulcerative colitis (granulomatous colitis)	Mostly in boxer dogs Weight loss may be severe. See Eosinophilic ulcerative colitis.	Nonregenerative anemia ±	Usually normal	Colonoscopy and colon biopsies—infiltration with PAS–positive macrophages
Idiopathic ulcerative colitis	See Eosinophilic ulcerative colitis.	Usually normal	Normal	Colonoscopy and colon biopsies

(continued)

TABLE 33-2. Characteristic Findings of Common Disorders Causing Diarrhea (*continued*)

Disease	Clinical Signs Other Than Diarrhea	Hematology	Biochemistry	Special Tests
Histoplasma colitis	Fever Depression Weight loss may be severe. See Eosinophilic ulcerative colitis.	See *Histoplasma* enteritis under Chronic small bowel diarrhea.	Normal	Colonoscopy and colon biopsies
Prototheca colitis	Fever Depression Severe weight loss Uveitis Tenesmus Hematochezia Mucus in feces	Neutrophilic leukocytosis with left shift	Normal	Examine rectal scrapings stained with Wright-Giemsa Colonoscopy with colonic biopsies
Rectal polyps	Tenesmus Hematochezia Mucus in feces Digitally palpable masses in rectum	Normal	Normal	Proctoscopy and rectal biopsies
Neoplasia	Variable weight loss Tenesmus Hematochezia Mucus in feces Palpable mass in colon or rectum	Normal	Normal	Colonoscopy and biopsies
Cecal inversion	See Neoplasia. Palpable mass in caudal abdomen ±	Normal	Normal	Survey abdominal radiographs followed by barium enema study

↓, decreased; ±, present or absent; PCV, packed cell volume; SAP, serum alkaline phosphatase; ELISA, enzyme-linked immunosorbent assay; ↑, increased; BUN, blood urea nitrogen; TCO_2, total carbon dioxide; PAS, periodic acid–Schiff

CHAPTER THIRTY-FOUR

Constipation

Michael D. Lorenz

PROBLEM DEFINITION AND RECOGNITION

Constipation is the infrequent or difficult passage of feces. Feces may be excessively hard, firm, or dry. Obstipation is intractable constipation and results in severe fecal impaction throughout the rectum and colon. Obstipated animals cannot eliminate the impacted fecal mass. Megacolon is a clinical disorder characterized by marked dilatation and hypomotility of the rectum and colon. Megacolon may cause obstipation and fecal impaction. In dogs and cats, the disorder is usually acquired; congential defects may cause megacolon in humans.

The clinical signs of constipation include tenesmus with little or no passage of feces. Defecation may be painful. The fecal mass can be palpated through the abdomen or by digital examination of the rectum.

PATHOPHYSIOLOGY

In dogs and cats, the colon absorbs water and electrolytes from ingesta passing from the small intestine. The colon stores fecal matter until it can be eliminated through the process of defecation. It is believed that the proximal half of the colon serves primarily an absorptive function, whereas the distal colon is more involved with storage. Rhythmic segmental contractions mix ingesta within the colon and increase the absorption of water and electrolytes. Segmental contractions thus tend to decrease the rate of movement of luminal contents through the colon. Occasionally, these contractions may weakly propel the fecal mass toward the rectum. The primary propulsive wave within the colon is a "mass movement." These movements occur only a few times each day and propel feces into the rectum, stimulating the desire to defecate.

When feces enter the rectum, a weak defecation reflex is stimulated. Distention of the rectal wall stimulates afferent signals that spread through the myenteric plexus to initiate mass movements in the descending colon and rectum. Neurologically coordinated relaxation of the anal sphincter allows the fecal column to pass through the anus. This intrinsic defecation reflex is enforced by a second reflex mediated via parasympathic nerves from the sacral spinal cord segments. This sacral reflex greatly enforces the strength of the colonic move-

Causes of Constipation

- Dietary
  - Foreign material
  - Hair
  - Bones
  - Rocks, sand
  - Low fiber
- Environment
  - Lack of exericse
  - Failure to provide adequate time
    and place for defecation
  - Dirty cat litter
- Colonic obstruction
  - Intraluminal
    - Foreign body
    - Neoplasia
    - Perineal hernia
  - Extraluminal
    - Healed fractured pelvis
    - Prostatic enlargement
    - Pelvic and perianal neoplasia

- Neurologic disease
  - Spinal cord disease L4–S3
  - Bilateral pelvic nerve injury
  - Idiopathic megacolon
- Perirectal pain
  - Anal sacculitis
  - Anal abscess
  - Perianal fistula
  - Anal stricture
  - Rectal foreign body
  - Pseudocoprostasis
- Metabolic and endocrine diseases
  - Hypothyroidism
  - Hyperparathyroidism
  - Pyrexia
  - Generalized debility
- Drug-induced
  - Anticholinergics
  - Antihistamines
  - Anticonvulsants
  - Barium sulfate
  - Opiates

ments and may allow complete evacuation of the colon. In house-trained pets, relaxation of the anal sphincter is voluntarily controlled by the cerebral cortex. Therefore, house-trained pets can inhibit the defecation reflex until they find an appropriate place.

Any condition or disease that promotes fecal stasis and increased water absorption may cause constipation (see Display, Causes of Constipation).[1] As feces are retained in the colon, they harden and dry due to water absorption. As the colon impacts with feces, the colonic wall is stretched and may develop irreversible degenerative changes. Megacolon may result from any disease that causes chronic constipation.

Idiopathic megacolon is a disease of unknown etiology that affects primarily adult dogs and cats. It is most likely a disease of altered myoneural function affecting the smooth muscle of the colon. Decreased motility causes chronic constipation, which causes further degeneration of the colonic wall. In this syndrome, there is no anatomic or inflammatory basis for the constipation. The perineal reflex is normal, and anal sphincter tone is usually good.

The sequelae of obstipation include weight loss, dehydration, anorexia, weakness, and depression. These signs have been ascribed to the absorption of toxins produced by colonic bacteria.[1] Paradoxic diarrhea may occur in some cases, perhaps due to hypersecretion by the colonic mucosa. The diarrheal feces can bypass the fecal impaction.

DIAGNOSTIC PLAN

The diagnotic plan for constipation is based on the cause. The diet, defecation habits, exercise patterns, drug therapy, and history of pelvic, lumbar, or coccygeal trauma should be recorded. The physical examination should emphasize palpation of the caudal abdomen, pelvis, tail, perianal tissue, prostate, and rectum. Neurologic examination with emphasis on the L4–S3 spinal cord segments should be performed. Survey radiographs of the abdomen and pelvis help establish the severity of fecal impaction and the presence of mechanical obstruction due to a fractured pelvis.

A complete blood count, urine analysis, and biochemical profile should be performed. These tests help evaluate the metabolic and endocrine status of the animal and also help evaluate the side effects of chronic constipation.

Colonoscopy and barium enema studies for the presence of intraluminal obstruction must be delayed until the constipation or fecal impaction is removed.

REFERENCE

1. Burrows CF: Diarrhea and constipation. In Ettinger SJ (ed): Textbook of Veterinary Internal Medicine, 2nd ed. Philadelphia, WB Saunders, 1983

CHAPTER THIRTY-FIVE

Flatulence

Michael D. Lorenz

PROBLEM DEFINITION AND RECOGNITION

Flatulence is distention of the stomach or the intestines with air or gases. Flatus is the gas expelled from a body opening. Ordinarily, the terms *flatus* and *flatulence* pertain to the expulsion of intestinal gas through the anus. The problem is easily recognized in house pets from the quantity or quality of gas expelled or by the constant rumbling noises created by gas movement in the intestines.

PHYSIOLOGY OF GAS PRODUCTION

Gas production or accumulation in the gastrointestinal tract is a normal physiologic event. Excessive production may not be indicative of any pathophysiologic event. However, in certain gastrointestinal diseases, the normal production of gas may be increased and excessive flatulence may result. Diagnostic plans and management are based on our current knowledge of intestinal gas production and composition.

Gas contained in the stomach is very similar to atmospheric air, whereas the composition of flatus is quite variable. Gastrointestinal gas comes from four primary sources: aerophagia (swallowed air), bacterial fermentation of substrates, diffusion of gas from the blood into the intestinal tract, and the reaction of acids with basic compounds in the upper intestinal tract. Generally, flatus contains mostly nitrogen (N_2) with far lesser quantities of hydrogen (H_2), carbon dioxide (CO_2), oxygen (O_2), and methane (CH_4). N_2 and, to a lesser extent, O_2 come from air swallowed into the intestinal tract. Since the concentrations of CO_2, CH_4, and H_2 in flatus are often greater than in atmospheric air, these gases are partially derived from other sources. CH_4 production by dogs and cats is thought to be very rare; 30% of the human population may be CH_4 producers.

In dogs, most of the H_2 and CO_2 in intestinal gas is produced by bacterial fermentation of nonabsorbable oligosaccharides, such as stachyose and raffinose. Soybeans contain large quantities of the nonabsorbable oligosaccharides. Production of H_2 and CO_2 is greatly increased in the intestinal tract of dogs fed a commercial diet high in soybean content.[1] The rapid growth of bacteria supporting this fermentation process is enhanced by diets high in soybean content.

289

The diffusion of gas from the bloodstream into the intestinal tract or the production of gas from acid-base reactions add only small amounts of gas to the total volume contained in the gastrointestinal tract. These reactions are not clinically important in small animals.

Diets that contain carbohydrates, such as the oligosaccharides in soybean meal, increase gas production. Diets high in fiber may cause poor carbohydrate digestion in the small intestine; thus, more of this fermentable substrate reaches the colon, where it is subject to bacterial fermentation. Diets that are low in fiber and easily digested produce less flatus than diets high in fiber, poorly digested carbohydrates, or fat. Diseases of the small bowel that cause maldigestion or malabsorption may cause flatulence, since increased amounts of carbohydrate are available for bacterial fermentation. Diseases that cause intestinal ileus, obstruction, or luminal stasis of ingesta may favor the rapid growth of fermenting bacteria such as clostridial species. The combined effects of luminal stasis and increased fermentation largely explain the gaseous distention of intestinal loops observed in these disorders.

The odor of flatus is attributed to minute quantities of ammonia, hydrogen sulfide, indole, skatole, volatile amines, and short-chain fatty acids. The major components of flatus are nonodorous.

DIAGNOSTIC PLAN

The presence of flatus is usually evident from the history. A thorough examination for other signs suggestive of digestive tract disease should be made (*e.g.*, vomiting, diarrhea, weight loss).

The owner should be questioned carefully concerning the patient's diet, eating habits, and bowel eliminations. Greedy eaters are subject to aerophagia and flatulence. Fecal retention or constipation may cause chronic flatulence. The diet should be closely inspected for the substrates that are potentially gas producers (*e.g.*, soybean meal, high fiber content).

If specific signs of digestive system disease are present, intestinal parasitism and malassimilation syndromes should be considered. The feces must be inspected for mucus, blood, fat, volume, and consistency. Microscopic examinations for parasites, fat droplets, muscle fibers, starch, and blood cells should be made. Rarely, dietary allergy may cause diarrhea and flatulence. A trial of hypoallergenic food is given for 2 to 3 weeks when dietary allergy is suspected. Diets containing large amounts of lactose may cause flatulence, especially in cats and puppies. In cats, hyperthyroidism may cause maldigestion, steatorrhea, and flatulence. Signs of restlessness, hyperactivity, weight loss, and polyphagia are usually apparent.

REFERENCE

1. Richards EA et al: Relationship of bean substrates and certain intestinal bacteria to gas production in the dog. Gastroenterology 55:502–509, 1968

CHAPTER THIRTY-SIX

Abdominal Pain

Laine A. Cowan

Abdominal pain may be the chief presenting complaint of the pet owner or, more frequently, may require a thorough history and physical examination by the veterinarian for detection. A painful abdomen may be the only indication of inflammation or organ dysfunction; hence, it is an important (though non-specific) finding.

Extraabdominal pain may mimic abdominal pain (Table 36-1). This may be due to the animal's similar response to pain (reluctance to move, anorexia, hiding behavior) in other locations.

Based on the tissue of origin and characteristics of the pain, abdominal pain can be subdivided into true visceral pain, deep somatic pain, and referred pain. In visceral pain, the abdominal organs, excluding the peritoneum, are the source of the noxious stimuli. Deep somatic pain, on the other hand, arises from the parietal peritoneum or the mesentery. Referred pain occurs when the stimuli is perceived as if it were coming from a site distant from the actual stimuli; it may accompany deep somatic or visceral pain.

PATHOPHYSIOLOGY

Abdominal pain usually is due to one of five basic mechanisms: (1) distention of a hollow viscus, (2) traction on the peritoneum or mesentery, (3) ischemia, (4) smooth muscle spasm, or (5) inflammation. Much less frequently, pain may be secondary to direct invasion of afferent neurons by a neoplasm[1] or by another infiltrative disease. In addition to the underlying etiology, inflammation or a decreased blood supply[6] may alter the pain by lowering the pain threshold (see Chapter 46).

The abdominal viscera are sparsely innervated and have no specific pain receptors. The low density of pain fibers may contribute to the poor localization of visceral pain.[1,4] Since localized visceral stimuli rarely cause pain, the presence of visceral pain usually is indicative of diffuse disease. This type of pain may be aggravated by movement (which causes torsion or tension on the peritoneum).

As detailed in Chapter 46, the sensory neurons from the viscera reach the spinal cord via splanchnic nerves, the pelvic nerve, and the mesenteric plexii and then travel in the lateral spinothalamic tract to the cerebral cortex.[6] In

TABLE 36-1. Conditions That May Mimic Abdominal Pain

Mimicking Condition	Basis for Differentiation from Abdominal Pain
Pleuritis	Auscultation of thorax, shallow respirations, thoracic radiographs
Severe pneumonia	Auscultation of thorax, thoracic radiographs
Spinal or paraspinal pain	Neurologic examination, careful digital palpation along the vertebrae, spinal radiographs, analysis of cerebral spinal fluid
Polyarthritis	Palpation, arthrocentesis, radiographs
Apprehensive patient	History, reevaluate without owner present
Myositis	Palpation, muscle enzymes, muscle biopsy
Vasculitis	Edema, hemorrhage, thrombocytopenia, vessel biopsy

humans, this type of pain tends to be a dull aching pain, and frequently, is felt at the skin surface. One explanation for the latter phenomenon is that visceral pain fibers, once in the spinal cord, utilize some of the same interneurons as skin pain fibers. This results in an animal feeling pain as if it were originating in the skin.[4] In solid viscera, pain commonly is due to a rapid stretching of the organ capsules.

The parietal peritoneum is innervated by spinal nerves; the afferents travel in the cerebrospinal pathways. Noxious stimuli to the parietal peritoneum or mesentery cause deep somatic pain. In humans, disease of the parietal peritoneum results in a very sharp, intense pain.[1,4]

Rigidity of the abdominal muscles is frequently associated with abdominal wall involvement or with deep abdominal pain. This abdominal splinting is due to a reflex of sustained muscle contraction. The prolonged muscle contraction and the resulting decreased blood supply to the muscles also may contribute to abdominal tenderness. Pain from hollow viscera, on the other hand, may not elicit the abdominal wall reflex.[8]

Specific Organs

See Table 36-2 for a list of diagnoses of abdominal pain caused by specific organ disorders.

Stomach. Gastritis, ulcers, dilatation-volvulus, and perforation may cause abdominal pain. Excluding the noxious stimuli of chemical irritation (ulcer) or distention, most gastric pain is due to muscular spasm, which results in decreased organ perfusion.[1] Gastric pain tends to localize in the cranial abdomen.

Intestine. Small intestinal pain is better localized than that in the large bowel.[6] The most common stimulus for pain in this organ is bowel distention. Enteroviruses may cause pain also, but usually it is of less severity. It may or may not be possible to localize pain in a specific region.

Pancreas. Pancreatic pain is multifactorial but its pathogenesis includes hypertension in the pancreatic duct and interstitium,[5] inflammation, and vascular spasms which cause ischemia. Cranial abdominal pain is one of the hallmarks of acute pancreatitis.

Hepatic and Biliary System. Hepatic pain is due to rapid distention of the liver, resulting in stretching of the liver capsule. Bile duct and gall bladder distention are noxious stimuli but are uncommon in the dog and the cat. In humans, hepatic pain is referred to the right scapular margin.[4] No such precise referral regions are reported in veterinary medicine.

Urinary Tract. Distention is the main cause of pain in the urinary tract. Acute renal parenchymal distention may occur in acute renal failure or in acute obstruction of urine flow. The resulting capsular stretching is the noxious stimulus. Renal pain may be referred to the paraspinal muscles ("flank pain"), but paraspinal pain is not recognized routinely in veterinary species with renal disease. Ureteral pain can be produced by the muscular spasms[3] occurring following a rapid increase in lumenal pressure and reflex peristalsis. In the urinary bladder, overdistention, irritation of the mucosa,[7] and subsequent muscular spasms are noxious stimuli.

In the prostate gland the parenchyma and the surrounding capsule are innervated.[2] Whether pain originates in the parenchyma or is secondary to stretch of the capsule is unknown.

DIAGNOSIS

Signalment

Younger animals tend to acquire more infectious diseases, more dietary indiscretion, and fewer malignancies in general than a similar older pet. Large dogs with deep chests may be predisposed to gastric dilatation, female miniature schnauzers may be predisposed to pancreatitis. Similar breed and sex predispositions occur for many abdominal disease syndromes.

History

The owner may notice trembling, reluctance to move, inappetence, crying, or abnormal posture, which may suggest that the animal is experiencing pain. An animal with peritonitis may refuse to move and have shallow respirations in an attempt to minimize peritoneal movement. Some animals assume specific postures in an attempt to relieve some of the discomfort. This is known as the "position of relief." The praying posture (extended outstretched forelimbs, normal standing position of hindlimbs, with head and neck resting on the forelimbs) has been described in dogs with abdominal pain.[9]

TABLE 36-2. Diagnosis of Abdominal Pain Caused by Disorder of Specific Organ

Organ	Location of Pain	Additional Clues to Suggest This Organ	Ancillary Diagnostic Tests	Commonly Associated Disease Processes (Less Common)
Pancreas	Cranial abdomen	Obese, high fat diet, vomiting, diarrhea, diabetes mellitus	Amylase, lipase, trypsinogen-like immunoreactivity, sonographic examination	Acute pancreatitis (Neoplasia)
Stomach	Cranial abdomen	Abdominal distention, vomiting, hematemesis, melena	Upper GI contrast studies, endoscopy, fecal occult blood	Dilatation/volvulus Nonspecific inflammation Gastric ulcer (Foreign body) (Toxin) (Neoplasia)
Small intestine	Midabdomen variable, diffuse	Vomiting, diarrhea, melena, history of garbage ingestion or inadequate vaccination	Endoscopy, serum folate and cobalamin, upper GI contrast studies, sonographic evaluation, rectal scraping	Fungal, bacterial, or viral infection Foreign body Parasites Intussusception (Neoplasia) (Toxin) (Torsion)
Large intestine	Middle to caudal abdomen	Tenesmus, diarrhea, mucus, hematochezia, constipation	Protoscopy, rectal scraping, barium enema	Inflammation Parasites (Obstruction) (Neoplasia) (Foreign body)
Liver	Cranial abdomen	Icterus, coagulopathy	Bilirubin (serum), bile acids (ammonia tolerance test), coagulo-	Idiopathic Infection (fungal, bacterial, viral)

Structure	Location	Clinical signs	Diagnostic procedures	Conditions
			gram, sonographic evaluation, biopsy	(Congestion) (Neoplasia) (Trauma)
Spleen	Cranial to midabdomen	Circulating nucleated red blood cells	Ultrasonography, cytologic examination of fine-needle aspirate	Neoplasia (Infection) (Torsion)
Kidneys/ureters	Cranial dorsal (canine) to midabdomen (feline)	Uremia, oliguria/anuria, polyuria, hematuria, pyuria	Urine analysis and culture Excretory urogram, sonographic evaluation, renal biopsy, angiogram	Infection Acute renal failure due to: Toxin Obstruction (Vascular) (Trauma)
Urinary bladder	Caudal abdomen	Anuria, stranguria, pollakiuria, hematuria, pyuria	Urine analysis, urine culture, cystogram, sonographic examination, cystoscopy	Infection Calculi Neoplasia Inflammation
Ovaries/uterus	Cranial dorsal to caudal abdomen	Estrous cycle, vaginal discharge, polyuria, polydipsia	Sonographic vaginal examination Vaginal cytology	Pyometra Endometritis (Granuloma) (Neoplasia)
Testicles	Variable if not descended—cranial dorsal to caudal abdomen	Cryptorchid	Sonographic, radiographic evaluation of abdomen	Neoplasia (Torsion) (Abscess) (Granuloma)
Prostate gland	Caudal abdomen	Tenesmus, urethral discharge, recurrent urinary tract infections	Cytology and culture of prostatic fluid (semen, prostatic massage, brush), sonographic examination, urethrocystogram, biopsy	Infection Abscess (Cyst) (Neoplasia)

GI, gastrointestinal

The owner should be questioned about the animal's environment and any history of emesis, diarrhea, melena, hematochezia, polyuria, dysuria, or other problems. Possible exposures to infectious diseases, toxins, or dietary indiscretions must be ascertained.

Duration, intensity, and the time sequence of the pain may be helpful. Unfortunately, even the most astute veterinarian may have difficulty in thorough characterization of the pain, due to its subjective nature and the lack of communicative ability of pets.

Physical Examination

A goal of a physical examination in a pet with apparent abdominal pain is to exclude the extraabdominal disorders that mimic abdominal pain (see Table 36-1). Once the problem is localized to the abdomen, the pain should be regionalized as specifically as possible. Dividing the abdomen into cranial, middle, and caudal regions may be helpful in determining the origin of the pain (Table 36-3). Not all pain, however, can be localized into just one region. Diffuse pain is seen with generalized peritonitis due to any cause. Sedation or analgesics may aid in palpation of the patient with a tender abdomen.

Findings that suggest abdominal pain include the animal crying out when lifted on to the examination table and splinting of the abdominal musculature during gentle palpation in a calm animal. Nonspecific findings such as body condition may suggest the nature of the disease process (*e.g.*, obesity may attend pancreatitis in the animal with the appropriate signalment; an animal with a chronic systemic disease process such as neoplasia may be emaciated). The presence of gas- or fluid-filled bowel loops, foreign bodies, intussusception, organomegaly, abdominal masses, organ displacement, lymphadenopathy, and ascites need to be specifically assessed during the physical examination. The abdominal examination must be complete (including a digital rectal palpation), and the extra-abdominal evaluation is essential.

Tests

The appropriate laboratory tests are dependent on the acuteness, severity, and localization of the pain (see Table 36-2). Other physical examination or historical findings also will influence the choice of tests. Acute, mild discomfort may only warrant observation of the pet initially. On the other hand, any severe or chronic pain of undetermined or unlocalized cause necessitates a complete blood count, chemistry profile (including BUN, creatinine, alanine aminotransferase, alkaline phosphatase, albumin, total protein, calcium, sodium, and potassium), and urine analysis. These laboratory test results will help rule out generalized inflammatory, infectious, and systemic disease processes. Abdominal radiographs may be of low yield if the abdominal palpation was unremarkable. However, even in those cases, radiographs can help confirm extravisceral

TABLE 36-3. Detection of Origin of Pain by Location in the Abdomen

Dorsocranial	Ventrocranial	Midabdomen	Caudal
Adrenals	Gallbladder	Intestines	Colon
Kidneys	Liver	Kidney	Lymph nodes
Liver	Pancreas	left (and right)	Prostate
Lymph nodes	Spleen	Lymph nodes	Testicle
Ovaries	Stomach	Ovaries (cat)	(retained)
Spleen		Spleen	Urinary bladder
Stomach		Testicle (retained)	Uterus
Testicle (retained)		Uterus	

diseases such as a small peritoneal effusion or diskospondylitis. Radiographs also are indicated when an abnormality was detected during palpation, or when a thorough palpation is impossible due to the pain elicited. Ancillary tests may include diagnostic peritoneal lavage, abdominal ultrasonographic evaluation, and more specific laboratory tests or diagnostic procedures (see Table 36-2).

REFERENCES

1. Asch D: Abdominal pain. In Blacklow RS (ed): MacBryde's Signs and Symptoms, 6th ed, pp 165–179. Philadelphia, JB Lippincott, 1983
2. Blacklock WJ: Surgical anatomy. In Chisholm GD, Williams DI (eds): Scientific Foundations of Urology, 2nd ed, pp 473–485. Chicago, Year Book Medical Publishers, 1983
3. Carlton CE: Initial evaluation including history, physical exam, and urinalysis. In Harrison JH, Gettes RF, Perlmutter A, et al (eds): Campbell's Urology, 4th ed, pp 203–221. Philadelphia, WB Saunders, 1978
4. Guyton AC: Somatic sensations: II. Pain, visceral pain, headache, and thermal sensations. In Guyton AC (ed): Textbook of Medical Physiology, 7th ed, pp 592–605. Philadelphia, WB Saunders, 1986
5. Karanjia ND, Reber HA: The cause and management of pain of chronic pancreatitis. Gastroent Clin N Amer 19:895–904, 1990
6. Menaker GJ: The physiology and mechanism of acute abdominal pain. Surg Clin North Am 42:241–248, 1962
7. Perlmutter AD, Blacklow R: Urinary tract pain. In Blacklow RS (ed): MacBryde's Signs and Symptoms, 6th ed, pp 181–194. Philadelphia, JB Lippincott, 1983
8. Ruch: Pathophysiology of pain. In Ruch TC, Patton HD, Woodbury JW, Towe AL (eds): Neurophysiology, 2nd ed, pp 345–363. Philadelphia, WB Saunders, 1965
9. Thrall DE, Bovee KC, Biery DN: Demonstration of a "position of relief" in dogs with lesions of the stomach or small bowel. J Am Anim Hosp Assoc 14:343–347, 1978

CHAPTER THIRTY-SEVEN

Icterus

Larry M. Cornelius

PROBLEM DEFINITION AND RECOGNITION

Icterus is a syndrome characterized by hyperbilirubinemia and deposition of bile pigment in tissues, including the skin and mucous membranes.

PATHOPHYSIOLOGY

Approximately 70% of bilirubin is derived from the death of senescent erythrocytes in reticuloendothelial cells, mainly in the spleen and liver; another 10% is derived from ineffective erythropoiesis in the bone marrow.[2] Most of the remaining bilirubin is derived from hepatic cytochromes, catalase, peroxidase, and myoglobin. Bilirubin is the only major breakdown product of heme that requires excretion. The protein and iron components of the heme molecule enter the body pool and are reused.

Newly formed unconjugated bilirubin is insoluble in water and bound to circulating albumin. In addition to allowing transport of bilirubin via the blood to the liver, binding prevents diffusion of the large bilirubin-albumin complex across cell membranes and thus tends to retain bilirubin in the vascular space. In humans, the plasma-binding capacity of albumin is about 20 to 25 mg bilirubin per deciliter.[1,10] Beyond this capacity, or if binding capacity is reduced, unbound bilirubin may cross cell membranes and enter tissues. Central nervous system toxicity termed *kernicterus* occurs in neonates whenever unconjugated bilirubin crosses the blood-brain barrier, but toxic effects in older patients are unknown. Bilirubin-binding capacity of albumin may be reduced by (1) decreased plasma albumin, (2) decreased binding sites on the albumin molecule caused by competition for sites by drugs (*e.g.,* sulfonamides or salicylates), and (3) decreased affinity of albumin for bilirubin, caused by acidosis.[1]

Bilirubin dissociates from albumin before entering the liver cell.[2] A carrier mechanism has been postulated but is unproven. The flow of bilirubin between plasma and liver is bidirectional, with approximately one-third of the unconjugated bilirubin that enters the liver cell ultimately returning unaltered to the plasma. Hepatic uptake of unconjugated bilirubin is apparently unaffected by severe impairment of hepatic conjugation or excretion of bilirubin.[2] Hepatic uptake of bilirubin is not affected by bile acids. Once inside the hepatocyte, specific proteins termed Y (or ligandin) and Z bind bilirubin. These proteins also bind other anions, such as drugs and steroids.[3]

Hepatic conjugation of bilirubin with glucuronic acid to form bilirubin monoglucuronide and diglucuronide is catalyzed by the enzyme glucuronyl transferase. The importance of conjugation is that bilirubin is transformed from a lipid-soluble to a water-soluble compound. Water solubility is mandatory for excretion of bilirubin in the urine. Lipid insolubility limits back-diffusion of bilirubin into hepatocytes and reabsorption from the intestine, causing it to be excreted through bile into the feces.

Conjugated bilirubin is excreted from the liver cell into the bile canaliculus by a system that appears to have the properties of active, carrier-mediated transport. The transport mechanism involved is different from that for hepatocellular secretion of bile salts. Hepatic excretion of conjugated bilirubin is the rate-limiting step in the overall capacity of the liver to move bilirubin from blood to bile. In contrast to uptake and conjugation, which are well preserved in the presence of hepatocellular injury, the excretory transport system is very sensitive to various types of liver damage. Hence, an increase in plasma conjugated bilirubin occurs early in the course of hepatocellular injury. However, total plasma bilirubin concentration may not increase until later in dogs with hepatocellular injury, because dogs have a low renal threshold for conjugated bilirubin, and significant bilirubinuria occurs soon after hepatocellular injury. Trace to 1 + amounts of conjugated bilirubin may also appear in the urine of normal dogs, especially in concentrated urine samples. In cats, the renal threshold for bilirubin is significantly higher. Bilirubinuria in cats is nearly always pathologic, indicating either cholestasis or hepatocellular damage.[8]

The bacteria of the lower intestinal tract reduce most of the conjugated bilirubin to a group of chromagens termed *urobilinogen*. Much of the urobilinogen is excreted in the feces, but some is reaborbed from the colon and carried via portal blood back to the liver. Most urobilinogen is subsequently reexcreted into bile, but a small amount may gain entrance to systemic circulation and be excreted in the urine.

Hyperbilirubinemia and Cholestasis

Bilirubin uptake, conjugation, and excretion are controlled by hepatocellular mechanisms that are separate from the conjugation and excretion of bile acids.[2] Disturbances in bilirubin transport are recognized by hyperbilirubinemia and icterus. Cholestatic syndromes (reduced bile flow) are characterized by marked bile acidemia, usually with normal to slightly elevated bilirubin levels. Severe cholestasis can, however, cause icterus. Measurement of serum bile acids is a reliable procedure for the detection of cholestasis and is also a sensitive test of hepatic function. Increased serum alkaline phosphatase and gamma glutamyl transpeptidase (GGT) activities also result from cholestasis.

Hyperbilirubinemia may be caused by increases in unconjugated or conjugated bilirubin in plasma. The van den Bergh test is sometimes used to fractionate plasma bilirubin into indirect (unconjugated) and direct (conjugated) reacting bilirubin. This test is of value only when total serum bilirubin is increased (greater than 1.0 mg/dl). One can generally observe a yellow color of plasma in a microhematocrit tube when total plasma bilirubin is increased. Other diagnostic procedures are now available that are more useful for distinguishing the different causes of icterus (see Diagnostic Plan below).

Unconjugated Hyperbilirubinemia. Increased plasma unconjugated bilirubin can result from increased pigment production (hemolysis or ineffective erythropoiesis) or impaired hepatic uptake or conjugation of bilirubin. Increased pigment production (hemolysis) probably accounts for most instances of unconjugated hyperbilirubinemia in icteric dogs and cats and is termed *prehepatic* icterus. The liver normally has a large reserve capacity for uptake, conjugation, and excretion of bilirubin (30 to 60 times basal rate[3]). It has been shown in humans that a plasma unconjugated bilirubin concentration in excess of 4 mg/dl suggests reduced hepatic bilirubin clearance (due to liver disease) irrespective of the presence or absence of hemolysis.[2] In hemolytic icterus, hyperbilirubinemia is initially characterized by a preponderance of unconjugated bilirubin. Three to 4 days after the hemolytic crisis, however, the plasma conjugated bilirubin concentration may equal or exceed unconjugated bilirubin (total serum bilirubin still being increased, although less than during the hemolytic crisis). Therefore, at certain stages of hemolytic icterus, relative concentrations of conjugated and unconjugated bilirubin may overlap those observed in hepatocellular disease and biliary obstruction. Although the process is incompletely understood, it has been suggested that increases in conjugated bilirubin later in hemolytic icterus may be due to compromise of the excretory system of a previously normal liver injured by anemic anoxia.[7] In this situation, it is assumed that hepatocellular uptake and conjugation of bilirubin remain relatively normal; the lack of excretion would lead to regurgitation from the hepatocyte into blood. Another possible explanation is that excessive hepatocellular production of conjugated bilirubin causes bile inspissation; this would result in intrahepatic biliary obstruction and regurgitation of conjugated bilirubin into blood.[7] It is doubtful that serum alkaline phosphatase activity would help differentiate these two possible mechanisms, since it takes 7 to 8 days of total biliary obstruction to produce maximum increases of serum alkaline phosphatase.[12] Patients with hemolytic icterus would be expected to have anemia characterized by signs of regeneration (reticulocytosis, anisocytosis, or poikilocytosis), provided that the bone marrow is functional and 3 to 5 days have elapsed since the hemolytic crisis. If hemolysis occurs intravascularly (rather than extravascularly in reticuloendothelial cells) and is sufficiently rapid, the plasma may be red because of the presence of increased amounts of free hemoglobin. Normally, a plasma protein termed *haptoglobin* binds the free circulating hemoglobin and prevents it from entering the urine. With rapid, massive hemolysis, all haptoglobin may be saturated with hemoglobin; the unbound hemoglobin is filtered by the glomerulus and appears in the urine, where it causes the urine to be red (port-wine colored). Few or no intact erythrocytes are present in the urine to account for the red color and strongly positive occult blood test results. One would not expect significant increases in serum levels of leaked enzymes (alanine aminotransferase [ALT]) or overproduced enzymes (alkaline phosphatases, GGT) in hemolytic disease. It is conceivable, however, that anemic anoxia might cause hepatocellular membrane damage and increases in serum ALT. It is possible that biliary obstruction due to bile inspissation, as previously mentioned, could eventually cause increases in serum alkaline phosphatase.

Conjugated Hyperbilirubinemia. Hepatocellular disease and biliary obstruction (intrahepatic or posthepatic) may result in an increase in plasma conjugated and unconjugated bilirubin, with the former predominating. It is not usually possible to distinguish icterus caused by hepatic disease from jaundice due to posthepatic biliary obstruction on the basis of laboratory data. Ongoing hepatocellular disease is often associated with marked increases in serum ALT. Other laboratory abnormalities that may be present with severe hepatic dysfunction include decreased serum concentrations of urea nitrogen, albumin, and glucose and increased serum bile acid and plasma ammonia levels. Conjugated bilirubin appears in the urine in increased amounts.

Studies in people,[13] rats,[6] and dogs[9] with chronic cholestatic icterus (hepatic or posthepatic causes) have proved the existence of a conjugated bilirubin fraction tightly bound (covalent binding) to albumin ("biliprotein" complexes). Since this albumin-bound conjugated bilirubin fraction is a large molecule and cannot be excreted in the urine, its elimination from the body is determined by the half-life of albumin (12 to 14 days). This results in a delay in clearance of circulating bilirubin and may explain why icterus persists in some patients after an improvement in hepatic function and a disappearance of bilirubin from the urine.[12,13] Since routine laboratory procedures for measuring plasma bilirubin do not separate covalently bound from noncovalently bound bilirubin, it is not accurate to assess the course of cholestatic jaundice by periodically measuring plasma bilirubin.[12] Biliproteins are generally low or not present in hemolytic jaundice.[12] The significance of biliproteins in cats is unknown.

Biliary obstruction is characterized by marked increases in serum alkaline phosphatase and GGT activities as a result of induction of synthesis of large amounts of alkaline phosphatase and GGT by hepatocytes and biliary epithelial cells.

Hepatocellular disease and partial biliary obstruction (usually intrahepatic) frequently coexist in patients with liver disease. Bacterial sepsis and endotoxemia may cause impaired hepatic secretion of conjugated bilirubin and decreased bile flow. Increased serum alkaline phosphatase activity and conjugated hyperbilirubinemia may result.[11]

Cholestasis. Cholestasis refers to decreased bile flow and is characterized by increased serum bile acid levels and alkaline phosphatase and GGT activities and, in more severe cases, by hyperbilirubinemia.[2] Causes of cholestasis include partial or complete biliary obstruction and drug administration. Drugs thought to cause cholestasis in dogs include corticosteroids and anticonvulsants (diphenylhydantoin [Dilantin], phenobarbital, and primidone). Their mechanisms have not been completely worked out, although it is known that corticosteroids induce a characteristic hepatopathy in most dogs, characterized by hepatocellular swelling due to accumulation of glycogen and water. Cholestasis probably results from intrahepatic partial biliary obstruction caused by diffuse swelling of hepatocytes.

DIAGNOSTIC PLAN

History and Physical Examination

Initially, one should make efforts to categorize icterus by cause as hemolytic (*prehepatic*), hepatocellular (*hepatic*), or obstructive (*posthepatic*), keeping in mind that combinations of these basic causes frequently occur in clinical disease states.[4] History and physical examination may sometimes suggest one of these categories, but laboratory evaluation is usually necessary (Table 37-1).

Laboratory Evaluation

Suggested initial laboratory tests include a complete blood count (CBC), reticulocyte count if anemia is present, platelet count, microfilaria check in dogs, urine analysis, and a biochemical panel including blood urea nitrogen (BUN), creatinine, total protein, albumin, glucose, total bilirubin, electrolytes (sodium, potassium, chloride, total CO_2, calcium) and a fecal examination for blood (Table 37-1).

Follow-up diagnostic plans for an icteric dog or cat depend upon which category or categories are suspected after results of initial tests are received (Tables 37-2, 37-3, and 37-4). With hemolytic icterus, a more in-depth history for toxin or drug ingestion is indicated. Careful examination for blood parasites should be done, as well as a Coombs' test, lupus erythematosus (LE) preparation, and antinuclear antibody titer if autoimmune disease is suspected.

Other Diagnostic Procedures

For hepatic disease, abdominal radiographs and sonograms are usually indicated. Serum bile acids (pre- and postprandial) and plasma ammonia, or the ammonia tolerance test, can be used to evaluate liver function. It is often helpful to repeat the CBC, serum biochemical analysis, and urine analysis to monitor the progress of hepatic disease.[5] If either no improvement or actual deterioration

TABLE 37-1. Initial Plan for Diagnosis of Icterus in Dogs and Cats

Data Base	Rule Out*	Most Common Findings
History (Hx), physical examination (PE), CBC, reticulocyte count, platelet count, microfilaria check (dogs only), urine analysis, biochemical profile including BUN, creatinine, ALT, SAP, total protein, albumin, glucose, total bilirubin, conjugated and unconjugated bilirubin ±, electrolytes (sodium potassium, chloride, TCO$_2$, calcium)	Prehepatic (hemolytic)	Hx and PE: Sudden onset of weakness and exercise intolerance, pale mucous membranes with slight yellow tinge, holosystolic mitral murmur common (anemic) Lab: PCV < 15, ↑ reticulocytes and NRBCs if 3–4 days since onset, WBC variable, slightly ↑ urine bilirubin, increased total bilirubin with >50% unconjugated (3–4 days after onset may have >50% conjugated), ALT normal or slightly ↑ (2–5× normal), rest of data base normal
	Hepatic	Hx and PE: Lethargy, anorexia, vomiting, diarrhea, dehydration, mild to marked icterus Lab: PCV normal or ↑, WBC variable, moderately to markedly ↑ urine bilirubin, increased total bilirubin with >50% conjugated, ALT moderately to markedly ↑ (5–50 times normal), SAP mildly to moderately ↑ (2–10× normal—dog, 2–5× normal—cat), total protein variable, albumin normal or ↓, globulin normal or ↑, BUN normal or ↓
	Posthepatic (obstructive)	Hx and PE: Mild to moderate lethargy, variable appetite, occasional vomiting and weight loss, mild to marked icterus Lab: PCV normal, WBC variable, moderately to markedly ↑ urine bilirubin, ↑ total bilirubin with >50% conjugated, ALT mildly to moderately ↑ (2–10× normal), SAP moderately to markedly ↑ (5–100× normal—dog, 5–15× normal—cat), rest of data base variable

*Combinations of these three basic types of icterus are frequently present in clinical cases. CBC, complete blood count; BUN, blood urea nitrogen; ALT, alanine aminotransferase; SAP, serum alkaline phosphatase; ±, present or absent; TCO$_2$, total carbon dioxide; PCV, packed cell volume; ↑, increased; ↓, decreased; lab, laboratory; NRBCs, nucleated red blood cells.

(Cornelius LM: Icterus. In Proceedings of the 49th Annual Meeting of the American Animal Hospital Association, 1982)

TABLE 37-2. Follow-up Plan for Icterus in Dogs and Cats

Rule Out	Data Base*
Prehepatic (hemolytic)	Further history, blood parasite check, Coombs' test, antinuclear antibody, blood cultures ±
Hepatic	Abdominal radiographs and sonograms, repeat biochemistry profile, serum bile acids (pre- and postprandial), plasma ammonia and ammonia tolerance test, serum amylase/lipase ±, feline leukemia virus test (cats only); consider blood cultures, biopsy liver (coagulogram first) by laparoscopy, sonographically guided needle, or celiotomy
Posthepatic (obstructive)	Abdominal radiographs and sonograms, repeat biochemistry profile, serum amylase/lipase ±, consider exploratory celiotomy

*May repeat all or part of initial data base (see Table 37-1)

(Cornelius, LM: Icterus. In Proceedings of the 49th Annual Meeting of the American Animal Hospital Association, 1982)

in clinical appearance or laboratory data is observed, liver biopsy is indicated. If the liver is noticeably enlarged, percutaneous needle biopsy (fine-needle aspiration with a 22-gauge, 1-inch needle or biopsy with a Vim tru-cut–type needle) is easy and relatively safe. If the liver is of normal or small size, biopsy via laparoscopy or celiotomy is preferred. Ultrasonography allows evaluation of liver size and consistency and permits accurate placement of the percutaneous biopsy needle. All liver biopsy procedures should be preceded by laboratory evaluation of clotting and a platelet count.

Follow-up plans for icterus due to suspected posthepatic biliary obstruction are similar to those discussed for hepatic disease. It is safer to perform biopsy via laparoscopy or celiotomy rather than risk bile peritonitis from puncture of a distended gallbladder or bile duct during blind percutaneous liver biopsy with a needle. Sonographic guidance of a percutaneous biopsy needle is also reasonably safe.

TABLE 37-3. Selected Causes of Icterus in Dogs and Associated Findings

Cause	History	Physical Examination	Laboratory Data
Prehepatic (hemolytic)*			
Autoimmune hemolytic anemia	Sudden onset of severe weakness and possible collapse in an adult dog	Very pale mucous membranes; icterus mild, when present; weakness, tachycardia, holosystolic murmur (anemic), splenomegaly	Severe anemia (PCV < 15) that is regenerative provided 3–4 days have elapsed since onset of hemolysis; leukocytosis with neutrophilia and left shift; spherocytes common; autoagglutination of erythrocytes possibly present, most Coombs' positive
Heartworm disease—postcaval syndrome	Sudden onset of weakness and collapse	Signs of shock; icterus mild to moderate; possibly evidence of impaired coagulation due to DIC (*e.g.*, petechiae, ecchymoses, melena)	May be positive or negative for microflariae; often positive on ELISA or fluorescent antibody test; leukocytosis, usually with stress leukogram, is present; hemoglobinemia (red plasma) and hemoglobinuria (port-wine–colored urine) may be marked; BUN and ALT may be markedly ↑; if DIC is present, see ↑ ACT, PT, PTT, TT, and fibrin degradation products and ↓ platelet numbers and fibrinogen; thoracic radiographs show enlarged right ventricle and pulmonary arteries and enlarged caudal vena cava ±.
Hemolytic bacteremia/ septicemia	Depression, anorexia, weakness; may have history suggesting a likely source of bacteria, such as bite wounds (other common sources are dental disease, bacterial endocarditis, prostatitis, diskospondylitis, and indwelling venous catheters).	Fever, depression, dehydration, possibly signs of shock; icterus usually mild; possibly signs of DIC	Nonregenerative anemia, neutropenia, and thrombocytopenia may be present; icteric plasma or hemoglobinemia may be found; mildly to moderately ↑ SAP (2–15× normal), ↓ albumin, and ↓ glucose are sometimes present; blood cultures may be positive; evidence of DIC may be found.

306

Incompatible blood transfusion	Depression, anorexia, occasional vomiting, history of multiple blood transfusions	Depression, icterus mild to severe	Mild to moderate anemia, usually nonregenerative, ↑ WBC with either a stress or inflammatory leukogram; SAP and ALT usually normal
Parasites *Babesia*	Weakness, depression, lethargy, exercise intolerance, anorexia, epistaxis	See History: fever, pale mucous membranes; periorbital edema ±, ataxia ±, splenomegaly, heart murmur (anemia) ±	Moderate to severe anemia (regenerative), stress leukogram, ↓ platelets, evidence of DIC, Coombs'-positive ±, see parasite in RBCs on Wright-Giemsa–stained capillary blood smear (from ear pinna) ±, indirect fluorescent antibody test—positive (>1:40) ±
Haemobartonella	History of prior splenectomy See *Babesia.*	Pale mucous membranes, weakness, depression, fever ±, heart murmur (anemia) ±	Moderate to severe anemia (regenerative), stress leukogram, Coombs'-positive ±, see parasite on Wright-Giemsa–stained capillary blood smear
Drugs or toxins Benzocaine	Weakness, depression, lethargy, history of benzocaine use	Pale mucous membranes, weakness, depression, heart murmur (anemia) ±	Moderate to severe anemia (regenerative), presence of Heinz bodies in RBCs, stress leukogram
Onions	Weakness, depression, lethargy, vomiting, history of onion ingestion	Pale mucous membranes, weakness, depression, heart murmur (anemia) ±	Moderate to severe anemia (regenerative), presence of Heinz bodies in RBCs ±, stress leukogram
Hepatic* Drugs or toxins Thiacetarsamide (Caparsolate)	Within a few hours of drug administration: depression, anorexia, vomiting	Depression, dehydration, mild to severe icterus in some cases	PCV and plasma total protein normal to ↑ (dehydration); WBC mildly ↑ with a stress leukogram, ALT markedly ↑ (15–50× normal), SAP normal to slightly ↑ (2–5× normal)

(continued)

TABLE 37-3. Selected Causes of Icterus in Dogs and Associated Findings *(continued)*

Cause	History	Physical Examination	Laboratory Data
Aflatoxins (molds from grain-type foods)	Chronic lethargy, anorexia, weight loss, sometimes polydipsia and polyuria	Depression, weight loss, dehydration, severe icterus, bloody vomiting, melena	PCV and WBC variable; slight ↑ ALT and SAP (2–5× normal); ↓ BUN, albumin, glucose, and cholesterol; evidence of DIC (↑ ACT, PT, PTT, TT, FDPs, and ↓ platelet numbers); high levels of aflatoxins in food
Mebendazole (Telmintic) Oxibendazole (Filaribits plus)	Within a few days of drug administration: anorexia, depression, dehydration, and vomiting	Depression, dehydration, moderate to severe icterus; in some, signs of hepatic failure (hepatic encephalopathy, bloody vomiting, melena)	PCV and plasma total protein normal to ↑ (dehydration), ↑ WBC with stress or inflammatory leukogram, ALT and SAP markedly ↑ (10–50× normal), serum bile acids ↑, plasma ammonia ↑ ±, bilirubinuria
Anticonvulsants—especially primidone	Takes 1–3 years of continuous therapy	Anorexia, weakness, ascites, no icterus or mild icterus	Albumin ↓, ALT and SAP moderately to markedly ↑ (5–30× normal), serum bile acids ↑; ascitic fluid—a low protein (<2.5 g/dl) transudate
Sulfonamides	Usually takes repeated exposure to the drug; anorexia, vomiting, depression; more common in large dogs	Depression, weakness, dehydration, moderate to severe icterus, signs of hepatic encephalopathy ±, signs of DIC ±	PCV and plasma total protein variable, ↑ WBC with stress or inflammatory leukogram; moderately to markedly ↑ ALT and SAP (5–50× normal), serum bile acids ↑, plasma ammonia ↑ ±

308

Disease	Clinical Signs	Laboratory Findings
Cholangitis/cholangiohepatitis	Depression, fever (103°–104.5°F), mild to moderate dehydration, and weight loss; mild to severe icterus; later, possibly signs of hepatic failure (stupor, head-pressing, apparent blindness, ascites, melena)	PCV and plasma total protein normal to slightly ↑, moderately ↑ WBC (20,000–30,000/cm³) with inflammatory leukogram. BUN may be ↓, albumin sometimes ↓, and globulin ↑, ALT mildly to moderately ↑ (2–10× normal), SAP moderately ↑ (5–15× normal), blood glucose may be ↓, serum bile acids ↑ (pre- and postprandial), plasma ammonia tolerance ↓, ascitic fluid, when present—a low protein (<2.5 g/dl) transudate
Hepatic copper accumulation (hereditary in Bedlington terriers and West Highland white terriers); also reported in Doberman pinschers, Skye terriers, and occasionally other breeds	May be asymptomatic; early, sporadic anorexia and vomiting with weight loss; later, severe depression, vomiting, and diarrhea	PCV and WBC usually normal (occasionally show severe hemolytic anemic crisis); ↑ ALT is earliest abnormality (2–100× normal); later, ↑ SAP (100–150× normal), ↓ albumin, ↓ BUN, ↓ glucose, ↑ serum bile acids, ↑ ammonia, or ↓ ammonia tolerance, and evidence of impaired coagulation (↑ ACT, PT, PTT, TT); ↑ hepatic copper (5–50× normal)

Chronic active hepatitis
Drug-induced
Infectious
  Viral
  Bacterial
Autoimmune
Copper accumulation
Idiopathic
	In most, no signs or only slight weight loss; later, severe depression, mild to severe dehydration, weight loss, icterus, ascites, melena, and signs of hepatic encephalopathy	PCV and WBC usually normal; ↑ ALT is earliest abnormality (2–100× normal); later, ↑ SAP (100–150× normal), ↓ albumin, ↓ BUN, ↓ glucose, ↑ serum bile acids, ↑ ammonia, or ↓ ammonia tolerance, and evidence of impaired coagulation (↑ ACT, PT, PTT, TT)

	Similar to hepatic copper accumulation; may have history of drug administration	See Hepatic copper accumulation.

(continued)

309

TABLE 37-3. Selected Causes of Icterus in Dogs and Associated Findings *(continued)*

Cause	History	Physical Examination	Laboratory Data
Hepatic fibrosis ("cirrhosis")	Chronic course of depression, decreased appetite, weight loss, sporadic vomiting and diarrhea; in some cases, polydipsia, polyuria, abdominal distention (ascites), head-pressing, stupor, apparent blindness, and seizures	Depression, weight loss, icterus (usually mild), ascites, melena; in some cases, signs of hepatoencephalopathy	Usually a mild nonregenerative anemia (PCV 20–30), WBC normal, BUN ↓, albumin severely ↓ (<1.5 g/dl), globulin normal to ↑, glucose ↓, ALT normal or mildly ↑, SAP normal to moderately ↑ (5–10× normal), ↑ serum bile acids, ↑ plasma ammonia or ↓ ammonia tolerance, clotting possibly abnormal, ascitic fluid—a low protein (<2.5 g/dl) transudate, liver is small radiographically, diffusely increased echogenicity sonographically
Bacteremia/septicemia ("reactive hepatopathy")	See Hemolytic bacteremia/septicemia.	See Hemolytic bacteremia/septicemia.	See Hemolytic bacteremia/septicemia. Some bacterial endotoxins (especially *Escherichia coli*) apparently interfere with hepatocyte secretion of conjugated bilirubin into the bile canaliculus.
Infectious canine hepatitis	Severe depression, vomiting, weakness, sometimes seizures or collapse	Depression, weakness, fever (103°–105°F), scleral injection, abdominal pain, hepatomegaly, "blue-eye" occasionally, evidence of DIC in some (e.g., petechiae, melena, hematuria); icterus uncommon	PCV variable, WBC ↓ (neutropenia), moderately to markedly ↑ ALT (10–50× normal), mildly to moderately ↑ SAP (2–10× normal), in some cases, ↓ blood glucose, ↑ serum bile acids, and ↑ plasma ammonia, proteinuria in the absence of cells, bilirubinuria, evidence of DIC

310

Hepatic neoplasia, primary or metastatic	Chronic course of lethargy, decreased appetite, moderate to severe weight loss, sporadic vomiting and diarrhea; in some cases, head-pressing, stupor, apparent blindness, and seizures	Depression, mild to moderate dehydration, mild to severe icterus, abdominal enlargement due to hepatomegaly, palpable intraabdominal mass, or ascites in some cases	Mild to moderate nonregenerative anemia (PCV 18–25). ↑ WBC with either inflammatory or stress leukogram, BUN variable, albumin variable, globulin may be ↑, ALT normal to mildly ↑ (2–5× normal), SAP normal to markedly ↑ (20× normal), ↑ serum bile acids, ↑ plasma ammonia or ↓ ammonia tolerance; abdominal radiographs showing hepatomegaly, abnormal masses, or ascites; abdominal sonograms showing hyper- and hypoechogenic areas in the liver; ascitic fluid—a high protein (>2.5 g/dl), modified transudate containing nondegenerate neutrophils, RBCs, macrophages and mesothelial cells, but rarely neoplastic cells
Posthepatic (obstructive) Acute pancreatitis—bile duct compression	Depression, anorexia, vomiting, restlessness, sometimes after a fatty meal	Often obesity, depression, mild to moderate dehydration, mild fever (103°–104°F), abdominal pain upon palpation in some cases, mild to moderate icterus	PCV and plasma total protein often ↑ (dehydration), fasting chylomicronemia in many cases, ↑ WBC with inflammatory leukogram, mildly to moderately ↑ BUN, mildly to moderately ↑ ALT (2–5× normal) and SAP (2–15× normal) in some cases, mild hypocalcemia, ↑ serum amylase or lipase, focal peritonitis, ileus, displaced bowel loops seen radiographically ±, dilated bile ducts and irregular hypoechoic areas seen sonographically in pancreatic areas in some cases

(continued)

TABLE 37-3. Selected Causes of Icterus in Dogs and Associated Findings *(continued)*

Cause	History	Physical Examination	Laboratory Data
Neoplasm compressing bile duct	Chronic course of lethargy, decreased appetite, weight loss, sporadic vomiting and diarrhea	Depression, weight loss, mild to moderate dehydration, severe icterus, possible palpation of abdominal mass	PCV variable, WBC normal to ↑, may be an inflammatory leukogram, mildly to moderately ↑ ALT (2–5× normal), markedly ↑ SAP (10–50× normal), ↑ serum bile acids, may see abdominal mass radiographically, mass and dilated bile ducts seen sonographically
Traumatic rupture of gallbladder or bile duct	History of trauma followed in 12–24 hours by depression, anorexia, and vomiting	Depression, fever (103°–105°F), icterus, abdominal pain	PCV and plasma total protein slightly ↑ (dehydration), ↑ WBC with inflammatory leukogram, moderately to markedly ↑ ALT (5–20× normal) due to hepatic trauma; SAP usually normal, ↑ serum bile acids, decreased contrast of serosal surfaces radiographically

		(peritonitis), mild fluid accumulation in abdomen in some cases, (high protein [>2.5 g/dl] nonseptic exudate with mostly neutrophils [nondegenerate]), bilirubin in abdominal fluid higher than in plasma
Cholelithiasis	May be asymptomatic Intermittent episodes of depression, anorexia, and vomiting	Most asymptomatic In some depression, dehydration, and moderate to severe icterus	PCV and plasma total protein sometimes ↑ (dehydration), WBC normal to ↑ with inflammatory leukogram, ALT normal to mildly ↑ (2–5× normal), SAP mildly to moderately ↑ (2–15× normal), may see cholelith radiographically and sonographically

*See Table 37-1 for general characteristics.

PCV, packed cell volume; DIC, disseminated intravascular coagulation; ELISA, enzyme-linked immunosorbent assay; BUN, blood urea nitrogen; ALT, alanine aminotransferase; ↑, increased; ACT, activated clotting time; PT, prothrombin time; PTT, partial thromboplastin time; TT, thrombin time; ↓, decreased; ±, present or absent; SAP, serum alkaline phosphatase; WBC, white blood cells; RBCs, red blood cells; FDPs, fibrin(ogen) degradation products

313

TABLE 37-4. Selected Causes of Icterus in Cats and Associated Findings

Cause	History	Physical Examination	Laboratory Data
		Major Characteristics and Associated Findings	
Prehepatic (hemolytic)*			
Haemobartonellosis	Lethargy, weakness, anorexia, often associated with stress such as fighting and abscesses	Fever (103°–105°F), depression, dehydration, pale mucous membranes; icterus mild, when present	Regenerative anemia (unless associated with feline leukemia virus), variable WBC, organisms seen in erythrocytes intermittently, mildly ↑ ALT (2–5× normal)
Drugs			
Acetaminophen	Depression, weakness, dyspnea, vomiting, drug administration	Severe depression; pale or cyanotic mucous membranes; icterus mild, when present; subnormal body temperature; dyspnea	Hemoglobinemia, stress leukogram, anemia (too acute for regenerative response), markedly ↑ ALT (5–20× normal), Heinz bodies in erythrocytes with methylene blue
Methylene blue			
Bacteremia/septicemia	Depression, anorexia, weakness	Subnormal temperature or fever; depression; dehydration; icterus mild, when present Sources of infection may be observed (*e.g.*, abscess, purulent vaginal discharge).	Nonregenerative anemia, neutropenia with inappropriate left shift, thrombocytopenia, mildly ↑ ALT (2–5× normal), mildly to moderately ↑ SAP (2–5× normal), ↓ albumin, ↓ glucose ±, positive blood cultures in some cases
Hepatic*			
Cholangitis/ cholangiohepatitis	Intermittent episodes of decreased appetite, lethargy, weight loss, occasional vomiting	Depression, unkempt appearance, icteric mucous membranes, thin, hepatomegaly ± (some are asymptomatic, except for mild, intermittent lethargy and anorexia) Fever ±, ascites ±	Mild nonregenerative anemia (PCV 20–25), WBC normal or ↑ (neutrophilia with left shift), moderately ↑ ALT (5–10× normal), mildly to moderately ↑ SAP (2–5× normal), in some cases ↓ al-

314

		bumin, ↑ globulin, ↓ BUN, ↑ serum bile acids, ↑ plasma ammonia or ↓ ammonia tolerance, and positive bacterial culture of bile ± (usually *Escherichia coli*); ascitic fluid—a transudate
Hepatic lipidosis Idiopathic	Chronic anorexia, history of obesity, lethargy, weight loss, stress	Depression, unkempt appearance, icteric mucous membranes, dehydration; may still be obese	Mild nonregenerative anemia (PCV 20–25), WBC normal, mildly to moderately ↑ ALT (2–5× normal), moderately to markedly ↑ SAP (5–15× normal), ↓ albumin, ↓ BUN, ↑ serum bile acids, ↑ plasma ammonia or ↓ ammonia tolerance, in some cases ↑ activated clotting time, ↑ prothrombin time, ↑ partial thromboplastin time, and ↑ thrombin time
Secondary to other disorders Diabetes mellitus Chronic anorexia or malnutrition associated with many different disorders Drugs or toxins Septicemia	Variable depending on the primary disorder. See Idiopathic under Hepatic lipidosis.	Variable depending on the primary disorder. See Idiopathic under Hepatic lipidosis.	Variable depending on the primary disorder; see Idiopathic under Hepatic lipidosis.
Feline infectious peritonitis	Chronic lethargy, decreased appetite, weight loss	Depression, dehydration, fever (103°–105°F), icteric mucous membranes, abdominal en-	Mild to moderate nonregenerative anemia (PCV 18–25), WBC variable, ALT and SAP

(continued)

Cause	History	Major Characteristics and Associated Findings	
		Physical Examination	*Laboratory Data*
		largement (ascites) and dyspnea (pleural effusion) in effusive form, anterior and posterior uveitis in some cases	normal, ↑ globulin (polyclonal gammopathy) in some cases, ascitic and pleural fluids—modified transudates with high protein (>3.0 g/dl), FIP titer variable, feline leukemia virus test positive in half of cases
Feline leukemia virus–associated diseases (lymphosarcoma, myeloproliferative disorders, immunosuppression with bacterial infection)	Lethargy, anorexia, vomiting, weight loss	Fever, depression, dehydration, icteric mucous membranes, sometimes hepatomegaly	Nonregenerative anemia, neutropenia with inappropriate left shift, neoplastic cells sometimes present in blood, thrombocytopenia, normal to slightly ↑ ALT (2–3× normal), ↑ SAP (3–10× normal), feline leukemia virus positive ±, neoplastic mass or effusion observed on radiographs ±; malignant lymphocytes possibly observed in the effusion with Wright-Giemsa stain.
Bacteremia/endotoxemia	See Bacteremia/septicemia under Prehepatic (hemolytic).		Hepatocyte secretion of conjugated bilirubin impaired, resulting in functional cholestasis; mildly to moderately ↑ SAP (2–5× normal), normal or mildly ↑ ALT (1.5–2× normal)

Drugs or toxins		
Acetaminophen	See Acetaminophen under Prehepatic (hemolytic).	
Tetracyclines	Anorexia, vomiting, depression within a few days of drug administration	PCV and total protein variable, ↑ WBC (inflammatory or stress leukogram), moderately to markedly ↑ ALT (10–50× normal), mildly to moderately ↑ SAP (3–5× normal), increased serum bile acids, bilirubinuria
Ketoconazole	See Tetracyclines.	
Neoplasia		
Feline leukemia virus–related (lymphosarcoma, reticuloendotheliosis)	See Feline leukemia virus–associated diseases under Hepatic.	
Others (primary or metastatic)	Depression, decreased appetite, weight loss, sporadic vomiting and diarrhea	Depression, weight loss, icteric mucosa, palpably enlarged liver ±, abdominal mass; ascites in a few
		Mild to moderate nonregenerative anemia (PCV 18–25), normal to ↑ WBC with either inflammatory or stress leukogram, ALT usually normal to slightly ↑ (1.5–2× normal), SAP normal to markedly ↑ (5–15× normal), neoplastic mass, ascites or hepatomegaly observed radiographically and sonographically in some; ascites—a modified transudate with moderate protein content (3.0–4.5 g/dl) and a preponderance of nondegenerate neutrophils

(continued)

TABLE 37-4. Selected Causes of Icterus in Cats and Associated Findings *(continued)*

Cause	Major Characteristics and Associated Findings		
	History	Physical Examination	Laboratory Data
*Posthepatic (obstructive)**			
Neoplasm compressing bile duct	Chronic course of lethargy, decreased appetite, weight loss, sporadic vomiting and diarrhea	Depression, weight loss, mild to moderate dehydration, severe icterus, possible palpation of abdominal mass	Mild to moderate nonregenerative anemia, WBC normal to ↑ (stress or inflammatory leukogram), mild to moderate ↑ ALT (2–5× normal), mildly to moderately ↑ SAP (2–5× normal), ↑ serum bile acids, radiographs possibly showing mass, possibly showing dilated bile ducts and mass
Trauma—ruptured gallbladder or bile duct	History of trauma or opportunity for trauma, depression, anorexia, vomiting	Fever 103°–104°, depression, dehydration, icteric mucosa, abdominal pain upon palpation	↑ PCV and total solids (dehydration), ↑ WBC with neutrophilia and left shift, moderately to markedly ↑ ALT

(5–20× normal), normal to slightly ↑ SAP (2× normal), abdominal fluid observed radiographically; fluid a moderate protein (3.0–4.5 g/dl), nonseptic exudate with a preponderance of nondegenerative neutrophils; bilirubin concentration of fluid higher than in plasma in acute stage

Cholelithiasis

Usually secondary to chronic cholestasis and bile inspissation associated with cholangitis/cholangiohepatitis (see above)

*See Table 37-1 for general characteristics and associated findings.

WBC, white blood cells; ↑, increased; ALT, alanine aminotransferase; SAP, serum alkaline phosphatase; ↓, decreased; ±, present or absent; PCV, packed cell volume; BUN, blood urea nitrogen; FIP, feline infectious peritonitis.

(Cornelius LM, Rogers KS: Finding the cause of jaundice in cats. Mod Vet Pract 66:166–170, 1985)

REFERENCES

1. Badley BWD: A physiologic approach to jaundice. Clin Biochem 9:144–148, 1976
2. Berk PD: Hyperbilirubinemia and cholestasis. Am J Med 64:311–326, 1978
3. Bissel DM: Formation and elimination of bilirubin. Gastroenterology 69:519–538, 1975
4. Cornelius LM: Icterus. In Proceedings of the 49th Annual Meeting of the American Animal Hospital Association, 1982
5. Dusol M Jr, Schiff ER: Clinical approach to jaundice. Postgrad Med 57:118–123, 1975
6. Gautam A, Seligson H, Gordon ER, et al: Irreversible binding of conjugated bilirubin to albumin in cholestatic rats. J Clin Invest 73:873–877, 1984
7. Maldonado JE, Kyle RA, Schoenfield LJ: Increased serum conjugated bilirubin in hemolytic anemia. Postgrad Med 55:183–190, 1974
8. Rogers KS, Cornelius LM: Feline icterus. Comp Cont Ed Pract Vet 7:391–399, 1986
9. Rothuizen J, van den Ingh T: Covalently protein-bound bilirubin conjugates in cholestatic disease of dogs. Am J Vet Res 49:702–704, 1988
10. Schmid R: Bilirubin metabolism in man. N Engl J Med 287:703–709, 1972
11. Utili R, Abernathy CO, Zimmerman HJ: Cholestatic effects of *Escherichia coli* endotoxin on the isolated perfused rat liver. Gastroenterology 70:248–253, 1976
12. Van Vleet JF, Albers JO: Evaluation of liver function tests and liver biopsy in experimental carbon tetrachloride intoxication and extrahepatic bile duct obstruction in the dog. Am J Vet Res 29:2119–2131, 1968
13. Weiss J, Gautam A, Lauff JJ, et al: The clinical importance of a protein-bound fraction of serum bilirubin in patients with hyperbilirubinemia. N Engl J Med 309:147–150, 1983

PART NINE

Urologic Problems

CHAPTER THIRTY-EIGHT

Abnormal Micturition: Dysuria, Pollakiuria, and Stranguria

Michael D. Lorenz

PROBLEM DEFINITION AND RECOGNITION

Dysuria is painful or difficult urination. Pollakiuria is frequent urination, and stranguria is slow and painful discharge of urine due to spasm of the bladder and urethra. These clinical signs are frequently encountered in small animals and are caused by disease of the lower urinary tract or genital tract. They must be differentiated from polyuria (increased urine volume). When in doubt, direct observation of the patient and quantitation of urine output should be performed early in the diagnostic process. Disease of the lower urinary and genital tract usually results in a combination of these three clinical signs. Throughout this chapter, dysuria is used to refer to all three clinical problems.

PATHOGENESIS

The urinary bladder is innervated by the pelvic and hypogastric nerves. The pelvic nerve originates from sacral cord segments S1, S2, and S3 and is composed of efferent and afferent parasympathic fibers. The efferent fibers innervate the detrusor muscle and provide motor function for coordinated voiding. The afferent fibers mediate the sensation to void, proprioception, and pain. The hypogastric nerve provides sympathetic innervation to the bladder; however, it has little influence on normal micturition. Sympathetic afferents provide some awareness of bladder distention and pain. Sensory receptors are located in the bladder mucosa and are most abundant in the ureterovesical junction and bladder neck. Mucosal inflammation may cause pain, urgency to urinate even though the bladder may be empty or partially filled, bladder wall spasm, or a burning sensation.

The urethra receives its nerve supply from the pudendal nerve, which arises from sacral cord segments. The pudendal nerve is a mixed somatic nerve that contains motor fibers to the external urethral sphincter. Stimulation of these

Causes of Dysuria

- Infection
  - Bacterial cystitis
  - Urethritis
  - Bacterial prostatitis
  - Prostatic abscess
  - Vaginitis
- Calculi
  - Cystic
  - Urethral
- Neoplasia
  - Bladder
    - Transitional cell carcinoma
    - Rhabdomyoma or sarcoma
  - Prostate
    - Carcinoma
    - Adenocarcinoma
    - Squamous cell carcinoma
  - Urethra
    - Transitional cell carcinoma
    - Transmissible veneral tumor
  - Vagina, penis
    - Transmissible veneral tumor
    - Fibromas
    - Sarcomas
- Trauma
  - Ruptured bladder, urethra
  - Urethral stricture
- Inflammation
  - Benign prostatic hyperplasia
  - Feline urologic syndrome
- Neurologic
  - Certain forms of incontinence (*e.g.*, vesicular-urethra asynchronization: reflex dyssynergia)

motor fibers contracts the urethral sphincter and maintains continence as the bladder fills with urine. During normal micturition, nerve impulses to the external urethral sphincter are inhibited, allowing the sphincter to dilate for the passage of urine. Sensory receptors within the urethra respond to flow, urethral distention, and thermal sensation. The awareness of voiding is from these urethral sensations and traction on the bladder neck and trigone. Irritation or inflammation of the urethra causes pain, burning sensations, and spasms of the urethral sphincter. In male dogs, disease of the prostate usually involves the urethra and bladder and produces dysuria by the mechanisms previously described.

CAUSES

Any disease of the lower urinary tract (bladder and urethra) or lower genital tract (prostate, vagina) that results in mucosal irritation or inflammation will produce dysuria. In addition, diseases that cause urethral or bladder neck obstruction also cause dysuria. The causes of dysuria are usually associated with hematuria or pyuria, or both, because of mucosal inflammation or infection. Hematuria is described in Chapter 39. Several causes of dysuria (calculi, neoplasia, and feline urologic syndrome) frequently cause urethral obstruction, a life-threatening emergency. Certain forms of urinary incontinence may also produce signs similar to dysuria (see Chapter 40).

DIAGNOSTIC PLAN

The initial data base includes a complete history regarding micturition characteristics and urine color, physical examination that emphasizes bladder and prostatic palpation, and midstream-voided and cystocentesis samples for urine analysis (Fig. 38-1). If the bladder is distended with urine, urethral obstruction should be strongly suspected. A catheter is passed to relieve the obstruction and obtain urine for analysis and culture. If the animal is depressed, anorexic, or vomiting, uremia may be present and should be confirmed with biochemical tests (blood urea nitrogen [BUN], creatinine, potassium, and total CO_2). In male dogs, rectal palpation for an enlarged or painful prostate gland identifies urethral obstruction due to prostatic disease.

If bladder distention is absent, the bladder is carefully palpated for calculi, neoplasia, or thickening of the wall. The prostate should be carefully palpated, since many dogs with prostatic disease are not obstructed. A voided midstream urine sample is collected for initial analysis. A second urine sample collected by cystocentesis is also analyzed. The results of these urine analyses are compared. The presence of blood, white blood cells (WBC), and bacteria in the cystocentesis sample suggests disease in the bladder or prostate; their absence from the cystocentesis sample, in animals with abnormalities in the voided sample, suggests disease in the urethra or lower genital tract.

The genital organs, vagina, uterus, penis, and testicles are thoroughly examined for pain, masses, or abnormal discharge. If traumatic rupture of the urinary tract is a possibility, the abdomen is carefully palpated for pain and the patient is assessed for uremia.

In male dogs with palpably abnormal prostate glands, the initial data base should be expanded to include cytologic and microbiologic examination of an ejaculate. Lower tract radiography and/or ultrasonography are also useful for estimating the extent and potential causes of the enlarged or painful prostate. Noninfectious inflammatory or neoplastic conditions may require prostatic biopsy to establish the definitive diagnosis.

In male dogs with normal prostate glands or in all nonobstructed small animals, the initial data base is expanded to further define the etiology of dysuria. A urine culture from a cystocentesis sample, urine cytology, double-contrast urethral and bladder radiography, ultrasonography, and vaginal endoscopy are indicated. If neoplasia or calculi are present, cystotomy and biopsy are indicated for therapeutic and diagnostic purposes.

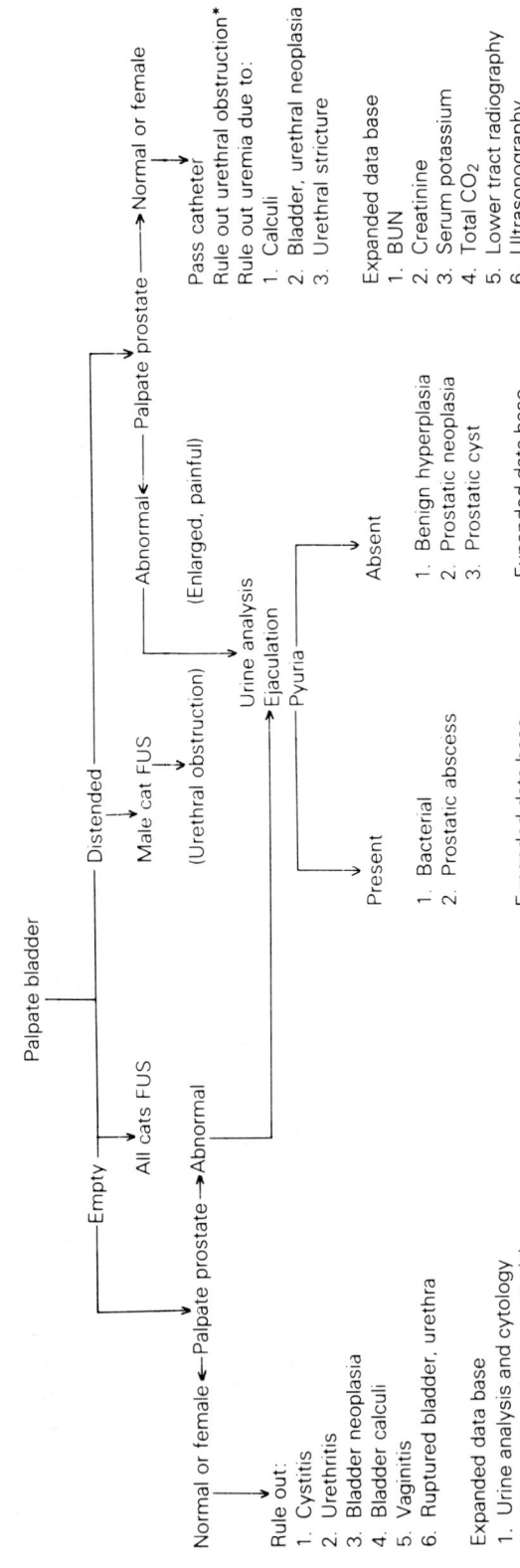

FIGURE 38-1. Algorithm for the differential diagnosis of dysuria.

* If no obstruction exists, pursue bladder detrusor or neurologic dysfunction. See Chapter 40.

If traumatic rupture of the bladder or urethra is likely, the initial data base is expanded to assess the patient for uremia (BUN, creatinine, serum potassium, total CO_2). Abdominal fluid collected by abdominocentesis is analyzed for creatinine concentrations. With intraabdominal rupture of the urinary tract, creatinine levels in abdominal fluid are usually higher than serum concentrations, since creatinine from urine leaking into the abdomen equilibrates rather slowly with intravascular fluid. Lower urinary tract radiography (positive contrast urethrocystogram) is also useful for identification of rents in the lower tract. The presence of normal urine from catheterization does not rule out urinary tract rupture.

Assessment of Urinary Tract Infection

Urinary tract infection (UTI) is a very common cause of dysuria and is often associated with urinary tract calculi or prostatitis. It is also a common complication with urinary incontinence and repeated bladder catheterization. For causes of UTI except urethritis, urine samples should be collected for analysis by cystocentesis. This is especially important for microbiologic studies. Urine should be placed in culture media within 30 minutes after collection to prevent the rapid growth of nonpathogenic, contaminating organisms. If possible, quantitative urine cultures should be performed. In properly obtained cystocentesis samples, organism numbers in excess of 1000 indicate probable UTI; this diagnosis should be verified by repeating the procedure or with appropriate therapy. Organisms in excess of 100,000 in quantitated culture of a cystocentesis sample indicate definitive UTI. Affected animals are treated accordingly.

The contraindications for cystocentesis include extreme bladder distention and possible necrosis of the bladder wall. Prolonged obstruction, detrusor muscle paralysis, or severe infection may result in abnormal urine leakage following cystocentesis.

Dysuria Versus Incontinence

In certain cases, dysuria as previously described may be difficult to distinguish from urinary incontinence due to detrusor muscle or neurologic dysfunction. When the previously described diagnostic plan for dysuria does not establish an etiologic diagnosis, the clinician should pursue incontinence as the probable problem. Incontinence is described in Chapter 40.

SPECIFIC DISEASES

The clinical and diagnostic characteristics of the specific diseases that cause dysuria are listed in Table 38-1.

TABLE 38-1. Summary of the Diseases That Produce Dysuria

Disease	Predominant Clinical Signs Other Than Dysuria	Hematology	Urine Analysis	Biochemistry	Special Diagnostic Tests
Bacterial cystitis (UTI)	Palpably thickened bladder wall in some cases	Usually normal unless associated with pyelonephritis	Hematuria Pyuria Bacteruria ↑Protein Alkaline pH	Normal	Cystocentesis for quantitative urine culture >1000 organisms/ml of urine on cystocentesis sample Thickened bladder wall on cystography
Feline urologic syndrome	In male cats, may result in urethral obstruction Inflammation of bladder and urethra	Normal	Hematuria ↑Protein Crystalluria	Normal	Urine cultures negative, unless sample contaminated or cat previously catheterized to relieve obstruction
Obstructive uropathy of any cause	Failure to void urine Severe stranguria Distended bladder Dribbling urine If prolonged, uremic signs	Early: normal Late: ↑PCV ↑WBC	Hematuria Pyuria ± Bacteruria ↑Protein Crystalluria	Early: normal Prolonged: ↑BUN, creatinine ↑Potassium ↑TCO₂ (acidosis)	Failure to easily pass catheter Positive double-contrast urethrocystography Urine culture positive in cases complicated by UTI
Cystic neoplasia	See Bacterial cystitis and Obstructive uropathy. Chronic hematuria despite appropriate therapy for UTI	See Bacterial cystitis.	See Bacterial cystitis.	Normal unless obstruction occurs	Cytology of urine sediment Positive double-contrast cystography Ultrasonography Urine cultures usually negative Abnormal excretory urogram (especially with transitional cell carcinoma of bladder neck)

328

Prostatitis, bacterial	Acute signs Fever Tenesmus Enlarged *painful* prostate	↑WBC	See Bacterial cystitis. (rarely, the urine analysis is normal)	Normal	Ejaculate or prostatic massage Cytology—septic exudate Culture—positive Positive contrast urethrocystography usually normal Ultrasonography *Brucella* titer
Prostatic abscess	Chronic signs Asymmetric prostatic enlargement Prostatic pain ± Tenesmus	↑WBC	See Bacterial cystitis.	Normal	Ejaculate or prostatic massage Cytology—septic exudate Culture—positive *Brucella* titer Positive contrast urethrocystography Ultrasonography Prostatic enlargement Dye reflux into prostate
Benign prostatic hypertrophy	Acute signs Symmetric prostatic enlargement Usually *nonpainful* Tenesmus	Normal	Hematuria or normal	Normal	Ejaculate or prostatic massage Cytology—hemorrhagic exudate Culture—negative
Prostatic cyst	Chronic signs Asymmetric prostatic enlargement *Fluctuant prostatic mass* Dribbling blood from penis Tenesmus	Normal	Hematuria, mild pyuria	Normal	Ejaculate or prostatic massage Cytology—hemorrhagic exudate Culture—negative Positive contrast urethrocystography: reflux of dye into cyst Ultrasonography Prostatic biopsy: squamous metaplasia

(continued)

329

TABLE 38-1. Summary of the Diseases That Produce Dysuria (*continued*)

Disease	Predominant Clinical Signs Other Than Dysuria	Hematology	Urine Analysis	Biochemistry	Special Diagnostic Tests
Prostatic neoplasia	See prostatic cyst *Firm palpable mass*	Normal	Hematuria	Normal	Ejaculate or prostatic massage Cytology—hemorrhagic exudate Tumor cells may be found Pelvic radiograph ↑Prostate ↑Sublumbar lymph nodes Ultrasonography Exostosis or lysis of pelvic brim Biopsy
Traumatic rupture of bladder or urethra	History of trauma or prolonged obstruction Abdominal pain Uremic signs	↑PCV ↑WBC	Normal or hematuria	Early: normal Late: ↑BUN, creatinine ↑Potassium ↓TCO$_2$ (acidosis)	Abdominocentesis Cytology—nonseptic purulent or hemorrhagic exudate Creatinine on fluid greater than plasma Positive contrast urethrocystogram—dye spillage into abdomen Abdominal radiography—evidence of peritonitis

Disease	Clinical Findings		Urinalysis		Diagnostic Tests
Urethritis (bacterial)	No consistent findings May see swelling or inflammation of urethral meatus Unknown incidence in dogs and cats	Normal	See cystitis	Normal	Difficult to confirm with special diagnostic tests currently available
Vaginitis	Vaginal discharge History of recent estrus Common in prepubertal bitches Rare in cats	Normal	Hematuria and pyuria on voided sample Normal on cystocentesis	Normal	Vaginoscopy—swelling, inflammation, or exudate Cytology—purulent exudate Culture—positive
Transmissible veneral tumor	Cauliflower-like growth on penis, in vagina, may involve urethra Persistent hemorrhagic penile or vaginal discharge	Normal	Hematuria	Normal	Vaginoscopy Exfoliative cytology Biopsy
Neurogenic-induced dysuria	Inability to void urine Distended bladder Various degrees of incontinence	Normal	Hematuria and pyuria if secondarily infected	Normal	Cystometrograms Urethral pressure profiles Lower tract radiography Neurologic examination (see Chapter 40)

UTI, urinary tract infection; $\uparrow$, increased; PCV, packed cell volume; WBC, white blood cells; $\pm$, variable; BUN, blood urea nitrogen; $\downarrow$, decreased; TCO_2, total CO_2

CHAPTER THIRTY-NINE

Discolored Urine

Michael D. Lorenz

Urine is yellow to amber in color. The depth of color is related to urine volume. Dark urine does not necessarily mean concentrated urine. Urine pigments, being rather large molecular structures, add little to urine osmolality. Therefore, urine pigments are assessed by strip reagents and specific gravity with a refractometer or hydrometer. The differential diagnosis and causes of discolored urine are listed in Figure 39-1. Simple diagnostic procedures (urine occult blood test, urine sediment examination, and urine bilirubin test) are required to complete this algorithm. In succeeding sections, the diagnosis of red and brown urine is discussed.

RED URINE

Many animals are presented for diagnostic evaluation of red urine. There are several basic causes of red urine and diverse etiologies for each of these basic causes. Figure 39-1 is a diagnostic plan for finding the basic cause of red urine. The initial step requires the collection of a voided urine sample and analysis for occult blood. The occult blood test will be positive for blood, hemoglobin, and myoglobin and negative for red pigments such as porphyrins, pyridium, or red dyes in some dog foods. The urine sample is centrifuged, and the supernatant and sediment are tested for occult blood. The sediment is also examined microscopically for red blood cells (RBCs). A negative occult reaction in the sediment coupled with the absence of RBCs suggests that hemoglobin or myoglobin is present. A positive occult test on the sediment with the presence of RBCs in the sediment confirms the presence of hematuria. Plasma in a capillary tube should be examined for the presence of a red color. The presence of hemoglobinemia further differentiates causes of red urine. Myoglobinemia does not impart any color change to plasma.

The color of urine containing different pigments of red hue is dependent on the amount of pigment and urine pH. Hemoglobin in an acidic urine is often brown or smoky; in an alkaline urine, the color is red. The causes of red urine are discussed in subsequent sections.

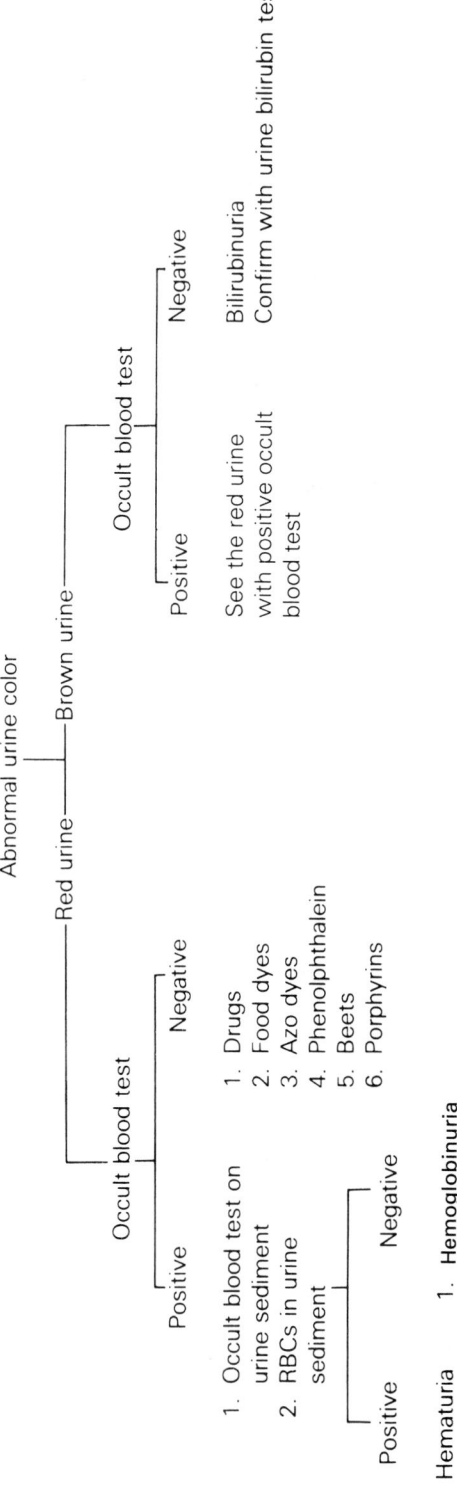

FIGURE 39-1. Algorithm for the diagnosis of discolored urine.

TABLE 39-1. Causes of Hematuria in Dogs and Cats Classified by Anatomic Site of Origin

Site	Diseases
Kidney	Pyelonephritis
	Glomerulopathy
	Neoplasia
	Calculi
	Renal cysts
	Infarction
	Trauma
	Benign renal bleeding
	Hematuria of Welsh corgis
	Dioctophyma renale
	Microfilariae of *Dirofilaria immitis*
	Chronic passive congestion
Bladder, ureter, urethra	Infection
	Calculi
	Inflammation—feline urologic syndrome
	Neoplasia
	Trauma
	Capillaria plica
	Cyclophosphamide
Any site	Coagulation disorders
	Heatstroke, DIC
Extraurinary causes (genital tract or spurious hematuria)	Prostate
	Neoplasia
	Infection
	Hypertrophy
	Uterus
	Estrus
	Subinvolution
	Infection
	Neoplasia
	Vagina
	TVT
	Trauma
	Penis
	TVT
	Trauma

DIC, disseminated intravascular coagulation; TVT, transmissible venereal tumor

Hematuria

Hematuria is the presence of blood in the urine. It occurs as a clinical sign in a variety of diseases affecting the urogenital tract (Table 39-1). The various types of hematuria are listed in the Display, Classification of Hematuria. In healthy animals, RBC excretion in urine is about 3000 per minute, which amounts to less than two to four RBCs per high-power field in the urine sediment. Because

Classification of Hematuria

- *Essential:* hematuria for which no cause can be identified after complete diagnostic evaluation
- *False:* redness of urine due to pigments other than blood
- *Macroscopic:* hematuria detectable by gross observation of the urine. Macroscopic hematuria occurs when more than 1 million RBCs are excreted per minute.
- *Microscopic:* hematuria detectable only by microscopic examination of urine. The finding of more than two to four RBCs per high-power field is abnormal.
- *Morphologic:* hematuria originating from a particular site:

Kidney	Urethra
Ureter	Prostate
Bladder	Genital tract

of the numerous potential causes for hematuria listed in Table 39-1, a systemic diagnostic plan must be followed if an accurate diagnosis is to be made.

Diagnostic Plan. There are three steps in the diagnostic plan for the problem of hematuria: (1) collection of the initial data base, (2) localization of hematuria to an anatomic site, and (3) identification of the cause. Figure 39-2 shows algorithms for the diagnosis of hematuria in the presence and absence of dysuria.

Initial Data Base. The initial data base includes a medical history, complete physical examination, observation of micturition, and analysis of the urine. The initial data base detects hematuria, helps localize the site of bleeding, and helps dictate further diagnostic procedures.

Historical information should include the duration and severity of hematuria; at what stage blood appears during urination; the presence of other urinary tract signs such as dysuria, stranguria, or pollakiuria; and any medication the patient may be taking. The owner's observations should be verified by the clinician. A complete physical examination is given; particular attention is given to palpation of the kidneys, bladder, prostate, and uterus. The animal is carefully searched for evidence of a generalized coagulation problem. The penis or vagina is carefully examined for evidence of bleeding, trauma, or tumors.

A urine analysis is performed early in the evaluation process, since subsequent diagnostic procedures are predicated in many cases on these findings. Urine collection techniques may affect the presence and amount of blood in the urine. The initial urine analysis should be a midstream voided sample, since no trauma is involved in collection and the urine has traversed the entire urogenital tract. However, blood, bacteria, and white blood cells may be contributed to urine by disease in the genital tract, and these findings may be confused with

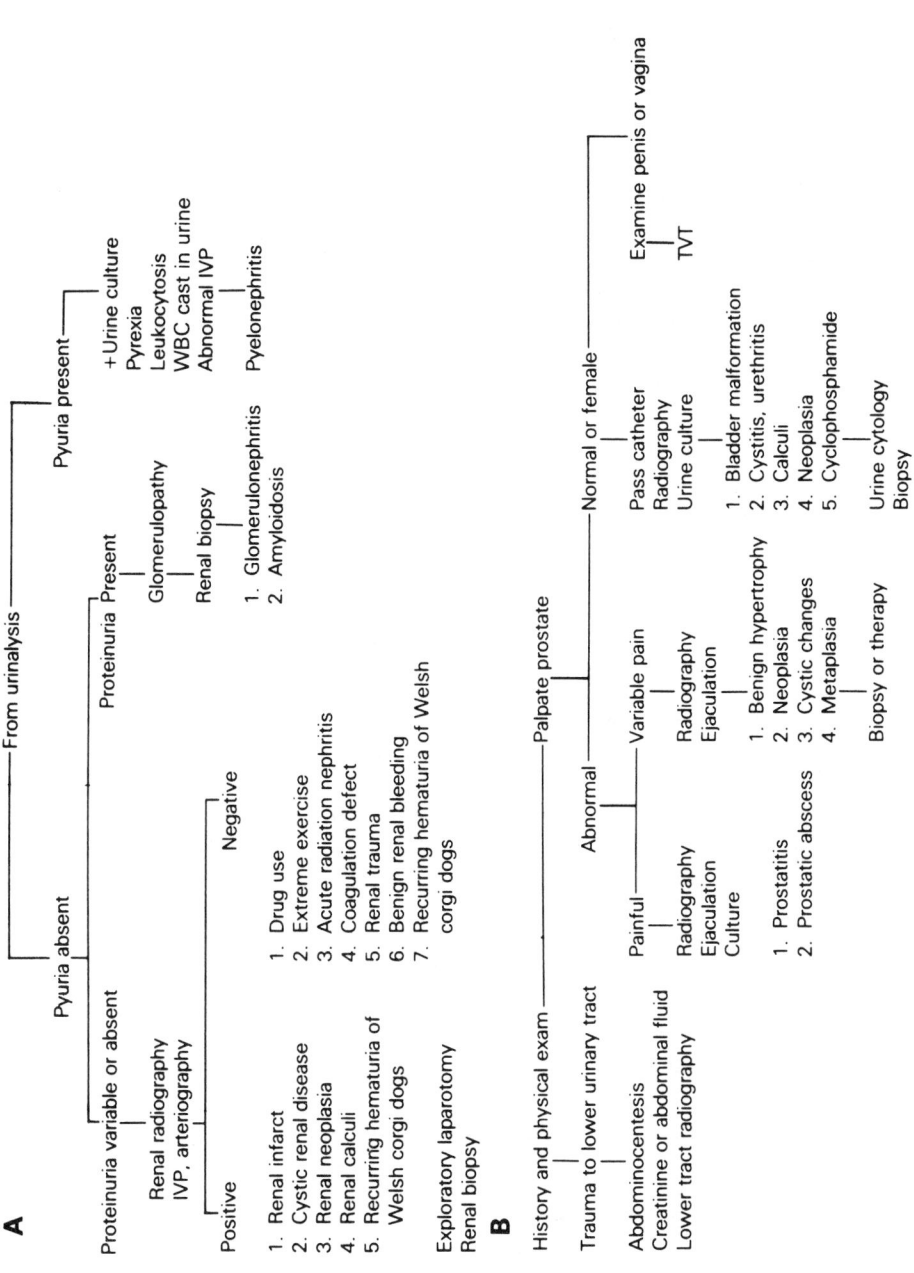

FIGURE 39-2. Algorithms for the differential diagnosis of hematuria when the animal does not have dysuria (*A*) and does have dysuria (*B*).

A

From urinalysis

Pyuria absent — Pyuria present

Pyuria absent

Proteinuria variable or absent

Renal radiography
IVP, arteriography

Positive

1. Renal infarct
2. Cystic renal disease
3. Renal neoplasia
4. Renal calculi
5. Recurring hematuria of Welsh corgi dogs

Negative

1. Drug use
2. Extreme exercise
3. Acute radiation nephritis
4. Coagulation defect
5. Renal trauma
6. Benign renal bleeding
7. Recurring hematuria of Welsh corgi dogs

Exploratory laparotomy
Renal biopsy

Proteinuria Present

Glomerulopathy

Renal biopsy

1. Glomerulonephritis
2. Amyloidosis

Pyuria present

+ Urine culture
Pyrexia
Leukocytosis
WBC cast in urine
Abnormal IVP

Pyelonephritis

B

History and physical exam

Trauma to lower urinary tract

Abdominocentesis
Creatinine or abdominal fluid
Lower tract radiography

Palpate prostate

Abnormal

Painful

Radiography
Ejaculation
Culture

1. Prostatitis
2. Prostatic abscess

Variable pain

Radiography
Ejaculation

1. Benign hypertrophy
2. Neoplasia
3. Cystic changes
4. Metaplasia

Biopsy or therapy

Normal or female

Pass catheter
Radiography
Urine culture

1. Bladder malformation
2. Cystitis, urethritis
3. Calculi
4. Neoplasia
5. Cyclophosphamide

Urine cytology
Biopsy

Examine penis or vagina

TVT

337

urinary tract disease. Collection of urine by catheterization or manual expression is not encouraged, since catheterization invites infection and some trauma, and manual expression usually produces some hematuria and is technically difficult in males. Cystocentesis is safe and does not produce significant iatrogenic hematuria if 22-gauge needles are used. The results of the voided urine analysis are compared with the cystocentesis specimen. The procedure helps localize the site of hematuria.

Urine specimens are examined within 30 minutes after collection, since RBCs begin to disappear within minutes after their addition to urine. Refrigeration of urine helps delay RBC degradation if examination must be delayed.

Localization of Hematuria to an Anatomic Site. Animals with gross hematuria can be divided into two groups, depending upon the presence or absence of dysuria, stranguria, and pollakiuria. The presence of these signs indicates disease of the bladder, urethra, prostate, or vagina. When dysuria is absent, disease of the kidneys or uterus is suspected. Blood that is present throughout urination indicates disease of the kidneys, ureters, or bladder, or prostatic reflex into the bladder. Hematuria at the beginning of micturition suggests disease in the prostate, urethra, penis, uterus, or vagina. Hematuria at the end of micturition is characteristic of bladder or prostatic disease. Hematuria detected in voided samples but absent in cystocentesis samples suggests disease of the urethra or genital tract. Although considerable overlap occurs among the various sites, the astute clinician is able to localize the source of hematuria to a general region of the urogenital tract.

Identification of the Cause of Hematuria. Following the procedures outlined in Figure 39-2, a clinical diagnosis is made after completion of radiographic, cytologic, microbiologic, and endoscopic procedures. These procedures constitute the expanded data base for the problem of hematuria. Table 39-2 lists the various causes of hematuria and characterizes them relative to clinical findings.

Hemoglobinuria

Hemoglobinuria, the presence of free hemoglobin in urine, arises from two basic sources: (a) hemoglobin filtered by the glomeruli and (2) hemoglobin released by the lysis of RBCs in dilute urine or aged urine. These two causes of hemoglobinuria are differentiated by examining the urine sediment for RBCs (hematuria causing hemoglobinuria). In this section, true hemoglobinuria is discussed.

Causes. Hemoglobin is a metalloprotein of molecular weight 64,500 and is barely small enough to pass the glomerular filter. True hemoglobinuria is caused by the intravascular destruction of RBCs with hemoglobin released into the plasma. When intravascular hemolysis is moderate to severe, free hemoglobin

Text continues on p. 343

TABLE 39-2. Causes and Differential Diagnosis of Hematuria

Disease	Clinical Sign(s)	Urine Analysis	Hematology	Biochemistry	Special Test(s)
Glomerulopathy Glomerulone- phritis SLE Amyloidosis	Early—no consis- tent signs Late—signs of chronic renal failure P&P Vomiting Ascites Edema	Primary pro- teinuria Hyaline casts Microscopic hema- turia Late—↓ specific gravity	Variable PCV, N or ↑ WBC, N or ↑	Early—normal Late ↓ Albumin ↓ BUN	24-hour urine pro- tein quantitation Urine electropho- resis Renal biopsy
Acute pyelone- phritis	Pyrexia Perirenal pain Vomiting P&P	Pyuria White cell casts or clumps Bacteruria ↓ Specific gravity Hematuria in acute cases	WBC ↑ (poly- morphonuclear leukocytosis)	Early—normal Late—↑ BUN	Urine culture IVP Renal function tests Ultrasonography
Renal calculi	Perirenal pain Late—may pro- gress to chronic renal failure	Hematuria—gross or microscopic Variable pyuria Variable bacteruria	Normal	Variable BUN, N or ↑	IVP Ultrasonography Exploratory lapa- rotomy Nephrotomy
Renal neoplasia	No consistent signs Perirenal pain Asymmetric renal en- largement	Hematuria—gross or microscopic	Normal	No consistent clues	IVP Ultrasonography Renal arteriogram Renal biopsy

(continued)

TABLE 39-2. Causes and Differential Diagnosis of Hematuria (*continued*)

Disease	Clinical Sign(s)	Urine Analysis	Hematology	Biochemistry	Special Test(s)
Renal cysts	No consistent signs May palpate enlarged kidneys	Hematuria—gross or microscopic	Normal	No consistent clues	IVP Ultrasonography Renal arteriogram
Renal infarction	Small infarcts—no consistent signs Large infarcts—may produce primary renal failure	Small infarcts—microscopic hematuria Large infarcts—gross hematuria	Variable—depends upon cause of infarction	No consistent clues	IVP Renal arteriogram
Recurring macroscopic hematuria of Welsh corgis	No apparent signs of illness	Hematuria—gross	Normal	No consistent clues	IVP Arteriogram Renal biopsy
Benign renal bleeding	No consistent signs Cause is unknown	Hematuria—gross	PCV, N	No consistent clues	IVP Arteriogram (negative) Biopsy
Dioctophyma renale infection	No consistent signs History of eating raw fish	Hematuria—gross Parasite ova in sediments	Normal	No consistent clues	None
Lower urinary tract disorders					
Cystitis	Dysuria Urethral obstruction	Gross hematuria Triple phosphate crystals	PCV, N ↑	BUN, N or ↑ K, N or ↑	Urine culture
Bladder calculi	Dysuria Bladder mass on palpation Incontinence	Gross hematuria Pyuria	Normal	Normal	Double-contrast cystography Pneumocystography

340

Disease	Clinical signs	Hematology	Blood chemistry	Diagnostic tests
Bladder neoplasia	See Cystitis.	Normal	Normal	See Cystitis. Urine cytology for neoplastic cells
Urethral diseases				
Urethritis	Edema or inflammation of urethral orifice / Blood dripping from urethra	Hematuria—gross	Normal	Normal	Voiding urethrocystogram / Urine culture / Cytology of urethral fluid
Urethral rupture	Depression / Abdominal pain / Vomiting / Subcutaneous fluid and inflammation of ventral abdominal skin	Gross hematuria	PCV	↑ BUN / ↑ Creatinine	Urethrogram / Abdominocentesis / Creatinine analysis on fluid
Urethral calculi / Urethral neoplasia	Stranguria / Urethral obstruction / Urinary incontinence	Hematuria—gross	Normal	Normal unless obstructed / Then: ↑ BUN / ↑ K	Catheterization / Retrograde urethrogram
Genital diseases				
Prostatic infection / Bacterial / Abscess	Palpably painful enlarged prostate / Pyrexia	Gross hematuria / Pyuria	WBC ↑ (neutrophilic leukocytosis)	No consistent clues	Ejaculation / Culture fluid / Cytology / Biopsy
Prostatic neoplasia	Prostate enlarged—surface may be irregular / Prostate adhered to pelvic structures	Gross hematuria at tip of penis	Normal	No consistent clues	See Prostatic infection. / Add retrograde urethrogram. / Ultrasonography

(continued)

341

TABLE 39-2. Causes and Differential Diagnosis of Hematuria *(continued)*

Disease	Clinical Sign(s)	Urine Analysis	Hematology	Biochemistry	Special Test(s)
Benign hypertrophy	Prostate enlarged, nonpainful Bleeding from tip of penis	Gross hematuria	Normal	No consistent clues	See Prostatic infection. Ultrasonography
Prostatic cyst	Prostate asymmetrically enlarged Palpatable fluctuating areas Usually nonpainful	Gross hematuria	Normal	No consistent clues	See Prostatic infection. Ultrasonography
Transmissible venereal tumor	Bloody vaginal or penile discharge Vaginal or penile masses	May be normal or show hematuria	Normal	No consistent clues	Vaginal examination Penis examination Exfoliative cytology

SLE, systemic lupus erythematosus; P&P, polydipsia and polyuria; ↓, decreased; PCV, packed cell volume; N, normal; ↑, increased; WBC, white blood cells; BUN, blood urea nitrogen; IVP, intravenous pyelogram

Causes of Hemolytic Anemia

- Intravascular hemolysis (more likely to cause hemoglobinuria)
  Bacteria
    Leptospira spp
    Clostridium spp
  RBC parasites
    Babesia spp
  Chemicals
    Phenothiazine
    Methylene blue
    Acetaminophen
    Copper
    Ricin
  Immune-mediated
    Neonatal isoerythrolysis
    Incompatible transfusion
  Hypoosmolality
    Cold-induced hemoglobinuria
- Extravascular hemolysis (less likely to cause hemoglobinuria)
  RBC parasites
    Haemobartonella spp
  Immune-mediated
    Autoimmune hemolytic anemia
    Systemic lupus erythematosus
    Cold agglutinin disease
  Intracorpuscular defects
    Pyruvate kinase deficiency
      Basenji
      Beagle
    Congenital porphyria—cats
    Hereditary stomatocytosis—malamute
  Fragmentation (microangiopathic disorders)
    Disseminated intravascular coagulation
    Cirrhosis of the liver

passes the glomerular filter and appears in the urine. Most of the free hemoglobin in plasma is probably excreted in urine as a dimer with a molecular weight of approximately 32,000. Since true hemoglobinuria results from intravascular hemolysis, the condition is usually accompanied by other clinical problems such as pale mucous membranes, rapid respiratory rate, rapid heart rate, and, in some cases, cyanosis. The presence of true hemoglobinuria necessitates an immediate search for the presence and cause of intravascular hemolysis. The causes of hemolytic anemia (see Display, Causes of Hemolytic Anemia) are discussed in Chapter 23. Hemoglobinuria results from hemolytic anemia only when RBCs are destroyed within the vascular system at a rate that exceeds the capacity for conversion of hemoglobin to bilirubin. Therefore, many patients with hemolytic anemia will not have hemoglobinuria but will have bilirubinuria and icterus (see Chapter 37).

Myoglobinuria

Myoglobinuria is characterized by brownish-red urine, a positive occult blood test, and no erythrocytes in the urinary sediment. Myoglobin does bind significantly to plasma proteins and is excreted in the urine before reaching levels that discolor the plasma. Myoglobin is released from muscle following severe muscle necrosis or trauma. Myoglobinuria is observed in generalized muscle diseases such as exertional rhabdomyolysis (greyhound cramps) and extensive crushing injuries to heavy muscle. It is rarely observed in acute polymyositis or generalized degenerative myopathies. The presence of myoglobinuria indicates the search for clinical or laboratory evidence of muscle disease. Generalized muscle pain, muscle weakness, muscle swelling, and elevated muscle enzymes (creatine phosphokinase, serum aspartate aminotransferase, and lactic dehydrogenase) are findings indicative of muscle disease. A muscle biopsy is often necessary for identification of the etiology.

BROWN URINE

Brown or reddish-brown urine suggests the presence of bilirubin, myoglobin, or heme products in acid urine. With the exception of bilirubin, these products give a positive occult blood test and have been previously discussed.

Bilirubinuria

Conjugated bilirubin is water-soluble and freely filtered by the glomeruli. Nonconjugated bilirubin does not pass the renal filter in quantities significant enough to be detected in urine. Reagent strips and the tablet method both employ the diazotization method for detection of bilirubin. Urine colors may interfere with reading the reagent strips; however, no interference occurs with the tablet method. Both tests are very reactive with conjugated bilirubin but insensitive to free bilirubin. Since bilirubin is oxidized on exposure to light, excessive delay in analysis may produce a negative test. Trace to +1 reactions are found in concentrated urine from normal dogs. Levels above this concentration or +1 reactions in dilute urine are abnormal. In cat urine, +1 reactions are always considered abnormal.

Causes. Bilirubinuria indicates the regurgitation of conjugated bilirubin into the blood. This may occur in hemolytic anemia, primary hepatocellular disease, or cholestatic disorders. Bilirubinuria may precede hyperbilirubinemia and clinical icterus. See Chapter 37 for a complete discussion of icterus.

CHAPTER FORTY

Urinary Incontinence

Jeanne A. Barsanti

DEFINITION

Urinary incontinence is defined as the lack of voluntary control of micturition. Incontinence must be distinguished from inappropriate urination, since they appear similar to the client. With inappropriate urination, urination occurs at the wrong place or time (as defined by the owner), but it is under the voluntary control of the pet. Problems associated with inappropriate urination include nocturia, dysuria, polyuria, urine spraying, submissive urination, and other behavioral problems. A thorough history or direct observation of the problem is necessary to determine whether the problem is incontinence or inappropriate urination. This chapter covers only incontinence (see chapters referring to the other problems listed.)

PHYSIOLOGY

Normal micturition requires storage and emptying phases. During the storage phase, the bladder slowly fills via the ureters as urine is produced by the kidneys. The detrusor muscle of the bladder adjusts to filling by stretching, with little increase in intravesicular pressure. The sympathetic system facilitates detrusor relaxation via beta-adrenergic receptors. Both an internal (smooth muscle) and an external (striated muscle) sphincter maintain continence during bladder filling by exerting a resting pressure, which can increase with sudden increases in intraabdominal pressure (*e.g.,* coughing). The smooth muscle of the internal sphincter is located in both the bladder neck and urethra and is innervated by the sympathetic system via alpha-adrenergic receptors. The striated muscle of the external sphincter is located in the urethra and is innervated by the pudendal nerve.

The emptying phase begins when stretch receptors in the bladder wall detect bladder fullness. Impulses are relayed via the pelvic nerves to the sacral segments of the spinal cord and up the spinal cord to the brain stem (Fig. 40-1). A reflex occurs at this level back down the spinal cord to the sacral parasympathetic nucleus. Impulses are sent via the pelvic nerve to the detrusor muscle. In the detrusor muscle, excitation spreads via tight junctions between muscle fi-

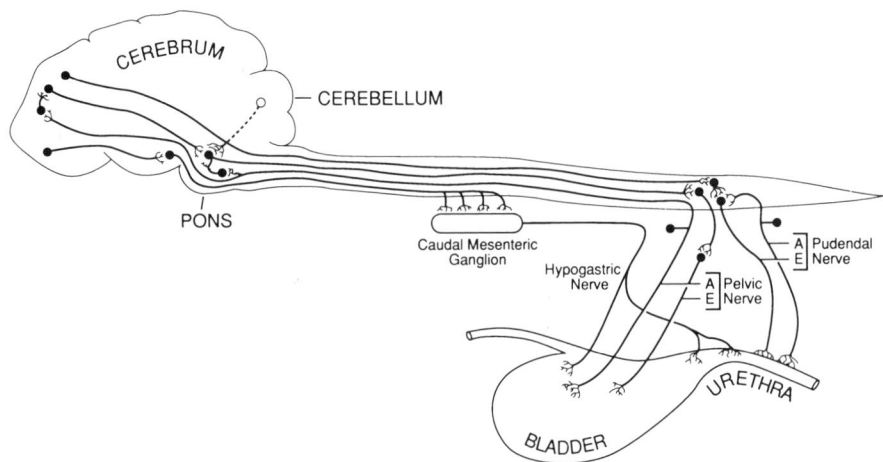

FIGURE 40-1. Neurophysiology of micturition. The cerebrum controls voluntary micturition by inhibitory and facilitory influences on the brain stem micturition reflex area. The cerebellum also has an inhibitory influence on the micturition reflex. The pelvic nerve (parasympathetic system) carries both afferent and efferent fibers between the bladder and the sacral spinal cord. The reflex between these fibers is in the brain stem. Efferent fibers are also carried by the hypogastric nerve (sympathetic system) and pudendal nerve. The hypogastric nerve supplies beta-adrenergic fibers to the bladder and alpha-adrenergic fibers to the bladder neck and urethra. The pudendal nerve innervates the striated muscle of the urethra. (Barsanti, JA: Problems of urine output and voiding. In Stone EA, Barsanti JA (eds): Small Animal Urologic Surgery. Philadelphia, Lea & Febiger, in press).

bers. Contraction pulls the bladder neck open. Simultaneously, the pudendal motor neurons and alpha-adrenergic sympathetic activity are inhibited, resulting in decreased urethral pressure. Urine is evacuated. When the bladder is empty, the afferent discharge from the pelvic nerve stops, the pelvic motor neurons cease their discharge, and sympathetic and pudendal motor activity again increase bladder neck and urethral pressure.

Voluntary control of this reflex pathway is via the cerebral cortex to the brain stem. The cerebellum has an inhibitory effect on the brain stem micturition center.

DIAGNOSTIC PLAN

The diagnostic approach to incontinence should start with a thorough history. The age of onset of the problem, reproductive status of the pet, relationship between the onset of incontinence and neutering, chronological course of the incontinence, associated urinary tract problems, history of other neurologic abnormalities, whether normal micturition occurs at all, and when incontinence occurs in relation to micturition are all important, as is any drug usage or dietary changes. Any drug or dietary change that stimulates a polyuria (*e.g.*, glucocorticoids, high salt diet) could precipitate a latent predisposition to incontinence by increasing the amount of urine the bladder must store.

A complete physical examination should follow. Special attention should be paid to the bladder. Is it large and distended, small and contracted, or normal? In a male dog the prostate gland should be palpated. Anal tone and the integrity of the perineal reflex should be evaluated. Any abnormal neurologic signs should be evaluated by a complete neurologic examination. Micturition should be observed and residual volume determined if there is any question about the ability of the bladder to empty. Residual volume has not been measured in large numbers of dogs and cats, but most have only a small residual volume, less than 10 ml. One must remember that some male dogs may want to mark territory repeatedly before the bladder is completely emptied. If complete micturition occurs, the emtpy bladder should be palpated for calculi, soft tissue masses, and wall thickness. If the bladder is not emptied, the urethra should be carefully palpated externally and per rectum in males and per rectum in females. Any yellow fluid found dripping from the urethra in male dogs should be compared with urine, since fluid from a prostatic cyst communicating with the urethra may have the same color as urine.

After the history and physical examination, the incontinence should be classified as neurogenic (associated with other neurologic problems) or nonneurogenic (see Display, Causes of Incontinence).

Causes of Incontinence

- Neurogenic
    - Cerebral lesions
    - Brain stem lesions
    - Spinal cord lesions (cervical, thoracic, lumbar)
    - Lesions of the sacral spinal cord, sacral spinal roots, pelvic or pudendal nerves)
- Nonneurogenic
    - Bladder distended
        - Urethral obstruction
        - Mass in the bladder neck area
        - Detrusor-urethral dyssynergia
    - Bladder not distended
        - Urethral incompetence
        - Ectopic ureter(s)
        - Mass in the bladder neck area
        - Patent urachus
        - Reduced bladder capacity

Neurogenic Incontinence

If neurologic abnormalities are detected, a complete neurologic examination is essential to localize the lesion site so that appropriate diagnostic tests can be chosen.

With cerebral lesions, micturition will be normal, except for loss of voluntary control. The pet cannot be house-trained or loses its former training. Associated neurologic signs might include change in mental attitude, possible loss of other cerebral functions, such as vision (with normal pupillary light responses) or hearing, and decreased postural reactions in spite of a normal-appearing gait. Segmental reflexes may be normal or hyperactive.

With cerebellar diseases, there is some loss of inhibition of micturition; thus, urination may occur at the wrong place or time. Signs of diffuse cerebellar disease, such as ataxia and intention tremors, should be present.

With brain stem and spinal cord lesions cranial to the first sacral spinal cord segment (fifth lumbar vertebra in the dog, and seventh in the cat), the micturition reflex is lost, but sphincter tone remains. The bladder fills, but the sensation cannot be relayed to the reflex center. As a result, the bladder overdistends with urine and bladder pressure markedly increases. When bladder pressure exceeds urethral pressure, some urine dribbles from the urethra. The detrusor muscle may attempt to contract intrinsically. These contractions occur against resting urethral tone. Such contractions are usually ineffectual in emptying the bladder. The bladder is distended on physical examination, and attempts to express it will be difficult because the sphincters do not relax. Passage of a urinary catheter is easy, since no anatomic urethral obstruction exists. With brain stem lesions, other neurologic abnormalities found may include changes in mental attitude, posture and gait, cranial nerve abnormalities, and postural reaction deficits in the limbs with normal or hyperactive segmental reflexes. With spinal cord lesions, mental attitude and cranial nerve function are normal, but postural reaction deficits are present in the limbs at or caudal to the lesion. See Chapter 47 for further help in localizing spinal cord lesions.

With sacral spinal cord lesions, bilateral sacral root lesions, and bilateral peripheral nerve lesions, the micturition reflex is lost and the external sphincter is atonic. The bladder overdistends, and urine dribbles out when bladder pressure exceeds urethral pressure. The detrusor muscle intrinsically contracts when stretched. Such contractions may be more successful in voiding urine, since resting urethral tone is decreased. However, complete voiding is rare, and loss of the tight junctions between detrusor muscle fibers by overdistention may prevent effective bladder contraction. On physical examination, the bladder is overdistended but relatively easy to express. Associated neurologic abnormalities may include decreased anal tone, fecal incontinence, loss of the perineal reflex, paralysis of the tail, decreased sensation in the tail, perineal area, and caudal back, and possibly evidence of sciatic nerve dysfunction, such as knuckling the paw, decreased stifle flexion, decreased flexor reflex, and loss of sensation in the limb—especially on the dorsal surface of the paw, which is solely innervated by branches of the sciatic nerve.

Once the lesion is localized by neurologic examination and characterization of the abnormality in micturition, further diagnostic tests could include skull and/or spinal radiographs, myelography, cerebrospinal fluid analysis, electromyography, electroencephalography, and other tests based on lesion localization (see Chapter 47).

Nonneurogenic Incontinence

Nonneurogenic incontinence is incontinence unassociated with other neurologic abnormalities on neurologic examination. Some etiologies that have a local neurologic cause (such as detrusor dysfunction) are included in this category. Nonneurogenic incontinence is best approached diagnostically by subdividing it into two categories on the basis of the physical examination: a distended bladder with inability to void or a normal bladder with ability to void (see Display, Causes of Incontinence).

Bladder Distended. A partial or complete urethral obstruction should be the first consideration in any animal with a distended bladder and inability to void, especially if the animal tries to urinate. In dogs, the urethra should be carefully palpated. This involves percutaneous palpation in males and rectal palpation in both males and females. After palpation, a urinary catheter should be passed as aseptically as possible. If an obstruction is encountered, it is characterized as to location and consistency. Survey and contrast radiographs are often necessary to further characterize the obstruction. Laboratory work, including blood urea nitrogen (BUN), serum creatinine, serum electrolytes, and urine analysis should be obtained to determine the degree of postrenal azotemia and to evaluate for the presence of urinary tract hemorrhage, inflammation, and/or infection. If a urolith is the cause of the obstruction, survey radiographs of the abdomen are necessary to determine if other uroliths are present in the kidneys, ureters, or bladder.

Ability to pass a urinary catheter to the bladder does not preclude the presence of an anatomic obstruction. An obstruction may prevent urine retrograde passage via bladder contraction, but not markedly inhibit antegrade passage of a catheter. Examples include prostatic diseases, masses in the area of the bladder neck and those partially obstructing the urethra, and small uroliths. Retrograde urethrography and contrast cystography are necessary to document such obstructions. Once the obstruction has been localized and characterized, a biopsy may be required to identify the cause precisely.

Once an anatomic obstruction has been *excluded,* two general etiologies are considered: (1) detrusor dysfunction and (2) failure of the urethral musculature to relax during detrusor contraction.

Detrusor dysfunction occurs most commonly as a result of loss of tight junc-

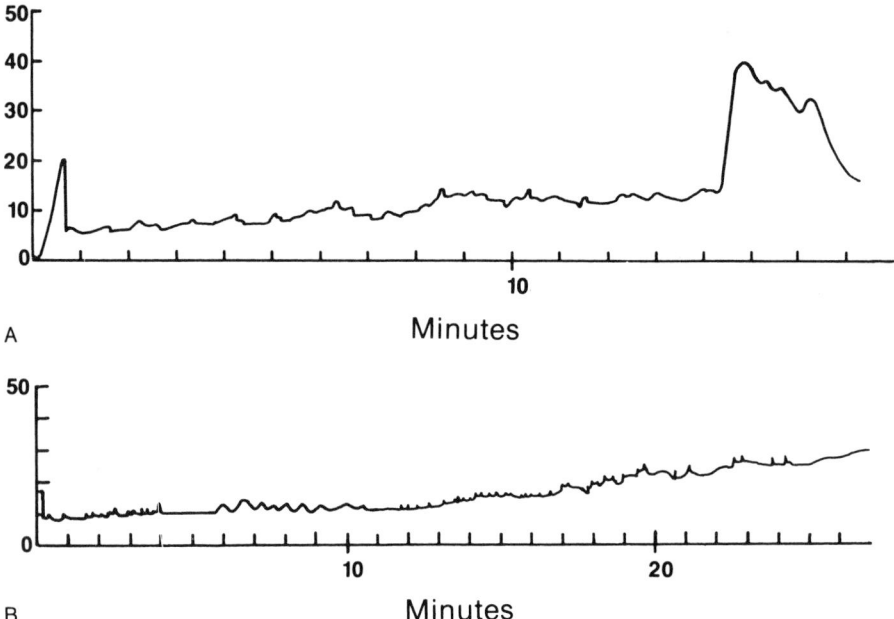

FIGURE 40-2. Comparison of a normal cystometrogram (*A*) with a cystometrogram (*B*) indicating detrusor dysfunction. Intravesicular pressure (cm H_2O) is on the vertical axis and time to contraction during CO_2 infusion (ml/min) is on the horizontal axis. The normal cystometrogram (*A*) shows little increase in pressure as the bladder fills. As the bladder contracts, intravesicular pressure rises dramatically and then falls as the CO_2 is expelled. The cystometrogram from a dog with detrusor dysfunction (*B*) shows a gradual rise in intravesicular pressure with no sharp increase in pressure, because the detrusor muscle could not contract even though the bladder filled.

tions from prolonged bladder overdistention. Bladder overdistention may result from urethral obstruction, from neurologic dysfunction (*e.g.*, intervertebral disk disease), with unwillingness to void with forced recumbency (*e.g.*, after pelvic trauma), and, we suspect, with development of polyuria in well house-trained dogs with limited access to the outdoors. One cause of detrusor atony in cats is feline dysautonomia, an autonomic polyganglionopathy (Key-Gaskell syndrome). The bladder dysfunction in this syndrome consists of an apparent inability to contract the bladder in spite of efforts to do so, although the bladder is easily expressed manually. Other signs such as persistent pupillary dilation, decreased tear production, chronic regurgitation due to megaesophagus, and constipation are more common than bladder atony. In some animals, the cause of detrusor dysfunction cannot be determined. Detrusor dysfunction is suspected on the basis of the history, physical examination, and the exclusion of an anatomic obstruction to urine outflow. Cystometry is necessary to confirm detrusor dysfunction (Fig. 40-2).

Lack of relaxation of the urethral musculature, preventing micturition despite detrusor contraction, is very difficult to confirm in veterinary medicine. There are two possible causes: (1) urethral spasm due to inflammation of any cause and (2) urethral dyssynergia, in which the urethra contracts rather than relaxes as micturition is initiated. The typical history with detrusor-urethral dyssynergia is that the dog initiates urination, but urination ceases immediately thereafter in spite of continued efforts to urinate. The condition has only been noted in male dogs. In humans, dyssynergia is documented at rest by urethral pressure profilometry, and during micturition in correlation with measurement of the volume and strength of the urine stream. The cause in humans is usually a spinal lesion, which may or may not be associated with other neurologic signs. A urethral pressure profile can also be performed in dogs. However, since it is performed at rest and not during micturition, it may be normal, even though a problem exists during micturition. The technique of uroflowmetry might be useful for diagnosing this problem in dogs, but it is relatively invasive and has only been described in normal dogs. Currently, dyssynergia is a diagnosis made by excluding anatomic urethral obstruction and detrusor dysfunction. If dyssynergia is suspected, spinal radiographs and a myelogram or epidurogram of the sacral area may be warranted.

Bladder Not Distended. If an animal is presented for incontinence and if the bladder is normal or empty on physical examination, there are two major possibilities to consider: (1) the urethral sphincter is not competent or is being bypassed or (2) the bladder is contracting involuntarily at low volumes.

The urethral sphincter may be bypassed with a patent urachus or an ectopic ureter, both usually congenital defects in young animals. A patent urachus should be recognizable on physical examination. In a puppy or kitten, an ectopic ureter is suspected when urine dribbling occurs in spite of apparent normal micturition. Female dogs are most commonly affected, but cases in male dogs and in cats of both sexes have been reported. The lesion may be unilateral or bilateral. The ureter may terminate in the urethra or in the vagina in females. Most cases are diagnosed by excretory urography in order to visualize the course of the ureters. Interpretation is difficult in some cases, since the ureters may enter the serosa at the normal site and then tunnel subserosally to enter the urethra. Positive contrast vaginourethrography can identify this defect. Cases in which the ureter exits into the vagina may be visualized by vaginoscopy. An advantage of excretory urography is that the kidneys and ureters can be examined for other associated problems such as hydroureter, pyelonephritis, and abnormal kidney size or shape. A complete blood count, BUN or serum creatinine, urine analysis, and urine culture should be performed prior to surgical correction of an ectopic ureter. Some dogs with ectopic ureters also have decreased resting urethral pressures, which can lead to continued incontinence after surgical correction of the ectopic ureter. A urethral pressure profile can be used to detect this defect. If a urethral pressure profile is unavailable, determining whether the bladder is easy or difficult to express manually may assist in evaluating urethral competence. In some puppies, the urethra will become more competent with maturity, while others will require medical or surgical therapy for urethral incompetence.

A urethral sphincter of decreased competence is the most likely cause of incontinence associated with neutering in dogs. Commonly called "spay incontinence," this also occurs in neutered males, in juvenile bitches of any breed, and in a few intact bitches, especially of the Doberman breed. Affected dogs have been found to have decreased resting urethral pressures on urethral pressure profilometry (Fig. 40-3). Diagnosis is usually made on the basis of history and physical examination. Suggestive historical findings include a neutered, medium- to large-breed female or male dog that leaks urine while sleeping or lying down, but otherwise urinates normally. Male dogs often have been neutered for treatment of a prostatic disease. The physical examination is normal, except for urine scalding in some cases. Affected adult dogs are often overweight. The urine analysis is usually normal, although some dogs develop a secondary urinary tract infection. The cause of the decrease in resting urethral pressure is not understood. It is known that reproductive hormone receptors are present in the urethral musculature and do increase resting urethral tone. In juvenile dogs, the problem may resolve with maturity. It is also known that incontinence in neutered dogs often responds to reproductive hormone replacement. Why only a small proportion of neutered dogs develop this problem is not understood, but studies to date have not shown any association with age of neutering. Some cases in bitches have been associated with an anatomically short urethra (i.e., intrapelvic bladder position on urethrocystography). However, intrapelvic bladder location can also be present in normally continent dogs. Rather than resulting from one cause in all dogs, the condition is more likely to be multifactorial, involving both physiologic and anatomic variables, and might depend on the severity of the abnormalities in these variables. For example, a neutered female dog with an intrapelvic bladder might be normally continent until she becomes overweight or develops polyuria. Urethral incompetence has also been mentioned as a rare sequela to urethral surgery, such as perineal urethrostomy in cats.

A similar type of incontinence occurs in cats of both sexes, neutered or not. The cat typically dribbles urine while relaxed but otherwise urinates normally. Physical examination may be normal, or the cat may have anisocoria. These cats are usually feline leukemia virus–positive, although the relationship of the viremia to the incontinence is unknown. Whether the incontinence is due to urethral incompetence or unrestrainable detrusor contractions at low bladder volumes, or both, has not been determined.

A mass in the area of the bladder neck may cause incompetence of the internal urethral sphincter. Diagnosis may be suspected by an associated history of dysuria or hematuria, a palpable abnormality (not always detectable), or abnormalities in the urine sediment (possibly hematuria, pyuria, or abnormal

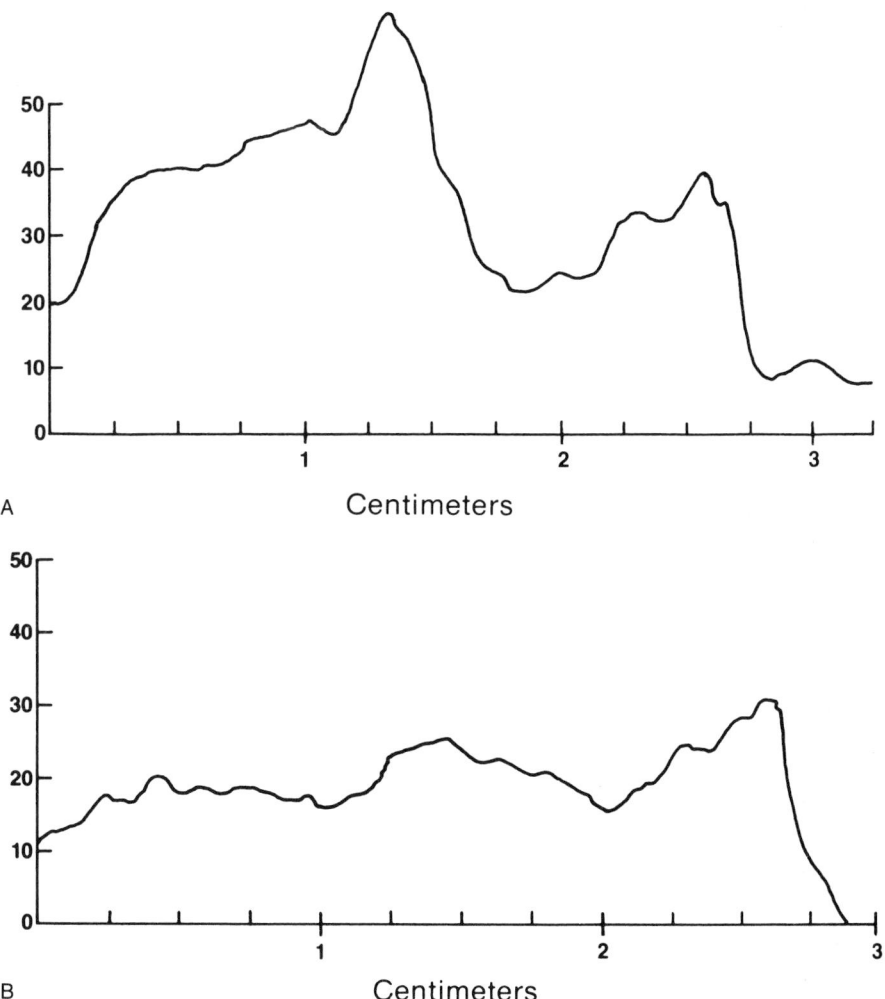

FIGURE 40-3. Comparison of a normal urethral pressure profile in a female dog (*A*) and a urethral pressure profile from a female dog with urethral incompetence (*B*). Profiles were recorded with xylazine restraint. Urethral pressure (cm H_2O) is on the vertical axis and urethral length on the horizontal axis. The abnormal urethral pressure profile (*B*) had markedly lower pressures than the normal profile (*A*).

cells). Cystography or retrograde urethrography is necessary to confirm the mass. A biopsy is usually required to determine its nature.

Unrestrainable detrusor contractions at low bladder volumes (urge incontinence) result in incontinence that appears very similar to urethral incompetence. Causes include severe chronic cystitis, bladder wall neoplasia, and prior cystectomy with markedly reduced bladder volume. Diagnosis is based on palpating an abnormal bladder, abnormalities on urine analysis, or an abnormal cystogram and a small bladder threshold volume on cystometry.

SUGGESTED READINGS

Barsanti JA, Downey R: Urinary incontinence in cats. J Am Anim Hosp Assoc 20:979–982, 1984

Downie JW: Bethanechol chloride in urology—a discussion of issues. Neurourol Urodynam 3:211–222, 1984

Holt PE: Urinary incontinence in the bitch due to sphincter mechanism incompetence: Prevalence in referred dogs and retrospective analysis of sixty cases. J Sm Anim Pract 26:181–190, 1985

Holt PE, Gibbs C, Latham J: An evaluation of positive contrast vagino-urethrography as a diagnostic aid in the bitch. J Sm Anim Pract 25:531–550, 1984

Lees GE, Moreau PM: Management of hypotonic and atonic urinary bladders in cats. Vet Clin N Am 14:641–647, 1984

Moreau PM, Lappin MR: Pharmacologic management of urinary incontinence. In Kirk RW (ed): Current Veterinary Therapy X, pp 1214–1223. Philadelphia, WB Saunders, 1989

Moreau PM, Lees GE, Gross DR: Simultaneous cystometry and uroflowmetry in dogs: Reference values for healthy animals sedated with xylazine. Am J Vet Res 44:1774–1781, 1983

Rosin AE, Barsanti JA: Diagnosis of urinary incontinence in dogs: Role of the urethral pressure profile. J Am Vet Med Assoc 178:814–822, 1981

Sharp NJH, Nash AS, Griffiths IR: Feline dysautonomia (the Key-Gaskell syndrome): A clinical and pathological study of 40 cases. J Sm Anim Pract 25:599–615, 1984

Wein AJ: Physiology of micturition. Clin Geriatr Med 2:689–699, 1986

PART TEN

Reproductive Problems

CHAPTER FORTY-ONE

Vaginal and Preputial Discharges

Jeanne A. Barsanti

DEFINITION AND RECOGNITION

Vaginal and preputial discharges are much more common in dogs than in cats. Such discharges can be normal or abnormal in dogs, but they are usually considered abnormal in cats unless associated with the recent delivery of kittens. Vaginal and preputial discharges can originate from the external genitalia, the reproductive system, or the distal urethra. To determine the cause of a discharge, a thorough history, a complete physical examination, and a cytologic study of the discharge are required.

In the history, the following are especially important: the amount, duration, and appearance of the discharge; the age of the animal when the discharge began; the breeding record; and, in the female, the relationship of the discharge to estrus or pregnancy. Establishing whether the affected animal has other systemic signs of illness or a change in attitude or activities is important, as is determining whether any medications have been given.

The entire reproductive tract should be examined as carefully as possible. In the male, the penis must be extruded for a thorough examination of the penis and prepuce; this may require sedation. The urethra should be thoroughly palpated from the os penis to the pelvis, and rectal palpation of the pelvic urethra and the prostate gland should be performed. In the female, the vaginal vault should be examined visually using a vaginal speculum or an endoscope. The normal canine vagina is narrow and long, 10 to 14 cm in medium-sized dogs. Sedation may be needed, depending on the dog's nature. The vaginal vault and the urethra can also be examined digitally per vagina and per rectum.

The discharge should be collected and applied to a slide, dried, stained, and examined microscopically. In the bitch, the discharge should be collected from the vagina, avoiding the clitoral fossa and the vestibule. In this chapter, the causes of vaginal and preputial discharges (see Displays, Rule Outs for Vaginal Discharge and Rule Outs for Preputial Discharge) are reviewed based on their cytologic characteristics. Discharges are classified according to whether they are primarily mucus, blood, or pus.

Rule Outs for Vaginal Discharge

Mucoid
  Normal
  Diestrus
  Late pregnancy
  Postpartum
  Intravaginal irritative lesion
Hemorrhagic
  Proestrus/estrus
  Postpartum
  Subinvolution of placental sites
  Neoplasia
  Cystic endometrial hyperplasia
  Coagulopathy
  Trauma
  Impending abortion
  Uterine torsion

Purulent
  Diestrus
  Vaginitis
  Acute metritis
  Pyometra

Rule Outs for Preputial Discharge

Hemorrhage
  Preputial or penile lesion
    Trauma
    Neoplasia
    Foreign body
  From urethral orifice
    Distal urethra
      Urethral prolapse
      Urolith
      Trauma
      Neoplasia
      Foreign body
    Prostate
      Cystic hyperplasia
      Bacterial prostatitis
      Neoplasia
      Trauma
  Coagulopathy

Purulent discharge
  Preputial or penile lesion
    Balanoposthitis
    Foreign body
    Neoplasm
  From urethral orifice
    Prostatic disease
      Acute prostatitis
      Chronic prostatitis
      Abscessation
      Neoplasia
    Urethral disease
Serous discharge
  Urethral
    Prostatic disease
      Prostatic cyst
  Preputial

CLASSIFICATION AND DIAGNOSIS

Vaginal Discharges

Mucoid. An occasional, mild mucoid discharge is normal in bitches, whether pregnant or not. A normal vaginal cytologic specimen contains epithelial cells, a few neutrophils, and bacteria. Usual numbers of bacteria are low, but higher numbers may be seen during estrus. A heavier mucoid discharge is normal in diestrus, in late pregnancy, and postpartum. In the first few days of diestrus, the mucus may contain large numbers of nondegenerate neutrophils. A heavier mucoid discharge may also be associated with an irritative lesion in the vagina, such as a tumor. Diagnostic plans for a heavy mucoid discharge in a nondiestral, nonpregnant bitch should include a thorough vaginal examination.

Hemorrhagic. A hemorrhagic discharge is normal during proestrus in the bitch and for up to 6 weeks postpartum. The normal postpartum discharge is nonodorous and greenish to greenish-red for the first 2 to 3 weeks. It gradually becomes more serosanguineous and decreases in amount, resolving within 6 weeks after parturition.

If a hemorrhagic discharge develops during pregnancy, abortion may be imminent. The animal should be closely confined to enforce rest and to permit observation for abortion. Dogs that abort should be checked for infection with *Brucella canis,* and cats for infection with feline leukemia virus.

If a hemorrhagic discharge persists for longer than 6 weeks postpartum in a dog, the most likely cause is subinvolution of placental sites. The affected bitch is usually young (less than 3 years) and is otherwise normal. The uterus may have palpable areas of nodular enlargement. Occasionally the hemorrhage is severe enough to cause blood-loss anemia and/or iron-deficiency anemia. Rarely, the uterine placental sites rupture. Diagnosis is made on the basis of history, physical examination, and vaginal cytologic findings. The condition is usually self-limiting, but supportive care for anemia may be required.

Neoplasia of the vagina, uterus, or distal urethra may cause a hemorrhagic or serosanguineous discharge. Neoplastic cells are rarely found in the discharge. The most common tumor of the vagina is a leiomyoma, which is predominantly found in older, intact bitches and queens. Another common vaginal tumor in some areas is transmissible venereal tumor. Transitional cell carcinoma of the distal urethra can cause a urethral discharge, which will be evident to the owner as a vaginal discharge. Diagnosis of neoplasia is based on identifying a mass by vaginal examination or uterine palpation and determining the type by cytologic study on an aspirate or impression smear, or by biopsy specimen. A transmissible venereal tumor is usually diagnosed by cytologic examination because of its characteristically large, round cells, which easily exfoliate.

In dogs that are intact but not frequently bred, cystic endometrial hyperplasia has been reported to cause a mild serosanguineous discharge with no other signs. This condition can be suspected only on the basis of history and by eliminating other causes of the discharge. Confirmation requires uterine biopsy.

An uncommon cause of a hemorrhagic vaginal discharge is uterine torsion. Major associated clinical signs are uterine distention and abdominal pain.

A coagulopathy should also be considered a possible cause for vaginal bleeding of unknown origin (see Chapter 19 for a diagnostic plan).

Purulent. A mucoid discharge with a large number of nondegenerate neutrophils is normal in metestrus in the bitch. Bacteria may be seen in a vaginal cytologic specimen from normal bitches at any time, and relatively high numbers may be present during estrus. Vaginal cultures are almost always positive (more than 98%) in normal bitches, and the organisms found are varied and include all the common pathogens of the reproductive and urinary tracts, with the exception of *B. canis*. Contrary to some breeders' understanding, organisms such as beta-hemolytic streptococci and Haemophilus can be cultured from normally fertile bitches and are only transiently transmitted to the stud dog.

With a purulent discharge in an intact female, it is important to determine whether the origin of the discharge is the vagina or the uterus. This differentiation is based on the history, physical examination, vaginal examination, and complete blood count (CBC). Ultrasonography of the abdomen and abdominal radiography may also be helpful.

The principal signs of vaginitis are a purulent vaginal discharge, vulvar licking, and, occasionally, attraction of males. Vaginitis does not result in any signs of systemic illness such as fever, depression, or leukocytosis. The usual cause is bacterial infection, although viral infection is also possible (*e.g.*, canine herpesvirus). Large numbers of degenerate and nondegenerate neutrophils and bacteria are found on vaginal cytologic studies in dogs with bacterial vaginitis. Mild vaginitis is common in puppies and usually resolves with the first estrus because estrogen stimulates the keratinization of mucosal cells. No further diagnostic work, other than a vaginal examination to exclude the possibility of a congenital defect causing prediposition to infection, is usually needed in puppies. In older bitches, a complete vaginal examination should be done to identify lesions and rule out a foreign body or a space-occupying mass, such as a neoplasm. A vaginal culture may also be indicated, although results will be difficult to interpret because of the normal vaginal flora. A culture should be taken by cleaning the vulva, inserting a sterile vaginal speculum, and passing a culturette through the speculum into the proximal vagina. The culture should be performed prior to a digital examination and before examination of the cranial vagina with an endoscope. An abnormal culture is identified when large numbers of a single organism are found. If a bacterial infection is confirmed or strongly suspected, a culture of urine collected by cystocentesis is indicated, since ascent of bacteria to the bladder is common.

Acute metritis and pyometra are uterine causes of a purulent vaginal discharge. Acute metritis is a bacterial infection of the uterus, which usually occurs early postpartum but can also occur postabortion or postbreeding. The usual causative organisms are gram-negative aerobic bacilli such as *Escherichia coli*, but anaerobes such as Bacteroides may also be causative agents. Factors causing predisposition to infection include prolonged labor, retained placental or fetal tissues, vaginitis, and improper manipulation or use of instruments. The discharge is usually copious and foul-smelling. The animal is usually systemically ill with fever, depression, and anorexia, and may neglect her young; sepsis may develop. The uterus is usually mildly enlarged and doughy. The white blood cell count indicates an inflammatory disease with either a regenerative or degenerative left shift. The diagnostic plan should include abdominal radiographs to ascertain the presence of retained fetal tissues and a *Brucella* titer if the problem follows abortion in a bitch.

Pyometra usually occurs several weeks postestrus or after estrogen or progesterone therapy. Pyometra is usually the final stage of the cystic endometrial hyperplasia/endometritis complex, which is common in intact, but not bred, bitches. Infection with *E. coli* is common but is secondary to the underlying changes in the uterine wall. Pyometra is referred to as "open" or "closed" in relation to the cervix. An open pyometra is accompanied by a profuse, purulent vaginal discharge; with a closed pyometra, no vaginal discharge is evident. Dogs with a closed cervix are usually very ill, while those with an open cervix may act relatively normal. Systemic signs with pyometra include depression, vomiting, dehydration, and anorexia. The enlarged uterus is usually palpable. A neutrophilic leukocytosis is common. Abdominal radiographs or sonograms may be necessary to distinguish pyometra from another illness in a dog that is pregnant.

Preputial Discharge

Hemorrhagic. The major causes of a hemorrhagic discharge are penile/preputial trauma, neoplasia within the sheath, distal urethral injury, neoplasia or urolith, and prostatic disease. The diagnostic plan should include a complete history and physical examination, including rectal palpation of the prostate in dogs and complete examination of the sheath. This involves protrusion of the penis and may require tranquilization.

The most common bleeding preputial lesions in dogs are trauma and neoplasia. The most common neoplasms of the prepuce and penis are transmissible venereal tumor, papillomas, and carcinomas. Transmissible venereal tumors can usually be diagnosed by finding the typical large round cells on an impression smear. Biopsy is usually required to diagnose the other types of tumors.

If the bleeding is from the urethral orifice, urethral diseases such as a urethral prolapse, neoplasm, urolith, trauma, and other disorders producing inflammation are possible causes. Urethral prolapse should be evident on physical examination. The other urethral diseases should be accompanied by additional signs, such as dysuria. A retrograde urethrogram may be necessary to further investigate these possibilities.

The most common cause of a hemorrhagic urethral discharge without other clinical problems, except perhaps hematuria, is cystic hyperplasia of the prostate. Other prostatic diseases, such as acute or chronic bacterial prostatitis and neoplasia, can also cause a hemorrhagic urethral discharge. History, physical examination, complete blood count, urine analysis, abdominal radiography, ultrasonography, and prostatic fluid and tissue evaluation may be needed to differentiate these possibilities. Prostatic cystic hyperplasia is predominantly characterized by blood in urine and prostatic fluid. The prostate is enlarged but nonpainful, and the enlargement is often mild to moderate and symmetric. The predominant finding with bacterial prostatitis is infection of the urine and the prostatic fluid. Systemic signs of illness may accompany acute prostatitis and prostatic abscessation. With prostatic neoplasia, the prostate is usually markedly enlarged and irregular, or contains firm nodules. Prostatic fluid often contains red and white blood cells but is usually not infected. The dog may be in pain, depressed, and anorectic. Because these signs may overlap, a tissue biopsy is often necessary for a definitive diagnosis.

Purulent. A purulent discharge from the prepuce should be determined to be preputial or urethral in origin by a careful physical examination. The entire sheath should be examined.

If the discharge is preputial, the most common cause is balanoposthitis. Balanoposthitis is characterized by a thick, yellow to green discharge associated with lymphoid follicular hyperplasia in the sheath. On cytologic examination, epithelial cells, neutrophils, and bacteria are noted. This condition is so common in dogs that a mild discharge is considered normal. First-time owners of male dogs need to be educated in this regard. If the discharge is copious, a careful physical examination is indicated to rule out foreign body or space-occupying masses such as a neoplasm, which may act as a source of irritation.

If the discharge is urethral, an inflammatory prostatic disease such as acute or chronic prostatitis, abscessation, or neoplasia should be considered. The diagnostic plan should include thorough prostatic palpation, complete blood count, urine analysis, urine culture, cytology and culture of prostatic fluid, and abdominal radiography or ultrasonography.

Urethritis as a cause of a purulent urethral discharge independent of other urinary tract disease is rarely recognized in dogs and cats.

Serous Fluid. Serous fluid may drip from the urethral orifice when prostatic cysts communicate with the urethra. This discharge is difficult to differentiate from urinary incontinence by visual examination alone. The diagnostic plan should include a ''urine analysis'' of the discharge and analysis of urine from the bladder to determine whether the two are identical.

SUGGESTED READINGS

Barsanti JA, Johnson CA: Genitourinary infections. In Greene CE (ed): Infectious Diseases of the Dog and Cat, pp 157–183. Philadelphia, WB Saunders, 1990

Barton CL: Canine vaginitis. Vet Clin N Am 7:711–714, 1977

Clemetson LL, Ward ACS: Bacterial flora of the vagina and uterus of healthy cats. JAVMA 196:902–906, 1990

Johnson CA: Vulvar discharges. In Kirk RW (ed): Current Veterinary Therapy X, pp 1310–1312. Philadelphia, WB Saunders, 1989

Kydd DM, Burnie AG: Vaginal neoplasia in the bitch: A review of forty clinical cases. J Sm Anim Pract 27:255–263, 1986

Ling GV, Ruby AL: Aerobic bacterial flora of the prepuce, urethral, and vagina of normal adult dogs. Am J Vet Res 39:695–698, 1978

Olson PN, Thrall MA, Wykes PM, et al: Vaginal cytology. Part II. Its use in diagnosing canine reproductive disorders. Comp Cont Ed 6:385–396, 1984

Wheeler SL: Subinvolution of placental sites in the bitch. In Morrow DA (ed): Current Therapy in Theriogenology 2, pp 513–515. Philadelphia, WB Saunders, 1986

CHAPTER FORTY-TWO

Abnormalities of the External Genitalia

Jeanne A. Barsanti

This chapter describes abnormalities of the external genitalia that are detectable by physical examination. Abnormalities of the vulva, mammary glands (see Display 1, Abnormalities of the Female External Genitalia), scrotal sac, and prepuce (see Display 2, Abnormalities of the Male External Genitalia) are presented. Abnormal discharges from the external genitalia are covered in Chapter 41.

VULVAR ABNORMALITIES

Small Size

A relatively small vulva can result from immaturity, neutering at a young age, or hypoplasia.

Swelling

A generalized swelling of the vulva can be characterized as turgid, soft, or pitting. The vulva is swollen and turgid in proestrus, occasionally with vaginitis or in association with perivulvar dermatitis. The vulvar swelling becomes softer with the onset of estrus and as a pregnant bitch nears parturition. Pitting edema of the vulva may be due to hypoalbuminemia. Diagnosis of the cause of generalized vulvar swelling can usually be made by establishing a history of the estrous cycle stage, by physical examination, and by vaginal cytologic examination. If pitting edema of the perineal area is present, a complete blood count, blood chemistry profile, and urine analysis are indicated.

Vaginal Mass

A mass protruding from the vulva may be vaginal prolapse, a vaginal neoplasm, or a prolapsed uterus. These diseases are documented in dogs, but they are very rare in cats.

Abnormalities of the Female External Genitalia

- Vulva
  - Small
    - Immaturity
    - Neutering at a young age
    - Hypoplasia
  - Generalized swelling
    - Proestrus
    - Vaginitis
    - Perivulvar dermatitis
    - Estrus
    - Nearing parturition
    - Edema
  - Mass
    - Vaginal prolapse
    - Vaginal tumors
    - Prolapsed uterus
  - Congenital
    - Anovulvar cleft
    - Vulvar stenosis
    - Clitoral hypertrophy
    - Trauma
- Mammary glands
  - Galactosis
  - Mammary hypertrophy/hyperplasia
  - Mastitis
  - Neoplasia

Abnormalities of the Male External Genitalia

- Scrotum
  - Dermatitis
  - Edema
  - Tumor
  - Trauma
  - Inguinal hernia
- Testicles
  - Cryptorchidism
  - Small testicles
    - Degeneration
    - Chronic inflammation
    - Atrophy
  - Enlarged testicles
    - Acute orchitis
    - Testicular torsion
    - Neoplasia
  - Trauma
- Epididymis
  - Epididymitis
  - Trauma
- Prepuce/penis
  - Balanoposthitis
  - Trauma
  - Tumors
  - Phimosis
  - Paraphimosis
  - Congenital defects
  - Urethral prolapse

Vaginal prolapse (vaginal hyperplasia) occurs during proestrus or estrus, principally in young, large-breed dogs. The edematous vaginal mucosa protrudes through the vulvar lips as a red fleshy mass. The amount of vaginal tissue that prolapses is variable, from just the ventral vaginal floor to the entire vaginal circumference up to the cervix. The dog's behavior is normal, except for possible licking at the mass and difficulty urinating. The condition typically regresses spontaneously and resolves at the end of estrus; however, it tends to recur with each estrous cycle.

Vaginal tumors may also protrude through the vulvar lips. Differentiation from vaginal prolapse in dogs can usually be made from history of estrous cycle stage, physical appearance of the mass, and impression smears; biopsy is occasionally required. The most common vaginal tumor is a leiomyoma, which is benign and often pedunculated. Other common benign tumors are fibromas, lipomas, and polyps. Diagnosis is usually based on excisional biopsy. Transmissible venereal tumors, which are common in some areas, can be diagnosed on impression smear by the characteristic uniform population of large round cells. The most common malignant tumor affecting the vagina is a transitional cell carcinoma arising from the urethra and invading the vagina at the urethral papilla. Transitional cell carcinomas in this location produce dysuria as the predominant clinical sign and are visualized by vaginoscopy.

A prolapsed uterus is uncommon in both dogs and cats. Prolapse occurs at or within 48 hours of parturition or abortion, when the cervix is open. Diagnosis is made from the history of recent parturition and physical examination. The entire uterus or only one horn may prolapse. Other clinical signs vary from straining and restlessness to hypovolemic or septic shock, depending on the severity and duration of the prolapse. In contrast to vaginal prolapse, uterine prolapse rarely recurs after the uterus is returned to its normal position.

Others

Other vulvar abnormalities that may be detected by physical examination include congenital defects, clitoral hypertrophy, and trauma. An anovulvar cleft results from incomplete closure of the skin from the dorsal vulvar commissure to the anus. Vulvar stenosis occurs at the junction of the vestibule with the labia as a result of incomplete fusion during fetal development. Clitoral hypertrophy occurs in hermaphrodites, pseudohermaphrodites, normal females receiving androgenic drugs, and, rarely, animals with hyperadrenocorticism.

MAMMARY GLAND ABNORMALITIES

Mammary gland enlargement can be due to milk accumulation, hypertrophy, inflammation, or neoplasia.

Galactosis

Galactosis refers to mammary accumulation of milk. Such accumulation is normal in advanced pregnancy and lactation. During weaning, in pseudopregnancy, and occasionally at the time of whelping, such accumulation may increase to the point that the mammae become painful and warm. There are no signs of systemic illness, and the white blood cell count is normal. Diagnosis is made from the history, physical examination, and cytologic examination of mammary fluid. Fluid expressed from the teats will look like milk; microscopically it contains variable numbers of neutrophils and macrophages with engulfed milk fat.

Mammary Hypertrophy/Hyperplasia

Mammary hypertrophy/hyperplasia is a hormone-dependent, dysplastic change in the mammary glands of cats. Young pregnant queens are most commonly affected, but the condition also occurs in nonpregnant intact queens and in neutered males or females receiving progesterone therapy such as megestrol acetate. In queens, the mammary enlargement starts in the first 2 weeks of pregnancy, rather than in late pregnancy as is normal.

Signs of mammary hypertrophy are painless, marked enlargement of one or more mammae. The overlying skin may ulcerate in severely swollen glands. There are no systemic signs of illness, except those related to the marked swelling, unless the ulcerated glands become secondarily infected. Diagnosis is based on the history and physical examination. The condition resolves with removal of the influence of progesterone such as the delivery of kittens, ovariohysterectomy, or discontinuation of progesterone therapy. In breeding queens the problem may recur in subsequent pregnancies, but it may not be as severe.

The major differential diagnosis is mammary adenocarcinoma, which is usually malignant in cats. If mammary swelling occurs in a cat that is neither pregnant nor receiving progestogens or if swelling does not resolve after the source of progesterone is removed, a biopsy is indicated.

Mastitis

Mastitis occurs 24 hours to 6 weeks postpartum. One or more mammae become hot, swollen, and painful. In severe cases, associated systemic signs include anorexia, depression, and fever. The bitch may fail to nurse and care for the puppies. The neonates may become systemically ill and die from bacteremia or toxemia or may fail to thrive because of starvation. The diagnosis is based on the history of recent parturition, physical examination, and cytologic examination of exudate expressed from the affected glands. The milk usually appears purulent or hemorrhagic with degenerative neutrophils and bacteria on cytologic examination. Affected bitches usually have an inflammatory hematologic response. The diagnostic plan should include bacterial culture and antibiotic sensitivity testing of the affected milk.

A condition that mimics mastitis in dogs is an inflammatory adenocarcinoma. Affected bitches are usually older animals, which may be neutered or intact. In intact animals, the onset occurs without association with whelping. Diagnosis requires a biopsy.

Neoplasia

Mammary gland neoplasia is common in older intact dogs (average age of 10 years) and is as often benign as malignant. Mammary neoplasia rarely occurs in bitches that had an ovariohysterectomy at or prior to the first estrus. Mammary gland neoplasia is less common in cats but is usually malignant. Affected cats are older (average age of 10 to 12 years). Ovariohysterectomy at a young age (6 months to 1 year) does not protect cats from tumor development; however, the incidence of mammary tumors is higher in intact cats.

Clinical signs include firm, nodular masses in one or more mammae, most commonly in glands 4 and 5 in dogs and in glands 1 and 2 in cats. The size of the inguinal and axillary lymph nodes should be assessed in an effort to detect possible metastasis. The affected female is otherwise normal, unless severe metastatic disease (such as lung metastasis) has already occurred. The differential diagnosis should include glandular fibrosis or chronic inflammation. Diagnosis usually requires excisional biopsy. The diagnostic plan should include thoracic radiographs to check for lung metastasis.

Occasionally, mammary nodules in dogs are associated with hyperemia, edema, and pruritus of surrounding mammary tissue. Such findings suggest aggressive, malignant neoplasia, and an aspirate or biopsy should be performed.

ABNORMALITIES OF THE SCROTUM

The most common lesions of the scrotum include dermatitis, edema, and neoplasia. An inguinal hernia may also affect the spermatic cord and scrotum.

Dermatitis

Scrotal dermatitis can be associated with a generalized dermatitis, due to local irritation, or secondary to orchitis. The sensitive scrotal skin may become inflamed by contact with soaps, dips, and disinfectants; by insect bites; or by abrasion. An underlying orchitis may result in scrotal licking and a secondary dermatitis. For this reason and because of its public health significance and contagious nature, infection with *Brucella canis* should always be considered in dogs with scrotal dermatitis.

Edema

Scrotal edema may result from local irritation or as part of a systemic tendency toward edema due to vasculitis or hypoalbuminemia. Examples of systemic causes are vasculitis due to Rocky Mountain spotted fever and hypoalbuminemia due to chronic hepatic failure or proteinuric renal diseases. Edema may be more evident in the scrotum than in other body parts of animals with these systemic causes.

Neoplasia

Certain tumors are prone to affect the scrotal skin. These include mast cell tumors, melanomas, and squamous cell carcinomas. Impression smears of ulcerated scrotal skin or aspiration of nodules should be performed to establish the diagnosis. A biopsy specimen should be taken from areas that are slow to heal and that yield nondiagnostic impression smears.

Inguinal Hernia

Tissues that herniate through the inguinal ring can enter the scrotal sac, leading to scrotal enlargement. The tissue involved can be omentum or a loop of intestine. In some cases it is possible to confirm the diagnosis by replacing the herniated tissues into the abdomen by palpation. In other cases adhesions prevent such replacement, and radiography, ultrasonography, or exploratory surgery is required for diagnosis.

TESTICULAR ABNORMALITIES

Cryptorchidism

Cryptorchidism (testicles within the abdomen or inguinal area rather than in the scrotum) is a common developmental defect, which is more often unilateral than bilateral. The testicles in dogs and cats generally descend into the scrotum within the first 7 weeks after birth; however, this time is variable. If both testicles have not descended to the scrotum by 6 months of age, the animal is considered cryptorchid. The condition is considered hereditary, and affected males should not be bred. Bilateral cryptorchid males are sterile because of thermal deterioration of spermatogenesis, but they will develop a masculine appearance and behavior, since testosterone production is normal. Diagnosis is based on physical examination. The risk of neoplasia is estimated to be 10 times greater in cryptorchid testicles. The risk of testicular torsion is also greater in intraabdominal testicles.

Small Testicles

A decrease in testicular size can be due to degeneration with aging, chronic inflammation and fibrosis, atrophy secondary to abnormal hormone production by a neoplastic testicle, or atrophy secondary to endocrinopathies such as hyperadrenocorticism, diabetes mellitus, and hypothyroidism. Sertoli cell tumors are commonly associated with atrophy of the other testicle. The diagnostic plan for small testicles should include thorough palpation for testicular tumors. If the dog is used for breeding, semen evaluation is indicated for evidence of inflammation or abnormal sperm production. A complete blood count, biochemical profile, urine analysis, and hormone assays are necessary to rule out an endocrinopathy.

Testicular Enlargement

An increase in testicular size can be associated with acute orchitis, torsion, tumors, or trauma.

Acute Orchitis. Acute orchitis can result from infection or trauma. Clinical signs include testicular swelling, pain, and heat. Signs of systemic illness may or may not be present. Diagnosis is based on history and physical examination. Infection with *B. canis* should always be considered and appropriate laboratory tests performed. The diagnostic plan should include urine analysis and urine culture, since infection can spread via the spermatic cord to and from the urinary tract. Sequelae can include abscesses, fibrosis, and decreased fertility.

Testicular Torsion. Testicular torsion is uncommon in intrascrotal testicles in dogs and cats. Clinical signs include pain, vomiting, lethargy, anorexia, diarrhea or constipation, tenesmus, and mild fever. The affected testicle becomes markedly swollen, and the scrotum may have mild edema. Diagnosis is based on the physical signs, but differentiation from acute unilateral orchitis may be difficult. An aspiration of the affected testicle may help rule out infection, but often it is not performed because of the degree of testicular pain.

Testicular Tumors. Testicular tumors are common in older male dogs (average age of 10 years) but very rare in cats. In dogs the usual types are interstitial cell tumors, seminomas, and Sertoli cell tumors. The rate of metastasis is low for all types, but Sertoli cell tumors and seminomas have the potential for malignancy. Growth is usually slow. Physical examination indicates an intratesticular nodule that is neither painful nor hot and that is very similar to fibrotic or chronic inflammatory nodules. Diagnosis is confirmed by histopathologic examination of testicular tissue removed by castration.

Approximately 50% of dogs with Sertoli cell tumors develop signs of feminization including loss of libido, pendulous prepuce, gynecomastia, contralateral testicular atrophy, and attraction of male dogs. Other signs that may develop include alopecia and hyperpigmentation, prostatic squamous metaplasia, and, rarely, bone marrow aplasia. Alopecia, hyperpigmentation, and pendulous preputce have also been reported with seminomas.

Testicular Trauma. Testicles are typically injured by bites, bullets, or contusion during blunt trauma. Vascular injury to the scrotum and testicles occurs as a result of the malicious placement of rubber bands or strings around the base of the scrotum. Testicular atrophy is a common sequela of testicular injury.

ABNORMALITIES OF THE EPIDIDYMIS

The most common problem with the epididymis is enlargement due to epididymitis. This is most often associated with orchitis. Diagnosis is by history, physical examination, semen cytologic examination and culture, and possibly aspiration or tissue evaluation. *B. canis* infection should always be evaluated by culture and serologic testing.

PREPUTIAL/PENILE ABNORMALITIES

The most common preputial/penile abnormalities are balanoposthitis, trauma, tumors, phimosis, paraphimosis, congenital defects, and urethral prolapse. The first three problems are discussed in Chapter 41.

Phimosis

Phimosis is the inability to protrude the penis due to a stricture at the preputial orifice. A stricture may be congenital or acquired as a result of trauma.

Paraphimosis

Paraphimosis is the inability to withdraw the penis into the prepuce. This may occur normally in male dogs with erection, usually after coitus or masturbation, and may be especially pronounced in young dogs. Such paraphimosis is of short duration. Abnormal paraphimosis occurs without erection or with prolonged erection. A small preputial orifice, prepuce of inadequate length, ineffective preputial muscles, or constricting preputial hairs may be predisposing factors. Prolonged exposure may lead to severe penile injury, desiccation, and necrosis, and to urethral obstruction.

Congenital Defects

Hypospadias is the most common developmental abnormality of the male external genitalia. It occurs when the urogenital folds fail to fuse, causing incomplete closure and formation of the penile urethra. On physical examination, the external urethral orifice is displaced to the ventral midline of the penis. The penis is underdeveloped, and the prepuce is incomplete ventrally. Urine scalding of the ventral abdomen may occur.

Other congenital defects include curvature of the os penis and a persistent penile frenulum. The penile frenulum is a fine band of connective tissue that attaches the penis to the prepuce ventrally. It usually ruptures prior to puberty; however when rupture does not occur, the dog may have pain on erection and may lick at the prepuce.

Other Disorders

Strangulation of the penis can occur from foreign bodies (*e.g.,* rubber bands) or a constricting ring of preputial hairs. The penis becomes swollen, necrotic, and painful. The dog or cat may lick the area and become dysuric.

Urethral prolapse appears as a small red pea-shaped mass at the end of the penis. Hemorrhage from the mass may occur. Urethral prolapse is most common in young, intact English bulldogs and Boston terriers.

SUGGESTED READINGS

Center SA, Randolph JF: Lactation and spontaneous remission of feline mammary hyperplasia following pregnancy. J Am Anim Hosp Assoc 21:56–58, 1985

Cox VS: Cryptorchidism in the dog. In Morrow DA (ed): Current Therapy in Theriogenology 2, pp 541–544. Philadelphia, WB Saunders, 1986

Hayden DW, Johnston SD, Kiang DT: Feline mammary hypertrophy/fibroadenoma complex: Clinical and hormonal aspects. Am J Vet Res 42:1699–1703, 1981

Johnston SD: Vaginal prolapse. In Kirk RW (ed): Current Veterinary Therapy X, pp 1302–1305. Philadelphia, WB Saunders, 1989

Johnston SD: Disorders of the external genitalia of the male. In Ettinger SJ (ed): Textbook of Veterinary Internal Medicine, pp 1881–1889. Philadelphia, WB Saunders, 1989

Loar AS: Tumors of the genital system and mammary glands. In Ettinger SJ (ed): Textbook of Veterinary Internal Medicine, pp 1814–1825. Philadelphia, WB Saunders, 1989

Madewell BR, Theilen GH: Tumors of the mammary gland. Veterinary Cancer Medicine, pp 327–344. Philadelphia, Lea & Febiger, 1987

Olson JD, Olson PN: Disorders of the canine mammary gland. In Morrow DA (ed): Current Therapy in Theriogenology 2, pp 506–509. Philadelphia, WB Saunders, 1986

Wood DS: Canine uterine prolapse. In Morrow DA (ed): Current Therapy in Theriogenology 2, pp 510–511. Philadelphia, WB Saunders, 1986

Wykes PM: Diseases of the vagina and vulva in the bitch. In Morrow DA (ed): Current Therapy in Theriogenology 2, pp 476–481. Philadelphia, WB Saunders, 1986

CHAPTER FORTY-THREE

Abortion, Abnormal Estrous Cycle, Infertility

Jeanne A. Barsanti

This chapter discusses two major reproductive problems in female dogs and cats, abortion and infertility, and one major problem in male dogs and cats, infertility.

ABORTION

Definition

Abortion refers to the expulsion of fetuses prior to term. Abortion is usually accompanied by abdominal contractions and a vaginal discharge. Diagnosis may be made by observing the abortion, by finding aborted material, or by confirming loss of pregnancy. It is possible for dogs and cats to abort some but not all fetuses and to carry the remaining fetuses to term.

Pathophysiology

The causes of abortion include maternal factors such as infection, trauma, and hormonal abnormalities, and fetal factors such as chromosomal abnormalities (see Display, Causes of Abortion in Dogs and Cats).

Viral, bacterial, protozoal, and possibly mycoplasmal infections can result in abortion. Viral causes in dogs include canine distemper and canine herpesvirus. Other signs of herpesvirus infection include vesicular vaginitis and mild rhinitis. Viral causes in cats include feline leukemia virus, feline panleukopenia, feline rhinotracheitis, and, possibly, feline infectious peritonitis. Of these, feline leukemia and feline panleukopenia infections are most important in natural, as opposed to experimental, infections. Feline leukemia typically causes abortion at 4 to 7 weeks of pregnancy.

Brucella canis is the major bacterial cause of abortion in dogs. Abortion typically occurs at 45 to 55 days of pregnancy. Other bacteria have also been sporadically associated with abortion in dogs, including beta-hemolytic streptococci type L, *Escherichia coli,* and *Leptospira* species. Bacterial metritis has also been suggested to be a cause of abortion in cats. *Toxoplasma* is the main protozoal

Causes of Abortion in Dogs and Cats

Maternal Factors	Cats
Infection	Viral
Dogs	Feline leukemia
Viral	Feline panleukopenia
Canine distemper	Feline rhinotracheitis
Canine herpesvirus	Bacterial
Bacterial	Trauma
Brucella canis	Endocrine disease
Beta-hemolytic streptococci	Hypoluteoidism
Escherichia coli	Hypothyroidism
Leptospira	
Protozoal	**Fetal Factors**
Toxoplasma	Chromosomal abnormalities

organism associated with abortion in dogs. Toxoplasmosis is not usually associated with abortion in cats. The role of mycoplasma in abortion in dogs and cats is postulated but not proven.

Abortion has been attributed to hypothyroidism in dogs. Hypoluteoidism has also been suspected as a cause of recurrent abortion in dogs and cats, but it has not been confirmed. Progesterone from the corpus luteum is essential for maintaining pregnancy to term in dogs but is only required in cats through days 42 to 45. Determining whether the inability to maintain progesterone concentrations leads to abortion in dogs and cats requires measuring progesterone concentrations near the time abortion occurs.

Trauma is a potential cause of abortion, but it is relatively infrequent.

Chromosomal abnormalities have been found in aborted fetuses in cases in which no maternal abnormalities could be identified.

Diagnostic Plan

Dogs. The diagnostic plan in dogs begins with a thorough history and physical examination. The physical examination should include a digital and visual vaginal examination. A complete blood count, vaginal cytologic examination, *Brucella* titer, and urine analysis should be performed. If the freshly aborted fetus is available, necropsy with histopathologic study of major body tissues and stomach culture for bacteria should be performed. The abortus can be karyotyped if no maternal causes for abortion are evident. All aborted material and discharges from the vagina should be handled carefully (wearing gloves), since *B. canis* is infectious to humans. If infection with bacteria is suggested by vaginal cytologic results or urine analysis, bacterial cultures should be performed on urine collected by cystocentesis and on discharge collected from the anterior vagina using a guarded culturette, such as a Tiegland swab. If the initial diagnostic tests are negative or normal, paired titers for toxoplasmosis are indicated. If no evidence of toxoplasmosis is found, testing of thyroid function with a thyroid-stimulating hormone (TSH) response test is indicated. If abortion has previously occurred with no apparent cause, serum progesterone concentrations should be monitored during the next pregnancy.

Cats. The diagnostic plan in cats also begins with a thorough history, physical examination and vaginal cytologic examination of the queen, and histopathologic study, culture, and possibly karyotyping of the abortus. A complete blood count and feline leukemia virus test are always indicated. If bacterial infection of the uterus is suspected, vaginal and urine (cystocentesis sample) cultures are indicated. If the queen has a history of repeated abortion of unknown cause, serum progesterone concentrations should be monitored during the next pregnancy.

ABNORMAL ESTROUS CYCLES AND INFERTILITY IN THE BITCH

Definitions

Normal onset of estrous cycles in the bitch occurs at 4 to 18 months of age. The marked variation in age is in part due to the variety of breed sizes, with smaller breeds cycling earlier and larger breeds later. In general, onset of estrus is not considered abnormal until the bitch is 2 years old or until 6 months after the growth plateau occurs.

The normal interestrous interval is 5 to 8 months, but individual variation is marked and a range of 4 to 14 months is considered acceptable. Variation does not seem to be related to breed size. Interestrous intervals normally increase in bitches over 8 years of age.

The estrous cycle consists of proestrus for 6 to 11 days, followed by estrus for 5 to 9 days, followed by diestrus for 56 to 60 days, followed by several months of anestrus. Again, individuals vary in the lengths of each phase of their cycles, particularly proestrus, estrus, and anestrus. For example, the average duration of standing estrus is 9 days, but the range is 3 to 21 days.

Most dog breeders place the male with the bitch at least twice, between 10 and 14 days after the onset of proestrus. The onset of proestrus is used because it is easy to detect: the vulva becomes swollen and turgid, and a hemorrhagic discharge is evident. Although this timing of breeding is successful for most dogs, it is not optimal for those whose cycles deviate from the average. Fortunately, sperm live a relatively long time (up to 7 days) in the bitch's reproductive tract, so the time of mating is not critical and can usually be based on the female's willingness to accept the male.

Estrous cycle abnormalities associated with infertility include the absence of estrous cycles in bitches 2 to 8 years of age; prolonged standing estrus; short, "split," or "false" estrus; prolonged proestral bleeding; very short interestrous intervals; and very long interestrous intervals. Infertility can also occur in bitches with normal-appearing estrous cycles.

Pathophysiology

The causes of infertility are subdivided into three categories: infertility with (1) a normal estrous cycle, (2) an abnormal estrous cycle but a normal interestrous interval, and (3) an abnormal estrous cycle with an abnormal interestrous interval (see Display, Causes of Infertility in the Bitch).

Normal Estrous Cycle. If a bitch is infertile but her estrous cycles are normal and she accepts the male, the major possible causes are bacterial uterine infection, reproductive tract obstruction, incorrect timing of breeding, failure to ovulate, and early fetal death and resorption.

One infectious cause of reproductive failure in a bitch with apparently normal cycles is early embryonic death due to *B. canis* infection. Because the normal vaginal flora contains many different potentially pathogenic bacteria, other bacterial causes of chronic bacterial metritis with subfertility are difficult to confirm without uterine biopsy or direct uterine culture. A presumptive diagnosis is usually based on cultures of the anterior vagina collected by a guarded swab (*e.g.,* Tiegland swab) during proestrus, on vaginal cytology, and on response to antibiotic therapy.

A vaginal or vestibular stricture preventing effective mating may also result in apparent infertility with normal estrous cycles. These strictures may be congenital or acquired as a result of injury, as might have occurred during a previous whelping. Congenital structures include persistent imperforate hymen and congenital atresia of the vagina. These abnormalities are usually identified with a carefully performed vaginal examination, although some unusual cases may require vaginography.

A uterine tumor might result in normal estrous cycles but failure to conceive. Diagnosis requires radiography or ultrasonography, plus celiotomy and biopsy.

Oviduct obstruction, if bilateral, may also result in subfertility or infertility. Diagnosis requires laparoscopy or celiotomy.

Hypoluteoidism also results in early reproductive failure. Diagnosis is based on the measurement of plasma progesterone concentrations 1 to 3 weeks after estrus. Normal values are greater than or equal to 5 ng/ml.

Abnormal Estrous Cycle, Normal Interestrous Interval. Certain causes of abnormal estrous cycles may be associated with a relatively normal interestrous interval. These include failure to stand (for acceptance of male for coitus), prolonged standing, and prolonged proestral bleeding.

Failure to stand during estrus may be due to vaginal/vestibular strictures that cause pain during penile penetration, dislike of the male, or inexperience. One

Causes of Infertility in the Bitch

Infertility Associated with a Normal Estrus

Infection
  Brucella canis
  Other bacteria
Uterine anomaly or tumor
Oviduct obstruction
Hormonal cause of early pregnancy failure

Abnormal Estrus, Normal Interestrous Interval

Failure to stand
  Vaginal/vestibular strictures
  Inexperience
  Inaccurate timing of estrus
Prolonged estrus
  Cystic ovaries
  Granulosa cell tumor
  Estrogen therapy

Abnormal Interestrous Interval

Short intervals
  Cystic ovaries
  "Split" estrous cycle
  Premature luteal regression
Prolonged intervals
  Endocrine diseases
  Nutritional problems
  Cystic endometrial hyperplasia
  Aging
Absence of cycles
  Endocrine disease
  Ovarian dysfunction
  Congenital dysfunction (intersex)
  Previous ovariohysterectomy
  Young or old age
  Drug therapy
  "Silent" estrus

must always consider human error in determining the time for breeding. Because of individual variation in length of proestrus and estrus, the bitch may be wrongly accused of failure to stand when the timing of breeding was inappropriately determined. The correlation of acceptance behavior with vaginal cytologic findings should detect this problem. Some bitches seem to have prolonged proestral-type bleeding into estrus. If the timing of breeding is based only on disappearance of bleeding, standing heat may be missed. Vaginal cytology and alternate-day exposure to the male after 9 days of proestrus may help detect this variation of normal estrus.

Acceptance of a male for over 21 days is considered abnormal. Prolongation of standing heat without conception usually indicates prolonged estrogen secretion with failure of ovulation. The usual cause is cystic ovaries.

Abnormal Interestrous Interval. An abnormal interestrous interval can be too short, too long, or due to absence of the estrous cycle.

A short interestrous interval is defined as one less than 4 months in duration. One cause is a "split" heat, which begins with vulvar swelling and a blood-tinged vaginal discharge that stops within a few days without progression to standing estrus. The cycle reverts to anestrus followed by a true, fertile estrus in 4 to 6 weeks. This is most common in young bitches. It may be caused by increased estrogen concentrations near the end of anestrus due to transient follicular growth. It is documented by measuring weekly estradiol and progesterone concentrations. The bitch should be bred according to her standing behavior and not according to the number of days from onset of bloody vaginal discharge. Other dogs may have short interestrous intervals without split heats. The cause is not known, but infertility may be associated. The infertility may be due to endometrial implantation failure, since complete endometrial desquamation and repair have not occurred.

An interestrous interval is considered prolonged when it is twice as long as usual for that bitch or for the breed, or is longer than 12 months. A long interval may be due to "silent heats," in which bleeding is not observed. This may be due to lack of owner observation. A long interval may be associated with hormonal abnormalities such as hypothyroidism, hypoadrenocorticism, and hyperadrenocorticism, cachexia or obesity, and cystic endometrial hyperplasia.

Absence of cycling can be associated with hypothyroidism, primary ovarian or adrenal dysfunction, intersex conditions, previous unreported ovariohysterectomy, and young (less than 2 years) or old (more than 8 years) age. Ovarian dysfunction can be congenital (hypoplasia) or acquired (neoplasia). In bitches that may have silent heats, only repeated vaginal cytology (or frequent reexposure to a male dog) will detect whether they are truly cycling. The reasons for silent estrous cycles are unknown.

Diagnostic Plan

The diagnostic plan must include a thorough history, including a complete breeding record with the dates of start of proestrus, time of mating, duration of standing estrus, duration of the interestrous interval, and the breeding record of the males involved. The general medical history, including current health and previous problems and treatments, should be obtained. In addition to a regular physical examination, special attention should be paid to abdominal palpation of the uterus and rectal examination of the pelvis and vagina. The vagina should also be examined digitally and then by vaginoscopy. It may be easier to detect a vaginal stricture by digital examination than by vaginoscopy.

A complete blood count, urine analysis (cystocentesis sample), and *B. canis* titer should be performed. If these tests are negative, a blood chemistry profile and thyroid response testing should be done. If the cause is still not evident and the dog is cycling, the next estrous cycle should be followed with vaginal cytologic examinations, characteristics of standing behavior, and determination of serum estradiol and progesterone concentrations. If the dog is not cycling, celiotomy for examination of the ovaries and uterus, and biopsy and culture of the uterus are indicated. The patency of the oviducts should be tested.

ABNORMAL ESTROUS CYCLES AND INFERTILITY IN QUEENS

Definition

Reproductive cycles in the normal queen begin between 5 months and 1 year of age. Queens cycle every 14 to 21 days when exposed to 14 hours of light per day. Cats kept outdoors are seasonally polyestrous in association with the length of daylight. Calling, rolling, rubbing, lordosis, and treading are the normal behavioral signs of estrus. Novice cat owners may conclude that their cat has developed a serious neurologic problem on first observing this behavior. In contrast to the dog, there is little vulvar swelling and no proestral bleeding. Otherwise vaginal cytologic findings are similar. The cat ovulates only in response to coitus. If a male is present, receptivity usually lasts 1 to 4 days. If no male is present, the estrous cycle lasts 7 to 10 days. A quiescent period occurs for 2 to 3 weeks, and then estrus recurs. These cycles are repeated throughout the breeding season, which seems to be determined largely by day length. An abnormal estrous cycle is failure to show estrus during the breeding season, and infertility is failure of conception in spite of normal estrous behavior and the presence of a male cat. Coitus is rarely observed, because it is rapidly completed in cats. The typical postcoital behavior of the queen (rolling and crying) may be observed by the owner.

Pathophysiology

There are two major categories for abnormal estrous cycles and infertility in cats: lack of apparent estrus and lack of conception despite apparently normal cycling and presence of male cats (see Display, Causes of Infertility in Queens).

Anestrus. If the cat does not cycle during the usual breeding season, the following should be considered: silent heats, use of progesterone-type drugs for other medical problems, congenital ovarian defects (dysgenesis), debility, en-

Causes of Infertility in Queens

Absence of Estrus	Failure of Conception
"Silent" estrus	Infertile cycles
Drug therapy	Cystic ovaries
Ovarian dysfunction	Cystic endometrial hyperplasia
Cachexia	Early embryonic death
Endocrine disease	Feline leukemia
Cystic endometrial hyperplasia	Cystic endometrial hyperplasia
Environment	
Previous ovariohysterectomy	
Young age (<1 year)	
Insufficient day length	
Lack of exposure to male cats	

dogenous hormonal imbalance, uterine (cystic hyperplasia) or ovarian (neoplasia, cystic change) disease, and environmental factors (lack of at least 12 hours of light per day, lack of exposure to other cats). A previous ovariohysterectomy unknown by the current owners should also be considered. Megestrol acetate, commonly used for dermatologic and behavioral problems in cats, can completely suppress estrus when used at 5 mg/day for 3 days and then 2.5 to 5 mg/week. These doses are well within usual therapeutic guidelines for dermatologic and behavioral problems.

Failure of Conception. Failure to conceive in cats that apparently cycle indicates either infertile cycles or early embryonic death. Lack of fertile cycles can be due to cystic ovarian follicles. These are most commonly reported in older, nulliparous queens. Cystic endometrial hyperplasia has also been associated with a poor conception rate. A remnant of ovarian tissue left from a previous ovariohysterectomy may cause estrus, with infertility due to the hysterectomy.

Early embryonic death is most commonly associated with feline leukemia virus infection. Cystic endometrial hyperplasia may cause early embryonic death.

Diagnostic Plan

As in the bitch, a good history may provide the key to problem resolution in the queen. This history should include (1) evidence of reproductive problems in the parents or littermates, (2) all medical problems of the queen, (3) vaccination status of the queen, (4) housing, nutrition, and contact with other cats, (5) the past or present use of hormonal therapy, (6) surgeries performed, (7) the dates and length of estrous cycles, (8) the characteristics of any pregnancy, (9) a description of sexual behavior, (10) the presence of any vaginal discharges, (11) breeding record of the male, and (12) the presence of any environmental stress factors.

A thorough physical examination should be performed with careful abdominal palpation of the uterus, visual examination of the vulva and vagina, and vaginal cytology. A feline leukemia virus test is essential. If no cause is determined, a complete blood count, blood chemistry profile, and urine analysis (cystocentesis sample) should be performed. Further tests to be considered include a TSH response test for thyroid function, reproductive hormone assays, and celiotomy with examination of the ovaries and uterine biopsy and culture.

INFERTILITY IN THE MALE DOG

Definition

Infertility in the male dog is usually identified by failure of conception in bitches bred to him. Semen analysis is the major diagnostic test used to further characterize the problem. In the normal dog, an ejaculate has 3 fractions produced in the order of (1) presperm, (2) sperm-rich, and (3) prostatic fluid. The presperm and sperm-rich fractions are often difficult to distinguish because of the small volume of the presperm fraction. These two fractions are usually considered together. The sperm-rich fraction is normally opalescent and milky white; prostatic fluid is clear. The total volume of an ejaculate can vary from 0.5 to 30 ml, mainly due to the amount of prostatic fluid collected, since prostatic fluid may be released for up to 30 minutes.

Sperm motility, numbers, and morphology are more closely related to fertility than is ejaculate volume. When checked on a warmed microscope slide after dilution with one drop of warmed normal saline, one drop of semen should contain greater than 75% motile sperm. Sperm numbers should be greater than 300×10^6/ml. Sperm numbers less than 100×10^6/ml are consistent with poor fertility. Over 80% of the sperm should be morphologically normal. If there are greater than 20% of sperm with primary (head and midpiece changes) or secondary (tail) abnormalities, disease of the testes or epididymis, respectively, should be suspected. Testicular sperm production is temperature-sensitive. Any increase in scrotal temperature can adversely affect sperm production, which is why cryptorchid testes are not fertile.

Pathophysiology

The major causes of infertility in the male dog can be grouped according to whether the problem is testicular, epididymal, prostatic, or with the penis and prepuce.

Testicular problems associated with decreased fertility can be congenital or acquired. Congenital problems include hypoplasia, cryptorchidism, chromosomal abnormalities in the germ cells, abnormal androgen or pituitary hormone production, and the immotile cilia syndrome. Acquired problems include inguinal hernia, testicular degeneration with aging, neoplasia, sperm granulomas, trauma, infection, toxins, systemic or metabolic disease, use of hormonal therapy for other diseases (*e.g.*, androgens, estrogens, glucocorticoids, antineoplastic agents, ketoconazole), sexual overuse, and environmental stress (especially high ambient temperatures). However, a recent study (Wong, 1985) indicated that dogs adapted to tropical climates did not have decreased sperm numbers. Sperm are not recognized as "self" by the body's immune system. Whenever an inflammatory, traumatic, or neoplastic process disrupts testicular structure and sperm come in contact with the immune system, an antigen-antibody reaction ensues. Sperm granulomas form by this mechanism and have been postulated to result in an autoimmune orchitis with sperm destruction.

Inguinal hernias of intestines and omentum into the scrotal sac have been associated with decreased testicular function due to increased heat and irritation from intestinal motility. Scrotal inflammation or trauma may also reduce testicular sperm production by generation of heat. Drugs and toxins associated with reduced sperm production include cadmium, cyclophosphamide, vinblastine, and amphotericin B. In some infertile male dogs, only oligospermia or azoospermia of unknown origin can be documented.

Congenital or acquired epididymal diseases can block the flow of sperm from the testicles. Congenital problems include aplasia of the epididymis. Acquired problems include trauma and infection such as canine brucellosis.

The deferent ducts may be congenitally aplastic or can become obstructed as they pass through a diseased prostate.

Prostatic infections have been suspected to cause subfertility, even in the absence of obstruction of the deferent ducts. This association has not been proved in men or dogs. The prostatic fluid is a transport fluid that is not essential for fertility. Recently in dogs, a role for prostatic fluid in sperm capacitation has been proposed.

Lesions of the penis and prepuce may prevent erection and/or mating (see Chapter 42).

Diagnostic Plan

The breeding history of the male should include (1) the breeding record of the bitches served, (2) the timing of each breeding, (3) the mating behavior of the male, (4) the number of bitches bred, (5) the number of bitches whelping, (6) the frequency of breeding, (7) housing and handling procedures, (8) all previous and current medical problems, (9) all previous and current drugs used. This history will usually determine whether the problem is congenital or has been acquired.

A semen evaluation should be performed prior to physical examination to minimize any anxiety or excitement. Behavior during ejaculation, appearance of the penis and prepuce during ejaculation, and semen color and volume should be recorded. Sperm motility, numbers, and morphology should be determined. Numbers of neutrophils should be noted.

Any scrotal, testicular, epididymal, spermatic cord, prostatic, preputial, or penile abnormalities should be detected by physical examination.

This diagnostic plan usually localizes the abnormality and determines the adequacy of sperm production. Further diagnostic tests to consider are complete blood count, blood chemistry profile, urine analysis, serum testosterone concentrations, thyroid function testing by TSH response, quantitative culture of semen, and biopsy of testicle or prostate. Serum testosterone concentrations have a wide normal range (0.5 to 5.0 ng/ml), making them difficult to evaluate. Possible contamination of semen samples by the normal bacterial flora of the distal urethra and prepuce during sample collection must be considered in interpreting results of semen culture. Semen cultures should be quantitative, and results should be correlated with the presence of inflammation on semen cytologic examination.

Prognosis

The prognosis depends on reversibility of the underlying cause. In idiopathic oligospermia or azoospermia, the prognosis is poor.

INFERTILITY IN THE MALE CAT

The causes of infertility in the male cat are similar to those in the dog. This section discusses the differences between the two species.

Pathophysiology

The major causes of infertility in the tom are congenital lesions, infection, trauma, and disturbances of territorial behavior. Endocrine diseases such as hypothyroidism are possible but not common. Administration of female reproductive hormones as therapy for other diseases may adversely affect fertility. Nutritional causes, such as malnutrition, obesity, and hypervitaminosis A, are also possible. Congenital defects described in the tom include testicular hypoplasia, segmental aplasia of the epididymis or deferent ducts, and chromosomal abnormalities. The major chromosomal abnormality described is the XXY trait found in tortoiseshell males. The major infectious causes of infertility in toms are bacterial orchitis as a result of cat bite wounds to the scrotum and feline infectious peritonitis granulomas. A hair ring around the base of the glans penis will inhibit mating. Territorial changes in relation to other toms may also inhibit mating.

Diagnostic Plan

A good history and physical examination, as described for dogs, are mandatory. Collecting semen for examination is difficult in that electroejaculation under anesthesia is required, unless the cat has been trained to allow collection in the presence of a queen in estrus. Normal semen volume is very small (0.03 to 0.5 ml), which further increases the difficulty in collection and analysis. More than 60% of the sperm should be motile, and more than 70% should have normal morphology. The normal number of sperm is greater than 10 million. The diagnostic plan may also include a complete blood count, blood chemistry profile, urine analysis, and feline leukemia virus test as well as thyroid function testing in cats in which no etiology for infertility can be found.

SUGGESTED READINGS

Banks DR: Physiology and endocrinology of the feline estrous cycle. In Morrow DA (ed): Current Therapy in Theriogenology, pp 795–800. Philadelphia, WB Saunders, 1986

Carmichael LE, Greene CE: Canine herpesvirus infection. In Greene CE (ed): Infectious Diseases of the Dog and Cat, pp 252–258. Philadelphia, WB Saunders, 1990

Concannon PA: Physiology and endocrinology of canine pregnancy. In Morrow DA (ed): Current Therapy in Theriogenology, pp 491–497. Philadelphia, WB Saunders, 1986

Dooley MP, Pineda MH: Effect of method of collection on seminal characteristics of the domestic cat. Am J Vet Res 47:286–292, 1986

Freshman JL: Drugs affecting fertility in the male dog. In Kirk RW (ed): Current Veterinary Therapy X, pp 1224–1227. Philadelphia, WB Saunders, 1989

Herron MA: Infertility from noninfectious causes. In Morrow DA (ed): Current Therapy in Theriogenology, pp 829–834. Philadelphia, WB Saunders, 1986

Johnson CA: Infertility in the bitch. In Morrow DA (ed): Current Therapy in Theriogenology, pp 466–468. Philadelphia, WB Saunders, 1986

Johnston SD: Spontaneous abortion. In Morrow DA (ed): Current Therapy in Theriogenology, pp 606–608. Philadelphia, WB Saunders, 1980

Olson PN, Behrendt MD, Weiss DE: Reproductive problems in the bitch: Formulating your diagnostic plan. Vet Med 82:482–496, 1987

Olson PN, Husted PW: Breeding management for optimal reproductive efficiency in the bitch and stud dog. In Morrow DA (ed): Current Therapy in Theriogenology, pp 463–466. Philadelphia, WB Saunders, 1986

Troy GC, Herron MA: Infectious causes of infertility, abortion and stillbirths in cats. In Morrow DA (ed): Current Therapy in Theriogenology, pp 834–837. Philadelphia, WB Saunders, 1986

Soderberg SF: Infertility in the male dog. In Morrow DA (ed): Current Therapy in Theriogenology, pp 544–548. Philadelphia, WB Saunders, 1986

Wong WT, Dhaliwal GK: Observations on semen quality of dogs in the tropics. Vet Rec 116:313–314, 1985

PART ELEVEN

Musculoskeletal Problems

CHAPTER FORTY-FOUR

Lameness

Jonathan N. Chambers

DEFINITION

Lameness is a dysfunction of the limb(s), creating a perceptible variation in movement or gait due to an alteration in one or more of the organs of locomotion.

PATHOPHYSIOLOGY

Lameness can be caused by pain alone, instability in the skeleton, or mechanical abnormalities. Pain is often encountered in combination with an instability or mechanical problem.

Acute inflammation due to minor trauma, localized infection, or a foreign body (thorn in the foot) is the usual cause of lameness when pain alone is involved. A recent fracture causes instability and pain from inflammation, whereas instability alone is the primary cause of lameness when the acute inflammatory process (pain) regresses and chronic nonunion (pseudarthrosis) of the fracture becomes established. Loss of joint mobility causes marked changes in limb mechanics and may or may not be accompanied by pain. An acute inflammatory process (and pain) of the joint or muscle-tendon unit usually precedes the development of a stiff nonpainful joint. Lameness can also be caused by neurologic dysfunction (discussed elsewhere in Chapters 47 and 48).

CLASSIFICATION

Once lameness has been identified as the problem, it should be classified by severity and course of onset, since this is helpful in establishing a list of possible causes, even before the thorough orthopedic examination is done. This is especially true if the lameness is spontaneous. The age, breed, and sex are also important to note. Many puppyhood problems are developmental and relatively breed-specific. Some of these common young-dog predispositions are given for the more popular breeds in Table 44-1.

TABLE 44-1. Predispositions to Causes of Lameness As Related to Dog Breeds

Predisposition	Hip Dysplasia	Panosteitis	Osteochondritis Dissecans of Shoulder	Osteochondritis Dissecans of Elbow/Fragmented Coronoid Process	Osteochondritis Dissecans of Tarsus	Osteochondritis Dissecans of the Stifle	Ununited Anconeal Process	Infraspinatus contracture	Hypertrophic Osteodystrophy	Lateral Patellar Luxation	Medial Patellar Luxation	Legg-Calvé-Perthes Disease
Sex	–	M	M	M	M	M	M	–	M?	–	F	–
Breeds												
Large	+	+	+	+	+	+	+	+	+	+	–	–
Small	–	–	–	–	–	–	–	+	–	+	+	–
Hunting	+	+	+	+	+	+	–	+	–	–	–	–
German shepherd	+	+	+	+	–	±	+	–	+	–	–	–
Labrador retriever	+	+	+	+	+	+	±	+	+	–	–	–
Golden retriever	+	+	+	+	+	–	–	–	+	–	–	–
Irish setter	+	+	+	–	+	–	–	–	+	–	–	–
Pointers	–	+	±	–	–	±	±	±	+	–	–	–
St. Bernard	+	+	+	+	–	±	+	–	±	+	–	–
Newfoundland	+	+	+	+	–	–	+	–	+	+	–	–
Irish wolfhound	–	+	–	–	–	+	±	–	±	–	–	–
Mastiff	+	–	+	–	–	+	+	–	–	–	–	–
Great Dane	+	+	+	–	–	±	±	–	+	–	–	–
Doberman pinscher	–	+	–	–	–	±	–	–	+	–	–	–

Breed												
Rottweiler	±	+	+	+	+	−	−	−	−	−	−	−
Chow	+	−	−	+	−	+	−	−	−	−	−	−
Boxer	+	+	+	−	−	±	−	−	+	−	−	−
Spaniels	−	−	+	−	−	−	−	+	−	−	−	−
Basset hound	+	+	−	+	−	−	+	−	+	−	−	−
Samoyed	−	+	+	−	−	−	−	−	−	−	−	±
Toy miniature poodle	−	−	−	−	−	−	−	−	−	−	−	+
Pekingese	−	−	−	−	−	−	−	−	−	−	+	+
Wire-haired fox terrier	−	−	−	−	−	−	−	−	−	−	+	+
West Highland terrier	−	−	−	−	−	−	−	−	−	−	−	+
Lakeland terrier	−	−	−	−	−	−	−	−	−	−	−	+
Cairn terrier	−	−	−	−	−	−	−	−	−	−	+	+
Yorkshire terrier	−	−	−	−	−	−	−	−	−	−	+	+
Boston terrier	−	−	−	−	−	−	−	−	−	−	+	±
Scottish terrier	−	−	−	−	−	−	−	−	−	−	+	±
Pomeranian	−	−	−	−	−	−	−	−	−	−	+	±
Chihuahua	−	−	−	−	−	−	−	−	−	−	+	±

±, There is no known report of predisposition, but body size and type are similar to those of breeds with documented predisposition.

Severity of Lameness

The degree of lameness may not correlate with the seriousness of the disease process, but it can usually be used to establish a rule out list. For example, a thorn in the foot pad and a bone cancer might both be included in the rule out list for a dog with a severe off-weight-bearing lameness. A I to IV grade system is suggested:

Grade I—Barely perceptible lameness

Grade II—Noticeable lameness, but weight bearing most of the time. This would be typical of a disease in the developing state, *e.g.,* degenerative joint disease or panosteitis; or recovery state, *e.g.,* healing traumatic injury.

Grade III—Severe lameness, with use limited to touching the paw to the ground for balance

Grade IV—No weight bearing; the limb is carried.

The more common causes of lameness can be classified by the most typical grade of severity at presentation (see Display, Typical Severity of Lameness at Initial Presentation). Some variation is seen, depending on the stage of a disease and pain tolerance of the individual.

Course of Onset

How quickly a lameness develops is often an indicator of the type of problem. Acute-onset lameness is typical of traumatic diseases and infections. These include foot lacerations and foreign bodies, blunt trauma, fractures, muscle strains, and sprains—including the most common sprain, rupture of the cranial cruciate ligament. The history of a patient presenting with chronic lameness must be scrutinized for an acute onset, which may indicate one of the aforementioned problems in a static or resolving stage.

A chronic, insidious onset without an acute initiation is most typical of degenerative problems, especially those involving the joints. These disorders include hip dysplasia, the osteochondroses, developmental patellar luxation, Legg-Calvé-Perthes disease, and the immune-mediated arthropathies. Several problems not only present as an insidious lameness but also have a cyclic or shifting nature. Included are panosteitis, infectious polyarthritis, and immune-mediated arthropathy or myopathy. A cyclic course may also indicate differing stages of a single disease. For example, puppies with developing hip dysplasia are often very painful at the age of 6 to 10 months as a result of stretching and microtrauma of the pliable tissues of the developing joint. The lameness appears to abate as the tissues mature, only to recur a few months later as secondary degenerative joint disease develops.

The more common causes of lameness are listed according to the most typical course of onset in the Display, Typical Clinical Onset of Common Lameness.

Typical Severity of Lameness at Initial Presentation

- Grade I
  - Minor trauma, contusion, laceration, strain, etc
  - Osteochondrosis of the distal femur
  - Biceps brachii tenosynovitis
  - Polymyositis
- Grade II
  - Degenerative joint disease (hip dysplasia)
  - Infraspinatus contracture
  - Panosteitis
  - Avulsion of long digital extensor tendon
  - Legg-Calvé-Perthes disease
  - Osteochondroses of shoulder, elbow, and tarsus
  - Developmental patellar luxation
- Grade III
  - Cranial cruciate rupture
  - Hypertrophic osteodystrophy
  - Infections
  - Bone neoplasia
  - Congenital patellar luxation
- Grade IV
  - Fracture
  - Luxation
  - Foreign body in foot
  - Snakebite

DIAGNOSTIC PLAN

Orthopedic Examination

After a thorough history (with a special note of the age, breed, and sex) is collected, the clinician will find a properly performed orthopedic examination to be the most valuable diagnostic tool. Once the clinician acquires a sound knowledge of normal anatomy, the skill needed to perform the orthopedic examination is gained only by examining many normal dogs and watching them gait.

The proper examination environment is essential. Grades III and IV lameness can usually be evaluated in the standard examination room. Ideally, all examinations for a more subtle lameness should be performed where there is enough space and solid footing to gait the patient at a run and a trot. Weather permit-

Typical Clinical Onset of Common Lameness

- Acute
    Trauma: fracture, luxation, sprain, etc
    Snakebite
    Foreign body in foot
    Panosteitis
    Hypertrophic osteodystrophy
    Cranial cruciate rupture
- Cyclic or shifting onset
    Panosteitis
- Chronic insidious
    Degenerative joint disease (hip dysplasia)
    Osteochondroses
    Infections
    Congenital and developmental patellar luxation
    Bone neoplasms
    Legg-Calvé-Perthes disease
    Infraspinatus contracture
    Biceps brachii tenosynovitis
    Immune-mediated arthropathy and myopathy
    Avulsion of long digital extensor muscle

ting, one should perform the entire examination in a large grassed area. The patient must be comfortable and relaxed; otherwise, results will be erroneous.

The patient is first walked, trotted, and run; the examiner watches from all angles. The exercise should be strenuous if the lameness is historically exercise-related. Next, the patient is observed and palpated in a standing position. Weight distribution among the limbs is noted. The palpation is started at the head and proceeds caudally; any swelling, atrophy, or pain is noted. The standing palpation of the forelimbs and then the hindlimbs is done simultaneously to check for gross or subtle changes in symmetry. Each limb is raised to check for the animal's willingness or reluctance to distribute the weight to the other three.

The next part of the examination is done with the patient in lateral recumbency. Each limb is thoroughly examined, palpated, and manipulated from the toes proximally. The patient is turned and the procedure repeated on the other side. An equivocal asymmetric finding, such as subtle pain or instability, is repeated as many times as necessary to confirm or refute its presence. Finally, the dog is gaited again, because a subtle lameness is often exacerbated after vigorous manipulation of the affected limb.

Physical Signs Related to Lameness

Almost all lameness involves inflammation in one stage or another. Therefore, the clinician is trying to detect the cardinal signs of inflammation (pain, swelling, heat, redness, and loss of function).

Lameness is synonymous with loss of normal limb function, but more specific signs of dysfunction are often present. Joints have a normal combination of mobility (range of motion) and stability. Abnormal mobility and stability (restrictive ankylosis) are both manifestations of loss of normal function. Atrophy of muscles is another indication of less-than-normal function and is a valuable localizing sign. Although the atrophy may be somewhat generalized in long-standing lameness, the most severe atrophy is often localized to the muscle group primarily responsible for moving the diseased (painful) joint or part, for example, the shoulder muscles in humeral head osteochondritis dissecans or the gluteal muscles in hip dysplasia.

Radiographic Examination

After the physical (orthopedic) examination, radiographs are the most common and useful aid for diagnosing lameness. Prior localization of the problem to a specific limb, and optimally to a part of the limb, limits the number of radiographs necessary for further definition. Standard views (craniocaudal and mediolateral) are taken first, followed by special techniques if necessary. The quality of the radiographs must be high because many lesions are quite subtle. Oblique projections may help to delineate some lesions; stress positioning of joints may help in documenting and defining a clinical instability. As in the physical examination, equivocal lesions should be further assessed, in this case by radiographing the opposite limb and checking for symmetry.

Special Diagnostic Aids

Additional diagnostic aids may be required to define the problem ultimately (see Display, Diagnostic Aids for Lameness). Common sense must prevail in deciding when a particular test is indicated. For example, fine-needle aspiration for cytology and culture is indicated in cases of localized soft tissue swelling, and arthrocentesis is indicated when the cause of a joint problem is not readily apparent from physical signs and radiographs. The indications for a more sophisticated test, such as a bone scan, are less apparent, and the probable value must be decided on a case-by-case basis. There are situations in which the most accurate, expeditious, and cost-effective method of diagnosis is exploratory surgery and biopsy.

Diagnostic Aids for Lameness

- Serial orthopedic examinations
- Radiography
  Routine
  Oblique views
  Stress view
  Arthrogram
  Radionucleotide (bone) scan
- Fine-needle aspiration
  Cytology
  Culture and sensitivity
- Arthrocentesis
  Cytology
  Culture
  Mucin clot
- Arthroscopy
- Immune profile
  Lupus erythematosus preparation
  Rheumatoid factor
  Antinuclear antibody
- Exploratory surgery and biopsy
  Muscle
  Joint capsule
  Other soft tissue
  Bone

CHAPTER FORTY-FIVE

Bone, Joint, and Periskeletal Swelling or Enlargement

James P. Toombs and William R. Widmer

Swelling is the transient abnormal increase in volume of a body part not caused by the proliferation of cells. Swelling may involve joints and periskeletal tissues, but not bone. Increased bone volume depends upon cellular proliferation and is more accurately described as bone enlargement. Enlargement is an increase in the size of an organ or body part attributable to hypertrophic, hyperplastic, metaplastic, or neoplastic processes. Enlargement may involve bone, periskeletal tissues, or joints.

PATHOPHYSIOLOGY

Bone Enlargement

The response of bone to injury or disease is limited to several basic processes: (1) production of new bone—osteogenesis and (2) resorption of existing bone—osteolysis. These processes are generally concurrent, although one or the other may predominate. Bone enlargement occurs when osteogenesis exceeds osteolysis. Osteogenic response to injury or nonneoplastic disease is most pronounced in animals that have not yet reached skeletal maturity and progressively declines from maturity to old age. Osteogenic response also depends on the region of the bone involved. Regions of bone that are predominantly cancellous (long bone epiphyses and metaphyses) are generally capable of greater and more immediate osteogenic response than regions of bone that are entirely cortical (long bone diaphyses). Bone enlargement associated with fracture healing involves periosteal, intercortical, and endosteal surfaces. Bone enlargement associated with disease frequently involves only the periosteal surface.

Joint Swelling or Enlargement

The essential components of synovial joints include articular cartilage, joint capsule, synovial membrane, and synovial fluid. Normal synovial fluid is a dialysate of plasma into which synovial membrane B cells secrete hyaluronate. This fluid is clear, highly viscous, relatively acellular, similar in glucose content to plasma, and slightly lower in protein content than plasma, and it has an albumin-to-globulin ratio of approximately 4 : 1. Its volume in normal synovial joints of dogs and cats is generally less than 1 ml.

Joint swelling (effusion) occurs when dynamics of the synovial membrane are altered by trauma or disease. It is associated with up to a 20-fold increase in fluid volume and qualitative changes dependent upon the disease process. Joint effusion may be serous, fibrinous, purulent, or hemorrhagic. It most commonly is secondary to inflammation of the synovial membrane (synovitis).

Joint swelling is often accompanied by joint enlargement. Joint enlargement involves hyperplasia; metaplasia; or neoplasia of the synovial membrane, joint capsule, articular cartilage, or periarticular bone.

Periskeletal Swelling or Enlargement

Swelling or enlargement of muscular and fascial tissues surrounding bones and joints may occur independently of or concurrently with similar processes involving the bones and joints themselves. Swelling may involve hemorrhage, edema, or inflammatory exudate, while enlargement of these tissues generally involves hyperplastic, metaplastic, or neoplastic processes.

For the remainder of this chapter, "swelling" will be used as a synonym for swelling or enlargement.

DIFFERENTIAL DIAGNOSIS OF MUSCULOSKELETAL "SWELLING"

History

Certain aspects of the medical history facilitate diagnosis of musculoskeletal "swelling." Information regarding signalment, previous geographic residence, diet, activities or events preceding onset of "swelling," and duration and progressing of "swelling" are critical to formulating a concise list of rule outs.

Signalment

Breed and sex predispositions to various diseases associated with musculoskeletal "swelling" are catalogued in Tables 45-1 through 45-3. While some diseases are usually confined to immature animals, others rarely occur except in mature, middle-aged, or older animals. In an 8-year-old large-breed dog with a swollen, painful lesion involving the distal tibial metaphysis, primary bone neoplasia might head a list of rule outs. Although neoplasia should not be totally dis-

Text continues on p. 403

TABLE 45-1. Predispositions of Diseases That Cause Bone Enlargement

Disease	Breed	Sex	Age	Common Anatomic Sites	Distribution
Bone cysts	Doberman, LB	M	I	Metaphyses, long bones	F or MC
Cartilage analogue of fibromatosis			A	Skull	F
Craniomandibular osteopathy	Terriers		I	Mandibular rami and tympanic bullae	MC, BS
Enostosis	German shepherd		I	Radius and ulna	U
Feline Maroteaux-Lamy syndrome	Siamese, Siamese-X		I	Costochondral junction of ribs and ends of long bones	MC
Fractures					F or MC
Fractures (humeral)	Spaniels		A	Distal humerus	F
Fractures (stress)	Italian greyhound		A	Distal radius and ulna	F
Hypertrophic osteodystrophy	LB, GB		I	Distal metaphyses—radius, ulna, and tibia	MC
Hypertrophic osteopathy			A	Distal extremities	MC, BS
Hypervitaminosis A	Cats		A	Cervical vertebrae	F or MC
Ossifying fibroma			A	Maxilla and mandible	F
Osteochondromatosis (canine)			I	Vertebrae, ribs, metaphyses—long bones and pelvis	F or MC
Osteochondromatosis (feline)			A	Ribs, scapulae, vertebrae, skull, and pelvis	F or MC
Osteoma			A	Bones formed by intramembranous ossification, especially skull	F
Osteomyelitis (fungal)				Long bone epiphyses	MC
Osteomyelitis (hematogenous-bacterial)				Long bone epiphyses or diaphyses	MC
Osteomyelitis (trauma-associated)			I		F or MC
Panosteitis	German shepherd, LB	M	I	Diaphyses—humerus and ulna	MC
Polyostotic fibrous dysplasia	Doberman		I	Distal metaphyses—radius and ulna	MC, UB
Tumors of bone (malignant primary)	LB, GB		A	Long bone metaphyses, skull, vertebrae, ribs, and pelvis	F
Tumors metastatic to bone			A	Vertebrae, ribs, and long bones, especially humerus and femur	MC

I, immature animals; LB, large breeds; M, male; F, focal (monostotic); MC, multicentric (polyostotic); A, adult, middle-aged, and older animals; BS, bilaterally symmetric; U, unilateral; GB, giant breeds; UB, unilateral or bilateral

TABLE 45-2. Predispositions of Diseases That Cause Joint Swelling or Enlargement

Disease	Breed	Sex	Age	Anatomic Sites	Common Features
Arthritis (feline progressive polyarthritis)		M	YA	Carpus, tarsus	b; E=e,g,h,k; L=n,o
Arthritis (immune-mediated secondary to chronic infectious diseases)				Major weight-bearing joints	b; E=e,g,h,k,m; L=o
Arthritis (infectious)					E=f,g,h,l; L=n,o
Arthritis (lupus)	German shepherd	F	YA	Elbow, carpus, stifle	b; E=e,g,h,k,m; L=o
Arthritis (rheumatoid)			A	Carpus, tarsus	b; E=e,g,h,k,m,n; L=o
Fractures (articular)					a,c; E=f,g,j; L=o,p
Fractures (physeal)			I	Long bone physes	a,c; E=f,g,j; L=o,p
Hemarthrosis					
Hypofibrinogenemia	St. Bernard				
Hemophilia A	*				
von Willebrand's disease	†	M	I	Major weight-bearing joints	b; E=f,g,h; L=k,m,n,o
Hemophilia B	‡				
Thrombasthenia	§				
Hip dysplasia	German shepherd, St. Bernard, LB		I	Hip	d; E=e,h,l; L=k,m,o,p
Legg-Calvé-Perthes disease	Terriers, TB		I	Hip	c; E=h,k,n; L=j,k,p
Luxations				Hip, shoulder elbow, hock	a,c; E=f,g,j; L=p
Luxations (lateral patellar associated with genu valgum)	Flat-coated retriever, great Dane, St. Bernard, Irish wolfhound		I	Stifle	d; L=e,k,p

Luxations (medial patellar)	TB	F	I	Stifle	d: L = e,k,p
Neoplastic joint disease			A	Elbow, stifle	a,c; E = f,g,h; L = i,m,n,o
Osteoarthrosis (primary DJD)	WB		A	Major weight-bearing joints	b,d; E = e,l; L = i,k,m
Osteoarthrosis (secondary DJD)			A	Major weight-bearing joints	E = e,l; L = i,j,k,m,o
Osteochondromatosis (synovial)		M	A	Hip, metacarpus	e,h,i,j
Osteochondrosis	LB, GB	M	I	Shoulder, elbow, stifle, hock	b,d; L = e,h,j,k,n,p
Subluxations				Carpus, tarsus, stifle	a,c; E = e,g,l; L = h,p
Subluxations (carpal)	Irish setter			Carpus	a,c; E = e,g,l; L = h,p

Breed: *Irish setter, German shepherd, collie, vizsla, sheltie, greyhound, poodle, Chihuahua, beagle, Labrador retriever, Weimaraner, schnauzer
†German shepherd, miniature schnauzer, golden retriever, Scottish terrier, Welsh corgi, Doberman
‡Cocker spaniel, St. Bernard, Cairn terrior, coonhound, Alaskan malamute, French bulldog
§Otterhound, basset hound, foxhound, Scottish terrier

LB, large; TB, toy; WB, working; G, giant

Sex: M, male; F, female

Age: YA, young adult; A, adult, middle-aged, and older; I, immature

Common features:

Distribution: a, usually monoarticular; b, usually polyarticular; c, usually unilateral; d, usually bilateral

Progression: E, early changes; L, late changes

Findings: e, mild to moderate joint effusion; f, marked joint effusion; g, extracapsular swelling or edema; h, joint capsule enlargement; i, joint capsule calcification; j, intraarticular radiodensities (chip fractures, Joint mice); k, periarticular osteophytes; l, normal subchondral bone; m, sclerotic subchondral bone; n, destruction (lysis) of subchondral bone; o, bone remodeling—juxtaarticular; p, possible progression to secondary degenerative joint disease

DJD, degenerative joint disease

401

TABLE 45-3. Predispositions of Periskeletal Enlargements

Disease	Breed	Sex	Age	Anatomic Sites	Common Features
Aneurysmal bone cyst	*		A	Sacral, iliac wing, and coccygeal regions	b,c,e,j,l
Fibrosarcoma			A	Cutaneous, subcutaneous, or oral	a,i,j,k,o
Granuloma					a,o
Hemangiomatosis				Skull, spine, extremities	b,c,e,f,j,o
Hemangiopericytoma			A	Extremities and chest wall	a,h,j,k,o
Hematoma				Fascial planes	a,d,l
Hematoma (subperiosteal)			I		b,d,l
Hygroma	LB, GB		A	Elbow region	a,e,k,m
Lipoma		OF	A	Subcutaneous tissues of thorax, abdomen, and upper portions of extremities	a,o
Myositis (fibrositis) ossificans				Muscles of gluteal and elbow regions	a,f,g,l
Nutritional myopathy (hypovitaminosis E)			I, YA	Muscles of extremities	a,g,m,n
Polymyositis (acute form)				Muscles of mastication	a,g,m,n
Spurious aneurysm				Extremities	a,e,g,l
Tumoral calcinosis			I, YA	Perispinal muscles of cervical region	a,f,o
Undifferentiated sarcoma			A		a,i,j,k,o

Sex: OF, obese females

Breed: LB, large breeds; GB, giant breeds; *, reported mainly in cats

Age: A, adult, middle-aged, or older; I, immature animals; YA, young adult animals

Common features: a, regional bone tissue generally unaffected; b, reactive periosteal new bone; c, regional bone destruction; d, acute extraosseus swelling; e, chronic extraosseus swelling; f, soft tissue calcification or ossification; g, muscular swelling or enlargement; h, nonmetastatic; i, potentially metastatic; j, locally invasive; k, locally recurrent; l, focal lesion; m, bilateral lesions; n, multicentric lesions; o, focal or multicentric counted in a large-breed puppy with the same lesion, hypertrophic osteodystrophy or osteomyelitis would be a more likely cause.

Geographic Residence

Some of the diseases that cause musculoskeletal "swelling" are endemic to specific regions of the United States. In a dog with a sclerotic diaphyseal lesion suspected to be osteomyelitis, coccidioidomycosis would be a likely cause if the dog lived in the Southwest, whereas blastomycosis would be suspected in a dog residing in the Midwest. In a dog with periskeletal swelling in the distal portion of a hindlimb, thromboembolism might be suspected if the dog is from an area where heartworm disease is endemic.

Diet

In animals maintained on commercially prepared balanced diets, certain diseases are unlikely to occur. In a cat with proliferative bony lesions involving the cervical spine, hypervitaminosis A would be suspected only if the cat was being fed a diet of raw liver or receiving vitamin A supplements. In a similar cat with a normal diet, osteochondromatosis would be more likely. Other diseases associated with musculoskeletal "swelling" in which an abnormal diet has been incriminated include hypertrophic osteodystrophy (hypersupplementation, especially with calcium), nutritional secondary hyperparathyroidism (all-meat diet—low calcium, excessive phosphorous), and nutritional myopathy (hypovitaminosis E).

Activity

In animals with known trauma, musculoskeletal "swelling" is often attributable to fractures, dislocations, ligamentous injuries, and associated hemorrhage and inflammation. In a sedentary house dog with a long bone fracture and no history of trauma, underlying metabolic or neoplastic disease should be considered. A sedentary older dog taken to the mountains for the weekend might present on Monday morning with a swollen, painful joint. Exacerbation of chronic degenerative joint disease by overactivity might be a likely explanation of this dog's problem. In contrast, a younger active dog with a similar history and signs would more likely have suffered an acute traumatic injury, such as rupture of the cranial cruciate ligament.

Duration and Progression

Fractures and other traumatic injuries are generally associated with extensive swelling of acute onset. Snake and insect bites and some bacterial infections often result in acute focal swelling. Chronic progressive "swelling" is more

TABLE 45-4. Periskeletal Swelling

Type	Physiologic Mechanisms and Causative Diseases

Hemorrhage	Traumatic vascular disruption
	Vascular disruption secondary to
	  Infection
	  Neoplasia
	Minor trauma and bleeding disorder
	  Congenital clotting factor deficiencies
	  Acquired clotting factor deficiencies
	  Platelet dysfunction

Edema	Lymphatic disruption or occlusion
	  Traumatic lesions
	  Inflammatory diseases
	  Neoplastic diseases
	  Anomaly—congenital primary lymphedema
	Increased capillary hydrostatic pressure
	  Cardiac failure
	  Thromboembolism
	  Allergic reactions
	Increased capillary permeability
	  Burns
	  Allergic reactions
	  Bacterial toxins
	Hypoalbuminemia
	  Excessive loss—renal, gastrointestinal, from burns or
	    open wounds, etc.
	  Decreased production—hepatic, pancreatic, or intestinal
	    disease or malnutrition

Inflammatory exudate	Reaction of tissues to irritants—dilation and increased
	    permeability of capillaries and release of chemical
	    mediators
	Infectious diseases
	Chemical poisons
	Mechanical and thermal injuries
	Immune reactions

commonly associated with neoplastic and certain metabolic and infectious musculoskeletal diseases.

PHYSICAL FINDINGS

Careful palpation may determine whether swelling or enlargement or both are present and whether bones, joints, periskeletal tissues, or some combination of these are involved. Swelling is usually fluctuant, and pitting may be noted following deep palpation. Rule outs and physiologic mechanisms for periskeletal swelling are listed in Table 45-4. Enlargements are firm and may be appreciated

TABLE 45-5. Rule Outs for Long Bone Lesions by Region

Epiphysis	Metaphysis	Diaphysis
Fractures	Bone cysts	Enostosis
Osteomyelitis (hematog-enous)	Fractures	Fractures
	Hypertrophic osteodys-trophy	Hypertrophic osteopathy
Joint diseases (see Table 45-6)	Osteochondromatosis	Panosteitis
Congenital	Tumors of bone (primary)	Tumors of bone (meta-static)
Infectious		
Immune-mediated		
Neoplastic		
Degenerative		

For predispositions of a specific disease, see Table 45-1.

as discrete masses or increased thickness of a part. Rule outs for enlargements have been tabulated by location: bone (see Table 45-1), joints (see Table 45-2), and periskeletal tissues (see Table 45-3).

Swelling is often accompanied by other cardinal signs of inflammation (redness, heat, and pain). Crepitance, laxity, and abnormal increases or decreases in range of motion are highly suggestive of fractures, dislocations, subluxations, or some combination of these.

Location and distribution of lesions are highly significant (see Tables 45-1 through 45-3). Some diseases are confined to a single focus, whereas others are almost always multicentric (polyostotic). Involvement of specific bones or joints, symmetry and asymmetry, and confinement of lesions to specific regions of bones are hallmarks of certain diseases (Tables 45-1 through 45-3 and Tables 45-5 through 45-9).

TABLE 45-6. Rule Outs for Subchondral Bone Lesions by Changes in Bone Density

Predominantly Sclerotic	Predominantly Lytic	Mixed Pattern—Sclerotic and Lytic
Hip dysplasia	Feline progressive polyar-thritis	Hemophilic arthropathy
Immune-mediated arthri-tis, polyarthritis sec-ondary to chronic infectious disease	Infectious arthropathy	Joint neoplasia
	Legg-Calvé-Perthes disease	Rheumatoid arthritis
Lupus arthropathy	Osteochondrosis	
Osteoarthrosis		
Primary DJD		
Secondary DJD		

For predispositions of a specific disease, see Table 45-2.
DJD, degenerative joint disease

TABLE 45-7. Rule Outs for Bone Lesions of the Axial Skeleton by Region

Skull or Mandible	Vertebrae	Ribs
Cartilage analogue of fibromatosis	Aneurysmal bone cyst	Feline Maroteaux-Lamy syndrome
Craniomandibular osteopathy	Fractures	Fractures
Feline osteochondromatosis	Hemangiomatosis	Osteochondromatosis
Fractures	Hypervitaminosis A	Osteomyelitis
Hemangiomatosis	Osteochondromatosis	Tumors metastatic to bone
Ossifying fibroma	Osteomyelitis	Tumors of bone
Osteoma	Tumoral calcinosis	(primary)
Osteomyelitis	Tumors (metastatic to bone)	
Tumors of bone (primary)	Tumors of bone (primary)	

For predispositions of a specific disease, see Tables 45-1 and 45-3.

DIAGNOSTIC IMAGING

Radiography

Radiographic examination is often the most efficient method of determining the cause of musculoskeletal "swelling." Radiographs of the swollen part should be made in two projections and should include the bones or joints proximal and distal to the area of interest.

TABLE 45-8. Rule Outs for Osteoproliferative Lesions by Distribution (Patterns of Increased Bone Density)

Polyostotic Lesions	Monostotic Lesions
Craniomandibular osteopathy*	Enostosis†
Feline Maroteaux-Lamy syndrome*	Healing fractures*,†,‡,§
Healing fractures*,†,‡,§	Ossifying fibroma*,‖
Hematogenous osteomyelitis*,†,§	Osteochondromatosis#
Hypertrophic osteodystrophy*	Osteoma*
Hypertrophic osteopathy*	Osteomyelitis*,†,§
Osteochondromatosis#	Subperiosteal hematoma*
Panosteitis*,†	Traumatic periostitis*
Tumors metastatic to bone†,§	Tumors of bone—malignant primary*,§,‖
	Tumors metastatic to bone†,§

*Periosteal new bone
†Endosteal new bone
‡Thickening of cortical bone
§Thickening and increased number of cancellous trabeculae
‖Soft tissue ossification
#Perichondrial new bone and cartilage

TABLE 45-9.   Rule Outs for Osteolytic Lesions and Pathologic Fractures
by Distribution

Generalized Loss of Bone Density—Entire Skeleton	Multicentric or Multifocal Osteolytic Lesions	Monostotic Focal Osteolytic Lesions
Hyperadrenocorticism	Bone cysts	Bone cysts
Hyperparathyroidism	Fibrous dysplasia	Fibrous dysplasia
Primary	Hemangiomatosis	Hemangiomatosis
Secondary	Multiple myeloma	Osteomyelitis
	Osteomyelitis	Tumors of bone—primary
	Tumors metastatic to bone	Tumors metastatic to bone

If bony lesions are detected, anatomic location and distribution should be initially considered. Rule outs for long bone lesions, according to whether they affect the epiphysis, metaphysis, or diaphysis are listed in Table 45-5. If the lesions predominantly affect subchondral bone, rule outs can be established by changes in bone density (see Table 45-6). Rule outs for lesions of the axial skeleton are listed in Table 45-7. Focal (monostotic) versus multicentric (polyostotic) distribution of lesions is considered in Tables 45-8 and 45-9.

The second step in condensing the rule out list for bony lesions is identification of the predominant pattern of change in bone density. Subchondral bone lesions are differentiated on the basis of osteoproductive (sclerotic), lytic, or mixed patterns of density (see Table 45-6). Bony lesions at other locations that are mainly osteoproliferative are listed in Table 45-8. Those that are mainly osteolytic are listed in Table 45-9. Presentation of an animal with osteolytic lesions is sometimes prompted by acute lameness attributable to pathologic fracture of the involved bone. Chronic pathologic fractures may manifest a mixed pattern of bone density changes—a lytic pattern attributable to the initial disease process and a proliferative pattern attributable with the body's attempt to heal the fracture.

Further condensation of the rule out list is benefited by evaluation of the pattern(s) of increased bone density (see Table 45-8) and the rate of expansion or change of the lesions (Table 45-10). Osteoproliferation may be manifested by cortical thickening, thickening or increase in the number of cancellous trabeculae, periosteal new bone, endosteal new bone, or some combination of these conditions (see Table 45-8). Radiographic appearance of bony lesions is often highly dependent upon their rate of expansion or change. Lesions that develop slowly are usually well-defined, have distinct borders, and are associated with smooth periosteal new bone formation. In contrast, rapidly developing lesions are poorly defined, have indistinct borders, often disrupt cortical continuity, and are associated with irregular periosteal new bone formation (see Table 45-10).

TABLE 45-10. Common Radiographic Characteristics of Bone Lesions by Rate of Expansion or Change

Slow Expansion or Change— Benign Lesions	Rapid Expansion or Change— Malignant Lesions
Well-defined zone of transition	Poorly defined zone of transition
Distinct margin	Indistinct margin
Sclerotic border	Motheaten border
Intact cortex	Broken cortex
Smooth periosteal new bone	Irregular periosteal new bone

Ultrasonography

Sonographic examination is a useful diagnostic tool for evaluating pathologic processes that cause "swelling" of superficial musculoskeletal soft tissue structures, including periosteum, tendons, ligaments, fascia, muscle bellies, synovial membranes, articular cartilage, and menisci. Its diagnostic use for periarticular and intraarticular problems that affect large synovial joints (*e.g.,* shoulder, elbow, knee, ankle) is well established in humans and is currently emerging in veterinary medicine. Ultrasonography can differentiate cartilage from subchondral bone, which may be useful in the detection of early or small lesions associated with osteochondrosis. Thickness of the synovial membrane can also be accurately quantitated using sonographic methods. Because of the large difference in acoustic impedance between soft tissue and bone, diagnostic ultrasonography is not useful for imaging bone "swelling."

Although often used as a supplement to radiographic examination, ultrasonography offers several distinct advantages over conventional radiographic methods:

(1) Ultrasonography is useful for distinguishing between solid versus fluid-filled periskeletal "swellings," and also for determining whether "swelling" is intra- or extraarticular. The tissue texture of a "swelling" also aids in determining the best method of biopsy (*i.e.,* punch biopsy versus fine-needle aspiration, etc.).

(2) Diagnostic ultrasonography can be used to identify periskeletal muscular swellings. Identification of tissue texture by this method may help to condense the rule out list. Edema or cellulitis is recognized by separation of muscle fibers by hypoechoic fluid; mature abscesses and organizing hematomas tend to have irregularly thickened walls that contain hypoechoic, hyperechoic or mixed-textured echoic material. With most abscesses and some hematomas, digital pressure may be used to produce swirling of fluid content that can be seen with real-time instrumentation. Cysts in the muscles have a hypoechoic to an anechoic internal content surrounded by smooth walls. Dystrophic mineralization causes a shadowing artifact, while gas accumulation from sepsis or open wounds produces bright evenly spaced echoes (reverberation artifact). Muscle

TABLE 45-11. Common Synovial Fluid Findings by Disease

Synovial Fluid (SF) Finding	Normal Joint	Noninflammatory		Inflammatory			
		Degenerative Joint Disease	Hemarthrosis	Rheumatoid Arthritis	Lupus Arthropathy	Neoplastic Joint Disease	Septic Arthritis
Color	C	PY	R	YBT	YBT	YBT	CCS
Turbidity	*	†	‡	§	§	§	‡
Viscosity	Normal	Normal	Reduced	Reduced	Reduced	Reduced	Reduced
Mucin clot	Good	Good	Fair	Poor	Fair	Good	Poor
RBCs	None	Few	Many	Moderate	Moderate	Moderate	Moderate
WBCs × 10³/μl	0.25–3	1–5	3–10	8–38	4.4–371	3–10	40–267
% PMNS	0–6	0–12	60–75	20–80	15–95	15–75	90–99
% Mononuclear cells	94–100	88–100	25–40	20–80	5–85	25–85	1–10
Ragocytes	–	–	–	+	–	–	–
LE cells	–	–	–	–	+	–	–
Neoplastic cells	–	–	–	–	–	+	–
Microorganisms	–	–	–	–	–	–	+
SF glucose (% of blood glucose)	100	80–100	100	50–80	50–80	50–80	<50

C, colorless; PY, pale yellow; R, red; YBT, yellow to blood-tinged; CCS, cream-colored to sanguineous
*, not turbid; †, slight turbidity; ‡, marked turbidity; §, moderate turbidity
–, absent; +, present

neoplasms have mixed texture and appear architecturally different from normal muscle. Tumor margins can usually be detected.

(3) Interventional ultrasonography enables constant, real-time visualization of a mass, the surrounding vasculature, and the tip of a biopsy needle without exposing medical personnel and the patient to ionizing radiation (as would be the case with fluoroscopy). This facilitates aspiration of musculoskeletal fluid accumulations, drainage of abscesses, and accurate biopsy of masses while minimizing the likelihood of vascular trauma during the procedure.

(4) Ultrasonography is more accurate than radiography in the detection and localization of radiolucent foreign bodies. Since the ability to detect an object on sonographic images is a function of the difference between the acoustic impedance of the object and the surrounding tissues, radiolucent foreign bodies can be imaged quite easily with ultrasonography. Penetrating foreign bodies such as wood splinters are identified during the acute or subacute stage as a hyperechoic line surrounded by a hypoechoic collection of sanguineous or purulent fluid.

DEFINITIVE DIAGNOSIS

In formulating rule outs for a lesion, the reader is encouraged to (1) evaluate the lesion by physical examination and diagnostic imaging, (2) based upon initial findings, consult pertinent areas of Tables 45-4 through 45-9, (3) make an initial rule out list, and (4) consult the appropriate disease catalogue (see Tables 45-1 through 45-3) and consider predispositions of suspected diseases in order to condense or rank order the rule out list. Final diagnosis may depend upon additional diagnostic aids, including sonographic techniques; needle aspirates for cytologic, microbiologic, and biochemical evaluation; incisional or trephine biopsies for histopathologic evaluation; skeletal survey radiography or bone scintigraphy to locate occult lesions in polyostotic diseases; and appropriate clinicopathologic testing to confirm or rule out certain systemic or metabolic diseases. Synovial fluid analysis and culture are especially helpful in differentiating various joint diseases. Synovial fluid findings for normal dogs are compared with findings commonly associated with different joint diseases in Table 45-11.

For additional information regarding the diseases listed in the tables of this chapter, the reader is referred to the texts listed below.

SUGGESTED READING

Bojrab MJ: Pathophysiology in Small Animal Surgery. Philadelphia, Lea & Febiger, 1981
Brinker WO, Piermattei DL, Flo GL: Handbook of Small Animal Orthopedics & Fracture Treatment, 2nd ed. Philadelphia, WB Saunders, 1990
Newton, CD, Nunamaker DM: Textbook of Small Animal Orthopedics. Philadelphia, JB Lippincott, 1985
Whittick WG: Canine Orthopedics. Philadelphia, Lea & Febiger, 1990

CHAPTER FORTY-SIX

Pain

Dennis N. Aron

PROBLEM DEFINITION AND RECOGNITION

Many diseases and disorders encountered in veterinary medicine cause pain. The ability to facilitate the diagnosis of many different diseases depends greatly on the veterinarian's knowledge of how to identify and localize the painful stimulus, understanding the physiology and disease mechanism of actual pain (projected pain), awareness that pain can be referred from one part of the body to another (referred pain), and knowledge of the different conditions that lead to pain. The treatment of pain for the relief of suffering is frequently overlooked in veterinary medicine because animals are unable to communicate abstract concepts. The veterinarian must recognize subtle behavioral changes that indicate that an animal has pain and must understand the diagnostic and therapeutic principles that afford pain resolution and control.

Pain is a concept that involves the mechanisms of the nervous system that transmit and integrate stimuli to the body and a psychologic component that includes affect, emotion, and memory. It is difficult to interpret human emotions and even more difficult to transpose these to animals. It is best to assume that animals perceive pain, react to stimuli, and respond to therapy in a manner similar to that of human beings. Fortunately, much research on pain is in animal models, and the results suggest that these assumptions are correct.

Terminology is not standardized, even in the research literature. Nevertheless, the following terms are defined for general use:

- Noxious stimuli—those that threaten or actually produce damage to tissues
- Nociceptors—sense organs that primarily respond to noxious stimuli
- Pain—the sensation caused by a noxious stimulus
- Hyperalgesia—increased sensitivity to noxious stimuli
- Hyperesthesia—increased sensitivity to stimulation, even that which is normally not noxious.

PATHOPHYSIOLOGY

The pain receptors (nociceptors) are free nerve endings that are especially numerous in superficial layers of the skin, cornea, anus, and internal tissues such as the periosteum, arterial walls, joint capsule, muscles, tendons, and the falx and tentorium of the cranial vault. Most of the other deep tissues are weakly supplied with pain endings, but widespread tissue damage can cumulatively cause pain in these areas. Three types of nociceptors exist in tissues: those responding to excessive mechanical stress, those responding to extreme heat, and those responding to abnormal chemicals. Different chemicals (*e.g.*, bradykinin, serotonin, histamine, potassium ions, acids, prostaglandins, leukotrienes, acetylcholine, and proteolytic enzymes) stimulate the chemosensitive receptors. These chemicals are highly concentrated in inflamed tissue. In contrast to most other sensory receptors of the body, nociceptors do not adapt to the initial stimulus. This mechanism keeps the animal appraised of the damaging stimulus. Similarly, nociceptors are capable of responding to a repeated stimulus by an attribute known as sensitization.

The viscera (unlike the skin, periosteum, and joints) contain only pain sensory receptors; localized damage to the viscera rarely causes severe pain. Conversely, any disease that results in diffuse stimulation of pain nerve endings throughout a viscus can result in extreme pain. In addition to true visceral pain, some pain sensations are also transmitted from the viscera through nerve fibers that innervate parietal peritoneum, pleura, or pericardium (parietal pain pathway).

Pain signals are transmitted from the periphery to the spinal cord by small type A-delta fibers at velocities between 6 and 30 meters/sec and by type C fibers at velocities between 0.5 and 2 meters/sec. In humans, the fast type A pain fibers conduct pain perceived as a pricking sensation, and the slower type C fibers conduct pain impulses perceived as a slow burning sensation. Most insults initially produce a sharp, pricking pain followed by a dull, burning feeling indicating pain is a complex mixture of sensations involving both the A-delta and C fibers. The slow burning sensation tends to become more painful over time, which gives the person the intolerable suffering of long-continuing pain.

Pain fibers enter the spinal cord through the dorsal roots and ascend or descend a few segments; the two fiber types terminate on neurons contained in separate sections in the dorsal horns of the cord grey matter. Most of the signals then probably pass through one or more additional short-fibered neurons, the last of which gives rise to long fibers that cross immediately to the opposite side of the spinal cord and appear to pass up the cord in the intermingled spinothalamic and spinoreticular tracts and dorsal column postsynaptic system. There is also a bilateral, multisynaptic, small-fiber pathway, possibly in the propriospinal system, that conducts pain. It is difficult to destroy: it survives hemisections of the spinal cord on opposite sides if they are spaced three to five segments apart. Lesions such as disk protrusion abolish proprioception, descending motor function, and cutaneous (superficial) pain sensation before eliminating all pain sensation. These multisynaptic small fiber tracts have been termed the *deep pain pathways*, referring to the stimulus to deep structures such as periosteum, which activate the system. The majority of fibers pass to the pontobulbar reticular system with ongoing pathways to the thalamus, hypothalamus, and mesencephalic areas. In humans, stimulation of the higher centers produces feelings of pricking pain, numbness and burning, and intense fear, along with autonomic signs associated with fear such as anguish, anxiety, crying, depression, nausea, and excessive muscular excitability. The thalamus reinforces the emotional aspects of pain; the reticular formation is involved in arousal and possibly in the conscious appreciation of pain.

Two related types of compounds with morphine-like actions are the enkephalins and endorphins. The enkephalins are found in areas of the brain associated with pain control, and the endorphins are concentrated in the hypothalamus and pituitary gland. The enkephalins and the endorphins act as excitatory transmitter substances that activate portions of the brain's analgesic system. Stress and fear cause the release of these substances, which act as analgesics. In part, this system works through descending pathways to the neurons in the dorsal horn of the spinal cord. As fear and anxiety subside, pain may increase due to decreased release of these endogenous analgesics.

Stimulation of large sensory fibers from the peripheral tactile receptors depresses the transmission of additional pain signals from the same area of the stimulus or even from areas located several body segments away. The feedback circuits from the large afferents and the descending pathways constitute the gating mechanism in the dorsal horn, which tends to limit the response to noxious stimuli. This response and simultaneous excitation of the central analgesic system are probably the basis for pain relief by acupuncture.

The source of pain may appear to be at a site considerably removed from the diseased tissues. This is "referred" pain, and it may confuse the localization of the diseased tissue. It is chiefly noted with pain initiated by one of the visceral organs and referred to an area of the body surface. Referred pain occurs because sensation from the viscera is conducted through some of the same neurons that conduct pain signals from the surface (excitatory convergence).

SPECIFIC MECHANISMS

Tissue destruction produces pain through stimulation of mechanosensitive, thermosensitive, and chemosensitive nociceptors. The presence and intensity of pain are dependent on several variables. First, it is necessary for the tissue to contain nociceptors; the central nervous system does not. Second, the density of nociceptors varies with the tissue. Skin, joint surfaces, and periosteum contain numerous receptors; hence, focal stimulation of these tissues may cause severe pain. Tissues with a lower density of receptors, such as the viscera, require diffuse stimulation of tissue, and therefore nerve endings, before the pain becomes severe. Third, even though the lowest intensity of stimulus that produces the sensation of pain (pain threshold) is constant across species, the tolerance of a painful stimulus varies widely, relative to the situation, within a single species.

Pain emanating from the joints can be an interesting phenomenon, as some conditions cause intense pain, while others cause a waxing and waning pain. Stimuli involving the joint capsule, ligaments, and synovium are very painful, because receptors are numerous in these components of the joint. With degenerative joint disease (DJD), pain can be variable and episodic. This is because DJD may not be particularly painful until the condition is exacerbated by stimulus of the joint capsule and ligaments through increased instability, pressure, or stimulus of the synovium through increased inflammation. With DJD, inflammation is created by excessive wearing of the joint surfaces, which leads to matrix degeneration, allowing mucopolysaccharides to leach from the substance of the cartilage, creating a painful chemical synovitis. Prolonged rest can be an effective treatment for painful DJD; rest reduces degeneration of the cartilage matrix, allowing the synovitis to abate.

Ischemia is an important cause of pain to most tissues of the body. The mechanism is the chemical stimulation of nociceptors. When blood flow to a tissue is disrupted, acidic metabolic end products (lactic acid) or tissue degenerative products (bradykinin, proteolytic enzymes, and others) are generated because of cell death. Both probably stimulate nociceptors. Ischemia of the spinal cord and brain does not produce pain, because there are no nociceptors in these tissues. In humans, muscle spasm is a very common cause of severe pain and is the basis of many clinical pain syndromes. This pain probably results partially from the direct effect of muscle spasm in stimulating mechanosensitive nociceptors and partially from the indirect effect of muscle spasm in causing ischemia and thereby stimulating chemosensitive nociceptors. Muscle spasm creating pain is uncommonly seen in dogs and cats but has been reported to occur with exertional rhabdomyolysis in racing greyhounds, status epilepticus producing exertional rhabdomyolysis in dogs, and muscle cramping in Scottish terriers during excitement of heavy exercise.

Any stimulus that excites pain nerve endings in diffuse areas of the viscera causes visceral pain. Such stimuli include ischemia of visceral tissue, chemical damage to the surfaces of the viscera, spasm of the smooth muscle in a hollow viscus, distention of a hollow viscus, and stretching of the ligaments. Two sources of pain result from visceral damage: (1) true visceral pain originates from structures in the thoracic and abdominal cavities, and (2) pain sensations are also transmitted from the viscera through nerve fibers that innervate the parietal peritoneum, pleura, or pericardium. The parietal surfaces of the visceral cavities are supplied mainly by spinal nerves that penetrate from the surface of the body inward. A disease that affects a viscus often spreads to the parietal wall of the visceral cavity. The wall is supplied with extensive innervation from spinal nerves, which include the "fast" type A fibers, producing a sharp pain. The kidney and ureters, being retroperitoneally located, are supplied by both visceral and parietal pain fibers and seem to be very painful when affected by abnormalities.

Clinically, certain lesions that involve the spinal column can be very painful (Table 46-1), but others may be nonpainful. Meningitis is usually highly painful

Text continues on p. 418

TABLE 46-1. Differential Diagnosis of Diseases That Produce Spinal Column Pain: Predispositions and Clinical Signs

Rule Out	Breed	Predominant Age and Sex	Localization of Pain	Predominant Clinical Signs
Cervical				
Atlantoaxial insta-bility	Miniature and toy dog breeds	6–18 months	Cranial	Cervical pain Neurologic deficits are variable.
Cervical malforma-tion, malarticula-tion (Wobbler)	Great Dane, Doberman pinscher (other large dog breeds)	Great Dane—young Doberman pinscher—middle age Male	Caudal and middle	Bilateral ataxia and paresis of pelvic limbs, occasionally thoracic limbs Cervical pain not marked
Diskospondylitis	German shepherds, great Danes (large dog breeds)	Middle age Male	Caudal	Anorexia, depression, fever Lameness Stilted gait Paresis Hyperesthesia, abdominal tenseness
Disk disease	Dachshund, beagle, toy poodle (chondrodystro-phoid and small breeds, in general) Cat—rare	Middle age Variable	Cranial (can occur at other sites)	Cervical pain
Fractures/luxation	Variable (dog and cat [rare])	Variable Variable	Cranial	Cervical pain Proprioceptive deficits, quadriplegia
Hypervitaminosis A	Cat	Variable Variable	Cranial	Lethargy, anorexia Hyperemia and edema of gums Abdominal distention Cervical pain Lameness Spinal exostosis History of exclusive liver diet or ex-cessive vitamin A concentration

(continued)

TABLE 46-1. Differential Diagnosis of Diseases That Produce Spinal Column Pain: Predispositions and Clinical Signs (*continued*)

Rule Out	Breed	Predominant Age and Sex	Localization of Pain	Predominant Clinical Signs
Meningitis	Variable (dog and cat)	Variable Variable	Diffuse	Pain ± Neurologic deficits Increased white cell count and protein of CSF
Tumors of spinal cord or vertebrae	Variable (dog and cat)	Middle, old age Variable	Variable	Cervical pain Radicular pain Weight loss, anorexia, lethargy ± Neurologic deficits Usually extramedullary if pain is produced
Back Diskospondylitis	Similar to cervical lesions with pain localized to the region involved—midthoracic spine, L2–L4 (plant migration), L7–S1 affected most commonly			
Disk disease	Dachshund, Pekingese, beagle, Welsh corgi, Lhasa apso, Shih tzu, (chondrodystrophoid and small breeds in general, but type II disk disease in nonchondrodystrophoid breeds occurs)	Chondrodystrophoid 3–6 years Nonchondrodystrophoid 6–8 years Variable	Upper	Neurologic deficits Pain

Fractures/luxations	Variable (dog and cat [rare])	Variable
		Variable
			Upper or lower	Upper
				  Pain
				  ± Paraparesis—paraplegia
				Lower
				  Pain

Disease	Breed	Age	Sex	Level	Clinical signs
					Proprioceptive deficits in hind limbs; Severe urinary and fecal incontinence; ± Paraparesis; ± Perineal and flexor hyporeflexia
Hemivertebrae	English bulldog, Boston terrier, pug ("screwtail" breeds)	Variable	Variable	Upper	Usually an incidental finding; Pain; ± Paraparesis
Lumbosacral stenosis	Toy or miniature poodle (small dog breeds)	Middle age	Variable	Lower	Same as lumbrosacral malarticulation, malformation; Lameness worsens with exercise; Paresthesia
Lumbosacral malarticulation, malformation	German shepherds (large dog breeds)	Middle age	Male	Lower	Pain; Proprioceptive deficits in hindlimbs; Urinary and fecal incontinence; ± Paraparesis; ± Perineal and flexor hyporeflexia
Meningitis	Similar to cervical lesion, diffuse pain is most common				
Progressive hemorrhagic myelomalacia	Variable	Variable	Variable	Upper; Diffuse	Painful, irritable, anxious; Pyrexia; Dysparity of radiographic focal lesion with diffuse clinical signs; No treatment—will die in 1–3 days of respiratory paralysis
Tumors of spinal cord or vertebrae	Similar to cervical lesion with pain localized to the region involved				

±, widely variable; CSF, cerebrospinal fluid

because of the diffuse involvement of the meninges (mechanism similar to that in pleuritis or peritonitis). Focal disk disease is severely painful because of the numerous tissues being stimulated. These tissues include the periostium—which is known to be especially dense with nociceptors, the dorsal nerve root, the meninges, and the anulus of the disk itself. Diskospondylitis is painful because of the diffuse stimulation of many of the same tissues.

DIAGNOSTIC PLAN

The recognition of pain in animals may be difficult; however, the localization of pain to a region, segment, or part of the body is often necessary for a correct diagnosis. Pain can be inferred from clinical signs such as lameness, dysphagia, and dysuria (see Chapters 31, 38, and 44). However, sometimes there is no functional impairment, for only behavioral changes are apparent. Initially, the animal may try to withdraw in an attempt to escape the painful stimulus. If this fails the animal often exhibits other behavioral responses such as vocalization, increased avoidance, pacing, guarding, and aggression. With acute sharp pain the animal usually bites or licks at the origin of the painful stimulus. Behavior seen with chronic low-grade pain includes changes in eating habits, lethargy, irritability, depression, reduced playfulness, dysuria, constipation, weight loss, and diminished grooming. Typical autonomic response to pain and stress is exhibited by the emotional reactions of increased blood pressure, heart rate, pupillary dilation, and changes in respiratory pattern. Even though an emotional response is usually associated with perception of pain, the absence of such a response is not an assurance that the animal has not perceived pain.

An algorithm for the localization of pain to a region, segment, or part of the body is given in a separate list (see Display, Localization of Pain by Region of Body). Identification and localization of long bone periosteal or joint pain is usually straightforward, whereas abdominal pain is difficult to localize beyond the cranial or caudal regions. Frequently, pain that seems to be emanating from the abdomen is actually referred from the spinal column and vice versa. Signs of abdominal pain include restlessness, panting, abdominal splinting upon gentle palpation, and possibly a "praying" posture.

Thoracic pain is uncommon and is usually associated with pleural diseases. The pain is usually referred directly to the overlying thoracic wall. The discomfort is greatly accentuated by inspiratory movement; this leads to splinting of the affected side of the thorax and rapid, shallow, and grunting respiration.

Pain affecting the appendicular skeleton is common and easily diagnosed because it almost always is reflected as lameness (see Chapters 44 and 45). Since any lesion involving the periosteum, ligaments, joint capsule, and synovium will lead to extreme focal pain, palpation of the lame limb usually leads to succesful localization of the site of the abnormality.

Generally, pain emanating from facial structures is exhibited by behavioral changes, but functional disturbances also occur. Painful corneal lesions cause the functional disturbances of blepharospasm, epiphora, and photophobia; pain

Localization of Pain by Region of Body

- Appendicular skeleton
    Long bone (see Chapters 44 and 45)
    Joint (see Chapters 44 and 45)
    Muscle
        Exertional rhabdomyolysis
        Muscle cramping (Scottish terriers)
        Myositis ossificans
        Polymyositis
        Status epilepticus
    Other
        Aortic thromboembolism
            (saddle thrombus—cat)
        Sensory polyneuropathy
- Facial
    Ocular (see Chapter 56)
    Oral (see Chapters 3, 30, and 31)
    Bone/muscle
        Craniomandibular osteopathy
        Fractures—maxilla or mandible,
            or both
        Myositis
        Temporomandibular joint
            disorders

- Cervical (see Table 46-1)
- Back
    Actual (see Table 46-1)
    Referred
        Acute pancreatitis
        Cholelithiasis
        Pyelonephritis
        Prostatitis
        Renal or ureteral calculi
- Thoracic cavity
    Pleuritis
- Abdominal cavity
    Actual (see Chapter 36)
    Referred
        Back trauma
        Disk disease
        Diskospondylitis
        Meningeal disease
- Perianal
    Anorectal trauma
    Anal/rectal cancer
    Anal sac abscess/impaction
    Perianal fistulas
    Rectal strictures

due to glaucoma is usually recognized as behavioral alterations. Painful oral lesions can be exhibited by excessive salivation and dysphagia along with behavioral changes.

Pain is a very useful localizing sign for cervical diseases and syndromes (see Table 46-1) and is the most prominent sign in cervical disk protrusions and meningitis. An animal with cervical pain holds its head and neck low and rigid. Cervical muscle spasms and a "walking on eggs" gait are common. Behavioral signs may consist of continuous crying or whining for no apparent reason and a reluctance to eat or drink. The animal may continuously or periodically resist any palpation or movement of the neck. Careful deep palpation of vertebrae may localize the pain to the cranial, middle, or caudal cervical segments. When the lesions involve the spinal cord, neurologic signs reinforce localization of the lesion (see Chapter 47). Even though pain from cervical disk protrusion is a common clinical sign, pain from thoracolumbar (cranial back) disk disease may be transient before profound neurologic deficits of paresis or paralysis occur. However, with more chronic cranial back syndromes, especially with disk disease, pain may be a constant sign. Terminal thoracic and lumbar spinal lesions (caudal back) may also cause generalized pain and arching of the back. With either cranial or caudal back syndromes, the animal may object to handling, walking up stairs, or jumping into a car. Frequent crying or whining, exaggerated tendon reflexes, and rigid limbs and dorsal musculature are also signs of back pain.

Generally, when evaluating the back for pain, the clinician should look for obvious reactions such as vocalization and aggressive or fearful behavior upon palpation and manipulation. More subtle responses may include resisting movement and tensing the muscles. By placing one hand on the abdomen and pressing on each vertebrae with the other hand, a tensing of the abdominal muscles can be felt as painful areas are palpated. This palpation is followed by pinching the skin with a hemostat or pricking the skin with an 18-gauge needle. The skin is pinched gently to avoid significant behavioral reaction in normal areas. Stimulating areas of hyperesthesia evokes an exaggerated skin twitch or behavioral response. This test should be conducted in a caudal to cranial direction, because areas caudal to the lesion will usually have decreased sensation. A level of normal or increased sensation can be determined by using this test. If a spinal lesion is present, the sensory area should have the conformation of a dermatome. As further confirmation of the level of thoracolumbar lesions, the cutaneous trunci (panniculus) reflex can be elicited with a needle in the same manner as for detecting hyperesthesia. The panniculus reflex is insufficient for localization of lesions when minor neurologic deficits are present and pain is the primary sign. The motor evaluation of the neurologic examination localizes the lesion to one of six regions of the spinal cord or to the brain, whereas the sensory evaluation should localize the lesion to within three segments of the spinal cord (see Chapter 47).

Painful perianal diseases and syndromes are often displayed by the behavioral signs of scooting, dragging, or rubbing the perineum on the floor, coupled with biting or chewing of the painful area. Functional disturbances common to problems of the perianal region include tenesmus, constipation, and dyschezia, along with intermittent diarrhea, constipation, and weight loss as the problem becomes progressive.

REFERENCES

1. Guyton AC: Somatic sensations. Part II. Pain, visceral pain, headache, and thermal sensations. In Guyton AC (ed): Textbook of Medical Physiology, 7th ed, pp 592–605. Philadelphia, WB Saunders, 1986
2. Kaplan M: Pain. In Ettinger S (ed): Textbook of Veterinary Internal Medicine, pp 39–45. Philadelphia, WB Saunders, 1983
3. Sackman JE: Pain: Its perception and alleviation in dogs and cats. Part I. The physiology of pain. Comp Cont Ed 13:71–75, 1991
4. Smith G, Covino BG: Acute Pain, pp 68–103. London, Butterworth, 1985
5. Wall PD: Defining "Pain in Animals." In Short CE and Poznak AV (eds): Animal pain, pp 63–79. New York, Churchill Livingston, 1992
6. Yoxall AT: Pain in small animals: Its recognition and control. J Sm Anim Pract 19:423–438, 1978

PART TWELVE

Neurologic Problems

CHAPTER FORTY-SEVEN

Paresis or Paralysis

John E. Oliver

PROBLEM DEFINITION AND RECOGNITION

Paralysis is the loss of motor function in a part of the body that is due to dysfunction of neural or muscular systems.[1] Paresis is partial paralysis. The most useful clinical definition of paralysis is loss of *voluntary* motor function. The term *paresis* is used in this chapter to include both partial and complete paralysis of a part of the body. Terms used to define the extent of paresis are monoparesis (one limb), pelvic limb paresis or paraparesis (both pelvic limbs), tetraparesis or quadriparesis (all four limbs), and paresis of specific structures (*e.g.*, facial paresis).[2]

PATHOPHYSIOLOGY

The final common pathway for all motor function is the lower motor neuron (LMN), the efferent neuron connecting the central nervous system to a muscle. All activity of the nervous system is expressed through LMNs located in the ventral and intermediate columns of the grey matter of the spinal cord and in the cranial nerve nuclei in the brain stem. The axons of these neurons form the peripheral spinal and cranial nerves. The LMN includes the nerve cell body, the axon, and the neuromuscular junction.

Dysfunction of an LMN prevents activation of the muscle (paresis), abolishes reflexes (areflexia), eliminates the normal tone in the muscle (flaccidity), and, in a short time, causes the muscle to atrophy. Paresis, areflexia, loss of tone, and early severe atrophy are the signs of LMN lesions.

The nervous system is arranged in a segmented fashion. Each spinal cord segment is demarcated by a pair of spinal nerves. The brain is less orderly in its segmentation, but anatomic and functional regions can be identified. Paresis of a muscle or group of muscles can be traced to a specific peripheral nerve, spinal nerve, or brain stem or spinal cord segment(s). Lesions of peripheral nerves cause severe LMN signs in all the muscles innervated. Peripheral nerves usually originate in several spinal cord segments; therefore, spinal nerve or cord lesions usually affect portions of the muscles rather than entire muscle groups. Brain stem lesions are more likely to affect all of the neurons in a nucleus and to appear as complete lesions.

Voluntary movement requires control from the brain. The LMN is under the

TABLE 47-1. Summary of Lower Motor Neuron and Upper Motor Neuron Signs

	Lower Motor Neuron Sign(s)	Upper Motor Neuron Sign(s)
Motor function	Paralysis of muscle or group of muscles	Paralysis or paresis of part of body
Reflexes	Hyporeflexia to areflexia	Normal or hyperreflexia
Muscle tone	Decreased	Normal to increased
Muscle atrophy	Early (weeks) and severe; affects all muscles denervated	Late (months) and mild; affects entire limb
Electromyography	Fibrillation potentials and positive sharp waves after 5–7 days	No change

control of motor pathways from the cerebral cortex and brain stem, the upper motor neuron (UMN). Cortical control is directed primarily through brain stem locomotor centers in the midbrain and pons. The pathways, which extend through the brain stem and spinal cord, are responsible for the initiation and maintenance of normal movements. Pathways from the vestibular nuclei maintain tone in the extensor muscles to support the body against gravity. The UMN includes the nerve cell in the brain and the axon forming the brain stem and spinal cord pathway.

Dysfunction of the UMN prevents voluntary movement (paresis) and may cause hyperactive reflexes, an increase in muscle tone, and abnormal reflexes (*e.g.,* crossed extensor reflex). Paresis, normal or exaggerated reflexes, normal or increased muscle tone, and abnormal reflexes are the signs of UMN lesions. Table 47-1 summarizes the characteristics of LMN and UMN signs.

DIAGNOSTIC PLAN

The diagnosis includes localization of the lesion, the anatomic diagnosis, and the cause (etiology) of the lesion.

Anatomic Diagnosis

The first step is to determine that the problem is neurologic in origin. Lameness and weakness may be caused by a variety of musculoskeletal and systemic problems. The neurologic examination, especially tests of postural reaction and reflexes in both spinal and cranial nerves, provides the necessary information. Abnormal proprioceptive positioning reactions or depressed reflexes are virtually always the result of neuromuscular disease.

Localization of peripheral spinal nerve lesions is summarized in Table 47-2. The examination must identify which muscles are paretic. Deficits of cranial nerves with motor function are summarized in Table 47-3, including the appro-
Text continues on p. 428

TABLE 47-2. Spinal Nerves: Distribution and Clinical Signs of Dysfunction

Nerve (Spinal Cord Origin)	Muscles	Function	Signs of Dysfunction
Brachial plexus—thoracic limb			
Suprascapular (C6–C7)	Supraspinatus Infraspinatus	Extends shoulder	Slight loss of shoulder extension Atrophy of muscles with prominent spine of scapula
Axillary (C6, C7, C8)	Deltoideus Teres major Teres minor	Flexes shoulder	Decreased shoulder flexion
Musculocutaneous (C6, C7, C8)	Biceps brachii Brachialis Coracobrachialis	Flexes elbow	Decreased elbow flexion at gait and on withdrawal Decreased sensation medial of medial forearm
Radial (C7–T1)	Triceps brachii Extensor carpi radialis Common and lateral digital extensors Ulnaris lateralis	Extends elbow, carpus, and digits	Loss of extension If triceps is involved, loss of weight bearing Decreased triceps and extensor carpi radialis reflexes Decreased sensation dorsal forearm and paw
Median (C8–T1)	Flexor carpi radialis Superficial digital flexor	Flexes carpus and digits	Decreased flexion of carpus and digits Decreased flexion of carpus on withdrawal
Ulnar (C8–T1)	Flexor carpi ulnaris Deep digital flexor	Flexes carpus and digits	Decreased flexion of carpus and digits Decreased flexion of carpus on withdrawal Decreased sensation of caudal forearm and fifth digit

(continued)

TABLE 47-2. Spinal Nerves: Distribution and Clinical Signs of Dysfunction *(continued)*

Nerve (Spinal Cord Origin)	*Muscles*	*Function*	*Signs of Dysfunction*
Lumbosacral plexus—pelvic limb			
Femoral (L4–L6)	Iliopsoas Quadriceps Sartorius	Flexes hip and extends stifle	Loss of extension of stifle, reduced hip flexion, unable to bear weight Decreased quadriceps (knee-jerk) reflex Decreased sensation medial surface of leg
Obturator (L4–L6)	Obturator externus Adductor Pectineus Gracilis	Adducts pelvic limb	Limb slides laterally on slick surfaces
Sciatic (L6–S2)	Biceps femoris Semimembranosus Semitendinosus	Extends hip and flexes stifle (see also Tibial and Peroneal)	Decreased flexion of stifle at gait and on reflex Decreased sensation below stifle
Tibial	Gastrocnemius Popliteus Deep digital flexor Superficial digital flexor	Extends hock and flexes digits	Decreased extension of hock Decreased sensation plantar surface of foot
Peroneal	Cranial tibial Peroneus longus Long and lateral digital extensors	Flexes hock and extends digits	Decreased flexion of hock and extension of digits Foot knuckles over Decreased sensation of dorsocranial surface of foot, hock, and stifle

TABLE 47-3. Cranial Nerves: Distribution and Signs of Motor Dysfunction

Nerve	Origin	Clinical Tests	Signs of Dysfunction
III oculomotor	Midbrain	Pupillary light reflex Voluntary and vestibular eye movements	Dilated, unresponsive pupil Ventrolateral strabismus, unable to move eye dorsally or medially
IV trochlear	Midbrain	Eye movements, difficult to detect	Rotation of eye, minimal deficit
V trigeminal	Pons	Jaw strength, palpate temporal and masseter muscles	Atrophy of temporal and masseter muscles
	Medulla	Sensory examination of face	Decreased jaw tone Loss of sensation on face
VI abducent	Medulla	Eye movements	Medial strabismus, unable to move eye laterally or to retract the eye
VII facial	Medulla	Observation of face, palpebral reflex, menace reaction, tone of facial muscles	Unable to move muscles of face Decreased blink reflex Asymmetry of lips, eyelids, and ears
IX glossopharyngeal	Medulla	Gag reflex	Dysphagia, weak gag reflex
X vagus	Medulla	Gag reflex, examination of larynx	Dysphagia, inspiratory dyspnea, altered vocalization
XI accessory	Medulla	Palpation of trapezius, sternocephalicus, and brachiocephalicus muscles	Atrophy of trapezius, sternocephalicus, and brachiocephalicus muscles
XII hypoglossal	Medulla	Examination of tongue	Atrophy of tongue; unable to lick in all directions; tongue deviates to side of lesion

TABLE 47-4. Signs of Lesions in the Spinal Cord

Location of Lesion	Clinical Signs
C1–5	Tetraparesis, UMN all four limbs
C6–T2 brachial plexus	Tetraparesis, UMN pelvic limbs, LMN thoracic limbs
T3–L3	UMN pelvic limb paresis; normal thoracic limbs
L4–S2 lumbosacral plexus	LMN pelvic limb paresis; normal thoracic limbs
S1–S3 pelvic plexus	LMN bladder and sphincters
Cd1–Cd5	LMN paresis of tail

UMN, upper motor neuron; LMN, lower motor neuron

priate tests. Localization of spinal cord or spinal nerve lesions is outlined in Table 47-4. Postural reactions and spinal reflexes provide the data necessary to recognize LMN and UMN signs. Lesions in the brain stem causing UMN signs in the limbs usually also cause cranial nerve signs, which are localizing. Lesions in the cerebrum or diencephalon may cause UMN paresis of the limbs without cranial nerve signs. Associated abnormalities of disease in these areas are listed in Table 47-5 (LMN signs are localizing to a small specific area). If only UMN signs are present, other findings are necessary to accuracy. The results of a sensory examination, including hyperesthesia and the ability to perceive superficial and deep pain, are useful in order to accurately localize the lesion. A single lesion is assumed until the examination clearly demonstrates a multifocal abnormality.

Etiologic Diagnosis

The etiology of the disease is derived from information obtained in the signalment and history, the location of the lesion, and ancillary studies such as hematology, serum chemistries, urine analysis, radiology, electrodiagnostic tests, and cerebrospinal fluid analysis.

The history provides data on the rate of onset and progression of the signs. Most diseases can be classified as acute nonprogressive, acute progressive, or chronic progressive. This information, plus the signalment and location of the lesion, usually narrows the cause of the problem to three to five general categories of disease. The diagnostic plans for most of the specific diseases in a category are usually the same. The major categories of disease are listed with their usual classification in Table 47-6. Diseases that may be acute or chronic in onset are listed twice, but the order of listing indicates the relative probability of occurrence.

The more common diseases are listed according to this classification in Tables 47-7 through 47-11. Diagnostic plans for the major categories of disease are listed in Table 47-12.[3]

Text continues on p. 435

TABLE 47-5. Signs of Lesions in the Brain

	Mental Status	Posture	Movement	Postural Reactions	Cranial Nerves
Cerebral cortex	Abnormal behavior, depression, seizures	Normal	Gait normal to slight hemiparesis (contralateral)	Deficits (contralateral)	Normal (vision may be impaired, contralateral)
Diencephalon (thalamus and hypothalamus)	Abnormal behavior, depression, seizures (endocrine and autonomic)	Normal	Gait normal to slight hemiparesis (contralateral) or tetraparesis	Deficits (contralateral)	II
Brain stem (midbrain, pons, medulla)	Depression, stupor, coma	Normal, turning, falling	Ataxia, hemiparesis, tetraparesis	Deficits (ipsilateral or contralateral)	III–XII
Vestibular central (medulla)	Depression	Head tilt, falling	Ataxia, hemiparesis, tetraparesis	Deficits (ipsilateral or contralateral)	VIII, may also affect V and VII, nystagmus
Vestibular peripheral (labyrinth)	Normal	Head tilt	Normal to ataxia	Normal, although may be awkward	VIII, sometimes VII, Horner's syndrome, nystagmus
Cerebellum	Normal	Normal	Ataxia, tremors, dysmetria	Normal, but dysmetric	Normal, deficit of menace reaction, nystagmus

(Oliver JE, Lorenz MD: Handbook of Veterinary Neurologic Diagnosis. Philadelphia, WB Saunders, 1983)

TABLE 47-6. Characteristics of Major Categories of Disease

Disease	Age	Onset	Course	Distribution
Degenerative	Young	Chronic	Progressive	Diffuse
Storage diseases	Young	Chronic	Progressive	Diffuse
Demyelinating diseases	Young	Chronic	Progressive	Diffuse
Neuronopathies	Young	Chronic	Progressive	Diffuse
Abiotrophies	Variable	Chronic	Progressive	Diffuse
Vertebral and disk diseases	Adult	Chronic	Progressive	Focal
Anomalous	Young	Birth	Nonprogressive	Focal
Brain malformations	Young	Birth	Nonprogressive	Focal
Hydrocephalus	Young	Birth	Progressive	Focal
Vertebral malformations	Young	Birth	Nonprogressive	Focal
Myelodysplasia	Young	Birth	Nonprogressive	Focal
Metabolic CNS signs secondary to other disorder (*e.g.,* liver, endocrine)	Variable	Variable	Variable	Diffuse
Neoplastic	Adult	Chronic	Progressive	Focal
Nutritional	Variable	Chronic	Progressive	Diffuse
Thiamine	Variable	Variable	Progressive	Diffuse
Vitamin A	Variable	Chronic	Progressive	Variable
Idiopathic	Variable	Variable	Variable	Variable
Inflammatory	Variable	Variable	Progressive	Diffuse
Viral	Adult	Chronic	Progressive	Diffuse
Viral	Young	Acute	Progressive	Diffuse
Bacterial	Variable	Acute	Progressive	Diffuse
Rickettsial	Variable	Acute	Progressive	Diffuse
Fungal	Variable	Chronic	Progressive	Diffuse
Protozoal	Variable	Chronic	Progressive	Diffuse
Toxic	Variable	Variable	Progressive	Diffuse
Traumatic	Variable	Acute	Nonprogressive	Focal
Vascular	Adult	Acute	Nonprogressive	Focal

TABLE 47-7. Etiology of Monoparesis

Category	Acute Nonprogressive	Acute Progressive	Chronic Progressive
Degenerative		Disk protrusion	Degenerative lumbosacral stenosis
Neoplastic			Nerve sheath tumor Other neoplasm
Immune Inflammatory		Brachial plexus neuritis Rabies Abscess	
Traumatic	Nerve injury Infraspinatus muscle contracture		
Vascular	Infarction		

TABLE 47-8. Etiology of Pelvic Limb Paresis

Category	Acute Nonprogressive	Acute Progressive	Chronic Progressive
Degenerative		Type I disk protrusion Hemorrhagic myelomalacia	Degenerative myelopathy Type II disk protrusion Myelopathy of Afghans Neuronopathy Demyelinating disease Degenerative lumbosacral stenosis
Anomalous	Myelodysplasia		Spinal dysraphism
Neoplastic		Primary Metastatic Vertebral	Primary Metastatic Vertebral
Nutritional			Hypervitaminosis A (cats)
Inflammatory		Canine distemper Bacterial Protozoal Diskospondylitis	Distemper Feline infectious peritonitis Fungal Granulomatous meningoencephalomyelitis Immune meningomyelitis
Traumatic	Spinal cord injury		
Vascular	Fibrocartilaginous or septic emboli Aortic thromboembolism Hemorrhage		

(Modified from Oliver JE, Lorenz MD: Handbook of Veterinary Neurologic Diagnosis. Philadelphia, WB Saunders, 1983)

TABLE 47-9. Etiology of Tetraparesis (Upper Motor Neuron)

Category	Acute Nonprogressive	Acute Progressive	Chronic Progressive
Degenerative		Type I disk protrusion	Cervical spondylopathy Type II disk protrusion Storage diseases Neuronopathy Demyelinating diseases
Anomalous	Myelodysplasia	Atlantoaxial luxation	Vertebral malformations Spinal dysraphism
Neoplastic			Primary Metastatic Vertebral
Nutritional			Hypervitaminosis A (cats)
Inflammatory		Canine distemper	Distemper Feline infectious peritonitis
		Bacterial, fungal, protozoal	Granulomatous meningoencephalomyelitis Fungal Immune meningomyelitis
Traumatic	Spinal cord injury		
Vascular	Fibrocartilaginous or septic emboli Hemorrhage Vascular malformations		

(Modified from Oliver JE, Lorenz MD: Handbook of Veterinary Neurologic Diagnosis. Philadelphia, WB Saunders, 1983)

TABLE 47-10. Etiology of Tetraparesis (Generalized LMN)

Category	Episodic Progressive	Acute Progressive	Chronic Progressive
Degenerative			Neuronopathies Myopathies Axonopathies
Anomalous		Myotonia	Demyelinating diseases
Metabolic	Polysystemic disorders: Hypoglycemia Hyperkalemia Hypercalcemia Hypocalcemia Hyperthyroidism		Diabetes mellitus Hypothyroidism Hypoadrenocorticism Hyperadrenocorticism Hypokalemia Hyperinsulinism
Nutritional			Thiamine deficiency Hypovitaminosis E
Inflammatory/ immune	Polymyositis Myasthenia gravis	Polyneuritis Polyradiculoneuritis Polymyositis Protozoal myositis and neuritis	Polyneuritis Polymyositis
Toxic		Tick paralysis Botulism Aminoglycosides	Lead Organophosphates Miscellaneous toxins

(Modified from Oliver JE, Lorenz MD: Handbook of Veterinary Neurologic Diagnosis. Philadelphia, WB Saunders, 1983)

TABLE 47-11. Etiology of Cranial Nerve Paresis

Category	Acute Nonprogressive	Acute Progressive	Chronic Progressive
Anomalous		Hydrocephalus (CN III,IV,VI)	Laryngeal paralysis (CN IX,X)
Metabolic			Hypothyroidism (CN V,VII,VIII,IX,X,XII)
Neoplastic			Brain tumors Direct compression (all CN) or secondary to tentorial herniation (CN III)
Idiopathic		Mandibular paralysis (CN V) Facial paralysis (CN VII) Megaesophagus (CN X)	
Inflammatory		Bacterial (retrobulbar CN III,IV,VI; labyrinth CN VII) Rabies (CN IX,X)	Polyneuropathies
Traumatic	Head injury (all CN)		
Vascular	Emboli or hemorrhage in brain stem (all CN)		

CN, cranial nerve

TABLE 47-12. Selection of Diagnostic Tests

		Diagnostic Tests	
Site	Disease Category	Useful	Usually Diagnostic
Brain			
	Degenerative	EEG, CSF	Biopsy
	Anomalous	Examination	Radiography
	Neoplastic	EEG, radiography	CT or MRI scans
Spinal cord			
	Degenerative	Myelography, CSF	None
	Anomalous	Radiography	Myelography
	Neoplastic	CSF, radiography	Myelography
Vertebrae			
	Degenerative	CSF	Radiography, myelography
	Anomalous	Examination	Radiography
	Neoplastic	CSF	Radiography, myelography
	Inflammation	CSF	Radiography, myelography
Peripheral nerve, muscle			
	Demyelinating	EMG, EDT	Biopsy
	Inflammation	EMG, EDT, CK	Biopsy
	Neoplastic	EMG, EDT	Biopsy
	Traumatic	EMG, EDT	Biopsy
	Toxic	EMG, EDT	Biopsy
Systemic or any site			
	Metabolic	History	Clinical laboratory profile
	Nutritional	History	Radiography
	Inflammation	History, examination	CSF, serology
	Traumatic	History, examination	Radiography
	Toxic	History	Clinical laboratory profile

(Oliver JE, Lorenz MD: Handbook of Veterinary Neurologic Diagnosis, 2nd ed. Philadelphia, WB Saunders, 1993)

EEG, electroencephalogram; CSF, cerebrospinal fluid; EMG, electromyogram; EDT, electrodiagnostic tests; CT, computed tomography; MRI, magnetic resonance imaging; CK, creatine kinase

PROGNOSIS

The prognosis depends primarily on the severity and duration of the paresis. Patients with complete LMN lesions usually have a poor prognosis. If the nerve cell in the central nervous system is destroyed it will not be replaced. Peripheral axons regenerate, but with complete lesions of those axons, recovery of normal function is unusual. The prognosis of patients with UMN paralysis is based on other findings. In lesions of the spinal cord between T3 and L3 producing pelvic limb paresis, the presence of sensation caudal to the level of the lesion is most important. If there is no response to a strong pinch of the digits of the pelvic limbs using a hemostat, it is assumed that the deep pain pathways are damaged and the prognosis is grave. If the lack of sensation persists for over 48 hours, there is little hope for functional recovery.

REFERENCES

1. Dorland's Illustrated Medical Dictionary, 27th ed. Philadelphia, WB Saunders, 1988
2. Oliver JE, Lorenz MD: Handbook of Veterinary Neurologic Diagnosis, 2nd ed. Philadelphia, WB Saunders, 1993
3. Oliver JE, Hoerlein BF, Mayhew IG: Veterinary Neurology. Philadelphia, WB Saunders, 1987

CHAPTER FORTY-EIGHT

Ataxia

John E. Oliver

PROBLEM DEFINITION AND RECOGNITION

Ataxia is incoordination of movements without spasticity, paresis, or involuntary movements, although each of these may be seen in association with ataxia. The animal usually has a wide-based stance. Limb movements are incoordinated. Truncal ataxia is swaying of the body.[2]

PATHOPHYSIOLOGY

Ataxia is caused by disorders of the conscious or unconscious proprioceptive systems (sensory ataxia), disorders of the cerebellum, and disorders of the vestibular system.

The proprioceptive systems provide information about the location of the parts of the body. Without this information the movements are poorly coordinated. Receptors for proprioception are located in the skin, joints, tendons, and muscles. The nerve fibers are large and heavily myelinated. The pathways in the spinal cord are primarily in the dorsal and dorsolateral columns, and also consist of large fibers. The pathways terminate in the cerebellum and cerebral cortex. These large-fiber pathways are susceptible to compression, so that compressive lesions of the spinal cord often cause ataxia as the first clinical sign. Paresis commonly follows. Localization is essentially the same as in paresis (see Chapter 47). For example, ataxia of the pelvic limbs with normal thoracic limbs indicates a lesion caudal to T3. Ataxia of all four limbs indicates a lesion cranial to T2 (see Table 47-4).

The cerebellum coordinates motor activity by comparing the intended action with the performance. It receives information from spinal pathways and from the cerebral cortex. The output of the cerebellum is to the brain stem and cortex. There are no direct cerebellar pathways to the spinal cord, and paresis is not seen with cerebellar lesions. Cerebellar ataxia has distinctive manifestations that are usually symmetric. Dysmetria is a disorder of the range of movements. They may be too long (hypermetria) or too short (hypometria). Clinically, hypermetria is easily recognized, since it causes a goose-stepping gait. Tremor, small oscillatory movements of the part, is common in cerebellar disease. Typically it

TABLE 48-1. Localization of Lesion Causing Ataxia

			Vestibular	
Clinical Sign	Sensory	Cerebellar	Central	Peripheral
Asymmetric ataxia	Usually no	No	Yes	Yes
Head tilt	No	No	Yes	Yes
Head tremor	No	Yes	No	No
Intention tremor	No	Yes	No	No
Proprioceptive deficit	Yes	No	Yes	No
Paresis	Often	No	Often	No
Nystagmus	No	Often tremor-like	Yes	Yes
Nystagmus altered in direction with head position	No	No	Yes	No

is an intention tremor, one that becomes worse as the animal starts a movement, and subsides at rest. Cerebellar disease usually causes dysmetria or tremor of the head, which distinguishes it from spinal tract disease (sensory ataxia). Nystagmus in cerebellar disease is usually a fine tremor of the eyes, especially as the animal shifts its gaze. Jerk nystagmus, with a fast and slow component as seen in vestibular disease, may be seen in lesions of the flocculonodular lobes, which are intimately related to the vestibular system. Generalized cerebellar disease frequently causes a deficit in the menace reaction, although vision and the palpebral reflex are normal.[1]

The vestibular system detects the position and movement of the head, providing the nervous system with information necessary to maintain normal posture. Ataxia associated with vestibular disease is usually asymmetric, with falling or rolling to one side. Head tilt and nystagmus are commonly seen in vestibular disease (see Chapter 49). The distinguishing characteristics of these three syndromes are listed in Table 48-1.

DIAGNOSTIC PLAN

The diagnosis of ataxia includes localizing the lesion and finding the cause of the disease.

Ataxia is usually a sign of nervous system disease. Generalized weakness may cause the gait to appear ataxic. Abnormal postural reactions indicate disease of

TABLE 48-2. Characteristics of Major Categories of Cerebellar Disease

Disease	Age	Onset	Course	Distribution
Degenerative	Young	Chronic	Progressive	Diffuse
Storage diseases	Young	Chronic	Progressive	Diffuse
Demyelinating diseases	Young	Chronic	Progressive	Diffuse
Neuronopathies	Young	Chronic	Progressive	Diffuse
Abiotrophies	Variable	Chronic	Progressive	Diffuse
Anomalous	Young	Birth	Nonprogressive	Focal
Cerebellar malformations	Young	Birth	Nonprogressive	Focal or diffuse
Metabolic CNS signs secondary to other disorder (*e.g.*, liver, endocrine)	Variable	Variable	Variable	Diffuse
Neoplastic	Adult	Chronic	Progressive	Focal
Nutritional	Variable	Chronic	Progressive	Diffuse
Thiamine	Variable	Variable	Progressive	Diffuse
Idiopathic	Variable	Variable	Variable	Variable
Idiopathic cerebellitis	Variable	Acute	Variable	Variable
Inflammatory	Variable	Variable	Progressive	Diffuse
Viral	Young	Acute	Progressive	Diffuse
	Adult	Chronic	Progressive	Diffuse
Bacterial	Variable	Acute	Progressive	Diffuse
Rickettsial	Variable	Acute	Progressive	Diffuse
Fungal	Variable	Chronic	Progressive	Diffuse
Protozoal	Variable	Chronic	Progressive	Diffuse
Toxic	Variable	Chronic	Progressive	Diffuse
Traumatic	Variable	Acute	Nonprogressive	Focal
Vascular	Adult	Acute	Nonprogressive	Focal

the nervous system. Sensory ataxia is characterized by deficits in postural reactions, especially in proprioceptive positioning. Determining the location of the lesion for proprioceptive deficits is similar to doing so for motor deficits (see Chapter 47; see also Table 47-4, substituting ataxia for paresis). Cerebellar disorders are characterized by dysmetria and intention tremor. Involvement of the head should be present if the cerebellum is involved. This is most obvious when the animal eats or drinks, as the head overshoots or undershoots the container. If paresis is present with cerebellar signs, motor pathways of the brain stem or spinal cord are involved in the disease. The signs of vestibular disease, head tilt, nystagmus, altered eye movements, and asymmetric ataxia are easily recognized. Vestibular disease is discussed in Chapter 49.

The general category of the etiologic diagnosis is suggested by the history. The onset, course, and location of the problem should indicate no more than three to five major categories; for example, acute, nonprogressive disorders are

TABLE 48-3. Etiology of Cerebellar Disease

Category	Acute Nonprogressive	Acute Progressive	Chronic Progressive
Degenerative	Cerebellar hypo-plasia (feline panleukopenia)		Storage diseases Spongiform degenerations Abiotrophies Neuroaxonal dystrophy Demyelinating disease
Anomalous	Malformation Dysmyelinogenesis		
Neoplastic			Primary Medulloblastoma Choroid plexus papilloma Glioma Meningioma
Nutritional		Thiamine deficiency	
Inflammatory	Idiopathic cerebellitis	Canine distemper Granulomatous meningoencephalitis Bacterial, fungal, protozoal	Distemper Feline infectious peritonitis Fungal Granulomatous meningoencephalomyelitis
Toxic		Heavy metals (lead) Organophosphate Hexachlorophene	Heavy metals (lead) Organophosphate Hexachlorophene
Traumatic	Occipital trauma		Brain herniations
Vascular	Infarction or septic emboli Hemorrhage		

(Modified from Oliver JE, Lorenz MD: Handbook of Veterinary Neurologic Diagnosis, 2nd ed. Philadelphia, WB Saunders, 1993)

almost always traumatic or vascular in origin. Chronic, progressive diseases are usually neoplastic, degenerative, or inflammatory, although some toxic, metabolic, or nutritional diseases may present in a similar manner. Characteristics of the major categories of disease are outlined in Table 48-2. The diagnosis is confirmed by appropriate laboratory, electrophysiologic, or radiographic studies. Tables 47-8 and 47-9 summarize the diseases causing sensory ataxia. Table 48-3 outlines the most important cerebellar diseases according to this scheme. Tables

49-1 and 49-2 list the diseases of the vestibular system. Table 47-12 lists the most useful tests for each category of disease.

PROGNOSIS

The prognosis depends on the cause, location, and severity of the disease. Sensory ataxia is similar to paresis, except that the lesion is often less severe and has a better prognosis (see Chapter 47). Cerebellar problems are often caused by untreatable diseases and have a poor prognosis. Exceptions include idiopathic cerebellitis and some toxicities. Patients with peripheral vestibular disease often have a good prognosis, while those with central disease usually do not (see Chapter 49).

REFERENCES

1. Holliday TA: Clinical signs of acute and chronic experimental lesions of the cerebellum. Vet Sci Comm 3:259, 1979/1980
2. Oliver JE, Lorenz MD: Handbook of Veterinary Neurologic Diagnosis, 2nd ed. Philadelphia, WB Saunders, in press

CHAPTER FORTY-NINE

Head Tilt

John E. Oliver

PROBLEM DEFINITION AND RECOGNITION

Head tilt is a postural abnormality, usually caused by an abnormality of the vestibular system. The head is twisted to one side on its long axis so that one ear is lower than the other; this is called a "roll." It must be distinguished from turning of the head and neck, with the head still parallel to the ground, a "yaw," which is usually caused by spasms of the cervical muscles or by brain stem disease. Animals with head tilt frequently have asymmetric ataxia and nystagmus.[4] Animals with acute otitis externa may tilt the head toward the affected side. There are no signs of neurologic disease.

PATHOPHYSIOLOGY

Head tilt is caused by an imbalance of tone in the cervical muscles, which are controlled in part by the vestibular system. The vestibular system includes the receptors in the inner ear, which detect changes in position of the head with respect to gravity and acceleration of the head, the vestibular nerve (cranial nerve VIII), the vestibular nuclei in the brain stem, the flocculonodular lobes of the cerebellum, and ascending and descending pathways. The vestibular system provides information that allows the animal to maintain a normal posture. Part of this is accomplished by the vestibulospinal tract, which provides tonic stimulation of the extensor motor neurons of the ipsilateral limbs. The vestibular system also controls some types of eye movements through connections in the medial longitudinal fasciculus to the nuclei of cranial nerves III, IV, and VI. This is the anatomic basis for physiologic nystagmus, the fast and slow movements of the eyes when the head is turned from side to side.[2]

Lesions of any part of the vestibular system produce one or more of the following signs: head tilt, usually to the side of the lesion; ataxia, which is usually asymmetric; falling or rolling to the side of the lesion; and nystagmus. It is important to differentiate central vestibular disease, which involves the brain stem, from peripheral disease involving only the receptors in the inner ear. Peripheral lesions disrupt normal posture through an imbalance of input to the nervous system. Central lesions may produce the same effect, but, in addition, usually damage some of the sensory (spinocerebellar tracts, medial lemniscus) or motor (reticulospinal, corticospinal, rubrospinal) pathways, causing ipsilateral proprioceptive deficits or paresis (see Chapters 47 and 48).[4]

DIAGNOSTIC PLAN

Anatomic Diagnosis

The signs of vestibular disease, head tilt, asymmetric ataxia, falling to one side, and nystagmus, are easily recognized. Differentiation of central lesions from peripheral lesions is essential for management. The most useful distinction is the presence of *postural reaction deficits* in central disease. Animals with acute vestibular syndromes may be difficult to test because of their severe disorientation. However, careful testing of the proprioceptive positioning reaction while the animal is supported usually produces normal responses in peripheral disease and abnormal responses in central disease. The character of the nystagmus may also be different. Nystagmus in peripheral disease is horizontal, with the fast phase away from the side of the lesion, or rotatory. It does not change direction when the head is held in a different position, although the severity of the nystagmus may change. Nystagmus in central disease may be in any direction and frequently changes direction when the head is held in a different position.

Other cranial nerves may be affected in vestibular disease. The facial nerve (cranial nerve VII) may be involved in both central and peripheral lesions. A Horner's syndrome (miosis, ptosis, and enophthalmos with prolapse of the third eyelid) is common with peripheral disease, because the sympathetic nerves pass through the middle ear; it is rare in central disease. Involvement of any other cranial nerves (*e.g.*, cranial nerves V, VI, IX, X) usually signifies central disease, unless there is a polyneuropathy. Normal physiologic nystagmus is produced when the animal's head is turned from side to side. This is a useful test of vestibular function as well as a test of cranial nerves III, IV, and VI and the connecting pathway in the brain stem. Either central or peripheral vestibular disease may produce a ventral strabismus of the eye on the affected side when the head is elevated.[2] Table 48-1 summarizes the signs of vestibular disease and compares these to cerebellar and proprioceptive ataxias.

Two less common vestibular syndromes are bilateral vestibular disease and "paradoxic" vestibular disease. Bilateral disease is characterized by a more symmetric ataxia, with swaying movements of the head. There is no nystagmus, including physiologic nystagmus. Paradoxic vestibular disease is caused by a lesion in the brain stem near the cerebellar peduncles.[3] It is paradoxic in that some of the signs indicate left-sided disease, while others indicate right-sided disease. If other cranial nerve deficits are present they indicate the side on which the lesion occurs.

TABLE 49-1. Etiology of Peripheral Vestibular Disease

Category	Acute Nonprogressive	Acute Progressive	Chronic Progressive
Anomalous	Congenital vestibular defects		
Metabolic			Hypothyroidism
Neoplastic			Neurofibroma or involving labyrinth
Idiopathic	Geriatric—dogs Feline		
Inflammatory	Otitis interna	Otitis media-interna	Otitis media-interna
Toxic		Drugs—aminoglycosides, metronidazole	Drugs—aminoglycosides, metronidazole
Traumatic	Labyrinth injury		
Vascular	Undocumented cause		

Etiologic Diagnosis

Most peripheral vestibular syndromes are caused by inflammation or are idiopathic. Idiopathic vestibular disease is diagnosed by exclusion of other causes. An increased incidence of peripheral vestibular disease, with or without facial paralysis, related to hypothyroidism has been recognized recently. Rarely, neoplasia, drug toxicity, trauma, or congenital anomaly is the cause (Table 49-1).[1,2,4]

Central vestibular syndromes may be caused by a variety of diseases. The history provides information on the rate of onset, course, previous illness, age, and previous medication. A few general categories of disease can be defined from this information (Table 49-2). Confirmation of the diagnosis requires additional tests. Infection of the middle and inner ear can spread to the brain stem via the vestibular nerve. Therefore, it is important to exclude peripheral infection, even if there are signs of central disease. A diagnostic plan is outlined in Table 49-3.

PROGNOSIS

Peripheral vestibular disease usually has a more favorable prognosis than central disease. Labyrinthitis can usually be treated effectively, although there may be a residual deficit. Most animals with idiopathic disease recover fully in several weeks, with or without treatment. Hypothyroidism can be corrected, and recovery of vestibular function usually occurs in 3 to 6 months. Degeneration of the receptors from toxicity is usually irreversible, but function improves through compensation.

TABLE 49-2. Etiology of Central Vestibular Disease

Category	Acute Nonprogressive	Acute Progressive	Chronic Progressive
Anomalous			Hydrocephalus
Metabolic			Hypothyroidism
Neoplastic			Neurofibroma or tumors of brain stem
Nutritional		Thiamine deficiency	
Idiopathic	Polyneuropathy		
Inflammatory		Viral, bacterial, rickettsial, fungal, protozoal Granulomatous meningoencephalitis Parasite migration	Viral, bacterial, rickettsial, fungal, protozoal Granulomatous meningoencephalitis Parasite migration
Traumatic	Brain stem		
Vascular	Infarction of brain stem		

TABLE 49-3. Plan for Management: Vestibular Signs

Signalment, history, physical and neurologic examinations
Signs of vestibular disease: ataxia, head tilt, nystagmus, positional strabismus
Otoscopic examination, radiographs of skull, including bulla ossea. If available, CT or MRI, tympanometry, auditory evoked-potential recording (helps localize central versus peripheral)

Signs of Peripheral Disease Only		Signs of Central Disease	
No postural reaction deficits, nystagmus in only one direction		Postural reaction deficits, nystagmus changes direction, abnormality of CN V, IX, X	
Otoscopic examination, myringotomy, radiographs		CSF, CT, MRI, EEG if available	
Positive:	Negative:	Positive:	Negative:
Otitis media-interna	History of ototoxic drugs: Discontinue drugs	Otoscopic (see Otitis media-interna)	Treat for inflammation and observe for changes
Treatment: Myringotomy with topical and systemic antibiotics	No history of drugs Idiopathic Otitis interna	Radiographs, CT, MRI Otitis media Neoplasia Trauma Hydrocephalus	
	Hypothyroidism Neuritis (CN VIII) Congenital		
		CSF Inflammatory Neoplasia	

CT, computed tomography; CSF, cerebrospinal fluid; CN, cranial nerves; EEG, electroencephalogram; MRI, magnetic resonance imaging

Many central diseases are progressive disorders that are unresponsive to treatment. Bacterial infections can be treated effectively if treatment is started early and appropriate antibiotics are used. Some central syndromes with an acute, nonprogressive history recover with little deficit. It is not known whether these are vascular lesions or lesions caused by some other mechanism. The key finding is the lack of progression of the signs.

REFERENCES

1. Chrisman CL: Problems in Small Animal Neurology, 2nd ed. Philadelphia, Lea & Febiger, 1991
2. de Lahunta A: Veterinary Neuroanatomy and Clinical Neurology, 2nd ed. Philadelphia, WB Saunders, 1983
3. Holliday TA: Clinical signs of acute and chronic experimental lesions of the cerebellum. Vet Sci Comm 3:259, 1979/1980
4. Oliver JE, Lorenz MD: Handbook of Veterinary Neurologic Diagnosis, 2nd ed. Philadelphia, WB Saunders, 1993

CHAPTER FIFTY

Collapse
(Seizures and Syncope)

John E. Oliver

PROBLEM DEFINITION AND RECOGNITION

There are three major types of sudden collapse: seizures, syncope, and narcolepsy-cataplexy. All are characterized by a sudden onset and usually by loss of consciousness. All are clinical syndromes with more than one cause.

Seizure, fit, and *ictus* are terms describing the stereotyped alterations in behavior resulting from paroxysmal abnormal brain function.[12] *Convulsion* usually refers to a seizure with generalized tonic-clonic muscle activity.[8] One or more of the following behavioral changes are present in a seizure: (1) loss or derangement of consciousness, (2) alteration of muscle tone or movement, (3) alteration of sensation, (4) disturbance of autonomic function, and (5) other psychic manifestations.[9] Epilepsy is a brain disorder characterized by recurring seizures.

Syncope is a sudden loss of consciousness caused by inadequate oxygen or glucose concentrations in the brain.[4] The episodes are usually brief, but they may recur. Severe oxygen or glucose deprivation can also cause convulsions.

Narcolepsy-cataplexy is a syndrome that includes excessive sleep (narcolepsy) and sudden loss of muscle tone (cataplexy).[1] Cataplexy is a prominent sign in affected animals. The animal suddenly drops to the ground and lies immobile for varying periods of time unless disturbed. Touching or calling the animal usually results in an immediate return to normal behavior.

PATHOPHYSIOLOGY

Seizures

The basic cellular event in seizures is paroxysmal discharge of a group of neurons, called the *seizure focus.* The focus may be single or multiple in any individual. Some neurons are capable of a large depolarization of the membrane (20 to 50 mV) that lasts 50 to 100 msec. The large depolarization may lead to multiple action potentials in a short time. This depolarization is called the paroxysmal depolarizing shift (PDS). Following the PDS the membrane usually has a prolonged afterhyperpolarization (AHP). The AHP tends to stabilize the population, preventing further discharge for a period. Some neurons have a prolonged afterdepolarization (ADP), which may lead to ictal behavior. Apparently, both synaptic and ionic changes contribute to these events. Alterations in inhibitory neurotransmitters such as gamma aminobutyric acid (GABA), may be a factor in the seizure mechanism as well.[3,7,15]

Spread of seizure activity from a focus is necessary for a seizure to occur. The activity can spread both locally to adjacent neurons and to other areas by axonal propagation. Eventually other seizure foci will develop. The reticular activating system (RAS) has a role in the genesis of seizures, although the exact mechanism is not clear. Many seizures occur during sleep when the RAS is least active. Experimentally, decreasing the output of the RAS increases seizure activity.[14]

Termination of seizure activity is primarily a function of the AHP and inhibitory feedback circuits from the cerebellum, thalamus, caudate nuclei and possibly other areas of the brain. The concept of "metabolic exhaustion" of the neurons is probably not valid.

Susceptibility to seizure activity varies among populations of neurons and among individuals. For example, the neurons of the hippocampus easily develop ictal activity, and the thresholds for seizures vary among individuals within a species. A genetic predisposition for seizures may be simply a low threshold. The threshold may also be lowered by a variety of internal and external factors, such as sleep and increased estrogen levels. Alterations in energy substrates, electrolytes, and many endogenous and exogenous toxins may precipitate seizures.

The occurrence of seizures increases the probability of additional seizures. The synaptic changes have been compared to "learning mechanisms" responsible for memory. There is also a pathologic change in neurons after seizures, primarily in the structure of the dendrites. These changes range from minor distortions, to the virtual absence of processes in the neuron, to the eventual death of the neuron. Prevention of these changes is a major consideration in the decision of whether to treat an animal with seizures.[14]

Seizures may be classified according to a modification of the international classification of human epilepsy (Table 50-1).[6] Differentiating partial seizures from generalized ones is important because partial seizures are caused by a focal brain lesion; therefore, they are acquired, not idiopathic. Generalized seizures involve the entire body at once. Partial seizures, also called focal seizures, have focal signs. Partial seizures may generalize secondarily; consequently, the seizure must be seen from the onset to ascertain the presence of a focal component. Idiopathic seizures are generalized, but not all generalized seizures are idiopathic. Idiopathic seizures may be inherited. Table 50-2 lists the breeds that have been studied by controlled breeding programs and those reported as frequently having idiopathic seizures.

Table 50-3 lists the major causes of seizure disorders in small animals.

TABLE 50-1. Classification of Seizures

Clinical Manifestation	Comments
Generalized seizures	Most common type
Tonic-clonic (grand mal, major motor)	May be caused by organic brain disease, toxins, or metabolic disorders
	Idiopathic form may be genetic
Absences with or without motor phenomenon (petit mal)	Rare in animals
Partial seizures	Focal signs during seizure may generalize to tonic-clonic seizure
Partial motor (focal motor)	Indicates an acquired brain lesion
Psychomotor	Complex behavioral activity that is stereotyped and similar each time
	Believed to be lesion of limbic system

Syncope

Transient loss of consciousness is caused by a temporary deprivation of oxygen or glucose supplies to the brain. It is usually of short duration but can lead to sudden death. Syncope is the result of (1) impaired cerebral circulation, (2) a transient decrease in cardiac output, (3) decreased systolic blood pressure, or (4) inadequate delivery of energy substrates to the brain.[2,4] The causes of syn-

TABLE 50-2. Breed Susceptibility to Collapse

Seizures	Narcolepsy	Syncope
Inherited	Inherited	Inherited
Beagle	Doberman	Pugs
Dachshund	pinscher	
German shepherd (Alsatian)	Labrador	
Horak's laboratory dogs		
Keeshond		
Tervuren shepherd (Belgian)		
High incidence	Reported cases	High incidence
Cocker spaniel	Afghan hound	Boxer
Collie	Airedale	Doberman pinscher
Golden retriever	Corgi	Miniature schnauzer
Irish setter	Dachshund	
Labrador retriever	Irish setter	
Miniature schnauzer	Malamute	
Poodle	Poodle	
St. Bernard	Springer spaniel	
Siberian husky	Wire-haired griffon	
Wire-haired fox terrier	Mixed breed	

TABLE 50-3. Causes of Seizures

Category	Diseases
Degenerative	Storage diseases
Anomalous	Hydrocephalus Lissencephaly
Metabolic	Hypoglycemia Hypocalcemia Renal failure Hepatic failure Hypothyroid (?)
Neoplastic	Brain tumors (primary and metastatic)
Nutritional	Thiamine Parasitism (multiple factors)
Idiopathic	Unknown Genetic
Inflammatory	Viral: canine distemper, rabies, feline infectious peritonitis Bacterial: any Mycotic: any Protozoon: toxoplasmosis, neosporosis, granulomatous meningoencephalitis, immune meningoencephalitis
Toxic	Heavy metals: lead Organophosphates Organochlorines Strychnine Tetanus Many others
Traumatic	Acute head injury Post-traumatic: weeks to months after injury
Vascular	Infarctions Arrhythmias

cope are summarized in Table 50-4. The various causes of syncope are discussed in detail in the chapters listed in Table 50-4.

Narcolepsy-Cataplexy

Narcolepsy is a disorder of the sleep mechanism of the brain. The primary complaint in humans, excessive daytime sleepiness, is not usually recognized in animals. However, it has been documented in laboratory studies.[5] Cataplexy is readily recognized in affected animals. The animal has a sudden loss of muscle tone, causing complete collapse. Usually consciousness is maintained and the animal is easily aroused by touch or noise.

TABLE 50-4.   Causes of Syncope

General Cause	Pathophysiology	Disease or Problem
Decreased cerebral circulation	Vascular obstruction or insufficiency	Thrombus, embolus, atherosclerosis, neoplasia, trauma

Decreased cardiac output	Abnormal heart rate or rhythm (see Chapter 21)
	Obstruction (see Chapters 21 and 22)
		Dysrhythmias
		  Impulse conduction
		  Impulse formation
		Congenital heart diseases
		Acquired heart diseases

Decreased blood pressure	Decreased blood volume (see Chapter 23) Increased vascular resistance (see Chapter 23)	Blood loss Postural, drugs, hyperventilation, carotid sinus
Metabolic	Decreased oxygen (see Chapters 23, 24, 26, 60, and 63) Decreased glucose (see Chapter 61)	Cardiopulmonary dysfunction, abnormal hemoglobin, anemia Insulin-secreting tumors, insulin overdose, glycogen storage disease, inadequate nutrition (mostly toy breeds, young animals)

The physiology of sleep is poorly understood, so it is not surprising that the pathophysiology of sleep disorders is still largely unknown. Normal sleep has two distinct stages, rapid-eye-movement (REM) sleep, and non–rapid-eye-movement sleep (NREM). REM sleep is characterized by atonic muscles, occasional fasciculation of distal and facial muscles, and rapid eye movements. The EEG is of low voltage with mixed frequency. NREM sleep has two components. Light slow-wave sleep is characterized on the EEG by higher-voltage slow waves, with at least one 10- to 14-Hz spindle per 30 seconds. Deep slow-wave sleep has even higher-voltage slow waves (less than 4 Hz) with spindles. REM sleep normally occurs after about 90 minutes of NREM sleep and recurs intermittently thereafter. It accounts for 11% to 13% of the sleep cycle.[1,16]

Narcoleptic dogs have significantly less REM sleep than normal dogs, but they have episodes of cataplexy that has some of the features of REM sleep. There are other changes in the pattern of sleep, suggesting that narcoleptic dogs have a disruption of the sleep-wake cycle, rather than hypersomnia.[1]

Most cases of narcolepsy are idiopathic. Inheritance has been established in Doberman pinschers and Labrador retrievers.[5] A variety of breeds of other dogs, horses, and ponies have been recognized to have narcolepsy (Table 50-2).

Data Base for Collapse

Minimum Data Base: One or More Episodes

Patient profile
  Species, breed, age, sex
History
  Environment
  Immunizations: kind, dates, by whom
  Previous or present illness or injury
  Description of collapse
    Age of onset
    Frequency, course
    General or partial; duration; aura; postictus; time of day; relation to
      exercise, food, sleep, or stimuli
  Behavioral changes
Physical examination
  Special attention to cardiovascular and nervous systems
  Funduscopic examination
Neurologic examination
  If collapse was within 24 to 48 hours and neurologic examination is
    abnormal, repeat in 24 hours.
Laboratory tests
  Complete blood count
  Urine analysis
  Chemistries (at least)
    Blood urea nitrogen
    ALT (serum glutamic-pyruvic transaminase)
    Aklaline phosphatase
    Calcium
    Fasting blood glucose
Others
  Electrocardiogram
  Blood lead

Complete Data Base

Seizures not controlled, evidence of central nervous system disease, or animal
    with first seizures at over 5 years of age
  Brain scan: computed tomography, magnetic resonance imaging
  Cerebrospinal fluid analysis: cell count, total and differential; protein levels
  EEG
  Skull radiographs

Modified from Oliver JE, Lorenz MD: Handbook of Veterinary Neurology, 2nd ed. Philadelphia, WB Saunders, 1993

DIAGNOSTIC PLAN

A data base for animals with collapse (see Display, Data Base for Collapse) should be adequate to differentiate syncope and narcolepsy from seizures.[13] The plan is based on the assumption that seizures are caused by three major categories of disease: (1) extracranial abnormalities, such as metabolic and toxic disorders; (2) intracranial disease, such as encephalitis, brain tumors, or trauma; and (3) idiopathic or primary generalized epilepsy.[10-12] The causes of syncope are extracranial: cardiovascular, pulmonary, or metabolic (hypoglycemia). Narcolepsy is considered idiopathic, although it may occur subsequent to a primary brain disorder.

The minimum data base should identify most extracranial causes of collapse. Some findings may be suggestive, requiring other specific tests in order to make a definitive diagnosis. Abnormal findings on the neurologic examination may necessitate the tests listed under "Complete data base" in the display. Brain tumor should be considered as a likely diagnosis in animals 5 years of age or older when seizures begin. Therefore, computed tomography or magnetic resonance imaging should be done before a cerebrospinal fluid tap is performed.

REFERENCES

1. Baker TL, Mitler MM, Foutz AS, Dement WC: Diagnosis and treatment of narcolepsy in animals. In Kirk RW (ed): Current Veterinary Therapy VIII: Small Animal Practice. Philadelphia, WB Saunders, 1983
2. Beckett SD, Branch CE, Robertson BT: Syncopal attacks and sudden death in dogs: Mechanisms and etiologies. J Am Anim Hosp Assoc 14:378–386, 1978
3. Bleck TP, Klawans HL: Convulsive disorders: Mechanisms of epilepsy and anticonvulsant action. Clin Neuropharmacol 13:121–128, 1990
4. Ettinger SJ: Weakness and syncope. In Ettinger SJ (ed): Textbook of Veterinary Internal Medicine. Philadelphia, WB Saunders, 1983
5. Foutz AS, Mitler MM, Dement WC: Narcolepsy. Vet Clin North Am 10:65–80, 1980
6. Gastaut H: Clinical and electroencephalographic classification of epileptic seizures. Epilepsia 10 (suppl): 512–513, 1969
7. Gloor P, Fariello RG: Generalized epilepsy: Some of its cellular mechanisms differ from those of focal epilepsy. Trends Neurosci 11:63–68, 1988
8. Holliday TA: Seizure disorders. Vet Clin North Am 10:3–29, 1980
9. Lennox WG: Epilepsy and Related Disorders. Boston, Little, Brown & Co, 1960
10. Oliver JE Jr: Protocol for the diagnosis of seizure disorders in companion animals. J Am Vet Med Assoc 172:822–824, 1978
11. Oliver JE Jr: Seizure disorders in companion animals. Comp Cont Ed Pract Vet 2:77–85, 1980
12. Oliver JE Jr, Lorenz M: Handbook of Veterinary Neurologic Diagnosis. Philadelphia, WB Saunders, 1983
13. Oliver JE Jr: Seizure disorders and narcolepsy. In Oliver JE, Hoerlein BF, Mayhew IG (eds): Veterinary Neurology, pp 285–302. Philadelphia, WB Saunders, 1987

14. Pedley TA, Traub RD: Physiology of epilepsy. In Swash M, Kennard C (eds): Scientific Basis of Clinical Neurology. Edinburgh, Churchill Livingstone, 1985
15. Russo ME: The pathophysiology of epilepsy. Cornell Vet 71:221–247, 1981
16. Wauquier A, Verheyen JL, Van Den Broeck WAE, Janssen PAJ: Visual and computer-based analysis of 24 H sleep-waking patterns in the dog. EEG Clin Neurophysiol 46:33–48, 1979

CHAPTER FIFTY-ONE

Coma

John E. Oliver

PROBLEM DEFINITION AND RECOGNITION

Altered states of consciousness vary, from depression to coma. The following definitions are used in this chapter:

Depression—The animal is lethargic and less responsive to its environment but still has the capability to respond in a normal manner.

Disorientation, confusion—Responses are inappropriate.

Stupor—The animal is asleep when undisturbed but can be aroused with strong stimulation.

Coma—The animal is unconscious and does not respond to any stimulus except by reflex activity.

Vegetative state—The animal lacks awareness of environment, although arousal is present.[1]

Depression has many causes, including systemic illness. Confusion, stupor, coma, and the vegetative state are always signs of abnormal brain function.[3]

PATHOPHYSIOLOGY

Consciousness is maintained by sensory stimuli acting through the reticular activating system (RAS). The reticular formation of the rostral brain stem receives input from most of the sensory systems of the body, including somatosensory (*e.g.*, touch, temperature, pain), visual, auditory, and olfactory pathways. Pathways from the reticular formation project diffusely to the cerebral cortex by way of the intralaminar nuclei of the thalamus, maintaining a background of activity mediated through cholinergic synapses on cortical neurons. A second pathway projects to the hypothalamus and basal forebrain.[4] Activity in the RAS is balanced by an adrenergic system from brain stem and diencephalic nuclei, which influence sleep (see Chapter 50). Any disorder that alters the activity of the RAS or interferes with its connections to the cortex can cause a change in the level of consciousness.

Coma is usually the result of one of four major categories of abnormality: (1) diffuse, bilateral cerebral diseases, (2) metabolic or toxic encephalopathies,

(3) compression of the midbrain or pons, or (4) destructive lesions of the midbrain or pons.[3]

Diffuse, bilateral cerebral hemisphere disease usually causes signs of depression or stupor, and only rarely coma. The vegetative state is seen in animals with severe cerebral disease. The animal will arouse, vocalize, and have brain stem reflex activity, including paddling movements of the limbs. However, there are no purposeful actions indicating cortical function. This state is most common after severe hypoxic episodes or cortical trauma. Metabolic disease, such as hepatic failure, may cause stupor or coma with preservation of brain stem function.

Lesions of the brain stem in the region of the midbrain or pons frequently cause coma. Head trauma often causes hemorrhage in this area. Typically, the animal is unconscious from the time of the injury and never regains consciousness. Other signs of brain stem dysfunction are present, including abnormal pupillary light reflexes, abnormal eye movements, other cranial nerve deficits, and postural abnormality. Brain stem function can also be compromised by compression, either directly from mass lesions or secondarily by tentorial herniation of the cerebrum. The brain is enclosed in an inelastic case, the skull. Any increase in volume in the skull must displace part of the contents. Increased pressure causes displacement of the cerebral hemisphere under the tentorium cerebelli, resulting in compression of the brain stem. Unilateral masses produce a herniation on the same side, whereas generalized pressure increases, such as in hydrocephalus or cerebral edema, cause a central or bilateral herniation.[2]

DIAGNOSTIC PLAN

Anatomic Diagnosis

Coma always indicates severe brain dysfunction. Structural damage to the brain stem is a grave prognostic sign, so the neurologic examination should be directed toward evaluating brain stem function. Motor function, pupil function, and eye movements are important parameters to assess. Table 51-1 outlines the findings in the most common syndromes. See Chapters 52 through 54 for details on assessing the pupils and eye movements.

Diffuse cerebral disease with a normal brain stem rarely causes coma. When it does, the animal is blind, but the pupils are either normal or constricted. Vestibular eye movements may be present. Extensor hypertonus is not present, as it is frequently in brain stem disease. Walking or paddling movements are often present. When this syndrome persists, it is called the vegetative state, and is seen most often after severe hypoxia, although it may occur with other metabolic problems such as prolonged hypoglycemia. Signs of diffuse cerebral disease are likely to be symmetric.

Metabolic or toxic encephalopathies may cause coma that is similar to the diffuse cerebral syndrome. However, many agents, such as barbiturates, also

TABLE 51-1. Clinical Signs in Coma

Location of Lesion	Motor Function	Pupillary Light Reflex	Eye Movements
Diffuse cerebral disease	Tetraparesis; may have locomotor movements, but postural reactions are abnormal	Normal	Normal, but no visual following
Metabolic or toxic encephalopathy	Tetraparesis; reflexes may be depressed	Normal or abnormal, depending on the cause	Normal or abnormal, depending on the cause
Bilateral tentorial herniation	Tetraparesis, increased extensor tone (decerebrate rigidity)	Dilated or midposition, unresponsive	Bilateral ventrolateral strabismus, poor to absent vestibular eye movements
Unilateral tentorial herniation	Hemiparesis or tetraparesis, increased extensor tone on affected side	Dilated ipsilateral	Ipsilateral ventrolateral strabismus, poor vestibular eye movements
Brain stem hemorrhage	Tetraparesis, increased extensor tone (decerebrate rigidity)	Midposition bilateral	No vestibular eye movements; may have bilateral ventrolateral strabismus

459

TABLE 51-2. Etiology of Coma

	Acute Nonprogressive	Acute Progressive	Chronic Progressive
Focal or lateralizing signs			
Neoplastic		Metastatic	Primary
Traumatic	Parenchymal hemorrhage	Epidural, subdural hemorrhage	Subdural hematoma (rare)
Vascular	Infarction, hemorrhage		
No focal or lateralizing signs, but evidence of meningeal irritation			
Inflammatory		Meningoencephalitis	
Traumatic	Subarachnoid hemorrhage		
No focal, lateralizing, or meningeal signs			
Degenerative			Storage diseases
Anomalous	Brain malformations		Hydrocephalus
Metabolic		Hypoglycemia, hepatic encephalopathy, heat stroke, hypoxia, diabetes, hypothyroid, uremic encephalopathy	
Nutritional		Thiamine deficiency	
Inflammatory		Encephalitis	Encephalitis
Toxic		Heavy metals (lead), barbiturates, narcotics, carbon monoxide	Heavy metals
Traumatic		Cerebral edema	

(Modified from Oliver JE, Lorenz MD: Handbook of Veterinary Neurologic Diagnosis, 2nd ed. Philadelphia, WB Saunders, 1993) affect the function of the brain stem, even though there is no structural damage. The animal has no voluntary activity and reflex activity is depressed (in contrast to most of the other syndromes, in which spinal reflexes are present). Signs are usually symmetric. An adequate history is critical for ascertaining the cause in these cases.

Brain stem lesions may be from compression or direct injury. The onset and course of the syndrome provide the key to differentiating the two. Most brain stem hemorrhages or contusions are the result of trauma; primary vascular disease is a relatively rare cause. The animal is usually comatose from the time of the injury, and the condition does not change. Herniations secondary to

TABLE 51-3.   Small animal coma scale.*

Coma Scale	
Motor activity	
Normal gait, normal spinal reflexes	6
Hemiparesis, tetraparesis, or decerebrate activity	5
Recumbent, intermittent extensor rigidity	4
Recumbent, constant extensor rigidity	3
Recumbent, constant extensor rigidity with opisthotonus	2
Recumbent, hypotonia of muscles, depressed or absent spinal reflexes	1
Brain stem reflexes	
Normal pupillary light reflexes and oculocephalic reflexes	6
Slow pupillary light reflexes and normal to reduced oculocephalic reflexes	5
Bilateral unresponsive miosis with normal to reduced oculocephalic reflexes	4
Pinpoint pupils with reduced to absent oculocephalic reflexes	3
Unilateral, unresponsive mydriasis with reduced to absent oculocephalic reflexes	2
Bilateral, unresponsive mydriasis with reduced to absent oculocephalic reflexes	1
Level of consciousness	
Occasional periods of alertness, and responsive to environment	6
Depression or delirium; capable of responding to environment, but response may be inappropriate	5
Stupor, responsive to visual stimuli	4
Stupor, responsive to auditory stimuli	3
Stupor, responsive only to repeated noxious stimuli	2
Coma, unresponsive to repeated noxious stimuli	1
Assessment	
Good prognosis	15–18
Guarded prognosis	9–14
Grave prognosis	3–8

(Modified from Shores A: Craniocerebral trauma. In Kirk RW: Current Veterinary Therapy X. Philadelphia, WB Saunders, 1989)

*Neurologic function is assessed for each of the three categories and a grade of 1 to 6 is assigned according to the descriptions for each grade. The total score is the sum of the three category scores.

increased pressure develop more slowly. They may be sudden in onset, but their signs show a definite progression. An early warning sign of tentorial herniation is one dilated pupil. The oculomotor nerve is vulnerable to compression by the herniating cerebrum as it crosses the petrosal bone. Tentorial herniation is likely to produce asymmetric signs, whereas brain stem hemorrhage is more likely to be symmetric.

Etiologic Diagnosis

The history and neurologic examination provide information to establish a small number of probable causes of coma. The onset and course of the syndrome are obtained from the history. Focal or diffuse signs are assessed from the neurologic examination. Signs of meningeal irritation, including hyperesthesia on deep palpation of the vertebral column, are also significant. Table 51-2 categorizes the most common causes of coma using these findings.

PROGNOSIS

The prognosis depends on the cause and the extent of brain damage. In head trauma, animals unconscious from the time of injury and remaining unconscious for more than 24 hours usually have brain stem hemorrhage with irreversible damage. Some regain consciousness, but they usually have severe deficits. If the onset is slower and progression can be reversed, the prognosis is more favorable. Use of a coma scale may be useful for measuring progression (Table 51-3).[5] Management of a comatose patient requires full-time nursing care. It is a major medical challenge.

REFERENCES

1. Cartlidge NEF: States of altered consciousness. In Swash M, Kennard C (eds): Scientific Basis of Clinical Neurology. Edinburgh, Churchill Livingstone, 1985
2. Kornegay JN, Oliver JE, Gorgacz EJ: Clinicopathologic features of brain herniation in animals. J Am Vet Med Assoc 182:1111–1116, 1983
3. Oliver JE, Lorenz MD: Handbook of Veterinary Neurologic Diagnosis, 2nd ed. Philadelphia, WB Saunders, 1993
4. Saper CB: Hypothalamus and brain stem. In Pearlman AL, Collins RC: Neurological Pathophysiology, 3rd ed. New York, Oxford University Press, 1984
5. Shores A: Development of a coma scale for dogs: Prognostic value in cranio-cerebral trauma. In Proceedings of the Sixth Annual Veterinary Medicine Forum, 251–253, Washington, D.C., 1988

PART THIRTEEN

Special Sensation Problems

CHAPTER FIFTY-TWO

Blindness

Charles L. Martin

PROBLEM DEFINITION AND RECOGNITION

Blindness, for purposes of this chapter, is defined as loss of vision in both eyes. The clinical tests that attempt to measure vision in veterinary medicine are crude, nonquantitative, and nonstandardized. They include navigation of an obstacle course in a strange environment, reacting to a menacing gesture, detection of movement (*e.g.*, a falling cotton ball), or optokinetic nystagmus and preferential vision testing. These tests are not specific, and lesions remote from the visual system may create deficits. Objective measurements such as visual evoked responses in the occipital cortex determine the integrity of the visual system, but they are not quantitative or widely available. The electroretinogram measures the function of the outer half of the retina but cannot be used as a quantitative test for visual function. Pupillary light reflexes (PLR) are not a visual function test, but when critically performed they are of benefit in localizing lesions that affect vision.

When examining the problem of blindness one has to consider the possibility of sequential events, for example, dissimilar lesions in each eye culminating in blindness, as well as simultaneous events such as progressive retinal atrophy. Moreover, an apparent acute blindness may only reflect a change in environment, an acute injury to one eye when the opposite eye has been chronically blind, or the final insult to an eye that has had chronically minimal function.

PATHOPHYSIOLOGY

Blindness can be produced by bilateral lesions in four general ways: (1) lesions that produce opacification of the clear ocular media, (2) failure of the retina to process the image, (3) failure to transmit or relay the message, and (4) failure in the final processing of the image.

The pathways for vision and the PLR are presented in Figure 53-1 (see Chapter 53 for a detailed interpretation). The two pathways are similar until just before the lateral geniculate body, where they diverge. These similarities and differences can be useful for lesion localization, but there are pitfalls. Although the pathways are initially similar, it must be remembered that vision is depen-

465

dent on not only the quantity but also the quality of light reaching the retina, whereas the PLR is dependent on quantity. Therefore, a lesion that causes a great deal of scattering of light (such as a cataract or any lesion of the clear media) may degrade the retinal image to the point of producing functional blindness but not be so obstructive to light as to interfere with the PLR. In addition, the pupillomotor fibers may be spared with some forms of retinal and optic nerve disease. Also, the efferent arm of the PLR is independent of vision and must be considered as the cause of pupillomotor dysfunction before the afferent arm of the reflex is used to localize the lesion. Finally the interpretation of a normal or abnormal response is subjective in most testing situations and depends on the examiner's experience, the patient's anxiety, brightness of the stimulus, contrast of the ambient light to the stimulus, and adaptation of the retina.

RULE OUTS

Blindness from Lesions of the Clear Ocular Media

As a group, lesions of the clear ocular media are the easiest to diagnose. Any opacity of the cornea, aqueous humor, lens, or vitreous or combinations of these opacities that are severe enough to block the light reflex from the tapetum can be considered severe enough to produce blindness, although the patient may be sensitive to light. Patients with a tapetal reflex and blurred fundus detail on ophthalmoscopy are usually functional; consequently, additional lesions should be suspected in the blindness evaluation. Lesions of the clear ocular media can be detected with only a penlight, and the patient will have *a normal PLR unless there is a concurrent lesion in the efferent arm of the pupillary light reflex.*

Blindness from Retinal Lesions

Diffuse bilateral lesions of the retina resulting in blindness also produce *dilated pupils under room light conditions.* In dogs blind from retinal disease, testing the PLR with a strong light often produces pupillary constriction, but the amount and speed of constriction is subnormal. The majority of patients blind from retinal causes have obvious abnormalities on ophthalmoscopy, but important exceptions exist (see Table 52-1). The obvious assumption is that the observer can accurately assess the normalcy of the ocular fundus. It is common for lesions of the clear media (cataracts, asteroid hyalosis) to coexist with advanced retinal lesions, and this possibility must always be evaluated, particularly if cataract surgery is being considered as a cure for the blindness. Ophthalmoscopic lesions typical of advanced retinal disease are retinal detachment, an attenuation in size and a decrease in number of retinal vessels, diffuse increases or decreases in tapetal reflectivity, and marked pigmentary disruptions and/or accumulations in the nontapetum or tapetum.

Etiologies of Bilateral Blindness

Opacification of the ocular media

Keratitis: keratoconjunctivitis sicca, immune-mediated, multiple ulcerative insults with scarring
Keratopathy: lipid dystrophy, endothelial dystrophy/degeneration
Aqueous turbidity: fibrin (anterior uveitis), lipid, hemorrhage from trauma or blood dyscrasia
Cataracts: genetic, metabolic, toxic, nutritional
Vitreous hemorrhage: blood dyscrasia, trauma, retinal disease

Diseases of the retina

Retinopathy
    Genetic: progressive retinal atrophy in dogs and cats, retinal pigment epitheliopathy (central retinal atrophy)
    Nutritional: taurine deficiency in cats, vitamin E deficiency, vitamin A deficiency
    Glaucoma
    Inborn errors of metabolism
    Sudden acute retinal degeneration syndrome (SARDS) in dogs, which is an idiopathic retinal degeneration
Retinal detachment syndromes
    Genetic: collie eye anomaly, retinal dysplasia
    Exudative: systemic mycoses, protothecosis, ehrlichiosis, toxoplasmosis, feline infectious peritonitis, feline leukemia–associated
    Transudative: hypertension, intravenous fluid overloading
    Neoplastic: metastatic
    Chorioretinitis: distemper, systemic mycoses, brucellosis, feline infectious peritonitis, toxoplasmosis, ehrlichiosis, granulomatous meningoencephalitis

Lesions of the conducting mechanism (optic nerve or tracts)

Hypoplasia of the optic nerves
Reticulosis or granulomatous encephalomyelitis
Distemper encephalitis
Feline infectious peritonitis meningoencephalitis
Systemic mycoses
Neoplasms involving the chiasm
Traumatic avulsion

Lesions of the occipital cortex

Hydrocephalus
Cerebral malformations (lissencephaly)
Distemper encephalomyelitis
Feline meningoencephalitis
Systemic mycoses
Reticulosis (granulomatous meningoencephalitis)
Hepatoencephalopathy
Inborn metabolic errors
Hypoxia
Vascular infarcts
Traumatic edema or hemorrhage

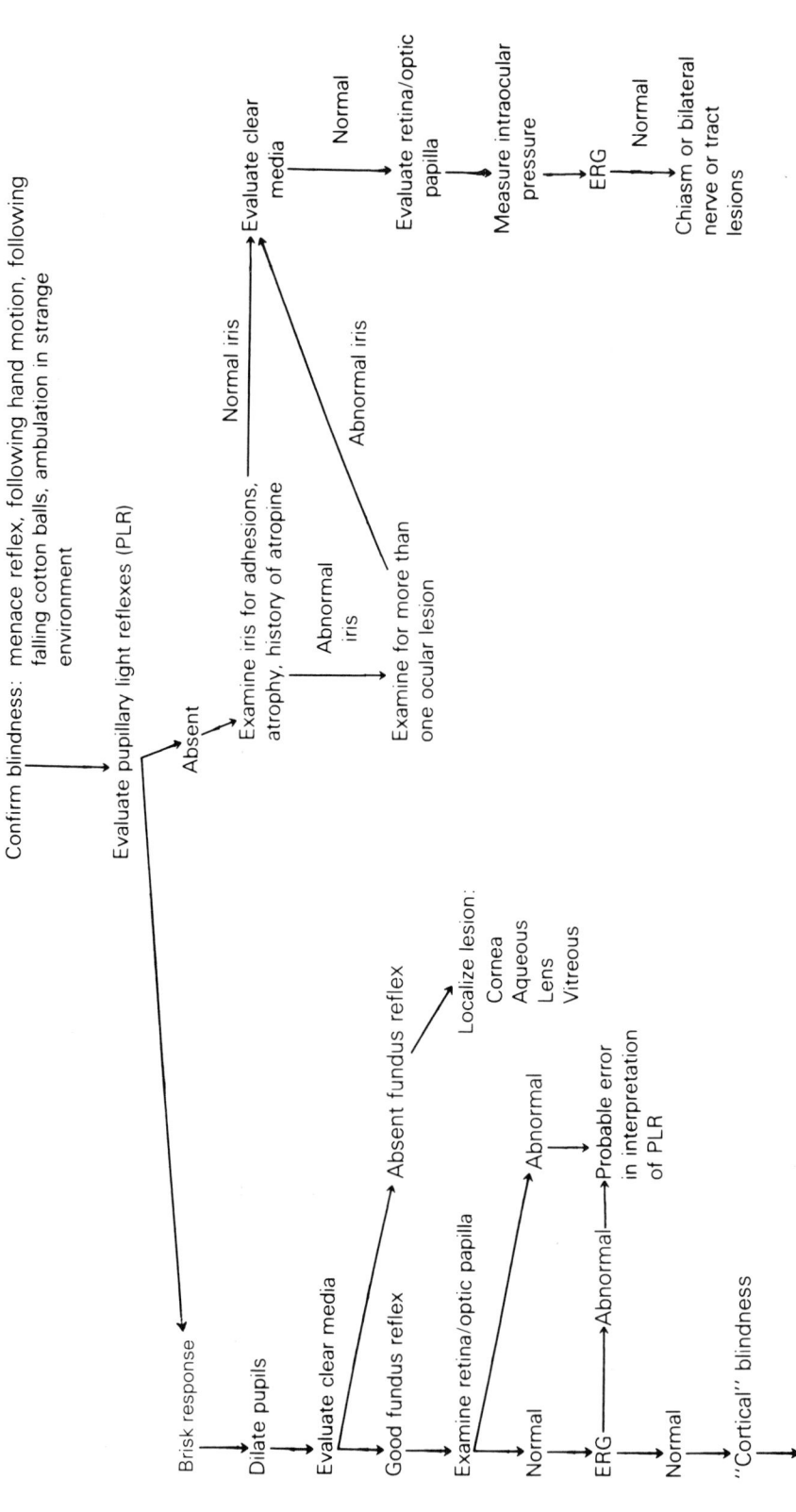

FIGURE 52-1. Diagnostic plan for evaluation of a blind patient. (ERG, electroreticulogram)

Blindness from Lesions in the Conducting System up to the Lateral Geniculate Body

With the exception of the optic disk, the conducting system cannot be directly observed without special radiographic techniques. Diagnosis is often made by exclusion, unless sophisticated electronics are available to perform electroretinograms and visual evoked responses. A lesion of the chiasm or bilateral lesions of the optic nerve or optic tracts will interfere with vision and the PLR. If the process extends to the optic disc, changes in color and elevation of the disk may be observed. Atrophy of the disk may be recognized in dogs by pallor, loss of myelin with scalloping of the disk border, and a decrease in elevation. Elevation of the disk may indicate papilledema or papillitis, clues as to retrobulbar involvement of the conducting system. Papillitis is accompanied by congestion of the retinal vessels, often with hemorrhages, peripapillary edema, and vitreous haze. Papilledema is quieter in appearance with less congestion, fewer hemorrhages and mild peripapillary edema. Papilledema *per se* does not produce blindness, although the process responsible for the edema may result in blindness.

Bilateral involvement of the conducting system below the lateral geniculate body produces blindness with loss of the PLR. Except for the optic chiasm, these pathways are distantly placed from one another, and bilateral involvement is usually produced by multifocal or diffuse lesions, which often produce accompanying neurologic signs (see Table 52-1).

Cortical Blindness

Lesions of the lateral geniculate body, optic radiations, and occipital cortex produce blindness with normal PLR and are usually consolidated under cortical blindness. The role of the occipital cortex in vision is "form recognition," whereas the dorsal colliculus in the midbrain is important in "pursuit" or "body orientation" to an object. Bilateral involvement of the occipital cortex may be produced by lesions such as encephalitis, hydrocephalus, or a metabolic or toxic encephalopathy, and is usually not selective; thus, a thorough neurologic examination is indicated (see Display, Etiologies of Bilateral Blindness).

DIAGNOSTIC PLAN

See Figure 52-1 for a diagnostic plan to evaluate the blind patient.

CHAPTER FIFTY-THREE

Problem-Oriented Ophthalmology: Anisocoria

Charles L. Martin

PROBLEM DEFINITION AND RECOGNITION

Anisocoria or unequal pupils can be broadly divided anatomically into ocular and neurologic causes. As the ocular causes can often be directly observed, it is usually expedient to eliminate ocular etiologies of anisocoria before proceeding to a neurologic explanation. If vision is impaired, the reader is also referred to Chapter 52. Determining which of the two pupils is abnormal is often difficult. If a pupil is immobile to either light or dark stimulation, or both, it is obviously the abnormal one of the two pupils. The normalcy of pupils that are not completely immobile must be judged by evaluating the range of the excursions, the briskness of the constriction, and the size of the pupil expected at a given ambient light and by utilizing the swinging light test. Anatomic abnormalities, such as an irregular pupil that may indicate a synechia or atrophy of the sphincter, may provide additional clues as to which pupil is abnormal.

PATHOPHYSIOLOGY

The pathways for the pupillomotor fibers and vision are illustrated in Figure 53-1.

The afferent arm of the pupillary light reflex (PLR) consists of three neurons: the bipolar cells, ganglion cells, and neurons in the pretectal nucleus. The afferent arm of the pupillomotor fibers courses with the visual fibers until just proximal to the lateral geniculate body. Seventy-five percent and 65%, respectively, of the dog and cat visual and pupillomotor fibers decussate, or cross, at the optic chiasm.[3] The majority of pupillomotor fibers then cross again in the pretectum to the original side.[7]

The efferent arm of the PLR consists of two neurons: the first originates in the parasympathetic nucleus of the oculomotor nerve (cranial nerve III) and remains ipsilateral to synapse in the ciliary ganglion; the second neuron passes

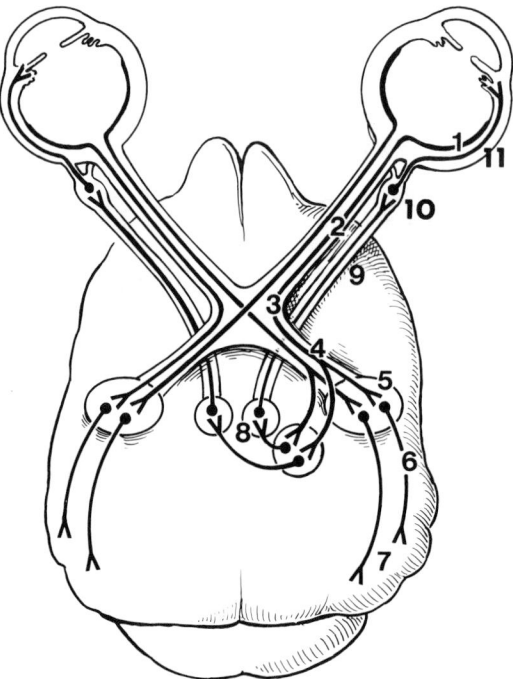

FIGURE 53-1. Pupillary light reflex and vision pathways. The two types of fibers have similar pathways until point 4, where they diverge. *1,* retina; *2,* optic nerve; *3,* chiasm; *4,* optic tract; *5,* lateral geniculate body; *6,* optic radiation; *7,* occipital cortex; *8,* parasympathetic nuclei of oculomotor nerve; *9,* oculomotor nerve; *10,* ciliary ganglion; *11,* short ciliary nerve. (Modified from Oliver JE, Lorenz MD: Handbook of Veterinary Neurologic Diagnosis, p. 255. Philadelphia, WB Saunders, 1983)

from the ciliary ganglion in the short ciliary nerves to the iris sphincter muscle. The short ciliary nerves differ in the dog and cat. In the dog multiple branches supply the globe, whereas in the cat only two branches are present.[7] Evaluation of PLR and dynamic anisocorias requires an appreciation of the differences in the proportion of optic nerve fibers that cross at the chiasm and subsequently the midbrain in the particular species examined. This lack of equal input to the eyes when the PLR is stimulated in one eye explains the dynamic anisocoria present in the normal dog; that is, the consensual reflex is not as strong or complete as the direct PLR. Data transposed from humans and primates in which 50% of the fibers cross are not completely applicable.

Sympathetic innervation to the iris provides the stimulation for dilation by relaxing the sphincter muscle and contracting the dilator muscle. The sympathetic chain is long and consists of three neurons. The first neuron originates in the hypothalamus passing with some descussation down the brain stem and cervical spinal cord to synapse at the level of thoracic segments 1, 2, and 3.

The second neuron passes through the rostral chest and up the neck in the vagosympathetic trunk to synapse in the cranial cervical ganglion. The third neuron traverses the tympanic bulla and joins the ophthalmic division of cranial nerve V in the cranial vault to reach the globe via the long ciliary nerve. Anisocoria can be classified as a static or dynamic inequality of pupils. Static anisocoria is manifested without stimulation of the PLR and is constant, whereas dynamic anisocorias become manifest during or immediately after stimulation of the PLR.[4]

TESTING THE PUPILLARY LIGHT REFLEXES

Direct and consensual reflexes are best determined in dim ambient light utilizing a strong stimulating light. The direct response is determined and the consensual response evaluated while alternately directing the light quickly from one eye to the other at 2- to 4-second intervals (swinging light test). The pupils will normally have minimal excursions when performing the swinging light test. An eye with an afferent defect in the PLR can be detected, even if an efferent arm lesion such as synechia or oculomotor paralysis is present. Afferent arm lesions are detected in the presence of efferent lesions with the swinging light test by the presence of further constriction of the opposite normal eye when the light is swung over to it. This is not as sensitive in animals because of the normal dynamic anisocoria that is present with the unequal decussation of the optic nerve. Afferent arm lesions are normally determined by pupil dilation when the light is shown in the abnormal eye on the swinging light test (Marcus Gunn pupil).

ANISOCORIA INDUCED BY OCULAR DISEASE

When evaluating an eye with anisocoria, one must note whether the pupil is capable of movement with either the direct or consensual PLR, whether vision is present, and the size of the immobile or relatively immobile pupil. An animal that has an immobile pupil creating anisocoria has a problem with the efferent arm of the reflex arc (oculomotor parasympathetic nucleus or nerve) or the target organ (iris).

Diseases of the Iris

Anisocorias associated with iris disease constitute an efferent arm defect. Several relatively common conditions involving the iris will produce static anisocorias: anterior uveitis, glaucoma, sphincter iris atrophy, iris hypoplasia, and pharmacologic blockade. Anterior uveitis (iritis) typically produces a miotic pupil, which is relatively resistant to mydriatic drugs (atropine, tropicamide). Additional signs of anterior chamber flare, iris color changes, iris texture changes and hypotony are usually present. Posterior synechiae frequently develop and are an additional cause for static anisocoria with anterior uveitis. Posterior synechiae are recognized by irregular pupil margins with pigment debris on the anterior lens capsule.

Iris atrophy near the pupil weakens the sphincter muscle function, resulting in a dilated pupil that is resistant to pharmacologic constriction. Sphincter atrophy may occur in otherwise normal eyes, but when it occurs with cataracts, evaluation of the preoperative cataract patient is difficult. The miniature and toy poodles frequently develop atrophy of the pupillary margin of the iris. The condition is usually bilateral, but if asymmetric in severity, it results in a static anisocoria. Atrophy of the sphincter is most reliably recognized by observing a scalloped pupillary margin, often with patches of iris that transilluminate against the tapetal reflex.

A "normal" mild anisocoria can be discerned in animals with heterochromia. The blue iris will be mildly dilated in relation to the darker iris.

Intraocular Pressure Elevation

Primary glaucoma usually manifests itself with a static anisocoria produced by a dilated pupil that is unresponsive to light. Once the intraocular pressure exceeds the diastolic blood pressure (about 50 mm Hg), the pupil becomes dilated if it is not adhered and is unresponsive to light or pharmacologic stimulation. Additional signs of increased firmness and globe size are typical of glaucoma. Anterior uveitis and glaucoma share the signs of conjunctival and episcleral injection and corneal edema. Secondary glaucoma from pupil occlusion and seclusion usually leaves the pupil immobile in the midposition.

Drug-Induced Anisocoria

Topical application of belladona alkaloids will produce a static anisocoria that may last for 4 to 5 days or longer after the last application. If the application was accidental, the history may not be helpful and the cause can be diagnosed only by the lack of ocular signs such as synechiae, increased pressure or iris atrophy, and the lack of response to direct-acting miotic drugs (pilocarpine). Improvement after several days aids in retrospectively diagnosing drug-induced mydriasis. Similarly, unilateral application of miotic agents may complicate diagnosis, although they have a shorter duration of action.

Anisocoria Induced by Corneal Disease

The pain of superficial corneal ulceration may produce a very strong miosis and static anisocoria. The miosis is atropine-resistant and mediated by antidromic impulses via the ophthalmic nerve (see Chapter 56).

Anisocoria Induced by Lenticular Disease

Mild anisocorias, either dynamic or static, may occur with lens subluxations, luxations, and hypermature cataracts that interfere with pupil mobility. Dyscoria or a misshapen pupil is often present with the latter conditions.

Anisocoria Induced by Retinal Blindness

Unilateral retinal and optic nerve blindness produce a mild static anisocoria with pupillary dilation in the involved eye in the dog and cat, as a result of the weaker consensual input to the blind eye. The blind eye exhibits a pupillary escape phenomenon or dilates when the light is moved from the visual eye to the blind eye during the swinging light test. The latter is termed a Marcus Gunn reaction.

ANISOCORIA ASSOCIATED WITH NEUROLOGIC DISEASE

Afferent Arm Lesions

Unilateral lesions of the afferent arm of the PLR produce mild static anisocorias due to the unequal distribution of crossed and uncrossed fibers in the dog. These will become more manifest with dynamic anisocorias upon PLR testing.

Optic Nerve Lesions. Unilateral lesions of the optic nerve produce a more dilated ipsilateral pupil that reacts consensually and exhibits a Marcus Gunn reaction with the swinging light test. Unilateral optic nerve lesions and retinal lesions manifest themselves in similar ways and are differentiated by ophthalmoscopy and electroretinopathy. Eyes with afferent arm lesions will dilate in the dark to equal pupil size.

Optic Tract Lesions. Unilateral lesions of the optic tract are more difficult to localize with the PLR because they contain a mixture of crossed and uncrossed fibers; in addition, the lesions may not be complete. A complete lesion becomes manifest with a mild static anisocoria, and the lesion is contralateral to the more dilated (abnormal) pupil. It may be differentiated from optic nerve and retinal lesions with the swinging light test by the lack of a Marcus Gunn response as a result of the intact uncrossed fibers.[7] Both pupils will dilate and be equal in darkness.

Efferent Arm Lesions

Lesions of the parasympathetic nuclei, oculomotor nerve, and ciliary ganglion produce an ipsilateral dilated pupil and static anisocoria. The anisocoria with efferent arm lesions is more marked than that with afferent arm lesions. Lesions that involve the parasympathetic nuclei usually also involve the motor nuclei and are often bilateral. Most oculomotor nerve lesions involve both the parasympathetic and motor fibers, creating an ocular deviation that, when acute, is lateral-ventral. The globe is immobile except for lateral and intorsional movements (lateral rectus muscle is innervated by cranial nerve VI, and dorsal oblique muscle by cranial nerve IV).[3] Oculomotor nerve involvement may arise intracranially, in the orbital fissure, or intraorbitally. In the dog, orbital lesions may involve both the oculomotor nerve and ciliary ganglion. In the latter instance, both the ocular parasympathetic and sympathetic fibers are damaged, producing a fixed midpoint pupil that does not constrict with light or dilate with darkness. In the cat, it is possible to have an isolated palsy of one of the two short ciliary nerves (postganglionic parasympathetic fibers). The latter event produces a D- or reversed-D–shaped pupil due to the hemidilation.[7]

Feline Dysautonomia (Key-Gaskell Syndrome). A syndrome of generalized dysautonomia with ocular manifestations of dilated pupils has been described in Great Britain. The etiology is unknown but does not appear to be related to the feline leukemia virus, as does the alternating anisocoria syndrome. Cats with dysautonomia may have an initial anisocoria, but subsequently the pupils are dilated and equal, the eyes are visual, the third eyelid prolapsed, and the tear secretions decreased. The signs are characteristic of an efferent arm parasympathetic lesion. Additional signs of dysautonomia are constipation, regurgitation, dry mucous membranes, bradycardia, and urinary incontinence.[6,8]

Paradoxic Anisocoria in Cats. In the cat a rather startling syndrome is observed in which a marked anisocoria develops that may alternate between eyes at irregular intervals of hours or days. The abnormal pupil may be dilated or constricted, or both pupils may be dilated or constricted. On ocular examination the eyes are normal, and although urinary incontinence may be a complaint, most cats are systemically normal.[1,5] Most affected cats are positive on feline leukemia testing and die within the next 6 months. Scagliotti has demonstrated the leukemia virus in the ciliary nerves and ganglion of involved cats.[7] The pupils do not respond predictably to pharmacologic testing.

Efferent Sympathetic Lesions

Interruption of the sympathetic fibers of the dog and cat produce a cluster of signs ipsilaterally known as Horner's syndrome. The signs of Horner's syndrome vary among species, but in the dog and cat consist of ptosis, miosis, prolapsed third eyelid, and enophthalmos or apparent enophthalmos. The anisocoria of Horner's syndrome is characterized by a miosis that will not dilate to be equal with the normal pupil. The anisocoria is most evident in dim light.

The ocular sympathetic neuron chain is long, and the location and type of lesion can be quite varied. Lesion localization is determined by association with

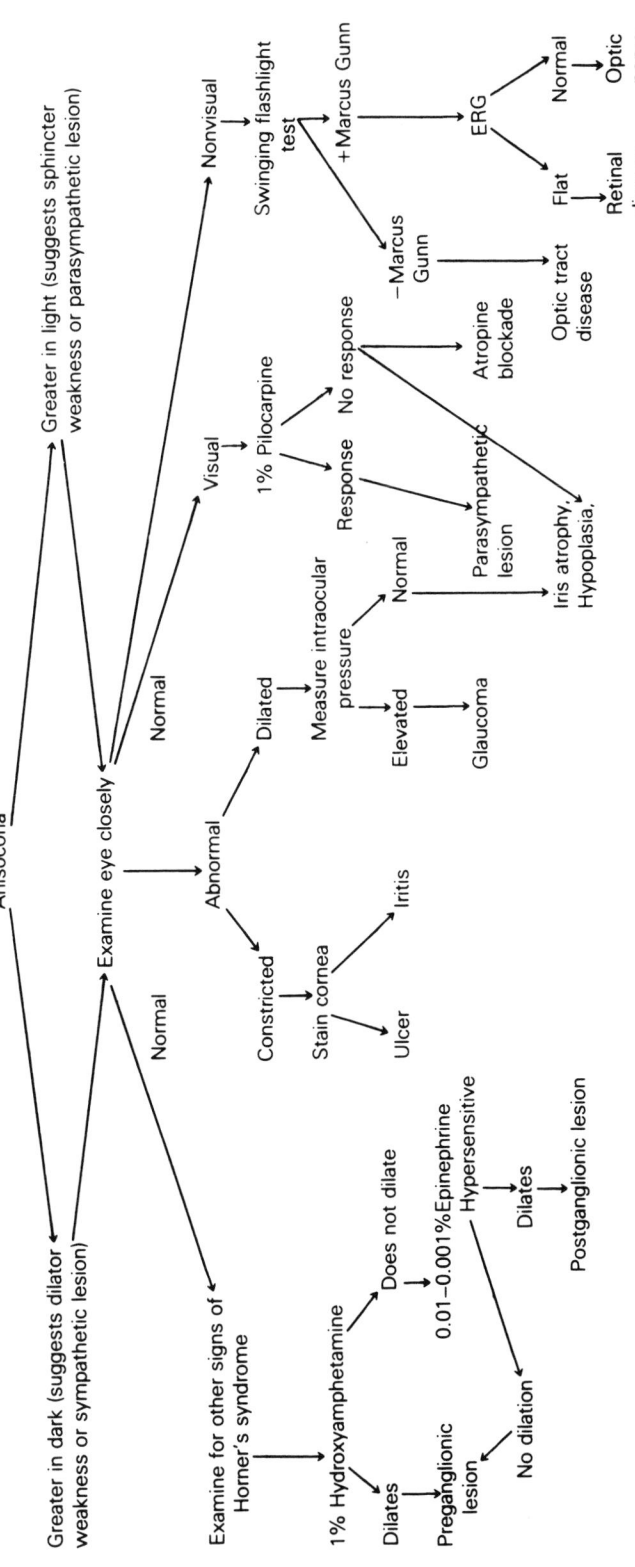

FIGURE 53-2. Algorithm for the diagnosis of anisocoria.

TABLE 53-1. Pharmacologic Lesion Localization in Horner's Syndrome

Drug	Normal	Central Lesion	Preganglionic Lesion	Postganglionic Lesion
1% hydroxamphetamine	+	+	+	0
1% phenylephrine	0	0	0	+
0.001% epinephrine	0	0	Mild +	+

+, dilates; 0, no response

other neurologic or systemic signs, pharmacologic testing, chest and tympanic bulla radiographs, ear examination, and palpation of the cervical region. Patients with Horner's syndrome of central nervous system origin usually have other neurologic complaints or deficits, which aid in lesion localization. Occasionally, a Horner's syndrome of central nervous system origin is prodromal to other neurologic signs, but the latter become manifest in days to a few weeks. Preganglionic lesions from the thoracic segments 1, 2, and 3 to the cranial cervical ganglion are common and may be detected by chest radiographs and palpation. The postganglionic chain is often affected by pathology of the middle ear, such as otitis media and interna. Associated signs of ipsilateral peripheral vestibular disease and facial nerve paralysis may be present with Horner's syndrome of otitis origin.

DIAGNOSTIC PLAN

Figure 53-2 outlines a diagnostic plan for anisocoria. Pharmacologic testing can be utilized, but a control eye, preferably the normal eye, should also be monitored because of variable responses. Pharmacologic testing employs the phenomenon of denervation hypersensitivity to the missing neurotransmittor if the third neuron is involved, and the intact response when stimulated with indirect acting drugs when the first or second neuron is destroyed. Third neuron disease of either the parasympathetic or sympathetic chain induces an exaggerated re-

TABLE 53-2. Pharmacologic Lesion Localization with a Dilated Pupil

Drug	Normal	Central Parasympathetic Lesion	Peripheral Parasympathetic Lesion	Iris Atrophy	Glaucoma	Atropine Blockade
1% pilocarpine	+	+	+ (hypersensitive)	0	0	0
0.01% phospholine iodide	+	+	0	0	0	0

+, constriction; 0, no response

sponse to acetylcholine (or other direct-acting parasympathomimetics) or epinephrine/norepinephrine (or other direct-acting sympathomimetics) because of the lack of uptake and neutralization of the neurotransmittors by the missing third neuron.[2] Indirect-acting parasympathetics and sympathetics act by stimulating the release of neurotransmittors or by interfering with the neutralization of the neurotransmittors and thus require an intact third neuron to release the neurotransmittors. Tables 53-1 and 53-2 list the pharmacologic testing and results of lesion localization. Preganglionic lesions require a thorough neurologic evaluation, and the prognosis is usually worse with either sympathetic or parasympathetic lesions.

REFERENCES

1. Barsanti J, Downey R: Urinary incontinence in cats. Anim Hosp Assoc 20:979, 1984
2. Bistner S, Rubin L, Cox T, Condon W: Pharmacologic diagnosis of Horner's syndrome in the dog. J Am Vet Med Assoc 157:1220, 1970
3. de Lahunta A: Visual system—special somatic afferent system. In Veterinary Neuroanatomy and Clinical Neurology, p 266. Philadelphia, WB Saunders, 1977
4. Duke-Elder S, Scott GI: The pupillary and ciliary systems. In System of Ophthalmology, Vol XII, p 613. London, Henry Kimpton, 1971
5. Martin C: Ocular signs of systemic disease, part I. Mod Vet Pract 1982, p 689
6. Rochlitz I: Feline dysautonomia (the Key-Gaskell or dilated pupil syndrome): A preliminary review. J Sm Anim Pract 25:587, 1984
7. Scagliotti R: Neuro-Ophthalmology. In Kirk R (ed): Current Veterinary Therapy VII, p 510. Philadelphia, WB Saunders, 1980
8. Sharp N, Nash A, Griffiths I: Feline dysautonomia (the Key-Gaskell syndrome): A clinical and pathological study of forty cases. J Sm Anim Pract 25:599, 1984

CHAPTER FIFTY-FOUR

Abnormal Ocular Movement and Position

Charles L. Martin

PROBLEM DEFINITION AND RECOGNITION

Abnormal ocular movements can be divided into ocular deviations (strabismus), paralysis of gaze, and nystagmus.[7] Nystagmus is defined as a rhythmic, involuntary movement of the eye(s) and may be in a horizontal, vertical, or rotary direction. The eye(s) may be in an abnormal position as a result of movement around its center of rotation or because of displacement of the globe within the orbit.[5] The latter movement is termed *translational* and may be active in domestic animals as a result of disorders of the retractor bulbi muscle or passive, resulting from changes in the orbital mass.

The term *duction* refers to movement of only one eye and is modified by a prefix to indicate the direction of movement. Adduction is movement of the eye medially in a horizontal plane, abduction is lateral movement, supraduction is dorsal movement, and infraduction is ventral movement. Torsional ductions include intorsion (incycloduction), in which the dorsal pupil rotates medially, and extorsion (excycloduction), in which the dorsal pupil rotates laterally (Fig. 54-1).[6]

Versions are the simultaneous movement of both eyes in the same direction (conjugate movement). Examples are the horizontal versions of dextroversion and levoversion, and the vertical versions of supraversion and infraversion. Vergence is the simultaneous and equal movement of the eyes in opposite directions, *i.e.,* convergence and divergence (Fig. 54-2).[6] The position of the frontally placed eyes when normally fixated on a distant object that is straight ahead is termed the *primary position* of the eyes. Eyes that have a manifest deviation are said to have a tropia (*e.g.,* exotropia, estropia). Eyes that have a latent deviation manifested when they are shielded from fixation are said to have a phoria (*e.g.,* exophoria, esophoria). A comitant trophia is one that is constant in all directions of gaze, whereas a noncomitant deviation varies with the direction of gaze.[3]

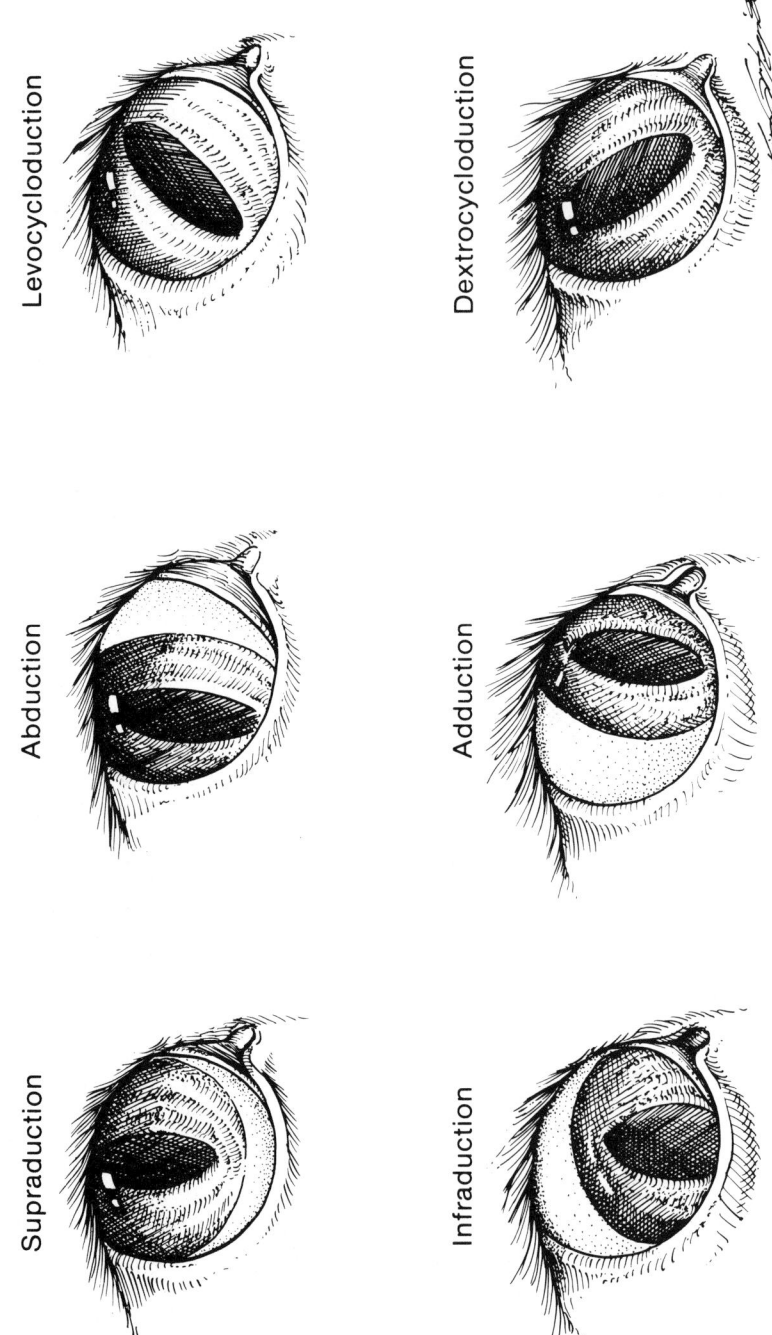

FIGURE 54-1. Ductional movements in a cat eye.

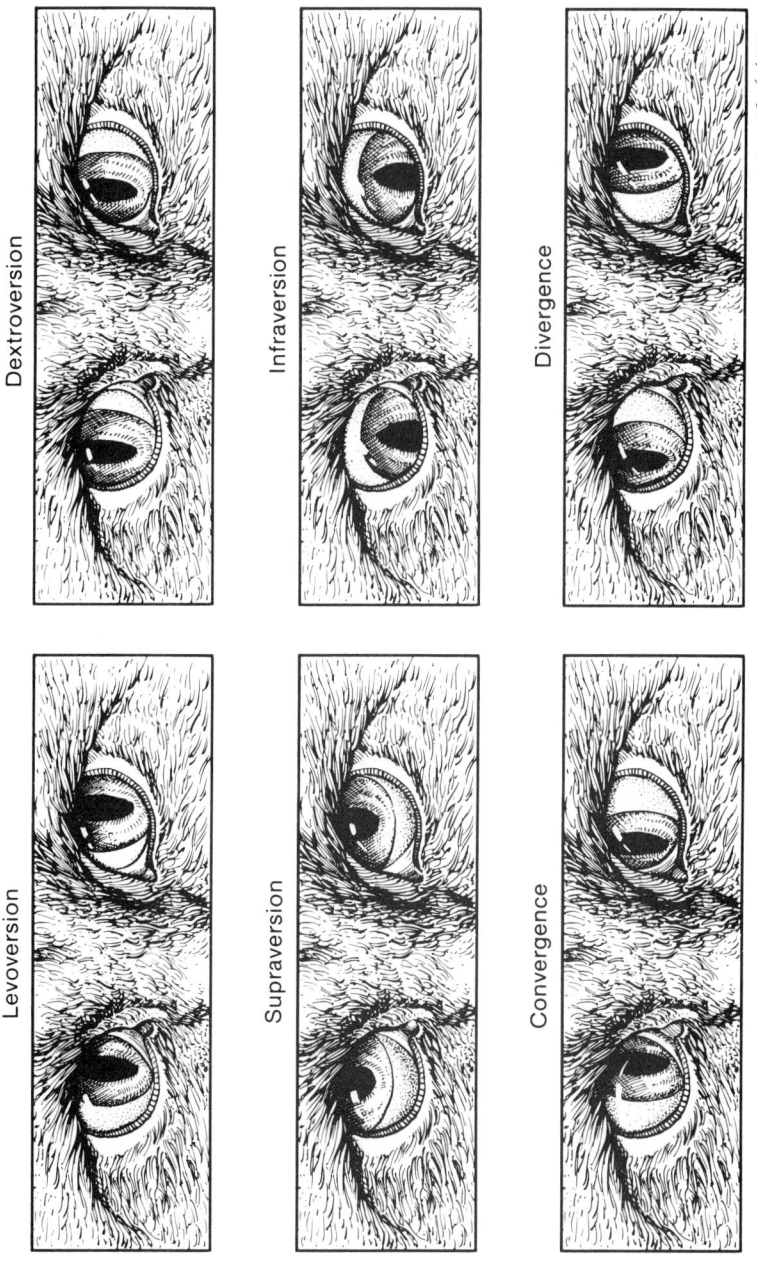

FIGURE 54-2. Version and vergence eye movements in a cat.

PATHOPHYSIOLOGY

The extraocular muscles of mammals are a type of skeletal muscle, but they differ from other skeletal muscle in having at least two fiber systems. One type of extraocular muscle fiber, usually found in skeletal muscle, is composed of well-organized myofibrils innervated with thick myelinated nerves and is responsible for the rapid eye movements, or saccades. The second type of fiber is not composed of definite myofibrils and is innervated by small myelinated nerves. These fibers are responsible for the smooth, slow contractions that hold the eyes in position or are used in following. The extraocular muscles are much more richly innervated than other skeletal muscle, which reflects their function in making rapid and fine adjustments in eye position.[5,8] Domestic animals generally have relatively limited ocular motility compared with that of humans. In general, the amount of exposed sclera in the palpebral fissure is directly related to the degree of ocular motility in the species. The lack of ocular motility is compensated by either the lateral positioning of the eyes or the increased ability to swivel the head, as in the owl.[7] The action of the individual extraocular muscles varies among species as a result of variable insertion sites. The main actions of the extraocular muscles are listed in Table 54-1. The deviations that would result from acute muscle or nerve function are given in Table 54-2, but in animals with a retractor bulbi muscle, compensation apparently occurs, and the acute ocular deviations are less apparent with time.

Figures 54-3 and 54-4 illustrate the extraocular muscles of the cat. The lateral rectus muscle and retractor bulbi muscle are innervated by cranial nerve VI, the dorsal oblique by cranial nerve IV, and the medial, ventral, and dorsal rectus and ventral oblique muscles by cranial nerve III. The pathways and control of ocular movements are complex and incompletely understood. Supranuclear pathways (above the cranial nerve nuclei) are involved with movement of the eyes in a coordinated manner, rather than contraction of an individual muscle.[4]

TABLE 54-1. Action and Innervation of Extraocular Muscles

Muscle	Action	Innervation
Dorsal rectus	Supraduction, adduction	CN III
Medial rectus	Adduction	CN III
Ventral rectus	Infraduction, adduction	CN III
Ventral oblique	Extorsion, adduction	CN III
Dorsal oblique	Intorsion, adduction	CN IV
Lateral rectus	Abduction	CN VI
Retractor bulbi	Retraction of glove	CN VI

CN, cranial nerve

TABLE 54-2. Acute Signs of Dysfunction of Extraocular Muscles and Cranial Nerves

Muscle/Nerve	Sign	Test
Dorsal rectus	Infratropia, inability to supraduct	Move head downward
Medial rectus	Exotropia, inability to adduct	Move head horizontally, visual following
Ventral rectus	Supratropia, inability to infraduct	Move head upward
Ventral oblique	Inability to extort eye	Rotate head
Dorsal oblique	Inability to intort eye	Rotate head
Lateral rectus	Esotropia, inability to abduct	Move head horizontally, visual following
Retractor bulbi	Inability to retract globe	Touch cornea
CN III	Extropia, infratropia, pupil dilated ±	
CN IV	No obvious signs (see Dorsal oblique)	
CN VI	Esotropia (see Lateral rectus)	

CN, cranial nerve; ±, may or may not be present

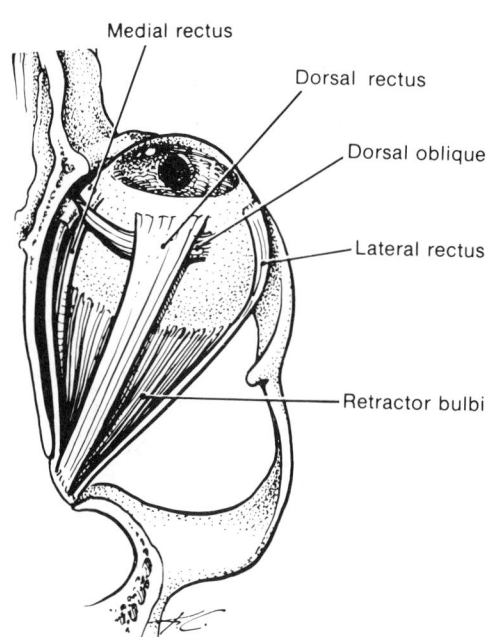

Medial rectus

Dorsal rectus

Dorsal oblique

Lateral rectus

Retractor bulbi

FIGURE 54-3. Dorsal view of the extraocular muscles of the cat.

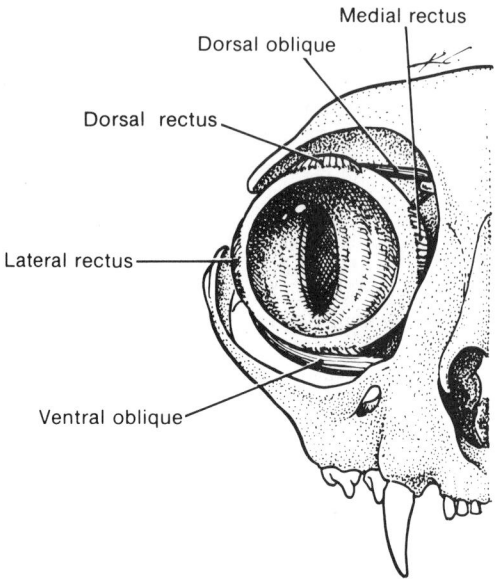

FIGURE 54-4. Anterior view of the cat eye and the extraocular muscles.

CORTICAL CENTERS FOR OCULAR MOVEMENT

The frontal cortex serves voluntary control of the ocular movements, while the occipital cortex serves movement of the eye in response to visual stimuli (optomotor). The optomotor stimuli produce slow, smooth following movements of the eye, while the voluntary movements produce rapid, jerky jumps, or saccades. Stimulation of the frontal cortex unilaterally produces lateral conjugate movements to the opposite side; thus, unilateral lesions of the frontal cortex produce transient paresis of conjugate gaze until the opposite cortex assumes bilateral control (a few weeks).[4]

The occipital cortex optomotor fibers pass down to the superior colliculus and subserve the function of keeping a moving target on the macula and orienting the body to a moving object. Connections between the frontal and occipital cortex are present, but the frontal eye reflexes predominate. Optokinetic nystagmus is the ocular movement produced by following a moving target going in one direction. The smooth following movement of the optomotor movements (occipital lobe) is followed by the rapid, jerky recovery saccade from the frontal cortex. A bilateral disease of the frontal cortex or a lesion interfering with the interconnection of the two cortices will produce a slow movement of the eyes without the rapid recovery phase.[4]

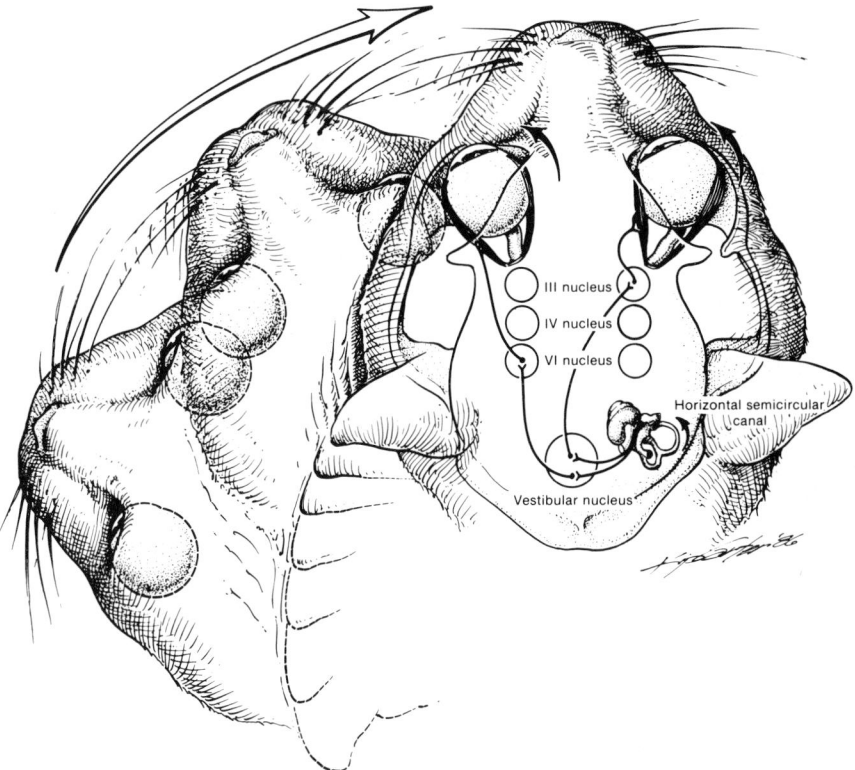

FIGURE 54-5. Connections of the horizontal labyrinth with the extraocular muscles and the stimulation of vestibular induced eye movement of the head.

VESTIBULAR (LABYRINTH) OCULAR MOVEMENTS

Vestibular reflex tonus coordinates changes in posture with movements of the eyes. These reflexes can be categorized into (1) static reflexes that respond to head position or gravitational changes and (2) kinetic reflexes that respond to movement such as acceleration or deceleration. Vestibular reflexes produce only conjugate movements (both eyes moving in the same direction). Each labyrinth exerts tone on the opposite lateral rectus and ipsilateral medial rectus via connections through the medial longitudinal fasciculus from the vestibular nucleus (Fig. 54-5). With a balanced input from both sides, the eyes are kept straight. Stimulation of one labyrinth produces a slow movement to the opposite side followed by a rapid saccadic movement that is a corrective movement from the frontal cortex. The direction of the nystagmus is named according to the rapid or cortical phase. Destruction of a labyrinth produces a slow drift to the affected side, due to the imbalanced input from the intact side. The fast phase movement (nystagmus) is to the contralateral side. The direction of the nystagmus with a unilateral lesion depends on whether the lesion is irritative (stimulating) or destructive.[4,8]

The otolith of the utriculus produces tonic sustained contractions of the extra-ocular muscles designed to keep the eyes fixed in position despite changes in the head position. They keep the eyes in a vertical position with tilting of the head to the side, and looking at the horizon with ventral or dorsal tilting of the head.[4]

NYSTAGMUS

Nystagmus may be characterized by the rate (rapid or slow), amplitude (coarse or fine), direction (horizontal, vertical, or rotary), and type of movement (pendular or jerk). The jerk nystagmus, such as vestibular nystagmus, has a fast and slow component, whereas with pendular nystagmus the eye movements in each direction are equal. The direction of the jerk nystagmus is by convention named after the fast component. Most cases of nystagmus are conjugate, with both eyes beating in the same direction. A few examples of nystagmus are relatively specific for lesion localization; however, many neurologic forms of nystagmus are nonspecific for lesion localization. Some forms of jerk nystagmus can be overridden by moving the head. The latter are indicative of peripheral vestibular disease.[3]

A congenital horizontal pendular nystagmus or flutter may be present with cerebellar disease (cerebellar flocculi) or with congenital ocular anomalies such as microphthalmos.[1-4]

DIAGNOSTIC PLAN

The evaluation of ocular position with the eyes in the primary position (straight ahead) is performed by placing a light on the midline about 2 feet from the eyes and determining whether the specular light reflex from the corneal surface lies in relation to each respective pupil. With normal alignment (orthophoria) the light reflex falls in the center of the pupil or just medial to the center. Constriction of the pupil allows for more critical evaluation of the location of the corneal reflex in relation to the pupil. Dissimilar positions of the light reflex in relation to the pupil are indicative of strabismus. This technique can be utilized for evaluating horizontal or vertical misalignments. Misalignment in positions of gaze other than the primary position is determined by eliciting following eye movements in attentive animals. Paresis of muscle action is determined by utilizing the vestibular ocular reflex and observing for deficits in horizontal, vertical, and torsional movement. Torsional deficits are most readily determined in species with an elongated pupil. In the dog, finding a landmark on the ocular surface and observing the fundus vessels or the tapetal-nontapetal junction are means of determining torsional movements.

Determining whether the deviation is similar in different planes of eye movement is an attempt to differentiate comitant from noncomitant strabismus. Comitant strabismus is constant through-movement of the eyes in all the planes of movement. Noncomitant strabismus is also termed *paretic strabismus* and varies depending on whether the gaze is in the direction of the paretic muscle or nerve. Two separate phenomena occur to create paretic strabismus: (1) lag due to weakness and (2) overreaction due to increased neural impulses going to the yoke muscle. The amount of deviation varies depending on which eye is fixating.

Translational movement of the globe is determined by observing the animal from the dorsal view and determining whether the corneal apices are equal in prominence. The latter observation combined with retropulsion of the globe in the orbit determines the presence of an orbital space-occupying lesion. The ease with which one eye can be pushed into its orbit is compared with that of the other. Acquired exophthalmos must be differentiated from buphthalmos (enlarged globe), and shallow orbits (brachycephalic breed). Translational movement of the eye forward in the orbit is often combined with strabismus when due to space-occupying masses that are outside the extraocular muscle cone. The direction of deviation is typically away from the location of the space-occupying lesion. Examination of the oral cavity for pain on opening the mouth, tooth root abscessation, and swelling or fistulas behind the last molar is indicated with orbital space-occupying lesions. Additional evaluation of the orbit with radiographs, ultrasonography, and fine-needle aspiration of localized lesions is indicated. Positive and negative contrast studies of the orbital spaces may provide additional information to characterize the noninflammatory lesions, but most require surgical exploration and biopsy for definitive diagnosis. Bony orbital involvement radiographically is typical of secondary orbital tumors that have invaded from the frontal sinus or nasal cavity.

Nystagmus is evaluated as to whether it is directional and, if so, in what direction and whether it can be overridden by closing the eyes. The presence of accompanying neurologic signs or ear pathology is determined. Jerk nystagmus that is horizontal or rotary and cannot be overridden is indicative of peripheral vestibular disease; the fast phase is toward the normal side (assuming that a destructive lesion is present).[3]

REFERENCES

1. Cogan DG, Chu FC, Feingold DB: Ocular signs of cerebellar disease. Arch Ophthalmol 100:755, 1982
2. de Lahunta A: Cranial nerve—lower motor neuron: General somatic efferent system, special visceral efferent system. In Veterinary Neuroanatomy and Clinical Neurology, p 89. Philadelphia, WB Saunders, 1977
3. Oliver JE, Lorenz MD: Handbook of Veterinary Neurologic Diagnosis. Philadelphia: WB Saunders, 1977

4. Parks MM: Supranuclear centers and pathways of the eye movements. In Duane TD, Jaeger EA (eds): Clinical Ophthalmology. Philadelphia, Harper & Row, 1985

5. Parks MM: Extraocular muscles. In Duane TD, Jaeger EA (eds): Clinical Ophthalmology. Philadelphia, Harper & Row, 1985

6. Parks MM: Eye movement and positions. In: Duane TD, Jaeger EA (eds): Clinical Ophthalmology. Philadelphia, Harper & Row, 1985

7. Prince JH, Diesem CD, Eglitis I, Ruskell GL: Anatomy and Histology of the Eye and Orbit in Domestic Animals, p 577. Springfield, IL, CC Thomas, 1979

8. Scott AB: Ocular motility. In Records RE (ed): Physiology of the Human Visual System. Philadelphia, Harper & Row, 1979

CHAPTER FIFTY-FIVE

Red Watery Eyes

Charles L. Martin

PROBLEM DEFINITION AND RECOGNITION

The problem of the red eye may refer to intraocular, corneal, episcleral, or conjunctival redness. Because most conditions that cause redness produce irritation or pain, reflex lacrimation is common, resulting in a watery eye.

PATHOPHYSIOLOGY

To understand the genesis of bulbar hyperemia or congestion, the anatomy of the vascular system of the eye and conjunctiva should be reviewed. The iris and ciliary body are termed the *anterior uvea* and the choroid the *posterior uvea,* and together they form the vascular tunic of the eye. The posterior uveal arteries enter the eye around the optic nerve; they consist of numerous short posterior ciliary arteries and two long posterior ciliary arteries. The retinal arterioles are branches of the short posterior ciliary arteries. The long posterior ciliary arteries course forward from the optic nerve to supply the anterior uvea. The anterior uvea is also nourished by arterial branches from the rectus muscles. These branches form the anterior ciliary arteries, which penetrate the anterior sclera to supply the episclera, limbus, and anterior uvea (Fig. 55-1). The bulbar conjunctival arteries originate as branches from the rectus muscle arteries and the palpebral conjunctival arcades from arteries supplying the eyelids.[2,5]

The venous returns from the anterior and posterior uvea and sclera freely communicate with each other. The anterior uvea drains anteriorly into the scleral venous plexus and posteriorly into the vortex veins. The choroid drains into the vortex veins, and the vortex veins and scleral venous plexus freely communicate. The scleral venous plexus not only drains the anterior uvea but communicates with the vasculature of the bulbar conjunctiva, episclera, and limbus.[1-5]

The selective conjunctival congestion with glaucoma is in part due to stretching of the thin equatorial sclera and the resultant collapse of the posterior communicating intrascleral channels; more drainage is directed into the anterior venous system. Anterior uveitis produces prostaglandin-induced conjunctival hyperemia.

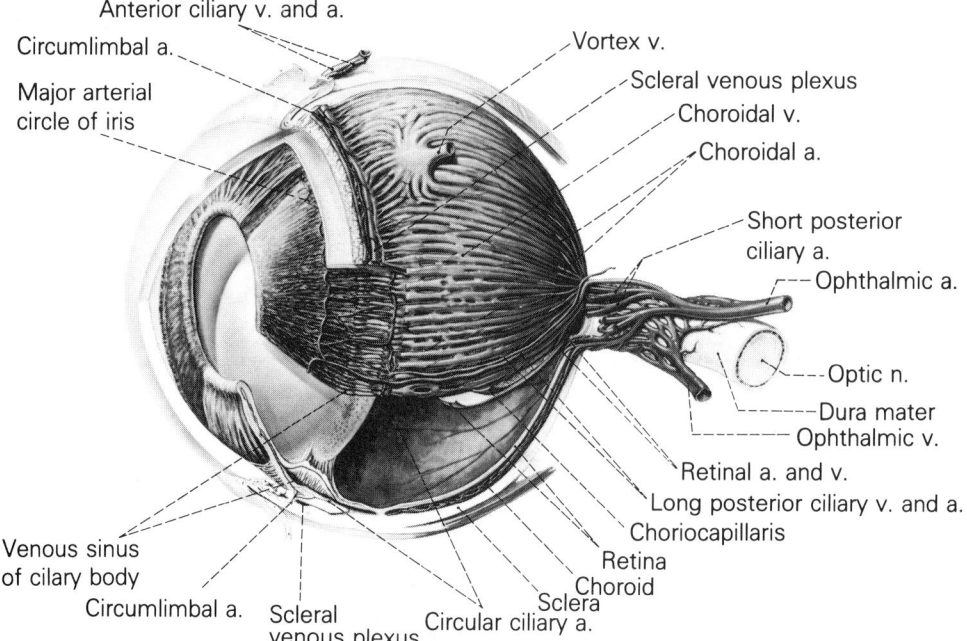

FIGURE 55-1. Vasculature of the canine eye.

RULE OUTS

Initially, redness should be categorized as intravascular or extravascular (hemorrhage), and as intraocular or on the ocular surface. Table 55-1 summarizes the rule outs for red eyes based on an anatomic diagnosis.

Intraocular Redness

Localization of intraocular redness requires differentiation of vitreal from aqueous hemorrhage, intraocular hemorrhage from intense corneal vascularization, and a normal nonpigmented atapetal fundus with a red reflection from hemorrhage. Vitreal hemorrhage is located behind the plane of the pupil, and all three of the Purkinje-Sanson images (cornea, anterior lens capsule, posterior lens capsule) are present. If the vitreous is liquefied (syneresis) the blood will be diffuse, but if it is a gel, the hemorrhage will be confined into discrete clots.

Hyphema, or hemorrhage, into the aqueous may be partial or complete, and clotted or liquefied. Hyphema obscures the iris to variable degrees. As the hemorrhage ages it becomes darker (eight-ball hemorrhage) and may, particularly with increased intraocular pressure, cause blood staining of the cornea. Severe blood staining of the inner cornea may be difficult to differentiate from simple hyphema without the aid of a slit lamp.

Determination of the etiology of intraocular hemorrhage is based on history,

TABLE 55-1.   Rule Outs for Red Eyes

Intraocular redness
  Hyphema
  Vitreous hemorrhage
  Normal albinotic fundus reflex
Ocular surface redness
  Conjunctivitis
  Subconjunctival hemorrhage
  Episcleritis/scleritis
  Prolapse of the third eyelid or its gland
  Corneal granulation/neovascularization, hemorrhage
  Superficial keratitis, such as pannus
  Corneal ulceration induced conjunctival hyperemia and corneal neovascularization,
    granulation
  Corneal neoplasia
  Anterior uveitis
  Glaucoma

ocular examination (both eyes), physical examination, and laboratory evaluation. Before diagnosing trauma-induced hemorrhage, a *definite* history of trauma
or choking and/or other evidence of trauma to the head, such as skin abrasions,
should be present.

Congenital ocular anomalies, such as the collie eye anomaly, persistent hyperplastic primary vitreous anomaly, or cardiac anomaly that induces cyanosis
with secondary polycythemia, may cause spontaneous intraocular hemorrhage.
If the underlying lesion is obscured by hemorrhage, its presence is inferred by
finding an anomaly in the opposite eye.

Ocular neovascularization is fragile and may spontaneously hemorrhage.
Uveitis and neoplasia-induced neovascularization should be ruled out as a cause
of spontaneous ocular hemorrhage. Primary ocular neoplasia is unilateral,
whereas secondary neoplasia is frequently bilateral. Ocular neoplasia is frequently masked by hemorrhage, inflammation, and glaucoma late in its course.
Previous degenerative conditions such as absolute glaucoma may develop spontaneous intraocular hemorrhage, as may eyes after therapy for glaucoma (in-
travitreal injections of gentamicin or cyclocryotherapy).

A physical examination should detect additional evidence of trauma, bleeding
or clotting disorders, systemic infections, and conditions associated with hypertension, hypervolemia, or hyperviscosity syndromes. Multiple hemorrhages or
those without an obvious cause should prompt laboratory evaluation for a blood
dyscrasia, clotting disorder, or vasculitis.

Ocular Surface Redness

Redness on or around the eye is the most common cause of the red eye problem.
Exophthalmic breeds have more exposed conjunctiva to observe, and individu-

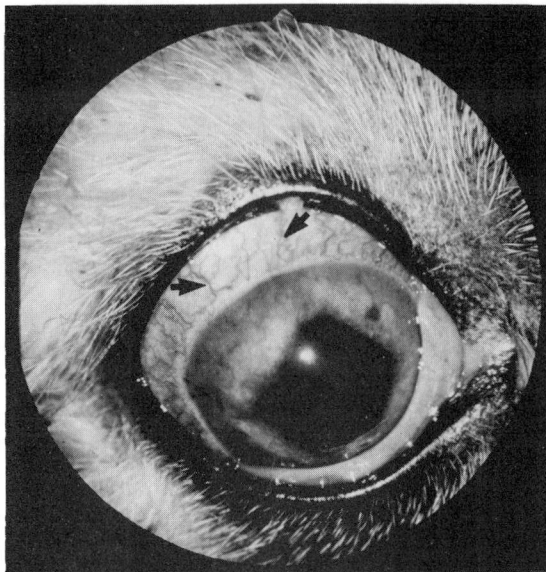

FIGURE 55-2. Selective bulbar conjunctival congestion (*arrows*) typical of anterior uveitis and glaucoma. The eye has a secondary glaucoma and an iris bombé associated with lymphosarcoma.

als in all breeds may lack pigmentation of the third eyelid and conjunctiva, giving the impression of increased redness. The three most common rule outs for bulbar conjunctival congestion are *conjunctivitis, anterior uveities (iritis, iridocyclitis), and glaucoma.* A fourth, less common, but sometimes difficult rule out is that of episcleritis/scleritis.

Bulbar conjunctival vascular injection can be either diffuse with capillary and large-vessel injection, or selective with only large-vessel injection. Intraocular diseases such as uncomplicated glaucoma and anterior uveitis characteristically have injection of the large conjunctival vessels as well as deep episcleral injection (Fig. 55-2). Conjunctivitis typically has a diffuse engorgement resulting

TABLE 55-2. Etiologies of Conjunctivitis and Diagnostic Testing

Etiology	Diagnostic Test(s)
Bacteria	Culture, cytology
Virus	Cytology, FA testing, systemic signs
Chlamydia	Cytology, response to tetracyclines
Tear deficiency	Schirmer tear test, rose bengal staining
Mechanical irritation	Examination with magnification, eversion of lids, history
Chemical irritation	History
Allergy	History, cytology, physical examination

FA, fluorescent antibody

TABLE 55-3. Etiologies for Anterior Uveitis

Etiology	Diagnostic Test(s)
Trauma	
Blunt	History, contusions
Perforating	Examination for full-thickness injury to cornea or sclera
Sterile or septic	Aqueous centesis—cytology, culture
Systemic infectious agents	
Dog	
Ehrlichia canis	Titers, blood smear
Rocky Mountain spotted fever	Titers, FA on skin biopsy
Infectious hepatitis	CBC, liver enzymes, history
Systemic mycoses	Titers, chest x-rays, needle biopsy, vitreous centesis
Aberrant parasites	Observation, removal and identification
Bacterial septicemia	Blood culture
Brucella canis	Titer, aqueous and blood culture
Leishmaniasis	Cytology, bone marrow
Prototothecosis	Vitreous centesis—cytology
Toxoplasmosis	Serum/aqueous titer—IgG, IgM
Cat	
Feline leukemia virus	FeLV testing
Infectious peritonitis	FIP titers, systemic signs, serum proteins
Feline immunodeficiency virus	FIV testing
Systemic mycoses	Titers, ocular centesis with cytology, bone marrow
Toxoplasmosis	Titer, biopsy
Sterile immune-mediated	
Phacoanaphylaxis	Aqueous cytology, history of injury
Phacogenic	Mature to hypermature cataract
VKH-like syndrome	Dermal depigmentation, breed
Idiopathic	Exclusion of other etiologies
	Sterile ocular fluid, cytology
Neoplasia	
Primary	Unilateral, observation of mass, ultrasonography, cytology, biopsy
Secondary	Often bilateral, observation of mass, cytology, physical examination, and history

FA, fluorescent antibody; CBC, complete blood count; FeLV, feline leukemia virus; FIP, feline infectious peritonitis; VKH, Vogt-Koyanagi-Harada

TABLE 55-4. Etiologies of Glaucoma

Etiology	Diagnostic Test(s)
Primary closed angle	Gonioscopy of both eyes
Primary open angle	Gonioscopy
Lens displacement	Lens in anterior chamber, aphakic crescent, gonioscopy
Intumescent cataract	Mature swollen cataract, shallow anterior chamber
Inflammation	Observation of synechia, iris bombé, gonioscopy, flare, keratic precipitates
Neoplasia	Observation of mass or infiltration, aqueous cytology, biopsy
Hyphema	Anterior chamber 3/4 full of blood

from dilation of capillaries between the larger vessels. Episcleritis is often focal or sectorial and nodular or elevated and produces conjunctival and deep episcleral injection similar to intraocular disease. Tables 55-2, 55-3, and 55-4 list etiologic rule outs for the anatomic diagnosis of conjunctivitis, anterior uveitis, and glaucoma.

The causes of bulbar conjunctival and episcleral injection must be differentiated to avoid undertreatment. Anterior uveitis and glaucoma often result in blindness, and misdiagnosing and treating the patient as for a conjunctivitis may be catastrophic for vision. Additionally, the therapies for glaucoma and anterior uveitis may be diametrically opposite, so an accurate diagnosis is critical.

Glaucoma and anterior uveitis, being intraocular diseases, are rarely presented with only the problem of ocular redness. Additional problems of corneal clarity, changes in pupil size and function, ocular enlargement, and changes in ocular pressure are usually present, whereas they are absent with conjunctivitis. Some forms of scleritis are very invasive and may result in intraocular signs, but a proliferative lesion on the scleral surface is usually present.

Subconjunctival hemorrhage presents as a red eye, but the blood is extravascular rather than intravascular. A simple subconjunctival hemorrhage should be differentiated from the more serious retrobulbar hemorrhage that has migrated forward. The latter will exhibit proptosis and decreased orbital compressibility on retropulsion of the eye.

DIAGNOSTIC PLAN

Determining the source of the redness, *i.e.*, conjunctival, corneal, or intraocular, is the initial step. A diagnostic plan for conjunctival redness is given in Table 55-5. If one investigates beyond the redness for intraocular signs, the risk of "underdiagnosing" a conjunctivitis should be minimal. As anterior uveitis fre-

TABLE 55-5. Diagnostic Plan for Red Eye

Diagnostic Plan	Anatomic Diagnosis				
	Conjunctivitis	Glaucoma	Anterior Uveitis	Episcleritis	Keratitis
Conjunctival injection					
Examine for diffuse or selective large-vessel injection.	Diffuse	Usually selective	Usually selective	Selective	Usually diffuse
Examine intraocular structures, pupil size and symmetry, iris color and texture, and aqueous flare.	Normal	Anisocoria, dilated, fixed flare ±	Anisocoria, constricted, irregular, darker, flare ±	Normal	May be miotic if ulcerative
Schirmer tear test / Topical anesthesia	↑ or ↓	Normal or ↑	Normal or ↑	Normal or ↑	↑ or ↓
Fluorescein stain	Normal	Normal	Normal	Normal	+ if ulcer
Measure IOP	Normal	↑	↓	Normal or ↓	Normal
Conjunctival cytology	Neutrophils, lymphocytes, inclusions ±	Normal	Normal	± Altered	± Altered

±, may or may not be present; ↑, increase; ↓, decrease; IOP, intraocular pressure quently precipitates or results in glaucoma, the diagnosis may be a complex of anterior uveitis and glaucoma.

REFERENCES

1. Martin C: Gonioscopy and anatomical correlations of the drainage angle of the dog. J Sm Anim Pract 10:171, 1969
2. Martin C, Anderson B: Ocular Anatomy in Veterinary Ophthalmology. In Gelatt K (ed): Philadelphia, Lea & Febiger, 1981
3. Troncosco MU: The intrascleral vascular plexus and its relations to the aqueous outflow. Am J Ophthalmol 25:1153, 1942
4. Van Buskirk M: The canine eye: The vessels of aqueous drainage. Invest Ophthalmol Vis Sci 18:223, 1979
5. Wong V, Macri F: Vasculature of the cat eye. Arch Ophthalmol 72:351, 1964

CHAPTER FIFTY-SIX

Ocular Pain and Blepharospasm

Charles L. Martin

PROBLEM DEFINITION AND RECOGNITION

The manifestation of ocular pain may be quite variable. Blepharospasm is an obvious manifestation of pain that brings immediate attention to the eye, but behavioral alterations distant from the eye are frequently not appreciated as having a causal relationship with the eye. Behavior alterations of sleeping excessively, hiding, decreased appetite, loss of playfulness, and worsening of disposition are often more subtle manifestations of ocular discomfort. The correlation of these subtle manifestations to ocular disease is often retrospective, once the animal has returned to its "normal" behavior.

PATHOPHYSIOLOGY

The sensory innervation to the cornea, conjunctiva, and uveal tract is the ophthalmic division of cranial nerve V (trigeminal). The cornea and the anus contain the most pain fibers of any areas of the body. The iris, ocular muscles, and optic nerve sheaths have marked pain sensation, whereas the retina, lens, and optic nerve have no pain sensation and the sclera has very minimal amounts. The pain from corneal and conjunctival stimulation is sharp, localized, and described as a foreign-body sensation, whereas pain from the iris and ciliary body is deep-seated, throbing and often radiates over the head to other regions innervated by the cranial nerve V.[2]

Corneal innervation is from two long posterior ciliary nerves that arborize in the anterior one-third of the cornea. The nerves lose their myelin sheath after entering the cornea and branch extensively, ending as single axons between the superficial epithelial cells. In comparison, the posterior cornea is poorly innervated. The clinical correlation is that a superficial corneal abrasion is typically more painful than the deep ulcer or descemetocele. The severe pain of a superficial ulcer may initiate an antidromic reflex manifested as a strong miosis and hyperemia of the conjunctiva and anterior uvea. This results in additional pain from vasodilation-induced ciliary muscle spasm. Topical atropine counteracts the ciliary muscle spasm of the antidromic reflex and thus decreases some of the discomfort associated with a corneal ulcer. The mediators of the antidromic reflex are thought to be substance P and calcitonin gene-related peptide.[2] These neuropeptide actions may be facilitated by prostaglandins. Atropine, prostaglandin inhibitors, and sympathetic denervation do not block the acute reflex when stimulated by chemical injury.[1]

Ocular pain can be aggravated by bright light. Photophobia may be present with corneal ulcers and anterior uveitis and results in additional ciliary muscle spasms. Corneal sensitivity may vary among breeds and individuals. "Old-World breeds," such as chows, Siberian huskies, and Samoyeds, are quite "eye-conscious" and readily develop blepharospasm with ocular pain. The triad of blepharospasm, prolapsed third eyelid, and retraction of the globe into the orbit can make ocular examination extremely difficult. Topical anesthesia facilitates examination in an animal with blepharospasm, but extreme examples may require regional anesthesia of the palpebral branch of the facial nerve, sedation, or occasionally general anesthesia.

RULE OUTS

Corneal Pain

All animals with blepharospasm should have fluorescein stain applied to the cornea to rule out corneal ulcers or abrasions. Only after eliminating corneal ulceration as the cause of the blepharospasm should the examiner feel confident in diagnosing other sources of ocular pain. If corneal ulceration, abrasions, erosions, or lacerations are present, the subsequent step is to search for a physical cause. These may vary from conformational faults to foreign bodies, and they may be obvious or very difficult to detect. Certain aspects of the ocular examination should be emphasized when one searches for a physical irritant: examining the unrestrained head for conformation, examining before and after topical anesthesia (occasionally after palpebral nerve block), examining with magnification (5 × or more), and everting the lids and third eyelid to visualize all conjunctival surfaces and cul-de-sacs. Following these guidelines minimizes the possibility of overlooking a physical cause for corneal pain.

Keratitis that is not associated with corneal ulcerations or anterior uveitis does not usually manifest with blepharospasm. Stromal keratitis is usually an extension of anterior uveitis, and discomfort is probably the result of ciliary spasm.

Conjunctival Pain

The degree of discomfort manifested with conjunctivitis varies among individuals, species, and causes. Cats manifest blepharospasm with conjunctivitis more consistently than dogs. In general, marked blepharospasm should not be attributed to conjunctivitis.

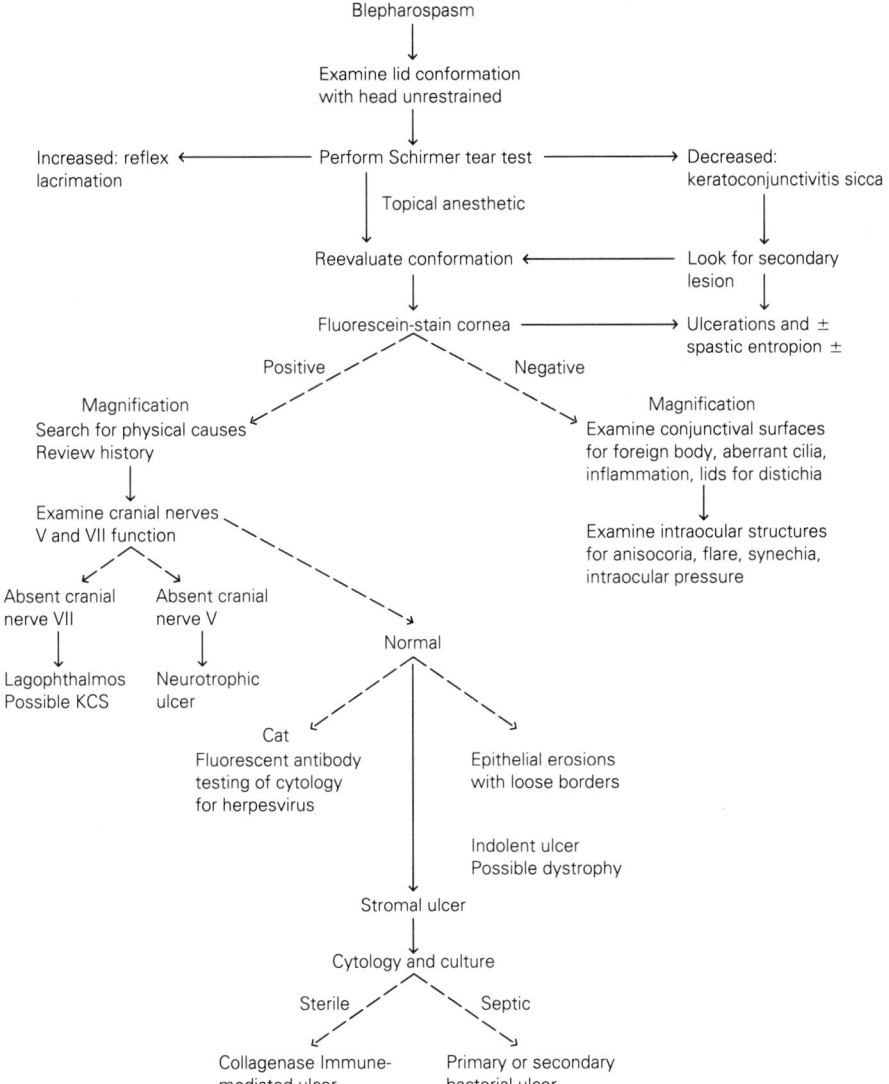

FIGURE 56-1. Diagnostic plan for blepharospasm.

Intraocular Pain

Animals with acute anterior uveitis and glaucoma are more likely to have blepharospasm and photophobia than animals with their chronic counterparts. Chronic anterior uveitis and glaucoma can be assumed to produce a deep-seated discomfort because mental status and activity typically improve when the conditions are corrected. The owners rarely appreciate the behavioral manifestations of pain.

Pure posterior ocular segment disease does not usually manifest pain. Inflammatory disease of the posterior uvea may cause discomfort, but as some degree of anterior uveal involvement is usually present, it is difficult to isolate the origin of the pain. Although clinically blind, optic neuritis patients seem photophobic to a strong examination light, and movements that stretch the inflamed nerve and meningeal sheaths produce discomfort. Some of the patients with optic neuritis also have other neurologic lesions, so it may be difficult to attribute mental depression, for example, to ocular pain. Figure 56-1 presents a diagnostic flow chart that may be used in evaluating ocular pain.

REFERENCES

1. Unger WG: Review: Mediation of the ocular response to injury. J Ocular Pharmacol 6:337, 1990
2. Waltman SR: The cornea. In Moses RA (ed): Adler's Physiology of the Eye: Clinical Application, 7th ed. St Louis, CV Mosby, 1981

CHAPTER FIFTY-SEVEN

Abnormal Cornea and Lens

Charles L. Martin

PROBLEM DEFINITION AND RECOGNITION

Corneal abnormalities are common, easily visible to the owner, and often secondary to lid conformational defects in many breeds. Problems of the lens are also common, since several popular breeds have inherited cataracts that lead to complete lenticular opacification. Because the cornea and lens are unique in their transparency, the most common sign of disease is opacification.

PATHOPHYSIOLOGY

Corneal Abnormalities

The most common problems of the cornea are changes in clarity or color, changes in smoothness or regularity, and combinations of those two types.

Corneal clarity and color may be altered by edema, vascularization, pigmentation infiltrates of leukocytes, deposits of lipids or calcium, and lack of smoothness. The normal cornea remains clear because of a combination of unique anatomic and physiologic features. The cornea normally lacks blood vessels and pigment that would obviously hinder transparency. The collagen lamellae of the stroma are arranged in a uniform parallel fashion; the fibrils are at a distance that produces mutual interference of light rays, and consequently light rays are not scattered.[12] The corneal stroma has a high water content (78%) that is attributed to hydrophilic nature of glycosaminoglycans that surround the collagen fibrils. The stroma has an affinity for even more water but is kept in a state of relative dehydration, despite being bathed in aqueous solutions, by the corneal endothelium and epithelium. The endothelium has an ATPase-activated Na/Cl pump that removes water from the stroma. In addition, on exposure to air the tear film becomes hypertonic, creating an osmotic gradient across the epithelium that draws water out of the cornea.[5] Loss of either the endothelium or epithelium results in increased stromal water or edema. The resultant stromal swelling results in disruption of the normal regular arrangement of the collagen lamellae and consequent scattering of light with opacification. Corneal edema is most marked with endothelial loss or dysfunction. In adults of most species, the endothelium has limited mitotic capability, and the dysfunction is often permanent.

The lack of corneal blood vessels or, conversely, the stimulus for neovascularization is incompletely understood. The inducement of corneal angiogenesis is mediated by chemical messengers, and morphologic features, such as tissue compactness, are probably of minor importance.[6] Corneal pigmentation is usually due to the migration of limbal melanocytes with corneal blood vessels.[1]

The smooth surface of the cornea is produced by the tear film filling small irregularities in the surface epithelium. The epithelial surface is hydrophobic, and the mucin layer on its surface is necessary in order for the aqueous phase of the tears to form a stable film. A lack of mucin results in the break-up of the aqueous phase and a dry irregular cornea.[10]

Breaks in the corneal epithelium are usually painful because of the concentration of nerve endings in the superficial cornea. Epithelial defects are detected by the retention of fluorescein stain. The aqueous fluorescein will not be retained by the intact epithelium, which is lipophilic, but diffuses into the hydrophilic stroma if an epithelial defect is present.

Lens Changes

The lens has the highest protein content of any tissue in the body (33%).[11] The proteins consist of water-soluble crystallins and water-insoluble albuminoids. The young lens is predominantly composed of crystallins, which shift with age to increasing amounts of albuminoids. The lens is also unique in its lack of vascularity, glycolytic energy metabolism, and high glutathione levels.[2] Lens fiber development occurs from an epithelial layer that lines the anterior capsule. Lens fibers are formed by the epithelium at the equator of the lens with successive new fibers pushing and condensing the older fibers toward the center of the lens (nucleus). This results in the newest fibers being present in the outer or superficial layers (cortex). The lens grows most rapidly, and increases in size, in the young dog. Later in life, new fiber formation persists, but the lens becomes denser from compacting rather than dramatically increasing in size. This increase in density is responsible for the grey haze of nuclear sclerosis that becomes manifest in the dog by 7 to 8 years of age. Vision is not significantly impaired with nuclear sclerosis, and this physiologic process should be distinguished from the pathologic process of senile cataracts.

Cataracts such as those induced by elevated glucose and galactase are initiated by a metabolic imbalance that produces an osmotic accumulation of water in the lens and subsequent scattering of light.[9] The initial vacuolar changes may be reversible, but if left unchecked they result in protein aggregation, which is not considered reversible.

Cataracts secondary to inflammation are thought to originate from a break-

TABLE 57-1. Prognosis for Cataracts Based on Anatomic Site of Involvement

Site	Prognosis
Anterior and posterior capsule	Usually nonprogressive
Fetal nuclear	Nonprogressive
Nuclear	Often static, may reduce in size with age
Sutures	Usually nonprogressive
Anterior and posterior cortex	Variable, most will progress
Equator	Usually progressive
Posterior axial subcapsule	Usually nonprogressive

(Modified from Gelatt K: Lens and cataract formation in the dog. Comp Cont Ed 1:175–180, 1979)

down of the blood-aqueous barrier that allows increased levels of plasma phospholipids, such as lysophosphatidyl choline, into the aqueous humor. Lysophosphatidyl choline then diffuses into the lens and lyses membranes of lens fibers.[3]

Many of the cataracts in dogs have a genetic origin, and their mechanism of formation is unknown.

The classification of cataracts can be based on age of onset, etiology, degree of opacification, location within the lens, and description of the opacity or on combinations of two or more of these classifications. Cataracts are described by age as congenital, neonatal, juvenile or developmental (up to 5 to 6 years), and senile or degenerative. Cataracts are described by degree of opacity as incipient (small, not outwardly visible), immature (severe, but with incomplete opacity and fundus reflex still visible), mature (swollen lens with complete opacification), and hypermature (late stages with shrinkage due to reabsorption of water). Anatomic descriptions are anterior and/or posterior, cortical or nuclear, capsular, equatorial, suture, and fetal nuclear. The location of the opacity may help to determine a prognosis and to date the onset of the injury, in lieu of considering the mechanism of lens growth (Table 57-1).

The etiologies of cataract formation are broadly categorized into genetic, metabolic, nutritional, traumatic, inflammatory, toxic, and radiation-induced. All are relatively common causes of cataracts in the dog except for toxicity and radiation. Species vary widely in the relative importance of the etiologies. Cats have comparatively few genetic cataracts and are resistant to diabetes mellitus–induced cataracts.[13] Intraocular inflammation is the most common cause of lenticular opacities in the cat.

Lens dislocations may occur from familial zonular defects, zonular degenerative changes, zonular ruptures from stretching with buphthalmos, and traumatic rupture. The latter is the least common etiology for lens dislocation. Zonular defects are most common in terrier breeds, but they have been observed in a wide variety of breeds in which they manifest as an eventual bilateral spontaneous displacement in a previously healthy eye.[4,7] A biochemical defect has not been identified in the dog with spontaneous lens displacements. Advancing cataracts may spontaneously dislocate as a result of concurrent degenerative changes in the capsular-zonular attachments, or in association with inflammatory cells digesting the zonules.[8,11] The increased globe circumference with buphthalmos is usually accompanied by a partial rupture of the zonules and some degree of lens displacement. While explosive traumatic ruptures of the globe frequently dislocate the lens or expel it from the eye, trauma without a loss of integrity of the fibrous ocular tunic is an uncommon cause of lens dislocation.

The lens may partially dislocate (subluxate) to either side or up and down, fall posteriorly into the ventral vitreous (posterior luxation), or move through the pupil into the anterior chamber (anterior luxation). The anterior luxations are most consistently symptomatic with a secondary glaucoma and corneal edema from touching the endothelium.

RULE OUTS

Corneal Disease

Corneal disease is frequently part of an intraocular process, and the latter should be ruled out for accurate therapy and prognosis. Chronic anterior uveitis eventually induces a deep stromal keratitis; anterior chamber fibrin, keratic precipitates, anterior luxated lenses, and glaucoma often compromise the corneal endothelium, resulting in corneal edema. Table 57-2 lists a variety of known causes for white corneal opacifications. Subtle corneal opacities are commonly observed, and their histopathologic corollary is usually unknown. Corneal edema is a common cause of white opacification, and the more common rule outs are given in Table 57-3.

Corneal pigmentation is stimulated by chronic keratitis with neovascularization. Corneal pigmentation due to a focal irritant such as trichiasis is limited to the area of corneal contact by the irritant, whereas that associated with diffuse keratitis from immune-mediated causes or keratoconjunctivitis sicca is progressive and diffuse. A second source of corneal pigment is from the anterior uvea,

---

TABLE 57-2.   Rule Outs for White Corneal Opacities

Stromal scar
Lipid accumulation—may be associated with stromal scar
Calcium—may be associated with stromal scar
Mucopolysaccharidosis—rare
Edema
Leukocyte infiltrates
Mycotic plaques
Descemet's membrane abnormalities—persistent pupillary membrane syndrome, anterior synechia
Inclusion cyst—rare

TABLE 57-3. Rule Outs for Causes of Corneal Edema

Epithelial ulceration
Endothelial dysfunction
  Anterior luxated lens
  Glaucoma
  Endothelial dystrophy—congenital (persistent pupillary membrane syndrome), senile
  Trauma
  Anterior uveitis
    Keratic precipitates
    Fibrin
    Anterior synechia
  Endotheliitis—autoimmune mediated?

which may leave deposits on the endothelial surface from anterior synechiae (congenital or acquired), ruptured iris cysts, and pigment dispersion with anterior uveitis.

Rule outs for a red proliferation on the cornea are given in Table 57-4. The most common cause of corneal irregularities is either extraneous mucus and hair on the surface or an ulcer. Proliferative lesions produce elevated irregularities. Etiologic rule outs for corneal ulceration are given in Table 57-5.

Lens Abnormalities

Opacities in the aqueous or vitreous may be confused with a cataract. Lipids or fibrin in the aqueous may simulate a cataract or an anteriorly luxated cataract on cursory examination. Congenital hyperplastic primary vitreal remnants, inflammatory clots, or fibrous proliferations in the anterior vitreous may be difficult to distinguish from a posterior cortical cataract. Quivering or movement of the opacity with ocular movement usually indicates the lens is loose in the vitreous, but a subluxated lens will exhibit phakodonesis (tremors of the lens).

The level of involvement of the opacity within the eye and within the lens is most accurately determined with a slit lamp (biomicroscope). A focal beam of light passing through the eye and observed from the side may suffice for

TABLE 57-4. Rule Outs for Proliferative Red Corneal Lesions

Superficial keratitis (pannus)
Corneal granulation in a healing ulcer
Fibrous histiocytoma—often in collies
Intense neovascularization, intrastromal hemorrhage
Hemangiosarcoma
Squamous cell carcinoma
Papilloma

TABLE 57-5. Rule Outs for Corneal Ulceration

Mechanical irritation
  Distichia, trichiasis, aberrant cilia, entropion, foreign body, dermoid
Trauma
Keratoconjunctivitis sicca
Epithelial bulla rupturing from corneal edema
Lagophthalmos: Results in trauma and focal keratoconjunctivitis sicca
                Shallow orbits
                Seventh cranial nerve paralysis
Neurotropic—cranial nerve V paralysis
Chemical injury—soaps, acids, alkalines
Viral—herpes in cats
Basal lamina defects—slowly healing epithelial erosions

lesion localization by determining where the opacity intercepts the light. The Purkinje-Sanson images will aid gross lesion localization. These images are three reflections from the optical interfaces that are observed when a light is projected into the eye. The first reflection is bright and arises from the anterior cornea, the second reflection is less bright and arises from the anterior lens capsule, and the third is dimmest and arises from the posterior lens capsule. Opacities can be localized by noting which images they obscure.

The genetic etiology of cataracts is frequently presumed from observing a certain type of lenticular opacity in a breed with a known defect. In most instances genetic cataracts are eventually bilateral in their involvement, but not symmetric as to time and degree of involvement of each eye. Trauma should be ruled out as an etiology for unilateral cataracts, but its effect may be nebulous, except with penetrating injuries. Cataracts of sudden onset with rapid progression should alert the examiner to consider diabetes mellitus as an etiology, but this history is not usual with the more common genetic cataracts. Many of the diabetic patients are also ketotic, and smelling the breath may be a rapid means of making a presumptive diagnosis. Large-breed dogs, particularly hunting breeds, presented with extensive cataracts usually have diabetes mellitus, retinal atrophy, or intraocular inflammation, rather than simple genetic cataracts. A blood glucose test and electroretinogram are routine preoperative screening tests to rule out complicating factors in a blind patient with mature cataracts.

Cataracts may stimulate inflammation (phakogenic uveitis) or be caused by intraocular inflammation (secondary cataract). Differentiation may often be made by the location of the cataract and examination of the opposite eye. Phakogenic uveitis is associated with advancing cataracts in the mature to hypermature stages. An advanced cataract with inflammation in one eye and a cataract with no inflammation in the opposite eye are presumptive evidence of phakogenic uveitis. A cataract secondary to uveitis typically has capsular and posterior subcapsular involvement.

REFERENCES

1. Bellhorn R, Henkind P: Superficial pigmentary keratitis in the dog. J Am Vet Med Assoc 149:173, 1966
2. Cotlier E: The lens. In Moses RA (ed): Adler's Physiology of the Eye: Clinical Application. St Louis, CV Mosby, 1981
3. Cotlier E, Baskin M, Kim JO, et al: Lysophosphatidyl choline and cataract uveitis. Arch Ophthalmol 94:1159, 1976
4. Curtis R, Barnett K: Primary lens luxation in the dog. J Anim Pract 21:657, 1980
5. Davson H: Physiology of the Eye. In Davson H (ed): Cornea, 5th ed. New York, Pergamon Press, 105, 1990
6. Ezra DB: Neovasculogenesis. Triggering factors and possible mechanisms. Surv Ophthalmol 24:167, 1979
7. Formston C: Observations on subluxation and luxation of the crystalline lens in the dog. J Comp Path 55:168, 1945
8. Gwin R, Samuelson D, Powell G, et al: Primary lens luxation in the dog associated with lenticular zonule degeneration and its relationship to glaucoma. J Am Anim Hosp Assoc 18:485, 1982
9. Kinoshita JH: Mechanisms initiating cataract formation. Invest Ophthalmol Vis Sci 13:713, 1974
10. Lemp M, Holly F, Iwata S, Dohlman C: The precorneal tear film: I. The factors in spreading and maintaining a continuous tear film over the corneal surface. Arch Ophthalmol 83:89, 1970
11. Martin C: Zonular defects in the dog: A clinical and scanning electron microscopic study. J Am Anim Hosp Assoc 14:571, 1978
12. Maurice DM: The structure and transparency of the cornea. Physiol 136:263, 1957
13. Schaer M: A clinical survey of thirty cats with diabetes mellitus. J Am Anim Hosp Assoc 13:23, 1977

CHAPTER FIFTY-EIGHT

Loss of Sense of Smell

John E. Oliver

PROBLEM DEFINITION AND RECOGNITION

The sense of smell (olfaction) is highly developed in dogs and cats. Dogs can detect some odors at 1/100 the concentration detectable by human beings.[5] The use of dogs for hunting, tracking, and seeking out drugs and explosives exploits this natural ability. Loss of the sense of smell (anosmia) is an uncommon complaint, although it probably occurs frequently. Unless the animal is used in one of the ways mentioned, the owner is unlikely to know that anosmia is present. Cats commonly quit eating when they have an upper respiratory infection, which may be in part from anosmia.[9] The most frequent clinical patient is the hunting dog.[4]

PATHOPHYSIOLOGY

The primary olfactory receptors are in the olfactory epithelium in the nasal mucosa at the caudal part of the nasal cavity.[2] The receptor cell is a bipolar neuron that acts as a chemoreceptor. Cilia projecting from the receptor cell are covered with secretion. Chemical substances (olfactants) dissolved in the secretion stimulate the cell. The axons of the olfactory neurons penetrate the cribriform plate of the ethmoid bone and form the olfactory nerve (cranial nerve I), which synapses on cells in the olfactory bulbs. Axons project from the olfactory bulbs to the cortex of the pyriform lobe. Connections are made to parts of the limbic system for behavioral reactions.[2]

A second olfactory system originates in the vomeronasal organ on the floor of the nasal cavity. It communicates with the oral cavity by the incisive duct.[3] The vomeronasal organ varies in size and function among species, but it is relatively well developed in dogs and cats. The vomeronasal nerves extend caudally to penetrate the cribriform plate and synapse on the accessory olfactory bulb. This system senses chemical stimuli important for sexual behavior in many species.[1,7]

A third system, through the trigeminal nerve (cranial nerve V), originates from the nasal mucosa. It is probably more sensitive to irritating substances. Although each of these systems is most sensitive to specific substances, it is probably impossible to stimulate only one system.[8]

Lesions of the epithelium, olfactory bulbs, or central pathways can affect the sense of smell. Diseases in the nasal cavity that affect the olfactory receptors in the epithelium are most common.[4,10] Receptor cells can regenerate from other receptor cells, which can be important in the prognosis of diseases that destroy part, but not all, of the receptor cells.[8]

DIAGNOSTIC PLAN

Proving that an animal has anosmia can be difficult. Simple tests involve presenting a noxious or rewarding odor and observing for a behavioral response. Food under a cover may be tried, preferably at home when the animal is more likely to respond normally. Hunters may recognize the loss of the sense of smell in a trained dog, but it is important to evaluate the animal carefully for other problems that may affect hunting performance.[9] Noxious odors that are recommended include cloves, alcohol, garlic, perfume, and a variety of chemicals. Eugenol is reported to be relatively specific for the olfactory receptors.[12] Newer tests using electrophysiologic techniques look promising for providing objective evidence of the function of the olfactory receptors.[9-12]

Functional anosmia can occur after exposure to some substances. Hunting dogs carried in the trunk of a car may have temporary anosmia, presumably from exposure to exhaust fumes.[4]

Anosmia can be caused by lesions of the nasal cavity or the brain (Table 58-1). The history, physical examination, and neurologic examination should identify one of these two sources. Nasal lesions usually cause sneezing, nasal discharge, difficult and noisy respiration, pawing at the nose, or deformity of the nasal or paranasal structures.[13] Lesions of the brain that affect the sense of

TABLE 58-1.   Etiology of Anosmia

Category	Nasal Cavity	Nervous System
Metabolic		Diabetes mellitus Hypoadrenocorticism Hypothyroidism
Inflammatory	Viral, bacterial, protozoal, and fungal infections	Viral, bacterial, protozoal, and fungal infections
Neoplastic	Adenocarcinoma Other tumors	Tumors near olfactory bulbs, usually meningiomas
Traumatic	Obstruction of airflow	Minor trauma, shearing of olfactory nerve Major trauma, direct damage to olfactory nerve, tracts, or cortex
Functional	Saturation of olfactory epithelium, temporary	

smell will usually cause behavioral abnormality, depression, seizures, compulsive pacing, or visual deficits.[6,14] Tumors or chronic infections can extend from the nasal cavity through the cribriform plate into the brain. Head trauma can cause shearing of the olfactory nerve, even when the trauma is not severe.

Supportive information on nasal lesions is obtained from hematology and serum chemistries, radiographs of the nose, cytologic and microbiologic examination of nasal secretions, and rhinoscopy. Both the rostral and caudal portions of the nasal cavity can be examined with fiberoptic endoscopes.[13] Brain lesions may require computed tomographic scans for confirmation.[14]

REFERENCES

1. Beaver B: Veterinary Aspects of Feline Behavior. St Louis, CV Mosby, 1980
2. De Lahunta A: Veterinary Neuroanatomy and Clinical Neurology, 2nd ed. Philadelphia, WB Saunders, 1983
3. Evans HE, Christensen GC: Miller's Anatomy of the Dog. Philadelphia, WB Saunders, 1979
4. Holloway CL: Loss of olfactory acuity in hunting animals. Auburn Vet 18:25–28, 1961
5. Houpt KA, Wolski TR: Domestic Animal Behavior for Veterinarians and Animal Scientists. Ames, IA, Iowa State University Press, 1982
6. Hutchison CP, Buxton DF, Garrett PD: Anatomic basis for the examination of olfactory and visual cranial nerve function in dogs. Comp Cont Ed Pract Vet 6:751–765, 1984
7. Ladewig J, Hart BL: Flehmen and vomeronasal organ function in male goats. Physiol Behav 24:1067–1071, 1980
8. Moulton DG, Beidler LM: Structure and function in the peripheral olfactory system. Physiol Rev 47:1–52, 1967
9. Myers LJ: Dysosmia of the dog in clinical veterinary medicine. Prog Vet Neurol 1:171–179, 1990
10. Myers LJ: Methods of diagnosis of disorders of special senses. Part I: The sense of smell. Auburn Vet 40:12–14, 1985
11. Myers LJ, Nash R, Elledge HS: Electro-olfactography: A technique with potential for diagnosis of anosmia in the dog. Am J Vet Res 45:2296–2298, 1984
12. Myers LJ, Pugh R: Thresholds of the dog for detection of inhaled eugenol and benzaldehyde determined by electroencephalographic and behavioral olfactometry. Am J Vet Res 46:2409–2412, 1985
13. O'Brien JA, Harvey CE: Diseases of the upper airway. In Ettinger SJ (ed): Textbook of Veterinary Internal Medicine, 2nd ed. Philadelphia, WB Saunders, 1983
14. Oliver JE Jr, Lorenz M: Handbook of Veterinary Neurologic Diagnosis. Philadelphia, WB Saunders, 1983

CHAPTER FIFTY-NINE

Deafness

John E. Oliver

PROBLEM DEFINITION AND RECOGNITION

Loss of hearing is difficult to detect in companion animals except in dogs trained to respond to verbal commands. Unilateral deafness is almost never recognized except in working dogs that may have difficulty orienting to the direction of the sound.

PATHOPHYSIOLOGY

The tympanic membrane separates the external ear canal from the middle ear. The auditory ossicles transmit air vibration of the tympanic membrane across the middle ear to the inner ear. The middle ear includes the tympanic bulla; the auditory ossicles; the auditory tube to the nasal pharynx; and sympathetic nerve fibers, which innervate the dilator muscles of the pupil. The inner ear, located in the petrosal bone, includes the vestibular receptor organs and the cochlea. The cochlea, which is the receptor organ for hearing, is the coiled portion of the bony labyrinth that contains perilymph. When sound waves move the tympanic membrane, which moves the ossicles, the last ossicle—the stapes—moves the oval window, imparting a waveform in the perilymph. The wave flow in the perilymph moves the basilar membrane causing movement of the hair cells of the spiral organ. Movement of the hair cells causes depolarization, which probably causes release of a neurotransmitter, activating the fibers of the cochlear nerve. The cochlear nerve joins the vestibular nerve to form the vestibulocochlear nerve. The cochlear division synapses in the cochlear nuclei in the medulla oblongata. Axons from the cochlear nuclei have two pathways into the medulla: (1) ventrally through the trapezoid body and (2) dorsally over the caudal cerebellar peduncle in the acoustic stria. The bilateral pathways proceed rostrally, with several synapses and projections to the contralateral side. Nuclei involved in the auditory pathway include the nuclei of the trapezoid body, nucleus of the lateral lemniscus, caudal colliculi, and the medial geniculate nucleus of the thalamus. Axons from the geniculate nucleus project to the temporal lobe of the cerebral cortex. Although the pathway is bilateral, most of the projection to the cortex is from the contralateral side.[8]

Total loss of hearing is rarely caused by lesions of the central nervous system. The auditory pathways are bilateral and multisynaptic in the brain, so lesions destroying them produce severe neurologic signs that would remove any concern for hearing loss. Peripheral hearing loss can be of two types: conduction (nonneural) and nerve deafness. Conduction deafness involves an abnormality of the transduction apparatus, including the tympanic membrane, middle ear cavity, or auditory ossicles. Punctures of the tympanic membrane, effusions in the tympanic bulla, or abnormalities of the auditory ossicles do not usually cause complete hearing loss. Acuity is decreased, but this is rarely recognized. Reduction in motion of the ossicles, a common change in aging humans, may account for the decrease in acuity in some older animals. In a study of nine older dogs with reduced hearing, all had degeneration of spiral ganglion cells and no evidence of conduction abnormality.[19] Complete hearing loss, either unilateral or bilateral, usually results from damage to the receptor in the inner ear or to the cochlear nerve. In acquired disease of these structures, abnormal vestibular function is common and is usually of more concern to the owner than deafness in one ear (see Chapter 49). Congenital deafness is usually a result of abnormal development or degeneration of the spiral organ, the receptor in the cochlea.[32] At least one report suggests that the defect is primarily in central structures, with the peripheral changes being secondary.[12] The cochlea can be damaged by various drugs and toxins, the most important being the aminoglycoside antibiotics.[24] Hypothyroidism also causes degeneration of the cochlea, as well as other neurologic abnormalities including vestibular and facial nerve dysfunction.[17,23]

DIAGNOSTIC PLAN

One of the most difficult tasks confronting clinicians is determining deafness in an animal. Results of simple clinical tests, such as making noises to alert the animal or having the owner give commands, are frequently equivocal. One of the best methods is to make a loud noise while the animal is asleep.[8] An animal usually stops panting briefly when alerted by noise; this is the basis of a potentially effective behavioral test.[34] Other tests involving electrophysiologic techniques are discussed later. The history supplied by the owner may be the most reliable data available.

Clinically it is useful to determine if the deafness is congenital or acquired. Congenital deafness is present from birth, although it is usually unrecognized until the animal is old enough to respond to sounds. Hearing is present in dogs by 10 to 11 days of age, and in cats by 5 days.[8]

Most congenital deafness is associated with a white or merle hair coat. Cats with a white coat and blue eyes are usually deaf.[32] If the cat has one blue eye, it may be deaf only on the side of the blue eye.[4] The gene for a white coat is autosomal dominant in cats, but it is incompletely penetrant for inner ear degeneration. Deafness shows high penetrance in the homozygote, but less in

TABLE 59-1. Hereditary Deafness—Additional Information Sources

Canine*	Reference	Feline	Reference
Akita	32	White, blue eye	5, 7, 10, 2, 22, 28
American Staffordshire	32		
Australian heeler	14		
Australian shepherd	14, 16		
Beagle	8		
Border collies	16		
Boston terrier	14		
Boxer	14		
Bull terrier	16		
Catahoula	32		
Cocker spaniels	14		
Collie	13, 20		
Dalmatian	15, 18, 33, 20, 21		
Dappled dachshund	32		
Doberman pinscher	35		
Dogo Argentino	32		
English bulldog	14		
English setter	14, 30		
Fox terriers	11		
Great Dane	13		
Great Pyrenees	32		
Maltese	32		
Miniature poodle	32		
Mongrel	32		
Norwegian dunkerhound	8, 15		
Old English sheepdog	14		
Papillon	32		
Pointer	31		
Rhodesian ridgeback	32		
Scottish terrier	11		
Sealyham terrier	1		
Shetland sheepdog	14		
Shropshire terrier	16		
Walker foxhound	1		
West Highland white terrier	32		

*Associated with white or merle color gene

the heterozygote. Total deafness is more often associated with long hair in white cats.[7] Dogs with a white or merle hair coat are at risk of congenital deafness (Table 59-1).[32] The highest incidence is in Dalmatians.[14] Hearing loss may be bilateral or unilateral in these dogs. For this reason, at-risk puppies should be screened with electrophysiologic tests, which can detect unilateral deafness.[32]

A complete physical and neurologic examination should be completed on animals presented for deafness. Special attention should be given to the ears,

---

Etiology of Deafness

- Acquired
    Degenerative—geriatric
    Metabolic—hypothyroidism, hypoxia
    Neoplastic—tumors of inner ear or cranial nerve VIII
    Idiopathic—unknown
    Inflammatory—otitis media or interna
    Toxic—aminoglycoside antibiotics, furosemide
    Traumatic—head injury
- Congenital
    Anomaly—hereditary aplasia, hypoplasia, or degeneration of receptor (see Table 59-1)

---

including a thorough otoscopic examination. The tympanic membrane should be intact, not inflamed, and translucent. Normally, it has a ground-glass appearance, and the promontory of the petrosal bone can be recognized in the middle ear. Effusions of the middle ear cause the tympanic membrane to be opaque, discolored, and, in many cases, bulging into the external ear canal. Radiographs of the tympanic bulla are useful as supportive evidence of middle ear disease, but are not as reliable as the otoscopic examination.[25] Other neurologic signs associated with middle and inner ear infections are Horner's syndrome, facial nerve paralysis, and vestibular disorders (see Chapter 49). The causes of hearing loss are listed in the Display, Etiology of Deafness. Infection of the external, middle, or inner ear is the most common acquired problem.[9] Geriatric hearing loss is also fairly common, but is usually not total. Hearing loss, sometimes associated with other neural deficits, occurs in animals with hypothyroidism. Some have responded to replacement thyroid hormone therapy.[6,17]

Several electrophysiologic tests for hearing are available at referral centers. The best test is the brain stem auditory evoked response (BAER). A computer signal averager is necessary to perform the test. Tone or click signals are introduced to each ear independently, and responses are recorded from scalp electrodes. The test is noninvasive, safe, and reliable; it can be used on immature animals; it tests each ear independently; and it does not require anesthesia. Function of the peripheral receptors and the brain stem pathway can be assessed.[29] The intensity of the stimulus can be varied to estimate hearing acuity.

Tympanometry assesses the integrity of the middle ear system.[27] The volume of the external ear canal is estimated by an acoustic impedance bridge. The change in volume with changing pressure measures the compliance of the tympanum. A reflex contraction of the stapedius muscle can be induced by a tone and causes a change in the compliance of the tympanic membrane, the acoustic (stapedial) reflex. The combination of these two tests (tympanometry and acoustic reflex) assess the integrity of the middle ear, hearing, and the facial nerve, which innervates the stapedius muscle.

Electroencephalographic (EEG) audiometry is performed on a conscious animal that is calm enough to demonstrate slow waves on the EEG or is asleep. A sound is introduced, which alerts the animal, causing a change in the EEG. Use of calibrated tone generators allows the quantitation of hearing.[26] Respiratory audiometry is based on the principle that animals change their respiratory patterns when alerted. It can be quantified and made more sensitive by recording respiratory patterns with a strain gauge around the abdomen or thorax.[3] These tests assess hearing but provide no information on the source of the problem.

The signalment, history, physical examination, and neurologic examination should differentiate congenital from acquired deafness. An otoscopic examination confirms infection in all but pure inner ear disease. If infection of the middle ear is found, a tympanotomy should be performed to obtain material for culture and to establish drainage. This can be done by aspirating material from the middle ear with a 22-gauge spinal needle and syringe. If the contents are too thick to aspirate, 0.25 to 0.5 ml saline can be injected into the middle ear and withdrawn. A larger opening can be made with a small intramedullary pin or an ear curette. Culture and assessment of sensitivity of exudate in the middle ear are recommended, because many infections are resistant to commonly used antibiotics. Radiographs are of less benefit in most cases, but they are recommended because of possible secondary changes, such as lysis of the bulla, which can affect the prognosis. Radiographs may detect fluid in the middle ear and tumors of the ear or surrounding structures that are occasionally responsible for hearing loss.

REFERENCES

1. Adams EW: Hereditary deafness in a family of foxhounds. J Am Vet Med Assoc 128:302–303, 1956
2. Bosher SK, Hallpike CS: Observations on the histologic features, development, and pathogenesis of the inner ear degeneration of the deaf white cat. Proc R Soc (Biol) Series B 162:147–170, 1965
3. Bradford LJ, McKinley JH, Rousey CL, Klein DE: Measurement of hearing in dogs by respiration audiometry. Am J Vet Res 34:1183–1187, 1973
4. Coulter DB, Martin CL, Alvarado TP: A cat with white fur and one blue eye. Calif Vet 34:11–14, 1980
5. Creel D, Conlee JW, Parks TN: Auditory brainstem anomalies in albino cats. I. Evoked potential studies. Brain Res 260:1–9, 1983
6. Crifo S, Lazzari R, Salabe GB, et al: A retrospective study of audiological function in a group of congenital hypothyroid patients. Int J Ped Otorhinolaryngol 2:347–355, 1980
7. Delack JB: Hereditary deafness in the white cat. Comp Cont Educ Pract Vet 6:609–616, 1984

8. de Lahunta A: Veterinary Neuroanatomy and Clinical Neurology, 2nd ed. WB Saunders, Philadelphia, 1983

9. Denny HR: The results of surgical treatment of otitis media and interna in the dog. J Sm Anim Pract 14:585–600, 1973

10. Elverland HH, Mair IWS: Hereditary deafness in the cat. Acta Otolaryngol 90:360–369, 1980

11. Erickson F, Leipold HW, McKinley J: Congenital defects in dogs—part 2. Canine Pract 14:51–61, 1977

12. Ferrara ML, Halnan CRE: Congenital brain defects in the deaf Dalmatian. Vet Rec 112:344–346, 1983

13. Gwin RM, Wyman M, Lim DJ, et al: Multiple ocular defects associated with partial albinism and deafness in the dog. J Am Anim Hosp Assoc 17:401–408, 1981

14. Hayes HM, Wilson GP, Fenner WR, Wyman M: Canine congenital deafness: Epidemiologic study of 272 cases. J Am Anim Hosp Assoc 17:473, 1981

15. Hudson W, Ruben R: Hereditary deafness in the Dalmatian dog. Arch Otolaryngol 75:312–319, 1962

16. Igarashi M, Alford B, Cohn A, et al. Inner ear anomalies in dogs. Ann Otol 81:249–255, 1972

17. Jaggy A: Neurologic manifestations of hypothyroidism to dogs. In: Proceedings Eighth Annual Veterinary Medicine Forum, pp 1037–1040. Washington, DC, 1990

18. Johnsson L, Hawkins J, Muraski A, Preston R: Vascular anatomy and pathology of the cochlea in Dalmatian dogs. In Darin de Lorenzo AJ (ed): pp 249–295. University Park, MD, University Park Press, 1973

19. Knowles K: Reduction of spiral ganglion neurons in the aging canine with hearing loss, Proceedings Eighth Annual Veterinary Medicine Forum, pp 105–108. Washington, DC, 1990

20. Lurie M: The membranous labyrinth in the congenitally deaf collie and Dalmatian dog. Laryngoscope 58:279–287, 1948

21. Marshall A: Use of brain stem auditory-evoked response to evaluate deafness in a group of Dalmation dogs. J Am Vet Med Assoc 188:718–722, 1986

22. Mattiasson A, Andersson K-E, Elbadawi A, et al: Interaction between adrenergic and cholinergic nerve terminals in the urinary bladder of rabbit, cat and man. J Urol 137:1017–1019, 1987

23. Meyerhoff WL: The thyroid and audition. Laryngoscope 86:483–489, 1976

24. Morgan JL, Coulter DB, Marshall AE, Goetsch DD: Effects of neomycin on the waveform of auditory-evoked brain stem potentials in dogs. Am J Vet Res 41:1077–1081, 1980

25. Oliver JE Jr, Lorenz M: Handbook of Veterinary Neurologic Diagnosis. WB Saunders, Philadelphia, 1983

26. Oliver JE, Hoerlein BF, Mayhew IG: Veterinary Neurology. Philadelphia, WB Saunders, 1987

27. Penrod JP, Coulter DB: The diagnostic uses of impedance audiometry in the dog. J Am Anim Hosp Assoc 16:941–948, 1980

28. Rebillard G, Rebillard M, Carlier E, Pujol R: Histo-physiological relationships in the deaf white cat auditory system. Acta Otolaryngol 82:48–56, 1976

29. Sims MH, Moore RE: Auditory-evoked response in the clinically normal dog: Early latency components. Am J Vet Res 45:2019–2027, 1984

30. Sims MH, Shull-Selcer E: Electrodiagnostic evaluation of deafness in two English setter littermates. J Am Vet Med Assoc 187:398–404, 1985
31. Steinberg SA, Klein E, Killens R, Uhde TW: Inherited deafness among nervous pointer dogs. Proceedings Seventh Annual Veterinary Medicine Forum, pp 953–956. San Diego, CA, 1989
32. Strain GM: Congenital deafness in dogs and cats. Comp Cont Educ Pract Vet 13:245–253, 1991
33. Suga F, Hattler K: Physiological and histopathological correlates of hereditary deafness in animals. Laryngoscope 80:80–104, 1970
34. van der Velden NA, Rijkse C: A practicable method of making audiograms in dogs. App Anim Ethol 2:371–377, 1976
35. Wilkes M, Palmer A: Congenital deafness in dobermans. Vet Rec 118:218, 1986

PART FOURTEEN

Laboratory-Defined Problems

CHAPTER SIXTY

Hematologic Problems

Craig E. Greene

ANEMIA

Anemia is a decrease in the hematocrit (less than 37 in dogs; less than 27 in cats) and has many causes. Diagnostic and therapeutic plans for anemia are predicated on the basis of the presence or absence of red blood cell (RBC) regeneration (Table 60-1). *Nonregenerative* anemias are caused by decreased bone marrow production of erythrocytes; *regenerative* anemias are caused by increased erythrocyte destruction (hemolysis) and blood loss (hemorrhage). Regeneration is best detected by examining blood films for the presence of reticulocytosis (by methylene blue stain) or polychromasia (by Wright's stain), or both. Only large aggregate (not punctate) reticulocytes should be used to assess the degree of reticulocytosis in cats. Other findings such as anisocytosis, Howell-Jolly bodies, and nucleated erythrocytes are *not* specific indicators of adequate RBC regeneration in dogs and cats. The reticulocyte count is normally expressed as a relative percentage of circulating erythrocytes and must be corrected for the hematocrit to accurately assess the degree of regenerative response. For instance, a 2% reticulocyte count with a hematocrit of 10 is less impressive than the same count with a hematocrit of 20. A simple correction and the clinical significance of a relative reticulocyte count is given in Table 60-2. As an absolute value, a given corrected reticulocyte percentage is indicative of more significant regeneration in the cat as compared with the dog.

Which clinical signs are associated with anemia depends on the degree of anemia, the rapidity of its development, the associated plasma volume loss, and cardiovascular dysfunction. The clinical signs of anemia are described in Chapter 23.

The diagnostic plan for regenerative anemia should differentiate blood loss from blood lysis. Plasma protein concentration should be determined as the first discriminatory measure. Plasma protein concentrations are normal with most hemolytic disorders and are decreased with hemorrhage. Body excretions (urine, feces, and vomitus) and body cavities should be examined for the presence of blood. Serum icterus, increased bilirubinuria, and hemoglobinuria (if present) are associated with hemolytic disorders. When hemolysis is suspected, additional diagnostic tests should include examination of blood films for the presence of Heinz bodies, stomatocytes, spherocytes, or blood parasites. These

TABLE 60-1. Causes of Anemia

Regenerative	Nonregenerative
Blood loss	Decreased erythropoietin
Surgery	Endocrine dysfunction
Trauma	Hypothyroidism
Gastrointestinal disorders	Hypoadrenocorticism
Ulceration	Renal failure
Parasites	Chronic disease
Hemostatic disorders	Inflammation
Urinary tract disorders	Neoplasia
Blood lysis	Cytotoxic marrow damage
Parasites	Chemical agents
Osmotic changes	Cytotoxic drugs
Metabolic defects	Fungal toxins
Malamutes—stomatocytes	Physical agents
Basenji—pyruvate kinase deficiency	Irradiation
Springer spaniels—phosphofructokinase deficiency	Immune-mediated cytotoxicity
Cats—porphyria	Pure red blood cell aplasia
Hepatic dysfunction	Myelophthistic diseases
Immune/infectious causes	Lymphocytic, granulocytic, or plasmacytic leukemias
Trauma	Nuclear division dysfunction
Microangiopathies	Sulfonamide drugs
Heartworms	Methotrexate therapy
Chemicals/toxins	Folic acid deficiency
Onions, acetaminophen, phenol, methylene blue, topical anesthetics, nitrates, copper, zinc	B_{12} deficiency
	Abnormal erythroid maturation
	Erythroleukemia
	Feline leukemia virus infection
	Feline immunodeficiency virus infection
	Heme synthesis interference
	Lead poisoning
	Chloramphenicol
	Microcytic iron deficiency

TABLE 60-2. Simple Corrected Reticulocyte Response

	Dog	Cat
Normal (%)	≤1	≤0.4
Slight (%)	1–4	0.5–2
Large (%)	5–20	3–4

Normal packed cell volume (PCV) for dogs is 45%; for cats, 35%.

Simple corrected response =

$$\frac{\text{Actual PCV}}{\text{Normal PCV}} \times \text{reticulocyte count (\%)}$$

Causes of Nonregenerative Anemia Based on Erythrocyte Size

- MCV <60—microcytic anemia
  - Iron deficiency
    - Deficient diet
    - Chronic blood loss
      - Gastrointestinal
      - Reproductive
      - Urinary
    - Pulmonary iron sequestration
    - Chronic intravascular hemolysis
    - Gastrointestinal malabsorption
- MCV 60–77—normocytic anemia (dog)
- MCV 35–55—normocytic anemia (cat)
  - Inadequate diet
  - Body protein loss
  - Decreased hormonal influence
    - Hypothyroidism
    - Hypoadrenocorticism
    - Chronic renal failure
  - Bone marrow intoxication
    - Chloramphenicol
    - Lead poisoning
    - Cancer chemotherapy
    - Estrogens

  - Chronic inflammatory diseases
  - Chronic infectious diseases
    - Feline leukemia virus infection
    - Feline immunodeficiency virus infection
  - Myeloproliferative disease
  - Chronic ehrlichiosis
  - Pure erythrocyte aplasia
- MCV >77—macrocytic anemia (dog)
- MCV >55—macrocytic anemia (cat)
  - Folic acid deficiency
    - Sulfonamides
    - Methotrexate
  - B_{12} deficiency

MCV, mean corpuscular volume

tests not only help confirm the presence of hemolysis but always provide valuable clues to the etiology of the hemolytic process. Urine that contains intact RBCs, myoglobin, or hemoglobin will be positive in the urine occult blood test. Urine sediment should also be evaluated. The absence of erythrocyte ghosts (phantom corpuscles) in the urine sediment of an anemic animal with a positive urine occult blood suggests hemoglobinuria from intravascular hemolysis or, less commonly, myoglobinuria due to severe muscle necrosis. When hemolysis has been proved, definitive tests to establish the etiology are indicated, including Coombs' test, feline leukemia virus (FeLV) test, heartworm test, and chest radiography. When hemorrhage is suspected, coagulation tests and platelet counts are needed to eliminate hemostatic disorders (see Chapter 19).

The diagnostic plan for nonregenerative anemia includes evaluation of the erythrocyte indices to determine RBC size (see Display, Causes of Nonregenerative Anemia Based on Erythrocyte Size, and Figs. 60-1 and 60-2). Macrocytic anemias are seen with diseases that inhibit nuclear division (vitamin B_{12} and folic acid deficiencies). Microcytosis occurs with disorders that inhibit heme synthesis (iron deficiency states). The relative numbers of leukocytes and plate-

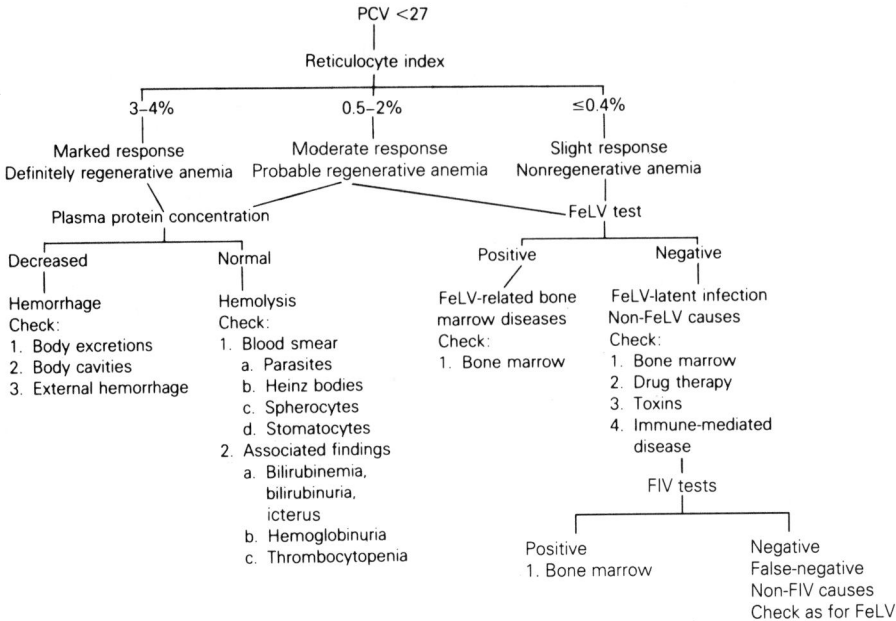

FIGURE 60-1. Diagnostic plan for feline anemia.

lets should be assessed, since certain diseases affect bone marrow elements in addition to the erythrocyte series. FeLV and feline immunodeficiency virus (FIV) testing is very important, since these diseases are common causes of nonregenerative anemia in cats. In dogs, serologic tests for ehrlichiosis may be necessary. The plasma protein concentration should be evaluated, since hypoproteinemia may suggest chronic blood loss associated with iron deficiency.

Feces should be examined for blood and the presence of helminth eggs or protozoal organisms that cause chronic gastrointestinal blood loss and iron deficiency. Many endocrine and metabolic diseases (*e.g.*, chronic renal failure) cause nonregenerative anemias of the normocytic normochromic type. Biochemical tests and urine analysis are indicated, since they may reveal the presence of these disorders. Bone marrow examination is indicated when hematologic tests, biochemical tests, urine analysis, and infectious disease serotests fail to substantiate a diagnosis. Bone marrow examination is also useful in the diagnosis and prognosis of cytotoxic damage, myelophthistic disease, abnormal erythroid maturation, and interference with heme synthesis (see Table 60-1).

LEUKOPENIA

Leukopenia (panleukopenia) involves a decrease in all leukocytes and is generally associated with severe white blood cell destruction, an overwhelming demand for leukocytes, or decreased bone marrow and lymphoid cell production.

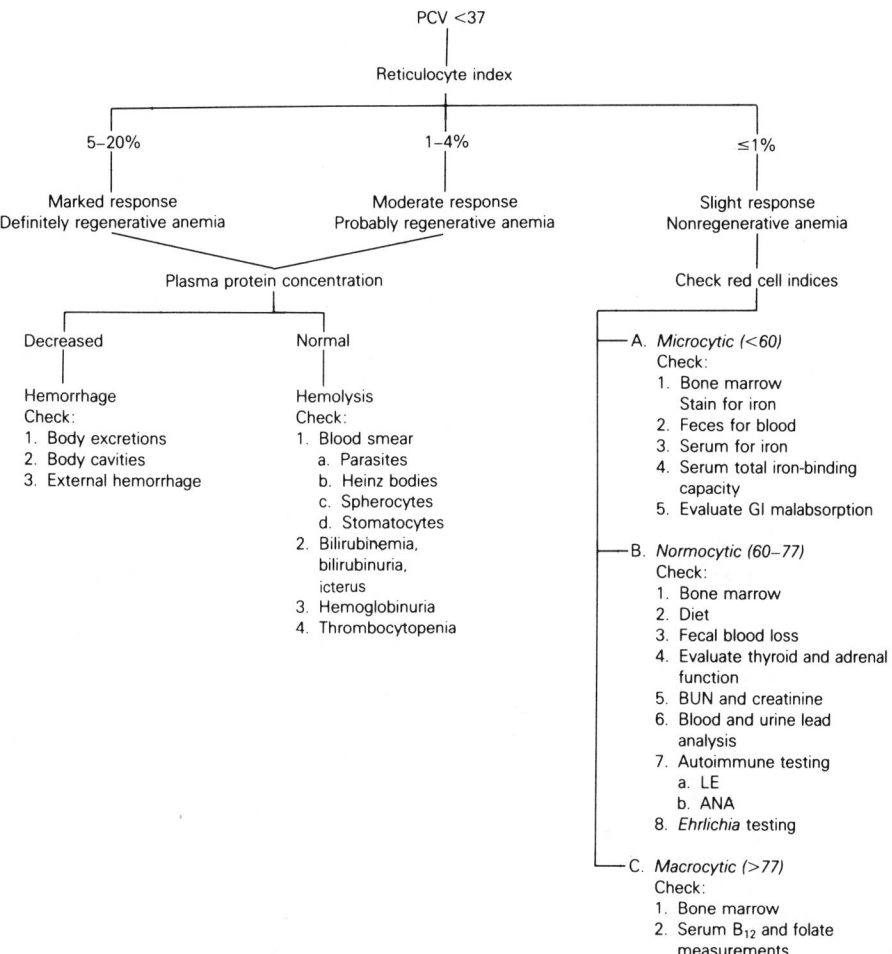

FIGURE 60-2. Diagnostic plan for canine anemia.

The usual causes of panleukopenia are listed in Table 60-3. In severe leukopenia, a second hemogram should be taken within 48 hours for comparison. If leukopenia persists, examination of the bone marrow is needed. Animals with persistent leukopenia are immunodeficient and frequently develop secondary bacterial infections. When hospitalized, they should be separated from other animals and should receive antimicrobial therapy if infectious complications develop. Bactericidal antibiotics are preferable to bacteriostatic antibiotics when severe leukopenia is present.

LEUKOCYTOSIS

Physiologic increase in leukocyte numbers are caused by epinephrine release from excitement, which is more common in cats than dogs (see Table 60-3).

TABLE 60-3. Leukocyte Abnormalities

Leukopenia	Leukocytosis	Neutropenia	Neutrophilia*

Toxins
  Irradiation
  Fungal (T-2)
Infections
  Ehrlichiosis
  Feline leukemia
  Feline panleukopenia
  Feline immunodeficiency virus infection
  Canine parvovirus infection
  Overwhelming sepsis
	Physiologic causes (epinephrine)
	Stress (glucocorticoids)
	Inflammation/infection (chronic)
		Increased usage or destruction
		  Peracute overwhelming infection
		  Cellulitis
		  Aspiration pneumonia
		  Endotoxemia
		  Peritonitis
		  Acute viral infections
		  Immune-mediated
		Decreased production
		  Infectious causes
		    Panleukopenia
		    Feline leukemia
		    Feline immunodeficiency virus infection
		    Ehrlichiosis
		    Canine parvovirus infection
		  Chemical causes
		    Fungal toxin
		    Estrogen intoxication
		    Anticonvulsants
		    Cytotoxic drugs
		    Radiation
		  Genetic disorders
		    Cyclic hematopoiesis
		  Myelophthistic disorders
		  Myeloproliferative diseases
			Physiologic disorders
			  Increased muscular activity
			  Increased blood pressure
			  Stress, epinephrine release
			  Glucocorticoid therapy
			  Cushing's disease
			Pathologic causes
			  Inflammation (especially local or chronic)
			  Immune-mediated diseases
			  Tissue necrosis
			Neoplastic disorders
			  Myeloproliferative diseases
			  Granulomatous and lymphocytic leukemias
			Hemorrhage or hemolysis

*>11,500 in dogs; >12,500 in cats

Diseases associated with endogenous glucocorticoid release can also cause leukocytosis, but lymphopenia and eosinopenia also occur. Chronic localized inflammatory or infectious processes are associated with an increase of all leukocyte types. In these cases, the body has control over the inflammatory process, and bone marrow production of leukocytes meets the demand.

NEUTROPENIA

Because neutrophils constitute a majority of leukocytes, neutropenia is usually associated with leukopenia and can be caused by increased utilization or decreased production of neutrophils. These causes can be distinguished in many cases, because increased utilization is associated with a shift to immature forms. Excessive utilization of neutrophils is associated with overwhelming tissue demand, as occurs with multisystemic or severe inflammatory or infectious processes (see Table 60-3). Decreased production of neutrophils is associated with many processes previously discussed under Leukopenia; however, many of these can be selective for the neutrophil series.

NEUTROPHILIA

Increased neutrophil counts are commonly associated with an infectious process. However, neutrophilia alone does not confirm the presence of infection, since noninfectious inflammatory processes such as acute pancreatitis or extravascular hemolysis or hemorrhage show similar neutrophil increases (see Table 60-3). Stress (glucocorticoid release) associated with many systemic disease processes is accompanied by neutrophilia in venous blood, resulting from decreased margination and emigration of the neutrophils. A left shift (increase in immature neutrophils), is usually absent in stress neutrophilia, unless the effect of endogenous glucocorticoids is superimposed on an existing inflammatory process. The degree of shift toward immature band forms correlates reasonably well with the severity of the infection or inflammatory process.

Neutrophilia without a shift may not always indicate that an animal is adequately coping with infection, although the highest counts and mature shifts usually correlate with abscess formation, or walling off of an infectious process. Defects in neutrophil function are commonly associated with a normal to increased neutrophil count without a shift in the presence of infection, because neutrophils are not effectively consumed in the inflammatory process.

MONOCYTOSIS

Increases in absolute monocyte counts are commonly found in conjunction with neutrophilia, eosinopenia, and lymphopenia when increased endogenous (stress) or exogenous glucocorticoid concentrations are present. Monocytosis may be an indicator of granulomatous disease, in which neutrophils have been unsuccessful in eliminating persistent intracellular infectious agents. Monocyte numbers are also increased in cases of neutrophilic defects or persistent neutropenia, when monocytes must perform primary phagocytic functions. A summary of the causes of monocytosis is presented in Table 60-4.

LYMPHOPENIA

Decreased circulating lymphocyte counts are associated with acute infectious or inflammatory processes as well as with stress or Cushing's disease (see Table 60-4). Selective lymphopenia is a feature of the viremic period of many acute systemic viral infections and of the period following modified live virus vaccination. Chronic persistent lymphopenia is a poor prognostic sign in any illness and usually indicates the body's inability to respond to the disease insult. Of the total number of body lymphocytes, only 10% are circulating. These are primarily T cells; therefore, absolute lymphocyte counts cannot always be directly correlated with the immunocompetency of the host.

LYMPHOCYTOSIS

Lymphocytosis, a common feature of chronic inflammatory diseases, occurs with neutrophilia and monocytosis (see Table 60-4). Chronic antigenic stimulation leads to proliferation of lymphoid precursors and, hence, circulating lymphocytes. Lymphocytosis may be found in cats infected with FeLV or in dogs with lymphosarcoma or lymphocytic leukemia. Atypical lymphocytes may also be seen. Cats, unlike dogs, have proportionally more lymphocytes than neutrophils in their peripheral circulation, so on a percentage basis, many cats appear to have a lymphocytosis.

EOSINOPENIA

Eosinopenia occurs during the acute stress of many disease states associated with endogenous glucocorticoid release, as with canine Cushing's syndrome (see Table 60-4). Exogenous glucocorticoid therapy also results in eosinopenia, the duration of which varies with the dosage and drug administered.

EOSINOPHILIA

In contrast to acute diseases, chronic infectious or inflammatory diseases result in eosinophilia rather than eosinopenia (see Table 60-4). The major tissues in which chronic inflammation results in eosinophil increases (*e.g.*, skin and re-

TABLE 60-4. Leukocyte Abnormalities

Lymphopenia	Eosinopenia	Monocytosis	Lymphocytosis	Eosinophilia	Basophilia
Glucocorticoids	Exogenous glucocorticoids	Stress (glucocorticoid)	Physiological disorders (especially cats)	Acute hypersensitivity	Chronic inflammation of mucosal and skin surfaces
Endogenous (Cushing's disease)	Endogenous glucocorticoids	Chronic inflammation	Chronic inflammation	Parasitism	Chronic fasting lipemia
Exogenous (drug therapy)	Stress	Internal hemorrhage/hemolysis	Lymphocytic leukemia	Gastrointestinal (hookworms, roundworms, whipworms)	Cushing's disease
Debilitating disorders	Cushing's disease	Persistent neutropenia	Lymphosarcoma	Pulmonary (lungworms)	Hypothyroidism
Chronic infections	Acute infections	Neutrophil function defect		Vascular (heartworms)	Eosinophilia
Metastatic neoplasia		Granulomatous diseases		Skin (fleas, *Demodex*)	Mastocytoma (especially pulmonary and systemic)
Renal failure		Neoplastic diseases		Specific syndromes	
Amyloidosis		Nonspecific malignancies		Gastrointestinal (eosinophilic infiltrates)	
Loss of lymphocytes		Monocytic leukemia		Lung (pulmonary infiltrates)	
Repeated chylocentesis				Muscle (polymyositis)	
Intestinal lymphangiectasia				Skin (miliary dermatitis, eosinophilic granuloma)	
Impaired lymphopoiesis				Soft tissues (eosinophilic infiltrates in dogs)	
Cancer chemotherapy				Neoplasia	
Prolonged use of glucocorticoids				Lymphosarcoma	
Irradiation				Mastocytoma	
Congenital T cell immunodeficiency				Metastatic types	
Acute infectious illnesses				Others	
Immunosuppressive viral infections				Estrus	
				Eosinophilic leukemia	
				Autoimmune disease	

spiratory, gastrointestinal, and genital mucosae) are those laden with tissue mast cells. Eosinophilia may also be noted with chronic fungal or protozoal infections, but it occurs more consistently in infections caused by metazoal parasites, such as fleas, roundworms, hookworms, heartworms, and lung-worms.

BASOPHILIA

Chronic antigenic stimulation of skin or mucosal surfaces causes an increase in IgE-mediated inflammatory processes. Basophils, the circulating equivalent of tissue mast cells, are increased in these processes, and their increase is usually associated with eosinophilia (see Table 60-4). Conditions associated with fasting hyperlipemia are also associated with basophilia, because basophils contain heparin, an activator of lipoprotein lipase. The basophilia may aid in the clear-ance of circulating lipids from the blood.

THROMBOCYTOPENIA

Platelets are produced by bone marrow elements, and any process that interferes with marrow production will lead to thrombocytopenia. Various causes of de-creased platelet production are listed in Table 60-5 and are discussed further in Chapter 19. Increased platelet removal and thrombocytopenia can occur as a result of immune or coagulatory consumption of platelets. Platelets also can be sequestered with splenomegaly that occurs in conditions such as portal hyper-tension, lymphosarcoma, and splenic torsion.

THROMBOCYTOSIS

Thrombocytes increase in the circulation whenever splenic contraction or sple-nectomy occurs, because the spleen is the major site of platelet storage in the body. Chronic iron deficiencies probably result in thrombocytosis because the marrow is stimulated by myelopoietic hormones to increase the production of erythrocytes. Diseases commonly associated with thrombocytosis are listed in Table 60-5.

HYPERLIPEMIA

Hyperlipemia, an increase in the amount of circulating lipid in the blood, may reflect a variety of diseases associated with altered fat metabolism (see Display, Causes of Fasting Hyperlipemia). Care must be taken to distinguish visible from invisible hyperlipemia when determining the cause of this syndrome. Visible

TABLE 60-5. Abnormalities in Platelet Numbers

Thrombocytopenia	Thrombocytosis
Decreased production	Reactive
Drugs	Splenectomy
Estrogens	Acute hemorrhage
Cancer chemotherapy	Trauma
Myelophthistic diseases	Fractures
Infections	Infections (chronic)
Ehrlichiosis	Malignancies
Feline infectious peritonitis	Iron deficiencies
Feline leukemia	Vincristine
Physiologic causes	Diabetes mellitus
Estrus	Autonomous
Sertoli tumors	Myeloproliferative disease
Increased destruction	
Immune-mediated	
Drugs	
Infectious	
Idiopathic	
Coagulatory	
Disseminated intravascular coagulation	
Endotoxin	
Sequestration	
Splenomegaly	
Portal hypertension	

hyperlipemia is caused by increased amounts of circulating chylomicrons derived from the digestive process. This normally occurs 1 to 3 hours postprandially. Delays of lipid clearance greater than 3 hours after eating usually reflect deranged lipid clearance and may indicate an increase in circulating invisible lipids. Invisible hyperlipemia, which can be assumed indirectly from the presence of visible hyperlipemia, must be substantiated by lipoprotein electrophoresis. Invisible hyperlipemia can also occur in the absence of fasting hyperchylomicronemia and, in such cases, is detected only if lipoprotein electrophoresis is

Causes of Fasting Hyperlipemia

- Hypothyroidism
- Hyperadrenocorticism
- Nephrotic syndrome
- Acute pancreatitis

- Steatitis
- Postprandial
- Idiopathic (familial)
  - Schnauzers
  - Dachshunds

performed. Serum sample analysis that involves colorimetric procedures is invalidated by the presence of visible lipemia. In some cases, lipemic samples may be cleared by high-speed ultracentrifugation following refrigeration or by the administration of heparin to the patient. A more accurate way to assess the lipemic state is to use noncolorimetric procedures (*e.g.,* enzymatic glucose test sticks) or not to feed the animal for 48 to 72 hours and repeat the analysis on samples taken after the plasma has cleared.

CHAPTER SIXTY-ONE

Abnormalities of the Standard Biochemical Profile

Larry M. Cornelius

DECREASED BLOOD UREA NITROGEN

Problem Definition and Recognition

A decreased blood urea nitrogen (BUN) level is defined as a BUN of less than 10 mg/dl.

Pathophysiology

Urea is produced in the liver from nitrogenous precursors such as ammonia and amino acids in portal blood. Dietary protein and blood in the intestinal tract are major sources of ammonia and protein. After entering the systemic circulation from the liver, urea is filtered through the glomeruli and excreted into the urine. Urea also enters the intestinal lumen, and a portion is converted to ammonia by bacterial ureases. Most of this ammonia is absorbed into the portal circulation and returned to the liver for resynthesis into urea.

A low BUN can occur because of decreased urea production or increased urea excretion (Fig. 61-1). Decreased production is most common with chronic hepatic dysfunction or long-term consumption of severely restricted protein diets. Increased urea excretion causing a low BUN is often observed in animals with significant polyuria.

Diagnostic Plan

History and Physical Examination. A history of the patient being on a severely restricted protein diet, such as Prescription Diet S-D (Hill's Pet Products, Topeka, KS), for several months or a history of chronic polyuria should alert the clinician to the possibility of a decreased BUN. Patients with chronic hepatic insufficiency and decreased BUN may have other signs of liver failure, such as vomiting, diarrhea, icterus, and ascites (see Chapter 37).

537

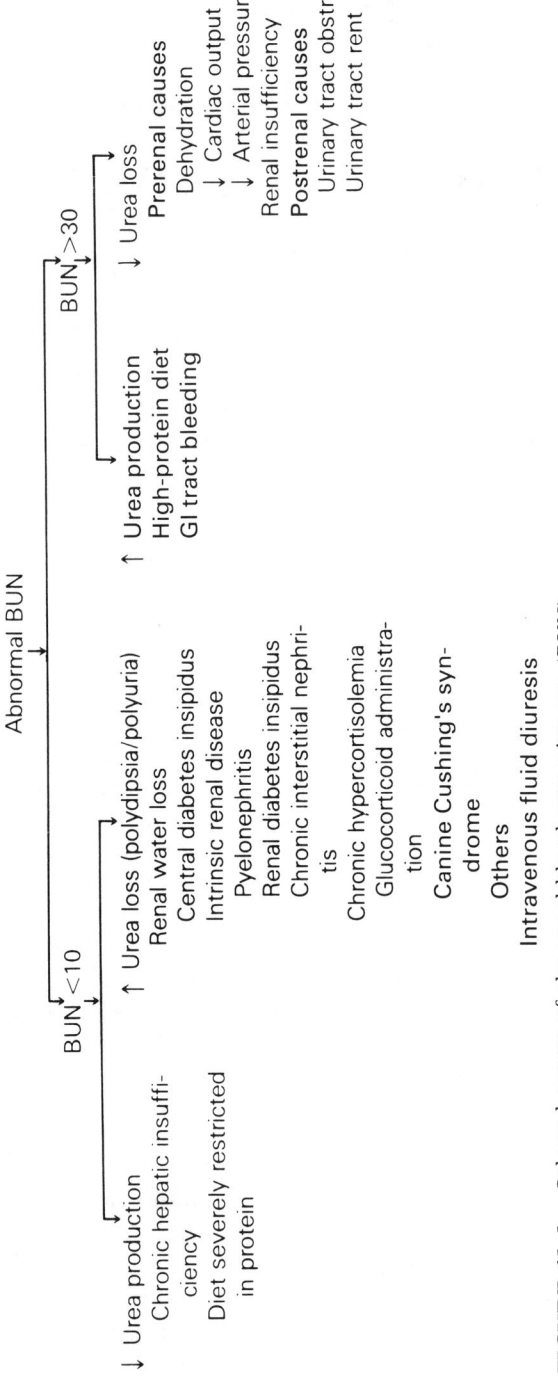

FIGURE 61-1. Selected causes of abnormal blood urea nitrogen (BUN).

538

Laboratory Evaluation. BUN is often determined as part of a standard bio-chemical profile of serum, which should include a serum creatinine. A urine specimen, preferably obtained prior to therapy and by cystocentesis, should be submitted for a complete urine analysis (including sediment examination). Follow-up laboratory procedures, including radiology and ultrasonography, will be determined by rule outs being considered after initial results are obtained.

INCREASED BLOOD UREA NITROGEN

Problem Definition and Recognition

An increased BUN level (azotemia) is defined as a BUN of greater than 30 mg/dl.

Pathophysiology

An increased BUN can be caused by increased urea production in the liver or intestinal tract, or both, or by decreased urea excretion by the kidneys (Fig. 61-1). Decreased renal excretion of urea is the most common cause of an in-creased BUN and may be due to decreased renal blood flow (prerenal), kidney failure (renal), or urinary tract obstruction or rent (postrenal). Signs of uremia are seen more often when the BUN exceeds 100 mg/dl. A more sudden increase in BUN is generally associated with a lower BUN concentration necessary to cause signs of uremia. Most reports indicate that urea is relatively nontoxic, but other wastes that always accompany increased BUN cause signs of uremia.

Diagnostic Plan

History and Physical Examination. As noted above, clinical signs of uremia (anorexia, lethargy, vomiting, melena, dehydration, and oral ulcers) are usually not observed until the BUN exceeds 100 mg/dl. With an increased BUN of 30 to 100 mg/dl (azotemia), dehydration or other signs caused by the primary disorder are usually observed.

Laboratory Evaluation. See section on laboratory evaluation under De-creased Blood Urea Nitrogen.

DECREASED CREATININE

There is no reported clinical significance of a decreased serum creatinine.

INCREASED CREATININE

Problem Definition and Recognition

Reported normal serum creatinine values vary depending on the particular labo-ratory procedure used. The upper range of normal is generally considered to be from 1.0 to 2.0 mg/dl.

Pathophysiology

Creatinine is formed largely in muscle, and its production is not significantly affected by dietary protein or blood in the gastrointestinal tract. Renal excretion of creatinine is affected by similar factors as renal urea excretion (see Pathophysiology of Decreased and Increased BUN). As is the case with urea, creatinine is not believed to be toxic but is accompanied by toxic waste products in conditions in which there is decreased renal excretion of creatinine (azotemia or uremia).

Diagnostic Plan

History and Physical Examination. Clinical signs are either those of uremia (see History and Physical Examination of Increased BUN) or of the primary disorder.

Laboratory Evaluation. See section on laboratory evaluation under Decreased Blood Urea Nitrogen.

HYPOALBUMINEMIA

Problem Definition and Recognition

Hypoalbuminemia is defined as a serum albumin concentration of less than 2.5 g/dl. Most normal adult dogs and cats have a serum albumin concentration of around 3.0 g/dl, whereas puppies and kittens have a slightly lower serum albumin level.

Pathophysiology

Albumin is synthesized in the liver from dietary amino acids. The normal half-life of serum albumin is about 10 days. Small amounts of albumin are normally lost in the urine and feces, but most albumin turnover is due to its use in various metabolic processes, such as tissue healing and repair. Albumin is normally not catabolized as a source of calories, but with sepsis, trauma, neoplasia, severe burns, and chronic starvation, albumin may be utilized for energy.

The primary functions of serum albumin are to maintain colloid osmotic pressure of plasma and to serve as a carrier for various compounds, both endogenous (*e.g.*, hormones, bilirubin, calcium) and exogenous (*e.g.*, drugs, toxins). With significant hypoalbuminemia, there is a decrease in plasma colloid osmotic pressure and an increased tendency for the formation of edema and body cavity effusions. Serum albumin must be severely decreased (less than 0.8 g/dl) before hypoalbuminemia alone will cause fluid accumulation. However, less marked hypoalbuminemia may contribute to the formation of edema and effusions whenever other potential causes of edema are present (vascular damage, increased blood pressure, lymphatic blockage, and increased sodium and water retention).

TABLE 61-1. Causes of Hypoalbuminemia

Globulin Decreased	*Globulin Normal or Increased*
Decreased production	
	Chronic hepatic insufficiency
	Chronic starvation
Increased loss	
Protein-losing enteropathies	Renal loss
Hemorrhage	Glomerulonephritis
	Amyloidosis
	Increased catabolism
	Sepsis
	Trauma
	Neoplasia
	Burns
Sequestration	
	Body cavity effusions
	Ascites
	Pleural effusion
	Vasculopathies
	Immune-mediated
	Infectious
	Endotoxemia/
	bacteremia
	Rickettsial diseases
	(*Ehrlichia;* Rocky
	Mountain spotted
	fever)
Dilutional	
Fluid therapy	

Causes of hypoalbuminemia may be classified as being due to decreased production, increased loss, sequestration, and dilution. It is helpful in the assessment of hypoalbuminemia to consider also the serum globulin level (Table 61-1).

Diagnostic Plan

History and Physical Examination. A variety of clinical disorders may cause hypoalbuminemia; therefore, the history and physical examination findings are variable. With severe hypoalbuminemia, evidence of peripheral edema, ascites, and pleural effusion may be observed. Although it would be expected that peripheral edema would be diffuse and symmetric, this is not always the case. In the early stages of edema due to hypoalbuminemia, only one leg may be involved. The exact reasons for this observation are not clear but may relate to other factors affecting circulation, such as the effects of gravity on the dependent limb.

Laboratory Evaluation. Serum albumin is usually determined as a part of a biochemical profile that includes measurement of serum total protein. Globulin is then determined by subtracting the albumin concentration from the total protein concentration. Albumin and globulin should each be interpreted independently. The albumin-to-globulin ratio is of little or no value in the assessment of clinical disorders. Follow-up laboratory procedures are determined by rule outs considered after initial results are obtained.

INCREASED SERUM ALBUMIN

Problem Definition and Recognition

An increased serum albumin is defined as an albumin concentration of greater than 3.8 g/dl.

Pathophysiology

See the section on pathophysiology under Hypoalbuminemia above. The only recognized cause of hyperalbuminemia is dehydration. The serum globulin concentration is also increased in dehydration (see section on hyperglobulinemia).

Diagnostic Plan

See section on hypoalbuminemia.

HYPOGLOBULINEMIA

Problem Definition and Recognition

Hypoglobulinemia is defined as a serum globulin concentration of less than 2.0 g/dl.

Pathophysiology

Most globulin is synthesized in plasma cells and lymphocytes as a part of the immunoglobulins, but the liver also makes globulin. The major functions of globulin are to act as antibodies in the humoral immune response and to bind certain compounds in the body, such as hormones, and to aid in their transport through the bloodstream to their sites of action. With severe hypoglobulinemia the animal may become more susceptible to various infections.

Causes of decreased serum globulin may be grouped: decreased globulin production, increased globulin loss, and dilutional causes. In addition, one should always consider the serum albumin in the assessment of the serum globulin concentration (see Table 61-1).

Diagnostic Plan

History and Physical Examination. The history and physical examination findings associated with severe hypoglobulinemia, when present, are the result of infection. Depression, fever, lymphadenopathy, and a variety of other signs may be observed.

Laboratory Evaluation. Serum globulin is usually determined indirectly by subtracting the serum albumin concentration from the total protein concentration. It is usually assessed as part of a standard biochemical profile. Follow-up plans are determined by the particular diagnoses considered.

HYPERGLOBULINEMIA

Problem Definition and Recognition

Hyperglobulinemia is defined as a serum globulin of greater than 3.8 g/dl.

Pathophysiology

Hyperglobulinemia may result from either increased globulin production or dehydration. Increased globulin production is usually the result of chronic antigenic stimulation, such as may occur with chronic inflammatory conditions (infectious or noninfectious), or neoplastic disorders associated with tissue necrosis. Some tumors involving cells of the humoral immune system (some lymphosarcomas and plasma cell myelomas) may also produce large amounts of globulin and cause hyperglobulinemia.

Diagnostic Plan

History and Physical Examination. A variety of disorders may be associated with increased globulin production or dehydration, or both; therefore, the history and physical examination findings are variable.

Laboratory Evaluation. See section on hypoglobulinemia.

DECREASED SERUM ALANINE AMINOTRANSFERASE

There is no known significance associated with a decreased serum alanine aminotransferase (S-ALT) level.

INCREASED SERUM ALANINE AMINOTRANSFERASE

Problem Definition and Recognition

An increased S-ALT level is defined as an S-ALT above the normal species reference range for the particular laboratory procedure being used.

Pathophysiology

Increased serum activity of the commonly determined enzymes is due to either increased cellular release or increased cellular production.[6] ALT is located in the cytosol of hepatocytes and is released whenever there is hepatocellular membrane injury or hepatic necrosis. ALT is generally considered to be liver-specific in dogs and cats, although results of a recent report indicate that ALT may be released from skeletal muscle of dogs during severe necrosis.[11] Other "release" enzymes, including aspartate aminotransferase (formerly glutamic-oxaloacetic transaminase [SGOT]) and lactate dehydrogenase (LDH), are found in other tissues besides liver and are not as useful for the evaluation of hepatic disease.

The magnitude of the increase in serum enzyme activity parallels the number of hepatocytes damaged but provides no information regarding the reversibility of the injury at the cellular level, the regenerative capacity at the tissue level, or the status of function at the organ level.[6] Neither S-ALT nor serum alkaline phosphatase determinations (see below) are liver *function* tests.

The duration of increased serum enzyme activity depends not only on leakage from hepatocytes but also on the rate of plasma disappearance. Inactivation of plasma enzymes involves stereochemical denaturation and subsequent loss of the enzyme's catalytic capabilities. The half-life of ALT injected into dogs is 2.5 hours. Renal excretion of hepatic enzymes is normally insignificant because of their large molecular size, which precludes glomerular filtration.

The magnitude of serum enzyme activity cannot be equated with reversibility of the hepatic injury. Any condition causing diffuse hepatocellular injury, such as hypoxia associated with shock, may result in markedly increased serum enzyme activity; however, all hepatocytes would be expected to recover. Organ function may remain near normal despite greatly increased serum enzyme values. On the other hand, hepatic failure may exist with normal serum enzyme levels. An example is severe hepatic cirrhosis in which it is likely that most enzyme-producing hepatic cells have been destroyed. Causes of an increased S-ALT are listed in Table 61-2.

Diagnostic Plan

History and Physical Examination. There are no historical or physical examination findings attributable to an increased S-ALT. However, signs of hepatic disease, such as icterus or ascites, are often associated with an increased S-ALT (see Chapter 37).

Laboratory Evaluation. S-ALT should be determined as part of a biochemical profile. The initial laboratory workup should include a complete blood count (CBC) and urine analysis. Follow-up laboratory evaluation will be determined by the diagnoses being considered after assessment of the initial test results.

TABLE 61-2.   Selected Causes of Increased S-ALT and/or SAP in Dogs and Cats

Dogs	*Cats*
Rule out:	Rule out:
Drug-induced	Drug-induced
Glucocorticoids	Acetaminophen
Anticonvulsants	Ketoconazole
Mebendazole	Tetracyclines
Oxibendazole	Others
Sulfonamides	Hyperthyroidism
Tetracyclines	Liver disorders (see Table 37-4)
Ketoconazole	Cholangiohepatitis
Thiacetarsamide	Feline leukemia virus–related
Others	Hepatic lipidosis
Diet-induced (Prescription Diet S-D*)	Idiopathic
Hyperadrenocorticism	Secondary to other disorders
Liver disorders (see Table 37-3)	Diabetes mellitus
Abdominal trauma	Chronic anorexia or malnu-
Hepatic necrosis	trition
Damaged biliary tract	Drugs or toxins
Diaphragmatic hernia with in-	Septicemia
carcerated liver lobe	Others
Acute pancreatitis	Abdominal trauma
Sepsis	Hepatic necrosis
Toxin (many)	Damaged biliary tract
	Diaphragmatic hernia with in-
	carcerated liver lobe
	Sepsis

*Hill's Pet Products, Topeka, KS
S-ALT, serum alanine aminotransferase; SAP, serum alkaline phosphatase

DECREASED SERUM ALKALINE PHOSPHATASE

There is no known significance to decreased serum alkaline phosphatase (SAP) activity.

INCREASED SERUM ALKALINE PHOSPHATASE

Problem Definition and Recognition

An increased SAP level is defined as an alkaline phosphatase above the normal species reference range for the particular laboratory procedure being used.

Pathophysiology

Certain enzymes can gain access to the extracellular fluid and blood without significant necrosis or damage to the membranes of the cells that produce the

TABLE 61-3. Comparison of Causes of Increased Serum Alkaline Phosphatase
in Dogs and Cats

	Magnitude of Increase (× Normal)	
Disorder	*Dogs*	*Cats*
Hypercortisolemia	1.5–200	Normal
Cholestasis	1.5–150	1.5–15
Anticonvulsants	1.5–5	Normal (?)
Bacteremia/endotoxemia	1.5–5	1.5–3
Osteoblastic activity	1.5–3	1.5–3
Neoplasia	Normal–100 (?)	Normal–10 (?)

enzymes.[6] Alkaline phosphatase and gamma glutamyl transpeptidase (GGT) are two such enzymes. Significant increases in SAP are caused by increased cell production of alkaline phosphatase and not usually by cell injury or necrosis.

Total SAP activity is composed of the action of all the isoenzymes of alkaline phosphatase. Tissues and cells known to produce these isoenzymes include osteoblasts, hepatocytes, biliary epithelial cells, intestine, placenta, kidney, and some neoplasms. Increased cellular production by any of these tissues may cause increased SAP activity. Cholestasis induces synthesis of large quantities of hepatic alkaline phosphatase isoenzyme in both dogs and cats (see below). Also, drug-induced (glucocorticoids, anticonvulsants) increases in SAP must always be considered (see below).

Hepatobiliary and osteoblastic alkaline phosphatase isoenzymes have significantly longer half-lives (3 days in dogs; 5 hours in cats) than intestinal, renal, and placental alkaline phosphatase isoenzymes (6 minutes in dogs; 2 minutes in cats). In dogs glucocorticoid-induced alkaline phosphatase isoenzyme has a half-life similar to that of cholestasis-induced alkaline phosphatase. Because of the significant differences in half-lives, increased SAP in adult dogs is usually due to either hepatobiliary disease or excessive glucocorticoids. In adult cats, increased SAP is generally caused by hepatobiliary disease (Tables 61-2 and 61-3).

Cholestasis, either intrahepatic or extrahepatic, is associated with increased alkaline phosphatase production by biliary epithelial cells and hepatocytes in both dogs and cats. Although neither the mechanism nor the reason for the increased production is known, the result is increased SAP activity. This increase may be detected prior to the onset and in the absence of hyperbilirubinemia. The magnitude of the increase in SAP activity varies between 1.5 and 200 times normal. The magnitude of SAP increase in cats with cholestasis is less, probably because of the shorter half-life of feline SAP (see Table 61-3). Normal feline SAP values are about one-third of normal canine values; therefore, even minor SAP increases in cats (1.5 to 2 times normal) are significant.

In dogs, excessive glucocorticoids are the most common cause of an increased SAP (Tables 61-2 and 61-3). Although the precise mechanisms are unknown, glucocorticoids have been reported to induce synthesis of a hepatic isoenzyme of alkaline phosphatase different from that caused by cholestasis. Glucocorticoids cause accumulation of glycogen and water in hepatocytes (so-called steroid hepatopathy), which may cause intrahepatic cholestasis, resulting in further induction of alkaline phosphatase synthesis (see below).

Increased SAP activity is commonly observed following glucocorticoid therapy and in Cushing's syndrome (hyperadrenocorticism) in dogs. Also, it appears that stress caused by a variety of serious chronic illnesses (*e.g.*, renal failure, pancreatitis) in dogs may result in chronic hypercortisolemia and increased SAP activity. The duration of the glucocorticoid-induced increase in SAP is unpredictable, but it can take several months for SAP to normalize. Cats are much more resistant to the hepatic effects of glucocorticoids, and there is usually no change in SAP following glucocorticoid treatment, hyperadrenocorticism, or stress of chronic illness.

It is now practical to differentiate the corticosteroid-induced alkaline phosphatase isoenzyme from the hepatic alkaline phosphatase isoenzyme produced as a result of cholestasis.[4,5] Corticosteroid-induced alkaline phosphatase is resistant to levamisole inhibition *in vitro* (less than 10% suppression), whereas the hepatic alkaline phosphatase isoenzyme induced by cholestatic disorders suppresses by more than 90%. Interestingly, the early increase in SAP (first 1 to 3 weeks) following glucocorticoid administration is the suppressible alkaline phosphatase isoenzyme. With more than 2 to 3 weeks of hypercortisolemia, the levamisole-resistant alkaline phosphatase isoenzyme is present.

Increases in SAP as a result of anticonvulsant therapy in dogs appear to be the result of increased levamisole-resistant alkaline phosphatase isoenzyme (see Display, Causes of Levamisole-Resistant Increased Serum Alkaline Phosphatase in Dogs).

The following examples illustrate the clinical utility of the levamisole-inhibition test in dogs.

Example 1	*SAP (IU/ml)*
Pre-levamisole incubation	2000
Post-levamisole incubation	180

The SAP increase is caused by either early effects of glucocorticoids (less likely) or hepatobiliary disease (more likely).

Example 2	*SAP (IU/ml)*
Pre-levamisole incubation	3000
Post-levamisole incubation	2700

In Example 2, the SAP increase is caused by chronic hypercortisolemia (more likely) or anticonvulsant therapy (less likely). Patients with increased SAP activity characterized by intermediate levamisole suppression probably have a mixture of the steroid-induced and cholestasis-induced alkaline phosphatase isoenzymes.

Some neoplasms reportedly may cause marked increases in SAP. In dogs,

> ### Causes of Levamisole-Resistant
> ### Increased Serum Alkaline Phosphatase in Dogs
>
> - Chronic hypercortisolemia (>2–3 weeks)
>   Glucocorticoid therapy
>   Hyperadrenocorticism (Cushing's syndrome)
>   Stress of chronic illness
> - Anticonvulsant therapy

adrenocortical adenocarcinomas, mixed mammary tumors, hemangiosarcomas, lymphomas, and oral carcinomas have been associated with increased SAP activity. Neoplasms are far more likely to cause an increased SAP when they involve the hepatobiliary system and cause cholestasis.

Increased osteoblastic activity and associated increases in SAP activity characterize normal bone growth of puppies as well as pathologic causes of increased osteoblastic activity, such as canine panosteitis. The magnitude of the increase in SAP activity associated with either a physiologic or a pathologic increase in osteoblastic activity is usually mild or on the order of 1.5 to 3.5 times normal SAP activity (see Table 61-3).

Diagnostic Plan

History and Physical Examination. There are no historical or physical examination findings attributable to an increased SAP. However, a history of administration of glucocorticoids or anticonvulsants to dogs is often associated with an increased SAP. Evidence of cholestasis, such as icterus, is often found in dogs and cats with an increased SAP.

Laboratory Evaluation. SAP should be determined as part of a serum biochemical panel. In addition, a CBC and urine analysis are usually helpful in the assessment of problems causing an increased SAP. Follow-up laboratory evaluation is determined by the rule outs being considered after assessment of the initial data.

HYPOGLYCEMIA

Problem Definition and Recognition

Hypoglycemia is a decrease in blood glucose concentration below 70 mg/dl.

Pathophysiology

Blood glucose concentration is a net result of glucose production and utilization in the body. Sources of blood glucose are exogenous (food intake) and endogenous (glycogenolysis and gluconeogenesis). When food is not available, continuing tissue glucose utilization necessitates endogenous glucose production. The liver, under hormonal influences, is the fulcrum of glucose homeostasis (glycogenolysis and gluconeogenesis), although the kidneys may synthesize significant amounts of glucose (renal gluconeogenesis) during prolonged fasting.[14]

During fasting, glycogenolysis in the liver maintains blood glucose for about 24 hours, after which hepatic glycogen is depleted. Thereafter, body proteins (mainly muscle) are the main sources of endogenous glucose via hepatic and renal gluconeogenesis. Glycerol derived from body fat breakdown is also utilized for gluconeogenesis.[10]

Several hormones (so-called stress hormones) increase blood glucose by promoting gluconeogenesis or glycogenolysis or by inhibiting cellular utilization of glucose. These include glucagon, glucocorticoids, catecholamines such as epinephrine, growth hormone, and progesterone. Insulin lowers blood glucose by inhibiting gluconeogenesis and causing uptake of glucose by insulin-dependent cells, primarily muscle and fat. Other cells, such as those in the central nervous system and kidneys, do not require insulin for glucose uptake.

Minute-to-minute regulation of blood glucose concentration is maintained quite efficiently by glucagon and insulin. Whenever blood glucose decreases, glucagon output from alpha cells in the pancreatic islets increases, and insulin secretion from pancreatic beta cells is suppressed. Hyperglucagonemia promotes glycogenolysis or gluconeogenesis, or both, resulting in increased blood glucose, which in turn suppresses glucagon secretion and enhances insulin output.

Hypoglycemia can result from decreased glucose production or increased glucose utilization (Fig. 61-2). Decreased glucose production occurs because of decreased food intake or decreased endogenous glycogenolysis or gluconeogenesis, or both. Unlike people, most normal dogs and cats do not become significantly hypoglycemic for days or weeks during fasting because of endogenous glucose production. This ability is probably necessary for survival in the wild, where the animal may not eat for many days. Exceptions are often encountered in puppies and toy breeds of dogs, in which hypoglycemia may occur within a few hours of fasting.

Increased glucose utilization occurs *in vitro* (delay in separating erythrocytes from serum) or *in vivo* due to hyperinsulinemia or increased uptake of glucose by various tissues.

Diagnostic Plan

History and Physical Examination. The history and physical examination will help rule out certain causes of hypoglycemia (Table 61-4). Short-term (24 to 48 hours) fasting in puppies and toy breeds of dogs often results in hypoglycemia. Endogenous glucose production is inadequate for unknown reasons. Chronic starvation results in cachexia and malabsorption and is characterized by

Text continues on p. 554

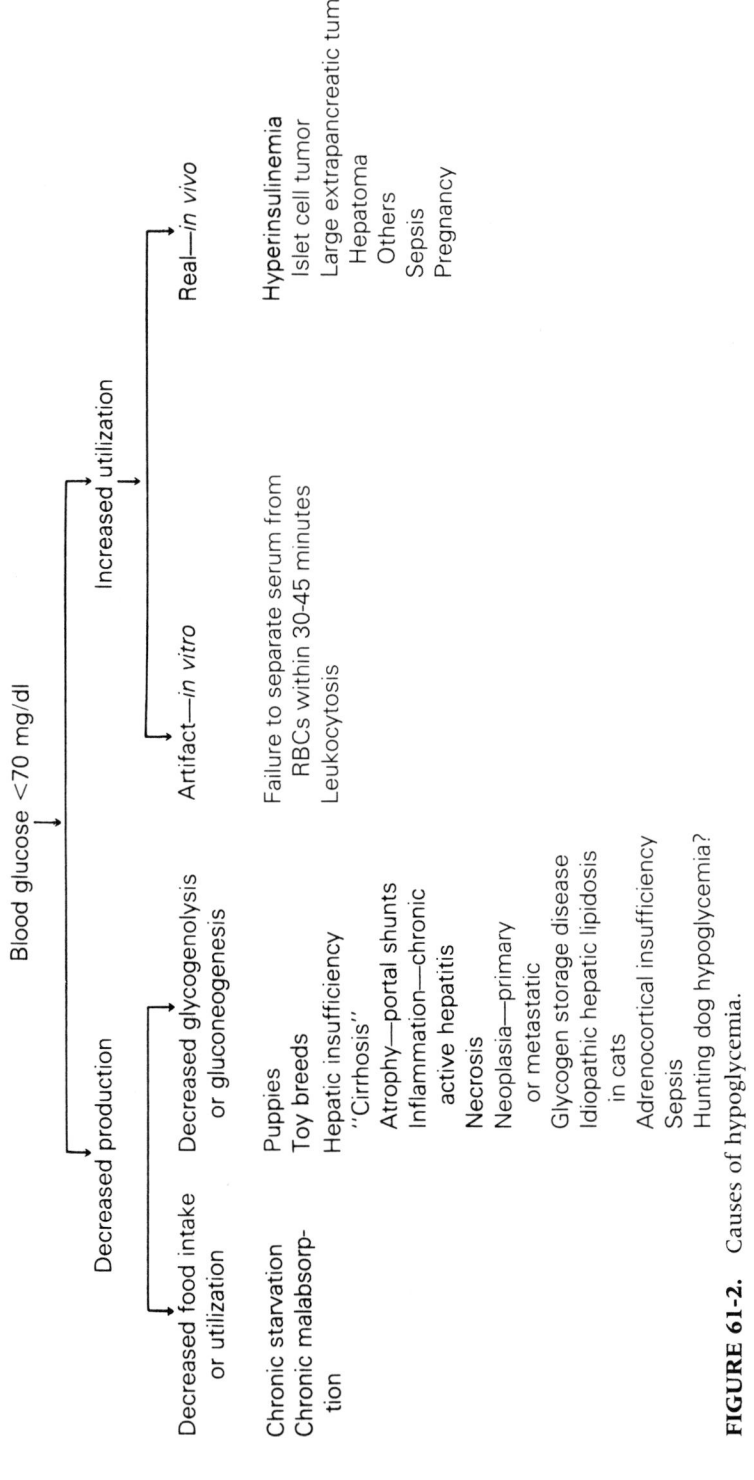

FIGURE 61-2. Causes of hypoglycemia.

Blood glucose <70 mg/dl

Decreased production

- Decreased food intake or utilization
  - Chronic starvation
  - Chronic malabsorption

- Decreased glycogenolysis or gluconeogenesis
  - Puppies
  - Toy breeds
  - Hepatic insufficiency
    "Cirrhosis"
    Atrophy—portal shunts
    Inflammation—chronic active hepatitis
    Necrosis
    Neoplasia—primary or metastatic
    Glycogen storage disease
    Idiopathic hepatic lipidosis in cats
  - Adrenocortical insufficiency
  - Sepsis
  - Hunting dog hypoglycemia?

Increased utilization

- Artifact—in vitro
  - Failure to separate serum from RBCs within 30-45 minutes
  - Leukocytosis

- Real—in vivo
  - Hyperinsulinemia
    Islet cell tumor
    Large extrapancreatic tumors
    Hepatoma
    Others
    Sepsis
    Pregnancy

TABLE 61-4. Characteristic Findings of Common Disorders Causing Hypoglycemia

Disorder	Clinical Signs Other Than Those of Hypoglycemia*	Hematology	Urine Analysis	Biochemistry Other Than Hypoglycemia	Special Tests
Decreased production Decreased food intake or utilization					
Chronic starvation	Weight loss	Normal or mild nonregenerative anemia	Normal	$\downarrow$ Albumin $\pm$	None; respond to feeding
Chronic malabsorption	Diarrhea Steatorrhea Cachexia	Mild to moderate nonregenerative anemia	Normal	$\downarrow$ Albumin $\downarrow$ Calcium	Chronic small bowel diarrhea (see Chapter 33)
Decreased glycogenolysis/gluconeogenesis					
Puppies	No other signs History of being off food >24–48 hours	Normal	Normal	Serum glucose <50 mg/dl	None; usually respond to intravenous glucose and feeding
Toy Breeds	Same as for puppies	Normal	Normal	Serum glucose <50 mg/dl	Same as for puppies
Hepatic insufficiency	Signs of hepatic failure Icterus Hepatoencephalopathy—stupor, coma, seizures, excessive salivation, head-pressing	Anemia, regeneration variable Stomatocytosis and microcytosis $\pm$ $\downarrow$ Plasma protein WBC variable	Hyposthenuria $\pm$ Ammonium biurate crystals $\pm$	$\downarrow$ Albumin $\uparrow$ Globulin $\pm$ $\downarrow$ BUN $\pm$ Serum glucose <70 mg/dl $\uparrow$ ALT and SAP $\pm$ $\uparrow$ Bilirubin $\pm$	$\uparrow$ Serum bile acids, pre- and postprandial $\uparrow$ Blood NH$_3$ or abnormal NH$_3$ tolerance Abnormal coagulogram $\pm$ Abnormal portal

(continued)

551

TABLE 61-4. Characteristic Findings of Common Disorders Causing Hypoglycemia *(continued)*

Disorder	Clinical Signs Other Than Those of Hypoglycemia*	Hematology	Urine Analysis	Biochemistry Other Than Hypoglycemia	Special Tests
	Ascites Melena Young dog or cat with hepatic atrophy due to congenital portal shunt				venography in portal shunt cases Abnormal liver biopsy
Adrenocortical insufficiency	Anorexia and lethargy Sporadic vomiting and diarrhea Bradycardia Dehydration Collapse—signs of shock	↑ PCV and total protein Eosinophilia and lymphocytosis ±	Usually normal Sometimes ↓ specific gravity	↑ Albumin and globulin (dehydration) Mild ↑ BUN ↓ Na, ↑ K (Na:K ratio <23:1)# ↓ TCO_2	ECG—signs of hyperkalemia Plasma cortisols—low baseline and little or no response to ACTH
Sepsis	Depression progressing to signs of shock Fever progressing to hypothermia Vomiting Diarrhea—melena	↑ PCV and plasma protein ± Neutrophilic leukocytosis with left shift progressing to leukopenia with inappropriate left shift Toxic neutrophils Thrombocytopenia	↑ Bilirubin ±	↓ Albumin ± ↑ Globulin ± ↑ SAP ± Mild ↑ bilirubin ±	Blood cultures ×3 at hourly intervals during febrile episode and when off antibiotics >48 hours
Hunting dog hypoglycemia	Weakness and collapse during hunting	Normal	Normal	Normal; hypoglycemia difficult to document	None; usually responds to high-protein feedings

Increased utilization					
Artifact—*in vitro*					
Failure to separate serum from RBCs within 30–45 minutes	No signs of hypoglycemia	Normal	Normal	Normal	Repeat biochemistry with proper handling of sample
Real—*in vivo*					
Hyperinsulinemia Islet cell tumor	Mostly in dogs >6 years old	Normal	Normal	Usually normal	High plasma insulin on a sample with a blood glucose <60 mg/dl
Large extrapancreatic tumors, *e.g.*, hepatoma, others	Mostly in dogs >7 years old ↓Appetite Weight loss Sporadic vomiting and diarrhea Palpable intraabdominal mass Others depending on organ involved	Mild to moderate nonregenerative anemia WBC variable	Normal or Bilirubinuria	↓Alubmin ± ↑Globulin ± ↑ALT and SAP ± ↑Bilirubin ±	↑Serum bile acids pre- and postprandial ↑Blood NH_3 or abnormal NH_3 tolerance Abnormal liver biopsy: neoplasia
Sepsis	See under Decreased production.				

↑, decreased; ±, present or absent; ↑, increased; WBC, white blood cells; BUN, blood urea nitrogen; ALT, alanine aminotransferase; SAP, serum alkaline phosphatase; PCV, packed cell volume; TCO_2, total CO_2; ECG, electrocardiogram; ACTH, adrenocorticotropic hormone

* Common signs of hypoglycemia include weakness, ataxia, collapse, hypothermia, and seizures.

‡ In some cases, only glucocorticoids are deficient and serum Na and K are normal.

diarrhea, steatorrhea, and weight loss. Hypoglycemia may be observed. Hepatic insufficiency severe enough to cause hypoglycemia is usually accompanied by other signs of hepatic failure such as icterus, ascites, melena, and central nervous system (CNS) disturbances (hepatoencephalopathy). Polydipsia and polyuria are sometimes observed in both adrenocortical insufficiency and hepatic failure. Whenever sepsis is the cause of hypoglycemia, other signs are generally obvious and may include depression, fever, "muddy" mucous membranes, "injected" sclera, dyspnea, and signs of shock. Extrapancreatic tumors causing hypoglycemia may be palpable and may cause other signs of organ dysfunction, such as weight loss, vomiting, diarrhea, and icterus. Islet cell tumors are small and generally cause few signs other than intermittent weakness, collapse, or seizures associated with hypoglycemia. Signs may occur during fasting, after exercise, or occasionally from 2 to 8 hours after eating as a result of excessive insulin output (insulin "overshoot") from the beta cell tumor.

Laboratory Evaluation. The laboratory workup of a hypoglycemic dog or cat will depend on associated clinical signs. A hemogram, a serum biochemical profile, and urine analysis are indicated for each animal. Follow-up diagnostic plans will depend on the assessment of results obtained (Table 61-4). In suspected cases of hyperinsulinism, plasma insulin concentration should be measured on a sample from which the blood glucose concentration is less than 60 mg/dl. In a normal patient with a low blood glucose, the plasma insulin is decreased below the normal range, whereas in an animal with an insulin-secreting tumor, the plasma insulin is high or occasionally in the high-normal range. Plasma insulin should be determined in a laboratory where the procedure has been validated for dogs and cats.

HYPERGLYCEMIA

Problem Definition and Recognition

Hyperglycemia is an increase in blood glucose concentration above 120 mg/dl. Mild hyperglycemia is frequently observed in dogs and cats, probably as a result of the effects of fear and struggling during blood collection.

Pathophysiology

Normal regulation of blood glucose concentration was discussed in the section on hypoglycemia. Hyperglycemia results from pathophysiologic mechanisms similar to those discussed for hypoglycemia, except in reverse (*i.e.*, increased glucose production or decreased glucose utilization) (Fig. 61-3).

Diagnostic Plan

Blood glucose levels should always be evaluated on blood samples obtained after a 12-hour fast. Although the blood glucose concentration after a meal

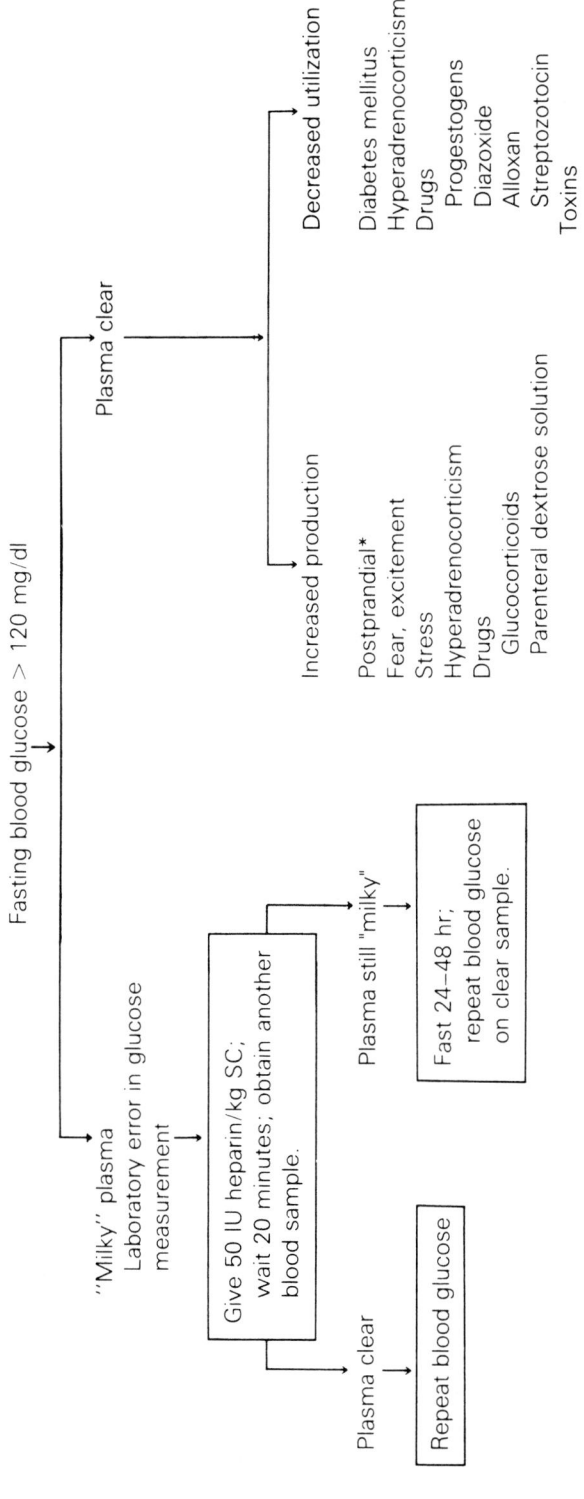

FIGURE 61-3. Causes of hyperglycemia.

* Blood glucose does not exceed renal threshold in normal animal.

should not exceed the renal threshold value (about 180 to 200 mg/dl) in a normal animal, postprandial hyperlipemia (due to circulating chylomicrons) may cause a significant error in some laboratory methods of measuring blood glucose, resulting in markedly increased glucose readings. If it is necessary to measure blood glucose from an animal with lipemia, subcutaneous administration of heparin (50 IU/kg) sometimes causes clearing of lipemia in about 20 minutes (by activating lipoprotein lipase, which breaks down chylomicrons). Some dogs, especially miniature schnauzers, may require 24 to 96 hours of fasting to clear chylomicronemia.

History and Physical Examination. The most common causes of mild to moderate hyperglycemia in dogs and cats are fear, excitement, and struggling associated with blood sample procurement and stress caused by a variety of medical and surgical disorders (Table 61-5). Fear and excitement cause catecholamine release, which results in hepatic glycogenolysis. Stress causes glucocorticoid secretion by the adrenal glands, which results in hepatic gluconeogenesis. Effects of stress on blood glucose are more dramatic in cats than in dogs. Blood glucose values from stressed cats may be as high as 300 mg/dl and be associated with moderate to marked glucosuria. In dogs, stress hyperglycemia seldom exceeds 180 mg/dl, and glucosuria is not present. History is usually sufficient to rule out these causes of hyperglycemia. It may be more difficult to decide whether marked hyperglycemia and glucosuria in a cat are due to stress or diabetes mellitus. Ketonuria may be present in either condition.

Diabetes mellitus usually occurs in obese or formerly obese cats with a history of marked polydipsia and polyuria. Similar signs are usually present in diabetic dogs. Concurrent disorders in a diabetic patient may cause other signs such as anorexia, depression, vomiting, and diarrhea. In diabetic dogs, acute pancreatitis, hyperadrenocorticism, ketoacidosis, and various infections are common. Ketoacidosis, hepatic insufficiency due to hepatic lipidosis, and infection are common in diabetic cats. Hyperadrenocorticism (canine Cushing's syndrome), either naturally occurring or iatrogenic, may cause mild hyperglycemia due to glucocorticoid-induced gluconeogenesis and inhibition of insulin action. Other signs of Cushing's syndrome, such as polydipsia, polyuria, alopecia, thin skin, abdominal distention, and hepatomegaly, may be present. Signs of hyperadrenocorticism may be easily overlooked in a diabetic dog. Large amounts of insulin (greater than 2.0 units/kg) may be necessary to normalize blood glucose in a diabetic animal with concurrent Cushing's syndrome, and blood glucose values may fluctuate markedly from day to day, even though insulin dosage, diet, and exercise are kept reasonably constant. Plasma cortisol values before and after adrenocorticotropic hormone (ACTH) stimulation and dexamethasone suppression are necessary to diagnose hyperadrenocorticism.

Laboratory Evaluation. The laboratory evaluation of a dog or cat with hyperglycemia will depend on associated clinical signs. A hemogram, a serum bio-

Text continues on p. 560

TABLE 61-5. Characteristic Findings of Common Disorders Causing Hyperglycemia

Disorder	Clinical Signs	Hematology	Urine Analysis	Biochemistry Other Than Hyperglycemia	Special Tests
Artifact					
Hyperlipemia	Usually normal or Obesity Abdominal pain, vomiting ± (acute pancreatis) Seizures?	Lipemia and hemolysis of sample ↑ Plasma protein by refractometry (artifactual) Neutrophilic leukocytosis with left shift ± (acute pancreatitis)	Normal	May interfere with other tests; consult clinical pathology text. ↑ Serum amylase and lipase ±, mild hypocalcemia ± (acute pancreatitis)	Usually none Blood lipid profile ±
Increased production					
Postprandial	Normal	Mild to marked lipemia Increased plasma protein by refractometry (artifactual)	Normal	Lipemia may interfere with other tests; consult clinical pathology text.	None
Fear, excitement, stress	Fear, nervousness, struggling during blood sampling Other signs associated with a variety of diseases leading to stress	Stress leukogram	Normal	↓ TCO_2 ± (↑ Lactic acid due to struggling)	None

(continued)

557

TABLE 61-5. Characteristic Findings of Common Disorders Causing Hyperglycemia (*continued*)

Disorder	Clinical Signs	Hematology	Urine Analysis	Biochemistry Other Than Hyperglycemia	Special Tests
Hyperadrenocorticism	Polydipsia and polyuria Alopecia Thin skin "Pot-belly" Hepatomegaly Others	Stress leukogram	↓ Specific gravity Bacteriuria ± Pyuria ± (numbers of WBC may be fewer than expected with infection)	↑ SAP ↑ ALT	Plasma cortisols before and after ACTH stimulation and low-dose dexamethasone suppression
Drugs Glucocorticoids	See Hyperadrenocorticism.				
Parenteral dextrose solutions	Usually normal Polyuria ±	Normal	Glucosuria	Normal	None
Decreased utilization Diabetes mellitus	Polydipsia and polyuria Obesity or weight loss Hepatomegaly Cataracts ± Others depending on complications Vomiting Abdominal pain Coma Others	Variable depending on complications	Glucosuria Ketonuria ± ↑ WBC and bacteriuria ±	Variable depending on complications	None for diabetes mellitus Depends on complications

	Clinical Signs	Urinalysis	Serum Chemistry	Diagnostic Test
Drugs Progestogens (megestrol acetate [Ovaban, Megase], medroxyprogesterone acetate [Depo-Proveral]) Others (diazoxide, alloxan, streptozotocin)	See Diabetes mellitus.			
Toxin Ethylene glycol (antifreeze)	Ataxia Depression, lethargy, progressing to stupor, coma Polydipsia and polyuria Vomiting and dehydration Seizures	↑ PCV and plasma protein (dehydration) ↑ WBC (stress leukogram)	↓ Specific gravity Calcium oxalate crystals ±	↑ BUN and creatinine ↓ TCO$_2$ Hypocalcemia Markedly ↑ anion gap	Blood ethylene glycol test
Diestrus—progesterone	Older unspayed female dogs See Diabetes mellitus.	See Diabetes mellitus.		

±, present or absent; ↑, increased; ↓, decreased; WBC, white blood cells; TCO$_2$, total CO$_2$; SAP, serum alkaline phosphatase; ALT, alanine aminotransferase; ACTH, adrenocorticotropic hormone; BUN, blood urea nitrogen chemical profile, and urine analysis are usually indicated. Follow-up diagnostic plans depend upon the assessment of results obtained. It is seldom necessary to do glucose tolerance testing to evaluate hyperglycemia in dogs and cats. Patients with diabetes mellitus usually have a blood glucose concentration greater than 250 mg/dl. With lesser degrees of hyperglycemia (blood glucose of 120 to 200 mg/dl), the cause of the increased blood glucose concentration can usually be determined without glucose tolerance testing.

HYPONATREMIA

Problem Definition and Recognition

Hyponatremia, defined as a decrease in serum sodium concentration below 140 mEq/liter, may occur with an increased, decreased, or normal extracellular fluid volume.

Pathophysiology

Sodium salts are primarily responsible for the osmolality of extracellular fluid and are the major determinants of extracellular fluid volume and distribution of water between extracellular and intracellular fluid.[10] Signs associated with deficit and excess states of sodium reflect its role in the regulation of extracellular fluid volume. Cell membranes are relatively impermeable to sodium but are freely permeable to water. Sodium ions that gain access to the cell interior are actively extruded back into the extracellular fluid by energy-requiring enzymatic "pumps" in the cell membrane. The sodium pump is coupled with potassium ions, and as sodium is extruded from cells, potassium is "pumped" into cells.[1] Potassium salts are mainly responsible for intracellular osmotic pressure. Since water rapidly equilibrates between extracellular and intracellular fluid, osmotic concentrations of both these major fluids are always the same.

Thirst receptors in the hypothalamus respond to increases in plasma osmolality to initiate water consumption, thereby helping to maintain body water. Supraoptic nuclei in the hypothalamus respond to increased plasma osmolality to cause secretion of antidiuretic hormone (ADH) from the posterior pituitary. ADH increases the permeability to water of the collecting ducts in the kidneys, causing reabsorption of water.

Sodium balance is closely regulated and maintained within narrow limits, despite large variations in dietary intake of sodium. Although sodium is excreted from both the gastrointestinal tract and kidneys, day-to-day regulation of sodium balance occurs primarily in the renal tubules. Several factors influence handling of sodium by the kidneys, including aldosterone secretion by the adrenal cortex. Decreased plasma sodium concentration causes decreased blood volume and blood flow to the kidneys. Renin is secreted by the renal juxtaglomerular cells, which stimulates aldosterone release. Aldosterone causes sodium and water reabsorption and potassium excretion in the renal tubules. The opposite changes occur whenever sodium intake is increased.

Hyponatremia can result from decreased intake or increased excretion of sodium, as well as from overhydration (Table 61-6). It is unusual for decreased sodium intake alone to cause hyponatremia because of the ability of the kidneys to reabsorb sodium so completely and to excrete free water. Hyponatremia is commonly due to combinations of the above mechanisms.

Any decrease in plasma sodium concentration following sodium loss is initially corrected by inhibition of both thirst and ADH secretion. Initially, plasma sodium concentration is preserved, but at the expense of extracellular fluid volume. With progressive sodium loss, extracellular fluid volume contracts; at a critical point, vascular volume receptors stimulate ADH production and thirst, causing a gain in water and a decrease in plasma sodium concentration. Thus, sodium loss may be characterized by signs of volume depletion (decreased skin pliability, weak pulse, or shock) and, unless sodium loss is abrupt, by hyponatremia.

On the other hand, hyponatremia is frequently associated with sodium gain and relative water excess. This occurs most commonly with conditions characterized by a decrease in effective circulating blood volume, such as congestive heart failure and hypoalbuminemic disorders (*e.g.*, cirrhosis and nephrotic syndrome). The kidneys respond to decreased perfusion by secreting renin, which causes aldosterone secretion, resulting in retention of sodium and water. Hyponatremia is worsened by stimulation of thirst and ADH output, owing to low effective circulating blood volume. Thus, hyponatremia may reflect sodium loss or sodium gain with water excess.

Pseudohyponatremia may occur due to the presence of hyperlipemia or marked hyperproteinemia. Excessive lipids or proteins cause hyponatremia because sodium is present only in the water portion of plasma; the laboratory measurement is taken from the lipid, protein, and water phases.

Osmotically active substances in plasma, such as glucose and mannitol, attract water from cells into the extracellular fluid, resulting in dilution of plasma sodium. Despite the fall in serum sodium concentration, plasma osmolality is normal or slightly increased.

History and Physical Examination. A history of administration of glucose solution or a history of disorders causing dehydration (*e.g.*, anorexia, vomiting, and diarrhea) may help initially categorize hyponatremia. Dehydration is usually associated with decreased skin pliability, dry mucous membranes, and decreased capillary refilling time (Table 61-7). Hyponatremic dehydration predisposes to early, severe vascular volume depletion and vascular collapse (shock).

Overhydration may be difficult to distinguish clinically from normal hydration. Generalized edema and ascites are sometimes present (see Table 61-7).

Text continues on p. 566

TABLE 61-6. Characteristic Findings of Common Disorders Causing Hyponatremia

Disorder	Clinical Signs	Hematology	Urine Analysis	Biochemistry Other Than Hyponatremia	Special Tests
Artifact Hyperlipemia	Usually normal Signs of acute pancreatitis ±	Lipemia Hemolysis ± Inflammatory leukogram ±	Normal	Usually normal ↑ Serum amylase and lipase ±	Consider blood lipid profile
Redistribution of fluid into extracellular compartment Hyperglycemia Hyperproteinemia	See Table 61-5 Dehydration Depression Other CNS signs and hemorrhagic tendencies associated with hyperviscosity	Nonregenerative anemia ± Malignant cells in circulation ± (multiple myeloma)	Proteinuria ± in myeloma	↑ Albumin and globulin (dehydration) Others depending on sites of tumor involvement	Skeletal radiographs for myeloma Others depending on sites of tumor involvement
Dehydration Vomiting	See Chapters 32 and 33.				
Adrenocortical insufficiency	Anorexia and lethargy Sporadic vomiting and diarrhea Bradycardia Dehydration Collapse—signs of shock	↑ PCV and plasma protein ± Eosinophilia and lymphocytosis ±	Usually normal—sometimes ↓ specific gravity	↑ Albumin and globulin (dehydration) Mildly ↑ BUN ↓ Na, ↑ K (Na:K ratio <23:1) ↓ TCO₂	ECG—signs of hyperkalemia See Table 61-10. Plasma cortisols—low baseline and little or no response to ACTH

562

Renal loss of Na Renal disease Diuretic use Polydipsia/polyuria Dehydration	↑ PCV and plasma protein	Low specific gravity Rest of urinalysis variable	↑ BUN ↑ Phosphorus Rest of biochemistry variable	Abdominal radiographs and sonograms Rest of workup variable, including renal biopsy
Overhydration Congestive heart failure Coughing Dyspnea Cyanosis Ascites—modified transudate Peripheral edema—rare Tachycardia Heart murmur	Normal	Normal	Normal or Mildly ↑ ALT and SAP	Thoracic radiographs ECG Low urine Na
"Cirrhosis" Ascites—transudate Icterus CNS signs (hepatoencephalopathy) Stupor Coma Head-pressing Others Melena Vomiting Polydipsia/polyuria Hemorrhagic tendencies	Anemia—regeneration variable Stomatocytosis ± Microcytosis ± ↓ Plasma protein WBC variable ↓ Platelets ±	Hyposthenuria ±	↓ Albumin ↑ Globulin ± ↓ BUN ± Mildly ↑ ALT and SAP ↓ Glucose ± ↑ Bilirubin ±	↑ Serum bile acids, pre- and postprandial ↑ Blood NH_3 or abnormal NH_3 tolerance Abnormal coagulogram ± Small liver on abdominal radiographs Low urine Na Abnormal liver biopsy

(continued)

TABLE 61-6. Characteristic Findings of Common Disorders Causing Hyponatremia *(continued)*

Disorder	Clinical Signs	Hematology	Urine Analysis	Biochemistry Other Than Hyponatremia	Special Tests
Nephrotic syndrome	Ascites Peripheral edema Lethargy Signs of renal failure ± Anorexia and vomiting Polydipsia/polyuria Others Hypercoagulation tendencies with thromboses Dyspnea, coughing (pulmonary thrombosis) Others	Nonregenerative anemia ±	↓ Specific gravity ± Proteinuria	↓ Albumin ↑ Cholesterol ↑ BUN	↑ Urine protein-to-creatinine ratio Coagulogram Abdominal radiographs and sonograms Renal biopsy ±
Iatrogenic water loading (5% dextrose therapy), especially for oliguric renal failure	Polyuria or Oliguria with renal failure	↓ PCV and plasma protein	↓ Specific gravity Glucosuria except in oliguric renal failure	↓ Albumin and globulin Slightly ↑ blood glucose ↑ BUN, ↑ K in oliguric renal failure	Abdominal radiographs to evaluate renal size

Disease	Clinical signs	Hemogram, PCV, plasma protein	Urinalysis	Serum chemistry	Special tests
Compulsive water drinking ("psychogenic polydipsia")	Polydipsia/polyuria	Normal or ↓ PCV and plasma protein ±	Hyposthenuria	Normal or ↓ Albumin and globulin	Water deprivation test; urine specific gravity <1.035 Low urine Na Urine osmolality may exceed serum osmolality Water intake >urine output High urine Na
Inappropriate ADH secretion	Signs of water intoxication—CNS Depression Weakness Confusion Focal neurologic signs Convulsions Coma Signs of primary disease (e.g., heartworms) Coughing Dyspnea Exercise intolerance Others	Normal or Changes due to the primary disease	Inappropriately hypertonic—see Special tests	Normal or Changes due to the primary disease	Normal plasma cortisols, pre- and post ACTH Water restriction and normal sodium diet correct hyponatremia

±, present or absent; ↑, increased; CNS, central nervous system; PCV, packed cell volume; ↓, decreased; BUN, blood urea nitrogen; TCO$_2$, total carbon dioxide; ECG, electrocardiogram; ACTH, adrenocorticotropic hormone; ALT, alanine aminotransferase; SAP, serum alkaline phosphatase; WBC, white blood cells

TABLE 61-7. Helpful Signs in the Evaluation of a Patient with Hyponatremia

Observation	Dehydration	Overhydration
Skin pliability	Decreased	Normal
Peripheral edema or ascites	Absent	Present
Capillary refilling time	Prolonged	Normal
Peripheral veins	Normal or collapsed	Normal or distended
Others	Tachycardia and weak pulse	Signs of congestive heart failure Pulmonary edema Ascites

Signs of water intoxication may be observed (CNS signs such as depression, weakness, confusion, focal neurologic signs, convulsions, and coma). Other signs depend on the specific disorder causing hyponatremia.

Laboratory Evaluation. Serum sodium levels should be evaluated on blood samples obtained after a 12-hour fast, because hyperlipemia may cause pseudo-hyponatremia. The initial laboratory workup of a dog or cat with hyponatremia should include a hemogram, a microfilariae check, a biochemical profile, and urine analysis. Dehydration frequently causes increased packed cell volume (PCV), total plasma protein, urine specific gravity, and sometimes BUN (prerenal). Depending on initial laboratory results, follow-up diagnostic procedures will vary (see Table 61-6). Measurement of urine sodium concentration sometimes helps differentiate causes of hyponatremia. Plasma aldosterone determination may be warranted in more difficult cases.

HYPERNATREMIA

Problem Definition and Recognition

Hypernatremia is defined as an increase in serum sodium above 155 mEq/liter.

Pathophysiology

As was discussed in the section on hyponatremia, sodium salts are primarily responsible for tonicity of extracellular fluid.[12] Therefore, hypertonicity may result from absolute or relative excess of sodium (as well as glucose). Urea freely diffuses across cell membranes and does not contribute to effective plasma osmotic pressure (tonicity), although it does affect measured osmolality. Effective plasma osmolality can be estimated from the following formula:

$$\text{Effective plasma osmolality} = 2(Na + K) + 18$$

Signs of CNS depression or coma may be observed when effective plasma osmolality is greater than 375 mOsm/liter. Theoretically, hypernatremia can occur as the result of excessive sodium intake, with or without excessive water loss, inadequate water intake, excessive water loss (usually with inadequate water intake), and losses of both water and sodium, with water loss predominating (Fig. 61-4; Table 61-8).

Diagnostic Plan

Causes of hypernatremia are shown in Figure 61-4 and Table 61-8. It is important to assess whether or not dehydration is present (as indicated by decreased skin pliability, dry mucous membranes, increased urine specific gravity, and increased BUN).

History and Physical Examination. Most patients with hypernatremia will also be dehydrated. Therefore, a careful history regarding water intake and conditions causing fluid loss (*e.g.*, vomiting, diarrhea, or polyuria) is warranted. Severe hypernatremia causes hypertonicity of extracellular fluid, which causes transfer of water out of brain cells (CNS desiccation). Severe weakness, depression, coma (hyperosmolal syndrome), and seizures may be observed.[9] Other signs depend on the primary disorder present (see Table 61-8). Severe hyperthermia and excessive panting typify heatstroke. A history of polydipsia and polyuria is usually present with diabetes insipidus and renal failure. Signs of uremia, including anorexia and vomiting, may also be present in patients with renal failure.

Laboratory Evaluation. The laboratory workup for hypernatremia is similar to that previously discussed for hyponatremia.

HYPOKALEMIA

Problem Definition and Recognition

Hypokalemia, as defined by a serum potassium concentration of less than 3.6 mEq/liter, may occur with an increased, normal, or decreased total body potassium.

Pathophysiology

Of the approximate 50 mEq of potassium per kilogram of body weight, almost 98% is intracellular at a concentration of about 150 mEq/liter. The remaining 2% that is in the extracellular fluid is closely maintained at a normal concentration of 3.6 to 5.6 mEq/liter. Thus, a large concentration gradient normally favors the transfer of potassium from cells into the extracellular fluid.[10] This situation is the opposite of that for sodium. The maintenance of high intracellular potassium

Text continues on p. 574

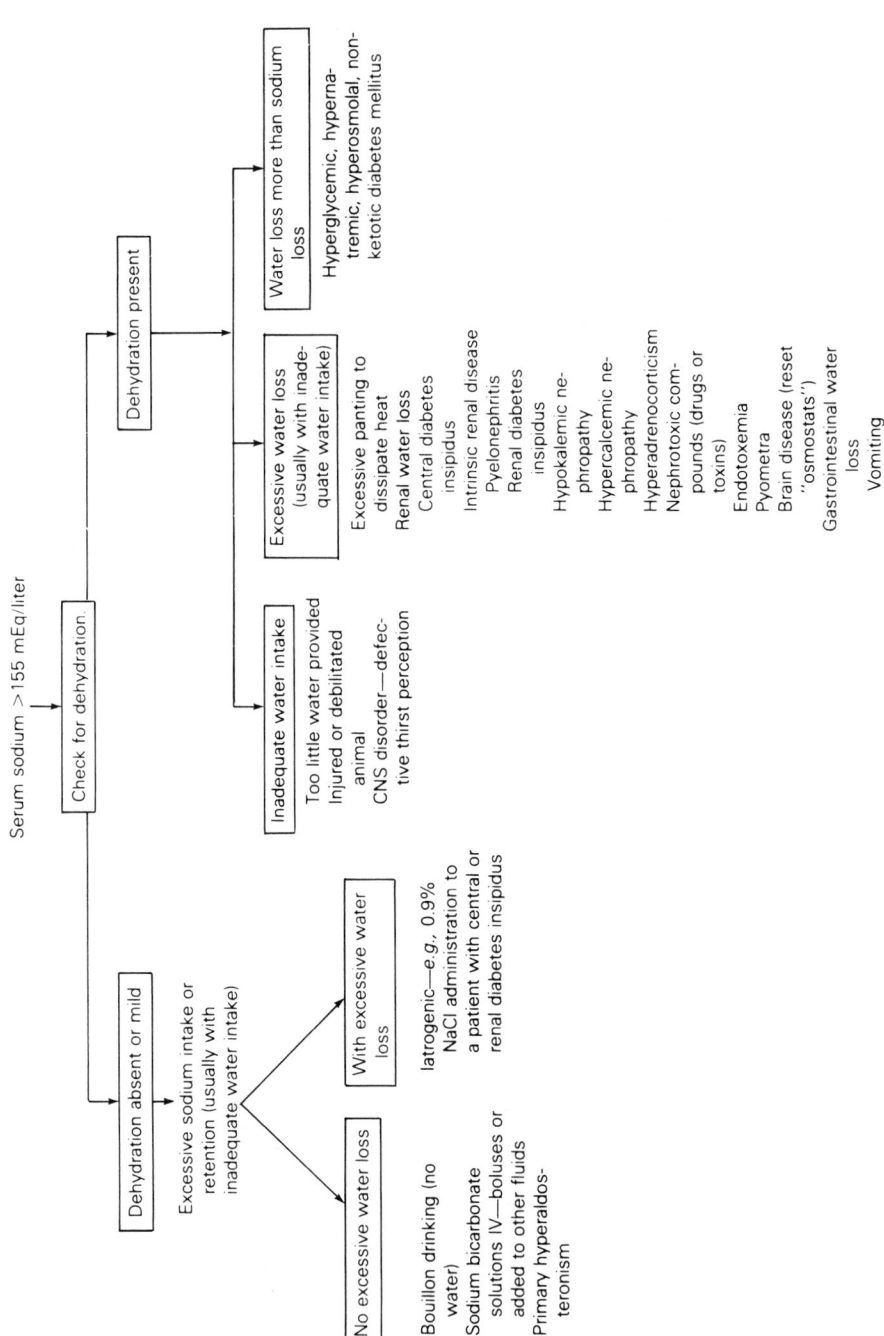

Serum sodium >155 mEq/liter

Check for dehydration.

Dehydration absent or mild

Excessive sodium intake or retention (usually with inadequate water intake)

No excessive water loss

Bouillon drinking (no water)
Sodium bicarbonate solutions IV—boluses or added to other fluids
Primary hyperaldosteronism

With excessive water loss

Iatrogenic—e.g., 0.9% NaCl administration to a patient with central or renal diabetes insipidus

Dehydration present

Inadequate water intake

Too little water provided
Injured or debilitated animal
CNS disorder—defective thirst perception

Excessive water loss (usually with inadequate water intake)

Excessive panting to dissipate heat
Renal water loss
Central diabetes insipidus
Intrinsic renal disease
Pyelonephritis
Renal diabetes insipidus
Hypokalemic nephropathy
Hypercalcemic nephropathy
Hyperadrenocorticism
Nephrotoxic compounds (drugs or toxins)
Endotoxemia
Pyometra
Brain disease (reset "osmostats")
Gastrointestinal water loss
Vomiting
Diarrhea

Water loss more than sodium loss

Hyperglycemic, hypernatremic, hyperosmolal, nonketotic diabetes mellitus

FIGURE 61-4. Causes of hypernatremia.

568

TABLE 61-8. Characteristic Findings of Common Disorders Causing Hypernatremia

Disorder	Clinical Signs	Hematology	Urine Analysis	Biochemistry Other Than Hypernatremia	Special Tests
Excessive sodium intake					
No excessive H$_2$O loss					
Bouillon drinking (no water)	CNS Depression Confusion Weakness Seizures Coma Mild dehydration	Mild ↑ PCV and total protein	Specific gravity >1.040	Mild ↑ albumin and globulin ↑ Cl	Urine Na ↑
Sodium bicarbonate solutions IV	See Bouillon drinking	Normal	Normal or Urine pH >7.5	↑ TCO$_2$	Urine Na ↑
Primary hyperaldosteronism	See Bouillon drinking	Variable	Variable	↓ K ↑ Cl ↑ TCO$_2$	↓ Urine Na ↑ Plasma aldosterone
With excessive water loss					
Iatrogenic, e.g., 0.9% NaCl administration to a patient with central or renal diabetes insipidus	Same as in No excessive H$_2$O loss	Same as in No excessive H$_2$O loss (above)	Specific gravity >1.030	Same as in No excessive H$_2$O loss	Urine Na normal to slightly ↑

(continued)

569

TABLE 61-8. Characteristic Findings of Common Disorders Causing Hypernatremia *(continued)*

Disorder	Clinical Signs	Hematology	Urine Analysis	Biochemistry Other Than Hypernatremia	Special Tests
Inadequate H$_2$O intake					
Too little water provided	Dehydration Thirst Later—depression, weakness	↑ PCV and total protein	Specific gravity >1.040	↑ Albumin and globulin ↑ Cl	Urine Na ↓
Injured or debilitated animal	Same as above and Signs of the primary injury or illness	Variable depending on injury or illness	Same as above	Variable	Urine Na ↓
CNS disorder—defective thirst perception	Depression, lethargy Decreased water intake Dehydration	Same as above	Same as above	Same as above	Urine osmolality-to-plasma osmolality ratio >4 No change in urine osmolality after ADH administration
Excessive water loss with inadequate water intake					
Excessive panting	Excessive panting to dissipate heat ↑ Body temperature ↑ Thirst Signs of heat stroke ±	↑ PCV and total protein Stress leukogram ±	Specific gravity >1.040	↑ Albumin and globulin Others if heatstroke is present	None

Condition	Clinical signs	Hematology	Urinalysis	Chemistry	Diagnostic tests
Renal water loss Central diabetes insipidus	Polyuria/polydipsia Rapid dehydration when water is denied Signs of hypertonicity when water is denied Depression, lethargy Weakness Stupor, coma, death	Normal or ↑ PCV and total protein	Specific gravity <1.005	Normal or ↑ Albumin and globulin ↑ Cl	Water deprivation test—little change in urine specific gravity ADH response test —urine specific gravity >1.030 Urine Na ↓
Intrinsic renal disease Pyelonephritis	Lethargy, depression Fever ± Abdominal pain Vomiting ±	Normal or Neutrophilic leukocytosis with left shift	↓ Specific gravity Pyuria and bacteriuria Hematuria, proteinuria, casts ±	↑ BUN ± If septic: ↓ Albumin ↑ SAP ↓ Glucose	Urine culture Excretory urogram Abdominal ultrasonography Renal biopsy
Renal diabetes insipidus	See Central diabetes insipidus Signs of renal failure ±	Variable	Specific gravity <1.012	↑ BUN ±	Water deprivation test—little change in urine specific gravity ADH response test —little change in urine specific gravity
Hypokalemic nephropathy	Polydipsia/polyuria Weakness Ileus ± Dehydration ±	Mild ↑ PCV and total protein ±	↓ Urine specific gravity	K <3.7 mEq/liter Others depending on cause of ↓ K	None

(continued)

571

TABLE 61-8. Characteristic Findings of Common Disorders Causing Hypernatremia *(continued)*

Disorder	Clinical Signs	Hematology	Urine Analysis	Biochemistry Other Than Hypernatremia	Special Tests
Hypercalcemic nephropathy	Polydipsia/polyuria Signs of renal failure ± Others variable	Variable	↓ Urine specific gravity	↑ BUN ± ↑ Ca Others variable	Variable depending on suspected cause
Hyperadrenocorticism	Polydipsia/polyuria Thin skin Bilaterally symmetric alopecia	Stress leukogram	↓ Urine specific gravity Pyuria and bacteruria ±	↑ SAP ↑ ALT ± ↓ K ± ↑ TCO_2 ±	Plasma cortisol panel—ACTH stimulation and low-dose dexamethasone suppression
Nephrotoxic drugs or toxins	Urine output variable Signs of renal failure ±	Variable	↓ Specific gravity Proteinuria ± Glucosuria ± Casts ±	↑ BUN Others variable	Usually none
Endotoxemia	Temperature variable Scleral injection Dehydration Signs of shock ± Others variable	WBC variable ↓ Platelets ±	↓ Specific gravity Others variable	↑ SAP ↓ Albumin ↓ Glucose	Blood cultures Others variable

Pyometra	Polydipsia/polyuria Enlarged uterus Vaginal discharge ± Depression and dehydration	Leukocytosis with neutrophilia and left shift Others variable	$\downarrow$ Specific gravity Pyuria and bacteriuria ±	See Endotoxemia.	Abdominal radiographs
Gastrointestinal H$_2$O loss Vomiting Diarrhea	See Chapter 32. See Chapter 33.				
Water loss more than sodium loss Hyperglycemic, hyperosmolal, nonketotic diabetes mellitus	Stupor or coma Dehydration Signs of shock ± History of polydipsia and polyuria	$\uparrow$ PCV and total protein Stress leukogram	Glucosuria Specific gravity variable	$\uparrow$ Albumin and globulin Marked hyperglycemia $\uparrow$ Cl Others depending on complications	Plasma osmolality >375 Others variable

CNS, central nervous system; $\uparrow$, increased; PCV, packed cell volume; IV, intravenously; TCO$_2$, total carbon dioxide; $\downarrow$, decreased; ADH, antidiuretic hormone; ±, present or absent; BUN, blood urea nitrogen; SAP, serum alkaline phosphatase; ALT, alanine aminotransferase; ACTH, adrenocorticotropic hormone; WBC, white blood cells and high extracellular sodium concentrations is accomplished with sodium-potassium "pumps" located in cell membranes (see section on hyponatremia).

Maintenance of the normal high intracellular and low extracellular potassium concentration is critical. Cellular potassium depletion may cause abnormalities in many biologic processes, including cell volume; acid-base status; electrophysiologic properties of cells; and synthesis of ribonucleic acid, protein, and glycogen.[7] Abnormal extracellular potassium concentration can cause derangements in acid-base status and electrophysiologic properties of cells.

The normal total body potassium content is determined by the balance between potassium intake and excretion (external potassium balance). Equally important is the distribution of potassium between extracellular and intracellular fluid (internal potassium balance).

External Potassium Balance. Daily ingestion of potassium in the diet equals or exceeds the amount of potassium in extracellular fluid. If potassium intake were not matched by excretion, fatal hyperkalemia would soon result. Since normal skin, salivary, and gastrointestinal potassium losses are minor, renal excretion of potassium is vital. Conversely, daily glomerular filtrate normally contains much more potassium than is present in extracellular fluid. Therefore, tubular reabsorption of potassium is critical to normal potassium balance. In health, the kidney efficiently maintains plasma potassium within a narrow range. However, in contrast to the kidney's ability to completely reabsorb sodium in hypovolemic conditions, small but significant amounts of potassium continue to be excreted, despite severe extrarenal potassium depletion.

Factors known to affect renal handling of potassium include (1) potassium intake, (2) renal tubular cell potassium concentration, (3) delivery of sodium and fluid to the distal tubule, (4) anions accompanying sodium to the distal tubule, (5) mineralocorticoid (mainly aldosterone) effects, and (6) functional integrity of the distal tubular cells.[8] Renal potassium excretion is caused by increases in potassium intake, delivery of sodium and fluid to the distal tubule, and relatively impermeable anions (such as bicarbonate) accompanying sodium to the distal tubule. Aldosterone is secreted in response to extracellular fluid volume reduction (increased adrenal output) and increased extracellular fluid potassium concentration. Aldosterone causes sodium reabsorption and potassium excretion in the distal tubules. The colon also responds to aldosterone by reabsorbing sodium and excreting potassium. Finally, distal tubular cell dysfunction can cause potassium retention, especially in oligoanuric renal failure. However, hyperkalemia is usually not observed in polyuric renal failure until the terminal stages of the disorder.

In disorders characterized by diarrhea or vomiting, potassium losses may be significant. With diarrhea, loss of large quantities of potassium in feces may occur. Gastric juice contains small amounts of potassium; nevertheless, metabolic alkalosis and extracellular fluid volume depletion due to the loss of gastric juice hydrochloric acid induce the loss of large amounts of potassium in the urine.

Internal Potassium Balance. Internal balance of potassium refers to the distribution of potassium between extracellular and intracellular fluid and is critically important in the control of plasma potassium concentration. As previously discussed, membrane-situated ion exchange pumps normally maintain extracellular-intracellular potassium distribution. When potassium intake temporarily exceeds renal excretory capacity, cellular potassium uptake prevents the accumulation of excess potassium in extracellular fluid. When renal or gastrointestinal potassium losses exceed potassium intake, transfer of potassium from cells into extracellular fluid helps to delay hypokalemia.

The most important factors modifying distribution of potassium between extracellular and intracellular fluid are (1) cellular integrity, (2) hormonal effects (mainly insulin and aldosterone), and (3) acid-base status. Severe tissue trauma, such as in crush injuries, may cause significant cellular release of potassium and hyperkalemia. Good renal function generally prevents marked hyperkalemia in the latter condition.

Evidence suggests that plasma potassium concentration influences secretion of both insulin and aldosterone and that feedback control exists for both hormones.[2] It appears that these two hormones are released in response to a potassium-rich meal. Insulin promotes cellular uptake of potassium, and aldosterone causes renal potassium excretion, thereby preventing large diet-induced changes in plasma potassium concentration. Reduced plasma potassium inhibits insulin and aldosterone release, although other factors (*i.e.,* plasma glucose concentration and extracellular fluid volume) take precedence in determining insulin and aldosterone release.

Accumulation of hydrogen ions in extracellular fluid (acidosis) causes transfer of hydrogen ions from extracellular to intracellular fluid. To maintain electroneutrality, potassium ions shift from intracellular to extracellular fluid. Acidosis also favors renal retention of potassium ions because less bicarbonate is presented to the distal tubules (see section on external potassium balance); thus, acidosis increases serum potassium concentration.

Hydrochloric and carbonic acids (as in respiratory acidosis), but not organic acids (*e.g.,* lactic acid and ketoacids), displace potassium ions from cells, thereby causing hyperkalemia. Hypokalemia is induced by metabolic and respiratory alkaloses.

Hypokalemia can occur because of decreased potassium intake, redistribution of potassium from extracellular to intracellular fluid, and loss of potassium from the body (mainly renal and gastrointestinal losses).

Diagnostic Plan

Causes of hypokalemia are shown in Figure 61-5 and Table 61-9. A thorough history is extremely important in the assessment of decreased potassium.

Text continues on p. 580

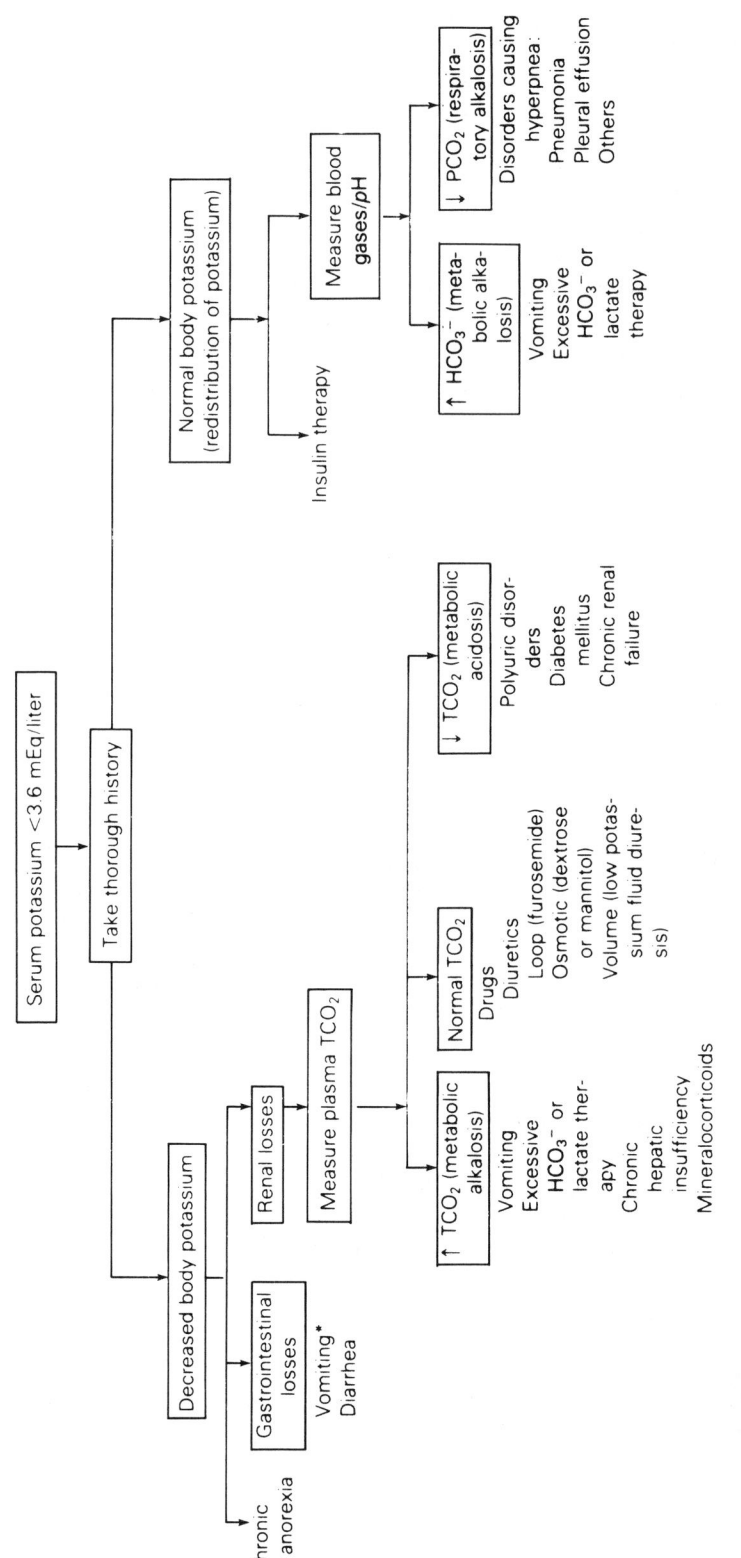

* Metabolic alkalosis causes renal potassium losses and redistribution of potassium from extracellular to intracellular fluid

FIGURE 61-5. Causes of hypokalemia.

TABLE 61-9. Characteristic Findings of Common Disorders Causing Hypokalemia

Disorder	Clinical Signs	Hematology	Urine Analysis	Biochemistry Other Than Hypokalemia	Special Tests
Decreased body potassium					
Chronic anorexia	Poor appetite Weakness Weight loss Others depending on cause	Mild to moderate nonregenerative anemia ±	Normal	↓ Serum albumin ±	None
Gastrointestinal losses					
Vomiting	Vomiting Anorexia, depression Weakness Dehydration Weakness Others depending on cause	↑ PCV and plasma protein ± Others depending on cause	Variable	Variable ↑ TCO_2	Depends on cause (see Chapter 32)
Diarrhea	Diarrhea Dehydration Weakness Others depending on cause	↑ PCV and plasma protein ± Others depending on cause	Variable	Variable	Depends on cause (see Chapter 33)
Renal losses					
Vomiting Excessive HCO_3 or lactate therapy	See Chapter 32. Weakness ± CNS depression ± (paradoxic CSF acidosis)	Normal	Urine pH >7.5	↑ TCO_2 ↑ Serum Na ±	None

(continued)

577

TABLE 61-9. Characteristic Findings of Common Disorders Causing Hypokalemia (*continued*)

Disorder	Clinical Signs	Hematology	Urine Analysis	Biochemistry Other Than Hypokalemia	Special Tests
Chronic hepatic insufficiency	Signs of hepatic failure Icterus Hepatoencephalopathy—stupor, coma, siezures, excessive salivation, head-pressing Ascites Melena	Anemia—regeneration variable Stomatocytosis ± Microcytosis ± ↓ Plasma protein WBC variable	Hyposthenuria ± Ammonium biurate crystals ±	↓ Albumin ↑ Globulin ± ↓ BUN ± Serum glucose <70 ↑ ALT and SAP ± ↑ Bilirubin ± ↑ TCO_2 ±	↑ Serum bile acids, pre- and postprandial ↑ Blood NH_3 or → NH_3 tolerance Abnormal coagulogram ± Abdominal radiographs show small liver Abnormal liver biopsy
Drugs Diuretics	Polyuria Dehydration ± Weakness ±	↑ PCV and plasma protein ±	↓ Urine specific gravity Glucosuria if dextrose is being used	↑ Albumin and globulin ↑ Blood glucose if dextrose is being used ↑ BUN ± ↑ Na ± ↑ TCO_2 ±	None
Mineralocorticoids Polyuric disorders	Weakness ±	Normal	Normal		None
Diabetes mellitus	Polydipsia/polyuria Obesity or weight loss Hepatomegaly Cataracts ± Others depending on complications	Variable depending on complications	Glucosuria Ketonuria ± ↑ WBCs and bacteruria ±	Blood glucose >200 mg/dl Others depending on complications	Depends on complications

Chronic renal failure	Polydipsia and polyuria Signs of uremia ± Depression, anorexia Dehydration Vomiting	Nonregenerative anemia ± Plasma protein ↑ ±	Specific gravity <1.025	↑ BUN and creatinine → TCO₂ → Anion gap ↑ Albumin and globulin ±	Small kidneys on abdominal radiographs ±
Normal body potassium (redistribution) Insulin therapy	Weakness Cardiac arrhythmias	Normal	Normal	Normal	None
Metabolic alkalosis Vomiting Excessive HCO₃ or lactate therapy	See Chapter 32. See Renal losses.				
Respiratory alkalosis (e.g., pneumonia, pleural effusion)	Tachypnea Others depending on cause	Depends on cause	Normal	↓ TCO₂ Others depending on cause	Blood gases/pH show respiratory alkalosis and usually ↑ arterial PO₂

±, present or absent; ↓, decreased; ↑, increased; PCV, packed cell volume; TCO₂, total carbon dioxide; CNS, central nervous system; CSF, cerebrospinal fluid; WBC, white blood cells; BUN, blood urea nitrogen; ALT, alanine aminotransferase; SAP, serum alkaline phosphatase; PO₂, partial pressure of oxygen

History and Physical Examination. Anorexia, vomiting, and diarrhea cause depletion of body potassium and account for most cases of hypokalemia in dogs and cats. Renal disease in cats is often associated with urinary potassium loss and hypokalemic polymyopathy. History and physical examination findings depend on the specific cause, but severe potassium depletion may result in muscular weakness, ileus, and polydipsia-polyuria due to a defect in renal concentrating ability. Hypokalemia and potassium depletion predispose the animal to digitalis intoxication, and cardiac arrhythmias are common. A history of the use of diuretics (loop, osmotic, or volume) may be noted in hypokalemic patients. Finally, polyuric disorders such as diabetes mellitus and chronic renal insufficiency may cause hypokalemia. History and physical examination findings will be typical of these two disorders.

Laboratory Evaluation. The laboratory workup of a hypokalemic patient usually depends on the cause of the disorder. A hemogram, a serum biochemical profile, and urine analysis are indicated. As previously mentioned, acid-base status affects extracellular potassium concentration. Measurement of blood gases and pH, or plasma total CO_2, may help in the interpretation of hypokalemia. Alkalosis causes reduction of serum potassium, and acidosis increases serum potassium. Measurement of total body potassium is impractical. Therefore, frequent measurement of serum potassium is necessary to assess response to treatment.

HYPERKALEMIA

Problem Definition and Recognition

Hyperkalemia is defined as a serum potassium concentration of greater than 5.6 mEq/liter.

Pathophysiology

Like the hypokalemic syndromes, those of hyperkalemia may occur with normal or altered total body potassium. However, since the electrophysiologic manifestations of severe hyperkalemia are potentially lethal (cardiotoxicity), only extracellular potassium concentration is considered to be clinically important. Theoretically, hyperkalemia may be caused by increased intake, decreased excretion (mainly renal), or redistribution of potassium from cells into the extracellular fluid. Clinically, important hyperkalemia is almost always associated with decreased urinary excretion (Fig. 61-6; Table 61-10).

Decreased urinary excretion of potassium can be due to (1) urinary tract obstruction or tear, (2) decreased delivery of sodium and fluid to the distal nephron, (3) acidosis, (4) severe distal tubule damage, (5) deficiency of aldoste-

Text continues on p. 584

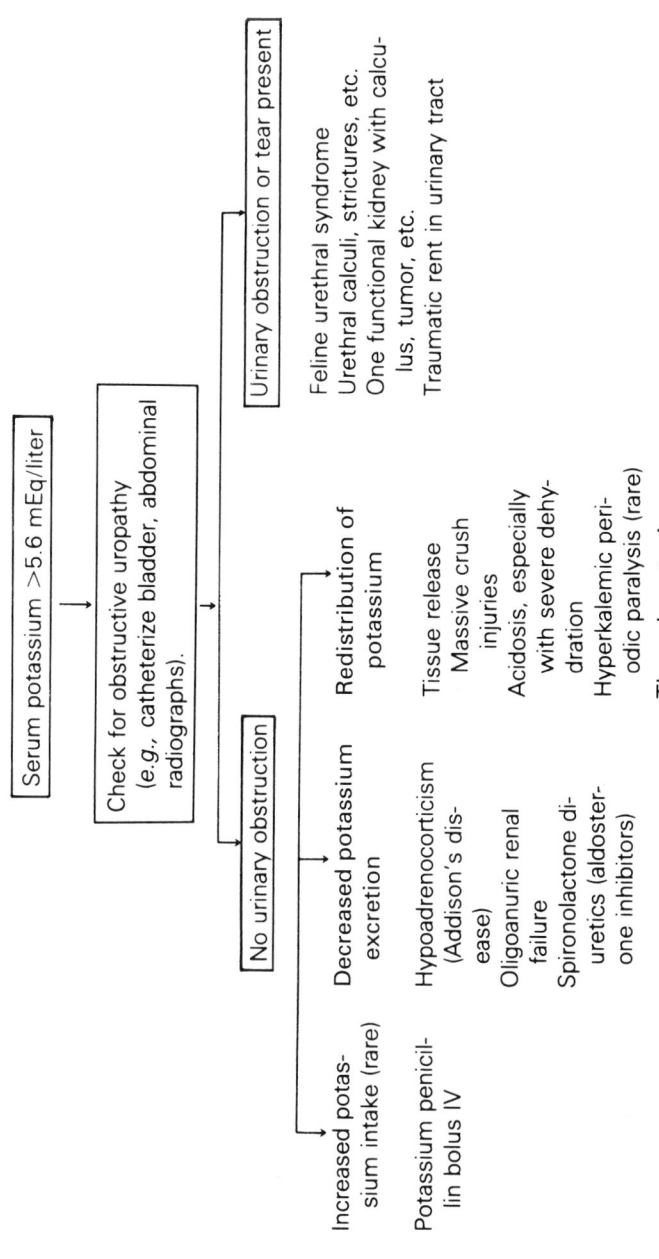

FIGURE 61-6. Causes of hyperkalemia.

TABLE 61-10. Characteristic Findings of Common Disorders Causing Hyperkalemia

Disorder	Clinical Signs	Hematology	Urine Analysis	Biochemistry Other Than Hyperkalemia	Special Tests
No urinary obstruction					
Increased potassium intake					
Potassium penicillin bolus IV	Bradycardia Acute death	Normal	Normal	Normal	ECG shows: Tall, peaked T waves Bradycardia Flattened P waves Atrial standstill Cardiac arrest
Decreased potassium excretion					
Hypoadrenocorticism (Addison's disease)	Chronic lethargy and anorexia Sporadic vomiting and diarrhea Weakness Dehydration Bradycardia Collapse, shock, death	↑ PCV and plasma protein Eosinophilia and lymphocytosis ±	Low urine specific gravity ±	↓ Na Na:K ratio <23:1 ↑ BUN ↓ Glucose ± ↑ Albumin and globulin (dehydration) ↓ TCO_2	ECG (see above) Plasma cortisols— low baseline and little or no response to ACTH
Oligoanuric renal failure	Depression, anorexia Vomiting Dehydration	↑ PCV and plasma protein Stress leukogram ±	May be anuric Variable depending on cause	↑ BUN ↑ Phosphorus ↑ Albumin and globulin ↓ TCO_2	Consider urine culture Abdominal radiographs ±
Spironolactone diuretics (aldosterone inhibitors)	Polyuria Dehydration ±	↑ PCV and plasma protein	↓ Specific gravity	↓ Na ↑ BUN	None

582

Condition	Clinical Signs	Hematology	Urinalysis	Biochemistry	Diagnostic Tests
Redistribution of potassium Tissue release, as with crush injuries	Signs associated with trauma	Associated with trauma Regenerative anemia Stress leukogram	Normal	Depends on injuries	Depends on injuries
Acidosis, especially with severe dehydration	Depends on specific cause Depression Dehydration Cardiac arrhythmia	Depends on specific cause ↑ PCV and plasma protein	Depends on specific cause Specific gravity >1.035 pH <6.0	Depends on specific cause ↑ Albumin and globulin	Depends on specific cause ECG may show arrhythmia or other signs of hyperkalemia (see Increased potassium intake)
Urinary obstruction present Feline lower urinary tract disease	Depression Vomiting Dehydration Grossly distended bladder Dysuria Later—collapse, bradycardia, shock, death	↑ PCV and plasma protein Stress leukogram	Gross hematuria Triple phosphate (struvite) crystals	↑ BUN ↑ Phosphorus ↓ TCO$_2$ ↑ Anion gap ↑ Albumin and globulin ±	None
Urethral calculi, strictures, and others	Similar to Feline lower urinary tract disease (above)				Abdominal radiographs—survey and contrast urethrography Abdominal ultrasonography
One functional kidney with ureteral calculus, tumor, etc. causing obstruction	Similar to Feline lower urinary tract disease (above)				Abdominal radiographs Excretory urogram Abdominal ultrasonography

ECG, electrocardiogram; ↑, increased; ±, present or absent; ↓, decreased; TCO$_2$, total carbon dioxide; ACTH, adrenocorticotropic hormone; PCV, packed cell volume; BUN, blood urea nitrogen rone (Addison's disease), and (6) use of aldosterone-inhibiting diuretics (spiro-nolactone).

Diagnostic Plan

Causes of hyperkalemia are shown in Figure 61-6 and Table 61-10. Whenever serum potassium exceeds 8.0 mEq/liter, primary attention should be devoted to quickly reducing serum potassium or antagonizing its effects, and diagnostic procedures should be temporarily delayed.

History and Physical Examination. Urinary tract obstruction should be ex-cluded initially. A history of dysuria with little or no urine being passed is suggestive. In most cases of urinary tract obstruction, the blockage is in the area from the neck of the bladder distally to the external urethral orifice. A distended bladder is palpable on physical examination. Occasionally, hyperkalemia caused by urinary tract obstruction is due to unilateral ureteral obstruction with only one functional kidney. In this situation, the bladder contains little or no urine, and dysuria is unlikely. Depending on the duration of urinary tract obstruction, signs of uremia (depression, dehydration, and vomiting) or hyperkalemia (bradycardia, cardiac arrhythmia, and collapse) may be observed.

With adrenocortical insufficiency (Addison's disease), a history of anorexia, severe lethargy, weakness, and sporadic vomiting and diarrhea followed by collapse is typical. Bradycardia, dehydration, and signs of shock may be ob-served. Similar history and physical examination findings may be present with oligoanuric renal failure.

Laboratory Evaluation. The initial laboratory workup for hyperkalemia is similar to that previously discussed for hypokalemia, except that electrocardio-graphic monitoring may be important. Radiographs of the abdomen may be needed to help assess the urinary system for an obstruction or a rent.

HYPOCALCEMIA

Problem Definition and Recognition

Hypocalcemia is defined as a total serum calcium concentration of less than 9.0 mg/dl.

Pathophysiology

Calcium has several important functions in both intracellular and extracellular fluid. In addition to its structural role in bone, intracellular calcium is critical for muscle contraction, nerve impulse transmission, and release of neurotrans-mitters. Calcium also serves as an intracellular messenger for a variety of meta-bolic functions. Extracellular calcium concentration is important for the intracellular functions mentioned above because of its influence on calcium pumps in cell membranes and its effects on cell membrane permeability to other ions.[3]

Calcium is present in extracellular fluid in three forms: (1) ionized, (2) protein-bound (mainly albumin), and (3) chelated with anions. Only ionized calcium is biologically active. Most laboratory methods for measuring serum calcium determine the sum of the three forms of calcium mentioned above (total serum calcium). Special equipment is needed to measure ionized calcium separately. Although the determination of total serum calcium may provide helpful information, it must be remembered that altered values, especially hypocalcemia, may be due to changes in the biologically inactive portions and therefore not dangerous to the patient. Examples include hypoalbuminemia and changes in blood pH. Decreased serum albumin causes hypocalcemia. The following formulas may be used to correct the hypoalbuminemia for calcium[3]:

1. Adjusted Ca (mg/dl) = Ca (mg/dl) − albumin (g/dl) + 3.5
2. Adjusted Ca (mg/dl) = Ca (mg/dl) [0.4 × total serum protein (g/dl)] + 3.3

These correction formulas do not account for the effects of blood pH on serum calcium. Alkalosis decreases ionized serum calcium, and acidosis has the opposite effect.

Causes of hypocalcemia in dogs and cats are listed separately (see Display, Causes of Decreased Total Serum Calcium in Dogs and Cats). The previously listed correction formulas should always be used before assessing a decreased serum calcium. Total serum calcium values above 5.0 mg/dl are usually not associated with clinical signs unless the ionized serum calcium is disproportion-

---

Causes of Decreased Total Serum Calcium in Dogs and Cats

- Hypoalbuminemia (see Table 61-1)
- Renal failure
- Eclampsia
- Acute pancreatitis
- Antifreeze (ethylene glycol) poisoning
- Dietary deficiency
- Malabsorption of calcium or vitamin D, or both
- Hypoparathyroidism
- Bone calcium uptake
  Adenoma removal
  Osteoblastic tumor
- Hyperphosphatemia
  Phosphate-containing enema
- Hypomagnesemia
- Inappropriate sample-handling
  Calcium-binding anticoagulant

ately low. Even though the animal is not showing clinical signs of hypocalcemia, the reduced serum calcium may be helpful in determining which clinical disorder is present in the patient.

Diagnostic Plan

History and Physical Examination. The classic clinical signs in a patient with hypocalcemia are muscle tremors and fasciculations, panting, nervousness, restlessness, seizures, and increased body temperature. Anorexia, depression, listlessness, aggressive behavior, and sensory abnormalities may be observed. These signs may sometimes be sporadic instead of constant.

Laboratory Evaluation. Serum calcium should be determined as a part of a standard biochemical panel, which should include measurement of serum phosphorus. As previously mentioned, most laboratories measure total serum calcium. Since there is variation from one laboratory to another, normal serum calcium values for dogs and cats should be determined in the same laboratory being used for patients.

HYPERCALCEMIA

Problem Definition and Recognition

Hypercalcemia is defined as a total serum calcium concentration of greater than 12.0 mg/dl.

Pathophysiology

Most of the abnormalities caused by hypercalcemia are attributable to its physiologic functions previously mentioned (see section on pathophysiology under Hypocalcemia). Because of calcium's role in muscle contraction and neuromuscular transmission, severe hypercalcemia (serum calcium greater than 16.0 mg/dl) may be fatal. Concomitant elevations in serum calcium and phosphorus with a calcium × phosphorus product of greater than 60 are more likely to cause soft tissue mineralization.[3] Severe renal damage is a likely consequence of renal calcification (see Display, Causes of Hypercalcemia in Dogs and Cats).

Diagnostic Plan

History and Physical Examination. Clinical signs of hypercalcemia may vary depending on the cause. Depression, anorexia, vomiting, constipation, weakness, polyuria, polydipsia, and arrhythmias may be observed.

Laboratory Evaluation. See section on hypocalcemia. Follow-up diagnostic plans will depend on the rule outs being considered after the initial results are assessed. In dogs, pseudohyperparathyroidism caused by lymphosarcoma is the

Causes of Hypercalcemia in Dogs and Cats

- Pseudohyperparathyroidism
  - Lymphosarcoma
  - Perianal carcinoma
- Renal failure
- Primary hyperparathyroidism
- Hypervitaminosis D
- Osteolytic lesions
- Hypoadrenocorticism
- Hemoconcentration/hyperproteinemia
- Immobilization

most common cause of hypercalcemia. A careful search for enlarged lymph nodes or organomegaly, including abdominal and thoracic radiography, is warranted. Fine-needle aspirates of enlarged structures should be obtained for cytologic examination. In some cases, the diagnosis must be established by excisional biopsy.

REFERENCES

1. Burke MD: Electrolyte studies: 1. Sodium and water. Postgrad Med 64:147–153, 1978
2. Cox M, Stems RH, Singer L: The defense against hyperkalemia: The roles of insulin and aldosterone. N Engl J Med 299:525–532, 1978
3. Finco DR: Interpretations of serum calcium concentration in the dog. Compend Cont Ed 5:778–788, 1983
4. Hoffman WE, Sanecki RK, Dorner JL: A technique for automated quantification of canine glucocorticoid-induced isoenzyme of alkaline phosphatase. Vet Clin Pathol 17:66–70, 1988
5. Mahaffey EA, Lago MP: Comparison of techniques for quantifying alkaline phosphatase isoenzymes in canine serum. Vet Clin Pathol 20:51–55, 1991
6. Moss DW, Butterworth PJ: Enzymology and Medicine. London, Pitman Medical Co, 1974
7. Nardone DA, McDonald WJ, Giard DE: Mechanisms in hypokalemia: Clinical correlation. Medicine (Baltimore) 57:435–446, 1978
8. Narins RG, Jones ER, Stoms MC: Diagnostic strategies in disorders of fluid, electrolyte, and acid-base homeostasis. Am J Med 72:496–520, 1982
9. Taclob LT, Needle MA: Hyponatremic syndromes. Med Clin North Am 57:1425–1433, 1973
10. Thier SO: The kidney. In Smith LH, Thier SO (eds): Pathophysiology—The Biological Principles of Disease, pp 799–920. Philadelphia, WB Saunders, 1981
11. Valentine BA, Blue JT, Shelley SM, et al: Increased alanine aminotransferase activity associated with muscle necrosis in the dog. J Vet Intern Med 4:140–143, 1990

CHAPTER SIXTY-TWO

Urine Analysis

Jeanne A. Barsanti

This chapter reviews each component of the urine analysis and its correct interpretation.

SAMPLE COLLECTION

Correct interpretation of a urine analysis is based on a knowledge of the method of sample collection. The method of collection should *always* be recorded. Samples collected by cystocentesis are usually preferred, since these avoid contamination from the urethra and external genitalia. The only disadvantage of cystocentesis is that some blood may be introduced into the urine during collection. For this reason, if the animal's problem is possible hematuria, a voided urine sample is taken first to confirm the presence of blood. The only contraindication to cystocentesis is a markedly distended bladder with a potentially ischemic or otherwise abnormal wall. Even under these conditions, cystocentesis is usually safe if the distention is relieved immediately thereafter. In fact, cystocentesis is often recommended just prior to relieving the animal of a urethral obstruction in order to remove the back-pressure from a full bladder.

If cystocentesis is unsuccessful, a catheterized sample is preferred in male dogs to avoid preputial contamination. Catheterization should always involve a sterile catheter and aseptic technique. Voided or expressed samples can be used in female dogs and cats when cystocentesis is unsuccessful, since catheterization is often difficult and can be associated with induction of infection in them, even when careful technique is utilized. This does not imply that catheterization should never be used to obtain a urine sample in female dogs. The information to be gained from the urine analysis may warrant risk of infection. For example, in a dehydrated female dog, urine specific gravity must be obtained prior to fluid therapy to correctly assess kidneys' ability to respond to dehydration. This information is *vital* to determining the cause of dehydration; if catheterization is necessary to obtain the sample, it should be performed.

COMPONENTS OF THE COMPLETE
URINE ANALYSIS

There is a strong tendency among veterinarians to consider a dipstick analysis a complete urine analysis. In doing so, they omit very important parts of a urine

Essential Components of a Routine Urine Analysis

Record of method of collection	Sediment examination
Specific gravity	Red blood cells
Dipstick analysis	White blood cells
pH	Bacteria
Protein	Casts
Ketones	Crystals
Glucose	Epithelial cells
Bilirubin	Miscellaneous
Occult blood	

analysis: determination of specific gravity and sediment examination. Without knowledge of the urine specific gravity, neither renal function nor the dipstick analysis for protein or bilirubin can be accurately assessed. Many cases of urinary tract disease are missed if the urine sediment is not examined. A prime example is urinary tract infection in association with canine Cushing's disease or steroid therapy. In these cases, hematuria is usually absent (negative occult blood), yet bacteruria may be marked. The essential components of a urine analysis are listed on page 590.

After urine has been collected, it should be examined as soon as possible. If not examined within 30 minutes, the sample should be refrigerated and examined within a few hours. Bacterial culture should be performed within 8 hours to avoid significant changes in bacterial numbers. Changes in pH, cellular deterioration, fragmentation and dissolution of casts, and precipitation of crystals can also occur during storage.

A urine analysis should always be interpreted in relation to any current or recent therapy or diagnostic tests the animal has received. For example, diuretics and glucocorticoids affect urine concentrating ability, and radiographic contrast agents affect urine specific gravity and urine protein and glucose determination.

INTERPRETATION OF THE COMPONENTS OF URINE ANALYSIS

Physical Properties

Urine is normally yellow, and its depth of color correlates with the degree of urine concentration; dilute urine is colorless to light yellow, and concentrated urine is dark yellow to amber. Abnormal colors include red to reddish-brown, which is associated with hematuria, hemoglobinuria, or myoglobinuria, and yellow-green to yellow-brown, which is associated with bilirubinuria. Other unusual colors may be caused by dyes ingested with food or drugs.

Urine is normally clear but may become cloudy because of the presence of cells, crystals, or mucus. Refrigeration may increase cloudiness because of precipitation of crystals at a lower temperature. Microscopic examination of the urine sediment is necessary to determine the cause of cloudiness.

Urine has a normal odor, which varies somewhat with species and diet. Urine may smell stronger as a result of concentration or changes associated with bacterial infection.

Urine Specific Gravity

In dogs and cats, any urine specific gravity may be normal. Because the kidneys maintain water balance, urine specific gravity varies with water and solute intake and body needs. In dehydrated dogs and cats, urine should be concentrated to a specific gravity greater than 1.035. Thus, specific gravity should always be interpreted in light of the animal's hydration status. Urine specific gravity is also greatly affected by administration of diuretics, corticosteroids, radiographic contrast agents, and fluid therapy. These treatments reduce the usefulness of specific gravity as an indicator of renal function. It is *essential* to collect urine prior to any treatment. Large amounts of protein or glucose increase specific gravity approximately 0.001 for each 0.3 g/dl glucose and 0.4 g/dl protein.

Specific Gravity Greater Than 1.045. A specific gravity of this magnitude in the dog indicates normal urine-concentrating ability. Normal dogs usually concentrate urine to greater than 1.045 when challenged with mild dehydration (5%).

A specific gravity of this magnitude may be associated with abnormal renal function in cats. In one experimental study, cats became azotemic as a result of renal insufficiency and still concentrated urine to greater than 1.045. A decrease in concentrating ability occurred with the onset of renal failure but was minimal and variable, even with mild azotemia. Thus, renal failure is ruled out in dogs, but not in cats, when urine specific gravity is greater than 1.045. To rule out renal failure in cats, blood urea nitrogen (BUN) or serum creatinine, or both, should be measured. If the cat is not azotemic and urine specific gravity is in this range, renal failure is ruled out (renal disease may still be present but is undetectable by routine laboratory tests).

Specific Gravity 1.030 to 1.045. In dogs and cats with no internal medical problems and with normal BUN, serum creatinine, and hydration, urine specific gravity in the range of 1.030 to 1.045 is considered normal. With dehydration or azotemia, values in this range are abnormal in cats. In dogs with dehydration or azotemia, or both, this range is more difficult to interpret and may indicate normal concentrating ability or a mild loss of concentrating ability. In general, no further diagnostic tests are indicated in relation to renal function for urine specific gravities in this range in animals that are otherwise normal.

Specific Gravity 1.013 to 1.029. Urine specific gravity in the range of 1.013 to 1.029 indicates some ability to concentrate urine. Such values may be normal if no stimulus for urine concentration exists; however, values in this range are abnormal if the animal is dehydrated or azotemic due to a prerenal or renal insult. (See Chapter 5 to review the causes of the inability to concentrate urine.)

Even if the animal appears normal and other laboratory work is normal, urine specific gravities in this range may warrant further diagnostic work to rule out conditions such as chronic renal failure. The tests indicated (besides complete blood count [CBC], blood chemistry profile, and complete urine analysis, which should be done first) are a water deprivation test and antidiuretic hormone (ADH) response test (see Chapter 5). A water deprivation test should be performed only on animals whose only problem is questionable urine-concentrating ability and who have otherwise normal laboratory tests (CBC, biochemistry profile, and urine analysis). A water deprivation test should always be performed under careful veterinary supervision and monitoring as described in Chapter 5 and not by having the client withhold water at home for a certain number of hours. A measure of glomerular filtration rate, such as exogenous or endogenous creatinine clearance, may also be used to further assess renal function.

Specific Gravity 1.008 to 1.012. Urine with a specific gravity in this range is called *isosthenuric,* meaning that no urine concentration has occurred (its specific gravity is equal to that of plasma). This value may be normal if no stimulus to concentrate is present. If a stimulus to concentrate, such as dehydration or azotemia of prerenal or renal origin, is present, values in this range are definitely abnormal. Routine laboratory workups including CBC, blood chemistry profile, and complete urine analysis should be performed. Even if routine laboratory results are normal and the animal is not dehydrated, urine specific gravities in this range may warrant further evaluation. Possible diagnostic tests include repeat urine specific gravities, water deprivation test, ADH response test, creatinine clearance measurement, and evaluation for endocrine diseases, such as hyperthyroidism in cats and hyperadrenocorticism in dogs. Water deprivation testing is potentially harmful, and precautions are indicated as noted in the previous section. Refer to Chapter 5 to review the causes of inability to concentrate urine.

Specific Gravity Less than 1.008. Urine specific gravities below 1.008 are hyposthenuric, indicating normal renal ability to dilute urine. Values in this range can be normal if the animal has a need to excrete extra water, but they are abnormal in animals with a need to retain water due to dehydration. Urine specific gravities in this range may be produced by primary polydipsia, lack of ADH, or inability of the kidney to respond to ADH (see Chapter 5). Hyposthenuria usually warrants further diagnostic testing because of profound polyuria and polydipsia. A CBC, complete blood chemistry profile, and complete urine analysis are indicated. If these are normal, water deprivation and ADH response tests should be performed. The water deprivation test must be performed cautiously as noted above.

Urine pH

Urine *p*H varies as the kidney maintains electrolyte and acid-base balances in relation to varying dietary intake; therefore, no specific urine *p*H is abnormal. Evaluation of urine *p*H is useful only as it relates to other findings on the urine analysis and in relationship to acid-base and electrolyte balances as a whole.

Urine *p*H Less Than 7.1. Urine *p*H in this range is acidic or neutral. Dogs and cats, as carnivores that eat relatively infrequently, generally have a urine *p*H in this range. If the *p*H is markedly acidic (less than 6.0), one should consider a systemic tendency to acidemia. Other causes of aciduria are acidifying drugs, increased protein catabolism, and paradoxic aciduria in metabolic alkalosis associated with chloride and potassium depletion. An acid urine *p*H does not rule out urinary tract infection, as most urinary tract pathogens do not affect urine *p*H *in vivo*.

Urine *p*H Greater Than 7.0. Alkaline urine is produced for several hours postprandially, to a degree dependent on diet. The most common disease condition that produces constantly alkaline urine is urinary infection with *Staphylococcus* or *Proteus*. These organisms produce the enzyme urease, which degrades urea to ammonia, causing alkalinity. Thus, when alkaline urine is identified, the rest of the urine analysis (especially the urine sediment) should be examined for evidence of bacterial infection. Consistently alkaline urine in the dog and cat can result in development of struvite uroliths. Monitoring urine *p*H for alkalinity is one method used to prevent recurrence of struvite uroliths.

Another cause of persistently alkaline urine is renal tubular acidosis. In this condition, metabolic acidemia results from the inability of the kidney to reabsorb bicarbonate (proximal renal tubular acidosis, type I) or secrete hydrogen ions (distal renal tubular acidosis, type II). Distal renal tubular acidosis is more commonly associated with alkaline urine than is proximal renal tubular acidosis. Both types of renal tubular acidosis are apparently rare in dogs and cats.

Alkaline urine may also be an appropriate renal response to metabolic or respiratory alkalosis.

Proteinuria

Proteinuria is usually assessed by dipstick analysis. This test is qualitative, not quantitative, and should be recorded as such (trace to 4 +). Various evaluations of laboratory technicians have indicated that the color change for protein on the dipstick is the most difficult color change to read consistently. This is another good reason for interpreting the result as relative and not absolute. Because of these problems with the dipstick plus its inability to detect Bence Jones proteins associated with plasma cell myelomas, many laboratories also utilize a precipitation test such as sulfosalicylic acid, trichloroacetic acid, or Roberts' reagent (nitric acid). These tests are also evaluated subjectively on a trace to 4+ basis. Precipitation tests for protein may become falsely positive in the presence of radiographic contrast agents.

To accurately interpret the significance of proteinuria, the urine specific gravity must be known. A small amount of protein might read as negative in dilute urine at 1.010, but as positive (1+) in urine concentrated to 1.040.

A small amount of protein in urine is normal. This protein is derived from small molecular weight proteins, which pass through the glomerulus and are largely but not completely reabsorbed in the proximal tubule, and from proteins produced within the urinary tract (e.g., Tamm-Horsfall protein). This amount of protein may register as negative at a specific gravity less than 1.035 or as trace to 1+ at a specific gravity greater than 1.035.

A protein of 2+ or more at a specific gravity greater than 1.035 or any amount of protein at a specific gravity less than 1.035 may be abnormal. As specific gravity decreases and urine protein levels increase, the evidence that the proteinuria is abnormal becomes more convincing. Marginal changes may be abnormal or normal because of the subjectivity of the tests involved. The next step in evaluating the proteinuria is to examine the rest of the urine analysis. First, evidence of hemorrhage should be sought. Bleeding into the urinary tract introduces red blood cells (RBCs) and serum proteins as well as the other constituents of blood. Since protein is present in blood in large quantities (g/dl) compared with the amount of protein in normal urine (mg/dl) and since the tests for proteinuria are designed for the small amount of protein in urine, blood in urine results in detectable proteinuria. One should also look for evidence of inflammation (pyuria), since inflammatory exudates also contain sufficient protein to result in significiant proteinuria.

When proteinuria is the only abnormality in the urine analysis, one should evaluate renal function by determining BUN, serum creatinine, and urine specific gravity. Serum albumin should be measured to determine whether the proteinuria is of sufficient magnitude to cause hypoalbuminemia.

The best method for determining the magnitude and clinical importance of proteinuria in urine with a normal sediment is protein quantitation. One method is to collect all urine produced for a known time period (usually 24 hours). The amount of protein in an aliquot of urine is quantitated (mg/dl). The amount of protein in the aliquot is then multiplied by the total urine volume to determine the amount of protein lost per day. Normal values in the dog and cat are less than 200 mg in our laboratory, although others have reported as much as 500 mg per day. Another test that can be used is the urine protein to urine creatinine ratio, in which protein and creatinine are measured in a single random urine sample. The ratio corrects for urine concentration changes. A normal ratio is less than 0.2, and an abnormal ratio is greater than 1.0. Values between 0.2 and 1.0 are indeterminate, and a timed collection should be performed. Quantitative urine protein determinations are only useful when there is no hemorrhage or inflammation.

If there is no evidence of hematuria or pyuria, then the cause of the proteinuria is usually one of the following: increased loss of serum proteins through the glomerulus as a result of glomerular disease or a change in glomerular dynamics, a decrease in renal tubular reabsorption of proteins, or excretion of increased quantities of a protein in the glomerular filtrate. An example of the latter is Bence Jones protein (light chain of an immunoglobulin molecule) formed by malignant plasma cells (plasma cell myeloma). This cause of proteinuria can be identified by markedly elevated serum protein concentrations and confirmed by serum and urine electrophoresis. Dipstick analysis for protein may not detect Bence Jones protein: turbidity tests are required.

A change in glomerular dynamics that can cause proteinuria is increased glomerular hydrostatic pressure. This can result from right-sided congestive heart failure or from increased intraabdominal pressure, as might be associated with ascites or a large neoplasm that partially obstructs the caudal vena cava. The degree of proteinuria is usually mild to moderate.

Tubular diseases do not result in severe proteinuria, because protein loss is due to failure of proximal tubular reabsorption of the small amount of small molecular weight proteins in glomerular filtrate. Tubular diseases do not cause hypoalbuminemia. Thus, if the protein loss is large and hypoalbuminemia is present, the cause is probably a glomerular disease, but if the loss is more moderate, further testing may be necessary to establish the cause as a tubular or glomerular disease. With failure of proximal tubular reabsorption, the proteinuria may be associated with glucosuria with a normal blood glucose. An example is the Fanconi syndrome described in basenji dogs. With chronic renal failure in general (chronic interstitial nephritis), mild proteinuria without glucosuria is characteristic.

Glomerular diseases are characterized by moderate to severe proteinuria. A renal biopsy is required to differentiate the two most common types of glomerular diseases in the dog: amyloidosis and glomerulonephritis. In cats, renal amyloidosis occurs but involves the medullary interstitium, more than the glomerulus, so protein loss is less marked. Glomerulonephritis in the cat is frequently associated with feline leukemia virus infection.

Ketonuria

Ketonuria is abnormal. False-positive reactions are uncommon but may occur in highly pigmented urine. The renal tubular reabsorptive mechanism for ketones is rapidly saturated, so ketonuria precedes detectable ketonemia. The most common cause of ketonuria is diabetes mellitus, in which ketonuria is associated with glucosuria and hyperglycemia. Other potential causes are starvation, chronic catabolic diseases, persistent fever, impaired liver function, and hypoglycemic syndromes. Young animals and those of very small body size apparently tend to develop ketonuria with anorexia faster than older, larger animals.

Glycosuria

Normal urine does not contain glucose, so any degree of glycosuria is abnormal. False-positive reactions can occur with dipsticks if urine contains an oxidizing agent such as H_2O_2 or chlorine. The most common cause of glycosuria is a blood glucose (greater than 180 mg/dl in dogs; approximately 300 mg/dl in cats) that exceeds the renal threshold for glucose reabsorption. The most common cause is diabetes mellitus. If blood glucose is normal, renal proximal tubular dysfunction, either specific for glucose or generalized should be considered. An associated finding in generalized proximal tubular dysfunction is mild proteinuria. Generalized renal proximal tubular dysfunction (Fanconi syndrome) can be congenital, as in basenji dogs, or acquired, as from nephrotoxicity due to drugs or heavy metals.

Bilirubinuria

Bilirubinuria can be normal in dogs but is abnormal in cats. In dogs, the degree of bilirubinuria should be compared with the urine specific gravity. A trace to 1+ bilirubin in concentrated urine (greater than 1.035) is normal. More marked bilirubinuria is abnormal.

Abnormal bilirubinuria indicates increased serum concentrations of conjugated bilirubin, since unconjugated bilirubin does not filter through the glomerulus. Increased concentrations of conjugated bilirubin may be the result of biliary obstruction (hepatic or posthepatic), cholestasis, or increased production secondary to accelerated hemolysis. Bilirubinuria precedes bilirubinemia in these conditions (see Chapter 37).

Positive Occult Blood

The occult blood reaction becomes positive in the presence of hemoglobin, myoglobin, or intact RBCs. To determine which is present, the rest of the urine analysis should be examined and the serum color should be determined. Hemoglobinuria can result from hemoglobinemia or from release of hemoglobin from RBC breakdown in urine. RBCs in the urine sediment plus a positive occult blood reaction indicate hematuria. If there are no RBCs in the urine, serum color should be examined for hemolysis. If the serum is not red, the positive occult blood reaction is unlikely to be the result of hemoglobinuria from hemoglobinemia. Other possibilities are the presence of hemoglobin in contaminants of urine (e.g., flea dirt in voided samples), complete RBC breakdown in urine, and myoglobin. Myoglobinuria is uncommon in dogs and cats and should be accompanied by clear serum and evidence of severe muscle disease. An ammonium sulfate precipitation test can be used to help differentiate hemoglobin from myoglobin.

Urine Sediment Results

Red Blood Cells. An occasional RBC per high-power field (hpf) is normal. Greater numbers are either iatrogenic or abnormal, except in a voided sample from a proestral bitch. To evaluate the RBCs, two questions must be asked: (1) Where is the site of bleeding? (2) What is the cause? One must know the method of urine collection to determine the site. If the sample was voided, the external genitalia and reproductive system as well as the entire urinary tract must be considered. If the sample was collected by cystocentesis or bladder catheterization, the bladder, kidneys, ureters, or prostate may be the origin. If the sample was collected by cystocentesis or catheterization, an iatrogenic injury during collection must also be considered. For this reason, if an animal is presented for evaluation of the problem of hematuria, a voided sample should be collected first to confirm the hematuria. Causes of hematuria include trauma, uroliths, infection, inflammation neoplasia, infarction, prostatic hyperplasia, parasites, toxins, and coagulopathies (see Chapter 39).

Pyuria. A few white blood cells (WBCs) in urine (less than 5/hpf) is normal. A greater number of WBCs indicates inflammation at or in advance of the sampling site. One exception is the prostate gland in the male dog, since prostatic fluid refluxes back into the bladder. If WBCs are found in a voided sample, they may be the result of contamination from the reproductive tract or external genitalia or they may indicate inflammation in the urinary tract. A sample collected directly from the bladder, preferably by cystocentesis, is *essential* to differentiating these possibilities. A conclusion that these cells are the result of contamination without an examination of urine from the bladder is *incorrect*.

Causes of inflammation within the urinary tract include infection, urolithiasis, neoplasia, trauma, toxins (including drugs such as cyclophosphamide (Cytoxan)), and idiopathic granulomatous diseases. Diagnostic tests, including urine culture and survey and contrast radiographs, may be necessary in addition to the history, physical examination, and urine analysis to differentiate these possibilities.

Bacteruria. As with pyuria, knowing the method of sample collection is essential for accurate interpretation of bacteruria. Urine from the bladder is normally sterile, but the distal urethra, vagina, and prepuce have resident bacterial populations. Thus, bacteruria is abnormal in urine collected by cystocentesis as long as contamination does not occur during or after collection and as long as sterile urine containers are used. Bacteruria in samples collected by voiding or catheterization may be normal or abnormal, depending on the degree of contamination from the urethra, vagina, or prepuce. If a voided sample is bacteruric, a sample should be collected by cystocentesis to determine if the bacteria are contaminants. If a catheterized sample is bacteruric, either a quantitative culture of the sample or a cystocentesis can be performed. More than 100,000 bacteria per milliliter in a catheterized sample usually indicate infection. Lesser numbers may be significant in male dogs and in cats (more than 10,000/ml). In female dogs, contamination may cause greater than 100,000/ml. This fact plus the possibility of inducing infection with catheterization in female dogs reinforces the importance of cystocentesis.

Estimation of numbers of bacteria on urine analysis often does not correlate with actual numbers. Some bacteria, especially cocci, are difficult to differentiate from amorphous debris with brownian movement. Bacteria are not reliably seen until numbers exceed 100,000/ml (cocci) or 10,000/ml (rods); therefore, absence of bacteruria does not rule out infection. A culture of bladder urine is the best method for establishing the presence or absence of infection.

Occasionally bacteria are seen, but a urine culture is negative. The possibilities are that the bacteria died or were killed prior to or during culturing or that the bacteria had unusual growth requirements (*e.g.*, anaerobes). Urinary tract infections are usually caused by common aerobic bacteria (*Escherichia coli*, staphylococci, streptococci, *Proteus*), so only aerobic cultures using common media are routinely done.

Cylindruria. A few granular casts (fine or coarse) are normally present in urine from turnover of renal epithelial cells. A few hyaline casts (precipitates of Tamm-Horsfall protein) may also be seen normally. Larger numbers of granular or hyaline casts and other types of casts are abnormal.

Increased numbers of granular casts indicate active renal tubular cell injury. The type of injury may be ischemic, toxic, infectious, immune-mediated, or traumatic. WBC casts indicate renal inflammation. RBC casts indicate renal bleeding. Absence of WBC or RBC casts does not rule out renal inflammation or hemorrhage, as these types of casts are uncommonly seen.

Hyaline casts are composed of Tamm-Horsfall protein, which precipitates in the presence of increased quantities of albumin; thus, hyaline casts are most often associated with glomerular proteinuria. Hyaline casts are also more apparent in very concentrated or very acidic urine. Hyaline casts dissolve in alkaline urine.

Waxy and broad casts are thought to be degenerate granular casts that form in collecting ducts and indicate current or previous slow urine flow rates (oliguria).

Crystalluria. Crystalluria may be normal or abnormal and primarily indicates the presence of the composing minerals in the urine. Struvite crystals are common in the urine of normal dogs and cats. However, in the presence of radiodense uroliths, urinary tract infection with staphylococci or *Proteus,* and alkaline urine, struvite crystals suggest that the uroliths are also struvite.

Biurate crystals are normal in dalmatian dog urine because of the reduced capacity of the liver of dalmatians to convert uric acid to urea. In the presence of uroliths in the Dalmatian dog with acid urine, no infection, and minimal radiodensity, the finding of biurate crystals suggests that the uroliths are uric acid. In dogs other than Dalmatians, the presence of biurate crystals suggests hepatic insufficiency. Tyrosine crystals also may indicate hepatic insufficiency.

Hippurate and oxalate crystals suggest ethylene glycol toxicity, especially when present in large numbers. Absence of these crystals does not rule out the diagnosis, since slow urine flow rates may keep the crystals in the kidney. Oxalate crystals are occasionally found in normal canine or feline urine and in association with calcium oxalate uroliths.

Bilirubin crystals can be normal in concentrated canine urine or abnormal in association with significant bilirubinuria. Cystine crystals suggest poor renal tubular ability to reabsorb cystine. Cystinosis predisposes dogs and cats to cystine calculi.

Epithelial Cells. Squamous epithelial cells usually enter urine as it is voided through the vagina or prepuce. Other epithelial cells found normally in urine in low numbers are transitional and renal. Renal epithelial cells are small, just slightly larger than WBCs. The size of transitional cells varies markedly. It is difficult to differentiate small transitional cells from renal epithelial cells. Caudate cells are small transitional cells with a tail-like appendage. Large numbers of transitional epithelial cells are present with infection, inflammation, injury, and neoplasia. If one suspects lower urinary tract neoplasia, the transitional cells should be examined closely for evidence of malignancy (mitoses, number of nucleoli). This can be a difficult determination to make with the normal variability of size and shape of transitional cells in urine.

Miscellaneous

Urobilinogen. So many problems exist in the dipstick measurement of urobilinogen that evaluation is not recommended. False-negative and false-positive results are common.

Parasites. The eggs of *Dioctophyma renale* (dog) and *Capillaria plica* (dog, cat) may be found in urine. Intestinal parasite ova may be found if the colon is inadvertently aspirated during cystocentesis.

Spermatozoa. Spermatozoa are often found in the urine of intact male dogs. Sperm migrate up the deferent ducts and enter the urethra at the prostate gland and then reflux back into bladder urine.

Fat. Lipid can be found in urine of normal cats.

Fungi. Fungi or yeasts are usually contaminants during collection, in transport containers, or in stain. Fungal urinary tract infection can occur but is rare. Some coliforms assume a markedly filamentous morphology in urine and may be mistaken for fungal hyphae.

SUGGESTED READINGS

Basanti JA, Finco DR: Protein concentration in urine of normal dogs. Am J Vet Res 40:1583, 1979

Biertuempfel PH, Ling GV, Ling GA: Urinary tract infection resulting from catheterization in healthy adult dogs. J Am Vet Med Assoc 178:989, 1981

Bovee KC, Joyce T, Blazer-Yost B, et al: Characterization of renal defects in dogs with a syndrome similar to the Fanconi syndrome in man. J Am Vet Med Assoc 174:1094, 1979

Carter JM, Klausner JS, Osborne CA, et al: Comparison of collection techniques for quantitative urine culture in dogs. J Am Vet Med Assoc 173:296, 1978

Chew DJ: Urinalysis. In Bovee KC (ed): Canine Nephrology, pp 235–274. Philadelphia, Harwal Publishing, 1984

Comer KM, Ling GV: Results of urinalysis and bacterial culture of canine urine obtained by antepubic cystocentesis, catheterization, and midstream voided methods. J Am Vet Med Assoc 179:891, 1981

Feeney DA, Walter PA, Johnston GR: The effect of radiographic contrast media on the urinalysis. In Kirk RW (ed): Current Veterinary Therapy IX, pp 1115–1118. Philadelphia, WB Saunders, 1986

Finco DR, Coulter DB, Barsanti JA: Procedure for a simple method of measuring glomerular filtration rate in the dog. J Am Anim Hosp Assoc 18:804, 1982

Hardy RM, Osborne CA: Water deprivation in the dog: maximal normal values. J Am Vet Med Assoc 174:479, 1979

Ihrke PJ, Norton AL, Ling GV, et al: Urinary tract infection associated with long-term corticosteroid administration in dogs with chronic skin diseases. J Am Vet Med Assoc 186:43, 1985

Kruth SA, Cowgill LD: Renal glucose transport in the cat (abstract). In: ACVIM Scientific Proceedings, p 78, 1982

Lees GE, Simpson RB, Green RA: Results of analyses and bacterial cultures of urine specimens obtained from clinically normal cats by three methods. J Am Vet Med Assoc 184:449, 1984

Ling GV, Ruby AL: Aerobic bacterial flora of the prepuce, urethra, and vagina of normal adult dogs. Am J Vet Res 39:695, 1978

Padilla J, Osborne CA, Ward GE: Effect of storage time and temperature on quantitative culture of canine urine. J Am Vet Med Assoc 178:1077, 1981

Ross LA, Finco DR: Relationship of selected clinical renal function tests to glomerular filtration rate and renal blood in cats. Am J Vet Res 42:1704, 1981

CHAPTER SIXTY-THREE

Abnormal Blood Gases, pH, and Anion Gap

Larry M. Cornelius

BLOOD GASES AND pH

Problem Definition and Recognition

The acidity of body fluids is expressed in terms of hydrogen ion (H^+) concentration or, more conveniently, as pH. The suffix -*emia* refers to the pH of blood. Acidemia (increased H^+ concentration) is defined as an acidic blood pH (less than 7.39), and alkalemia is an alkaline blood pH (greater than 7.51). The terms *acidosis* and *alkalosis* refer to processes that cause acid and alkali to accumulate and that, if not halted, will cause a change in blood pH.[6]

Pathophysiology

Body fluid pH is normally maintained within narrow limits; this occurs despite the continuous addition of large quantities of metabolic acids synthesized via intermediary metabolism from dietary precursors and the addition of carbon dioxide (CO_2) from complete cellular oxidation of carbohydrates, fats, and proteins. Three different types of mechanisms defend against large changes in the pH of body fluids:

1. *Chemical buffers* include proteins and phosphates (mostly intracellular), hemoglobin (erythrocytes) and HCO_3^- (mostly extracellular). Buffers are compounds that can absorb or donate H^+ ions and thereby minimize changes in pH. Since all blood buffers act as if they were in functional contact with a common pool of H^+ ions, the assay of both members of any blood buffer should reflect blood pH. The HCO_3^-/H_2CO_3 buffer system is especially important to the clinician and is discussed later.
2. *Ionic shifts* between extracellular and intracellular fluid help protect extracellular pH. When acid or base is added to extracellular fluid, approximately one-half of the added ions eventually diffuse into cells, where they are buffered chemically.[5] In order for electroneutrality of extracellular and intracellular fluid to be maintained, other ions of the same charge diffuse in the opposite direction or ions of opposite charge accompany the diffusing ions.

3. *Organ-mediated compensatory responses* include renal and respiratory mechanisms. The kidney can either retain or excrete acids and bases. Respiratory regulation of acid-base balance occurs through the retention or excretion of CO_2 via changes in the rate and depth of respiration. Disturbances of acid-base homeostasis may be simple or mixed.

Classification of Simple Acid-Base Disturbances[1]

Disease states that initially alter blood PCO_2 are termed *respiratory acidosis* or *alkalosis,* whereas those initially affecting plasma HCO_3^- concentration are termed *metabolic acidosis* or *alkalosis.* Changes in blood *p*H are determined by changes in the ratio of plasma HCO_3^-/H_2CO_3.* This ratio (and therefore *p*H) is stabilized by the ability of primary respiratory disorders to initiate offsetting metabolic changes and the ability of primary metabolic disorders to effect countervailing respiratory changes. Thus, the secondary increase in HCO_3^- induced by primary respiratory acidosis and the secondary decrease in HCO_3^- caused by primary respiratory alkalosis tend to return the HCO_3^-/H_2CO_3 ratio toward normal. Generally, the compensatory processes do not completely normalize *p*H, since to do so would remove the stimulus to compensation. These countervailing responses are physiologic consequences of the primary or initiating disturbance and are termed *secondary* or *metabolic compensation* for primary disturbances. The terms *acidosis* and *alkalosis* should not be used to describe compensatory changes in HCO_3^- and PCO_2 but should be reserved for primary pathologic processes.[10]

Respiratory Acidosis. Whenever CO_2 production in body tissues exceeds the rate of its removal by the lungs, blood PCO_2 increases and the patient is said to have respiratory acidosis. Based on clinical experience, primary respiratory acidosis is less common than primary respiratory alkalosis in nonanesthetized animals. Depression of the medullary respiratory center by anesthetic agents, when accompanied by inadequate assisted ventilation, frequently causes respiratory acidosis and acidemia (Table 63-1). CO_2 rapidly diffuses across the blood-brain barrier and combines with water to form H_2CO_3, thus lowering cerebrospinal fluid (CSF) *p*H. CSF acidosis causes central nervous system depression and even coma in human patients.[5] Lower airway disorders such as pneumonia and pulmonary edema are more commonly associated with either respiratory alkalosis or normal PCO_2 values; however, severe pneumonia or pulmonary edema may cause respiratory acidosis. Two other causes of respiratory acidosis are largyngeal or tracheal obstruction and diaphragmatic paralysis. Increased PCO_2 (hypercapnia, hypercarbia) may also occur as a compensatory response to metabolic alkalosis (Table 63-1).

---

*HCO_3^- and H_2CO_3 are used as representatives of all body fluid buffers. The kidneys regulate HCO_3^- concentration, and the lungs regulate PCO_2 (and therefore H_2CO_3) concentration.

TABLE 63-1.   Causes of Abnormal Arterial PCO_2

Increased PCO_2	*Decreased PCO_2*
Compensation for metabolic alkalosis	Compensation for metabolic acidosis
Respiratory acidosis	Resiratory alkalosis
CNS depression	Mild or moderate lung disease
Sedation or anesthesia	Pneumonia
Damage to respiratory center	Pulmonary edema
Airway obstruction	Mild or moderate restrictive airway
Foreign body	disease
Laryngeal paralysis	Pleural effusion
Severe tracheal collapse	Pneumothorax
Enlarged left atrium with left heart	Diaphragmatic hernia
failure	Anxiety/panting
Severe lung disease	Mechanical ventilation
Severe pneumonia	Fever/sepsis/endotoxemia
Pulmonary edema	Hepatic encephalopathy
Restrictive airway disease	
Pleural effusion	
Pneumothorax	
Diaphragmatic hernia	
Thoracic cage limitation/flail chest	
Neuromuscular disorder	
Phrenic nerve paralysis	
Botulism	
Coonhound paralysis	

CNS, central nervous system

Defense mechanisms against acidemia due to CO_2 retention include chemical buffering by blood and cellular proteins (limited magnitude) and renal compensation (retention of HCO_3^-, excretion of H^+ ions).

Respiratory Alkalosis. Whenever CO_2 removal by the lungs exceeds its production by body tissues, decreased PCO_2 (hypocapnia, hypocarbia) results. Decreased PCO_2 due to a primary disease process is termed *respiratory alkalosis*. As previously stated, respiratory alkalosis is relatively common in lower respiratory disorders such as pneumonia and pulmonary edema. It is theorized that lowered arterial PO_2 in these disorders becomes the driving force for respiration, resulting in hyperventilation and excessive exhalation of CO_2. Respiratory alkalosis frequently results from hyperventilation caused by use of a mechanical ventilator. Hypocarbia is also observed as a compensatory response to metabolic acidosis.

Defense against alkalemia due to hypocarbia consists of chemical buffering by hemoglobin and other blood proteins (acute respiratory alkalosis), renal excretion of HCO_3^-, and renal retention of H^+ ions. Chronic respiratory alkalosis appears to be unique among the simple acid-base disorders in its ability to induce compensatory responses that return blood pH completely to normal.[6] The cause of enhanced buffering in chronic respiratory alkalosis is unexplained.

TABLE 63-2. Causes of Abnormal Plasma HCO_3^-

Increased HCO_3^-	*Decreased HCO_3^-*
Compensation for respiratory acidosis	Compensation for respiratory alkalosis
Metabolic alkalosis	Metabolic acidosis
Vomiting of mostly gastric contents	Diarrhea
(see Chapter 32)	Renal failure
Pyloric or upper duodenal ob-	Diabetic ketoacidosis
struction	Lactic acidosis
Gastric foreign body	Drugs of toxins
Pyloric hypertrophy/hyperplasia	Ammonium chloride
Neoplasia	Ethylene glycol
Acute pancreatitis	Others
Others	
Sequestration of fluid in stomach	
Gastric atony	
Gastric volvulus	
Fluid or drug therapy	
HCO_3^-	
Lactate	
Citrate	
Furosemide	

Metabolic Acidosis. Reduction in plasma HCO_3^- due to accumulation of H^+ ions from acids other than H_2CO_3 or from actual loss of HCO_3^- ions from the body is termed *metabolic acidosis*. Whether or not blood pH is actually decreased (acidemia) depends upon the severity of the primary disturbance, the buffering capacity of blood and tissues, and the efficiency of respiratory compensation. Metabolic acidosis is the most common acid-base disturbance in dogs and cats. Various causes include diarrhea (loss of HCO_3^-), severe azotemia (renal H^+ ion retention), diabetic ketoacidosis (ketones are acids), and circulatory collapse (shock) (Table 63-2).

Compensation for metabolic acidosis occurs as the chemoreceptors in the respiratory center of the medulla respond to increased H^+ ion concentration and cause increased ventilation and loss of CO_2 from the lungs. This respiratory response to metabolic acidosis is apparently sluggish, often requiring 12 to 24 hours for a maximal response to develop.[6]

Metabolic Alkalosis. An increase in plasma HCO_3^- due to loss of H^+ from noncarbonic acids or from excessive alkali therapy is defined as metabolic alkalosis. As is true for each acid-base disorder, whether or not blood pH is changed depends upon the severity of the primary disturbance and the efficiency of body defense mechanisms. Causes of metabolic alkalosis include profuse vomiting, accumulation of gastric juice in the stomach (gastric atony, pyloric obstruction), and overzealous alkali administration (see Table 63-2). Metabolic alkalosis is usually more severe when vomiting is caused by a lesion near the pylorus, resulting in loss of mostly gastric juice with its high content of hydrochloric acid (HCl).

Body defense against pH increase (alkalemia) due to metabolic alkalosis is principally respiratory. Hypoventilation and retention of CO_2 in response to metabolic alkalosis occur but are reportedly somewhat erratic.[6] The kidney would be expected to maximize H^+ ion retention and HCO_3^- excretion, resulting in an alkaline urine; however, in metabolic alkalosis due to profuse vomiting, acidic urine is frequently observed. The precise mechanism of paradoxic aciduria during severe vomiting is not fully understood, but it may be a consequence of the body's necessity to retain equivalent quantities of cations and anions.[4] Since large amounts of chloride are lost in gastric juice, HCO_3^- is required to match quantities of sodium reabsorbed in the renal tubules. The result is an acid urine nearly devoid of HCO_3^-.[4] An additional factor that can impair body defenses against alkalemia during metabolic alkalosis is potassium depletion.[10] Hypokalemia causes relatively more H^+ ions to be available for secretion into the urine, thus enhancing paradoxic aciduria and worsening metabolic alkalosis. Furthermore, hypokalemia causes potassium to diffuse out of cells into extracellular fluid in exchange for H^+ ions, which move into cells. This exchange further enhances metabolic alkalosis (see Chapter 61).

Mixed Acid-Base Disorders

Recalling the definition of acidosis and alkalosis given earlier—processes that cause acid and alkali to accumulate in the body—it should be clear that mixed acid-base disturbances are common in clinical disorders. For example, a patient with pyloric outlet obstruction resulting in vomiting will probably have metabolic alkalosis due to loss of HCl in gastric juice. The expected compensatory response would be hypoventilation and a resultant secondary increase in PCO_2. If this patient develops aspiration pneumonia, hypoxemia may result in hyperventilation and subsequent respiratory alkalosis. This would be an example of mixed metabolic alkalosis and respiratory alkalosis. It is possible that metabolic acidosis may also develop in this animal. Metabolic acidosis could be a result of (1) hypoxemia (from aspiration pneumonia) severe enough to cause increased cellular anaerobic metabolism and lactic acid production, (2) dehydration severe enough to cause prerenal azotemia and retention of inorganic acids, and (3) enhancement of glycolysis by alkalosis with increased lactic acid production.[6] This is an example of a so-called triple acid-base disorder[6] (metabolic alkalosis, metabolic acidosis, and respiratory alkalosis). In this clinical example, blood *p*H and plasma HCO_3^- may be increased, decreased, or normal, depending upon the relative severity of the opposing processes causing accumulation of acid and alkali. Despite a normal or near normal arterial *p*H, recognition of mixed disturbances is very important because each process requires appropriate corrective therapy. The treatment of one process without attention to the other can result in severe alkalemia. Although mixtures of metabolic disturbances may occur, it should be apparent that mixed respiratory acid-base disorders are impossible because CO_2 cannot be concurrently overexcreted and underexcreted by the lungs. An in-depth discussion of mixed acid-base disorders is beyond the scope of this chapter.

Diagnostic Plan

History and Physical Examination. The history may provide information concerning the type of acid-base disturbance present in a patient. By considering the severity of the signs of the primary disorder, it may be possible to predict whether the acid-base disorder is mild or severe. Physical examination is notoriously unreliable in predicting the type and severity of acid-base disturbances.

Laboratory Evaluation. The most reliable information about acid-base status is gained from laboratory data. All that is necessary for initial acid-base evaluation is a routine set of serum electrolytes (sodium, potassium, chloride, and calculated HCO_3^-) and blood pH and PCO_2. Calculation of the anion gap from serum electrolyte values is also helpful in the assessment of acid-base balance (see selection on anion gap). A hemogram, a serum biochemistry profile, and a urine analysis are also helpful in evaluation of the patient. Ideally, arterial blood should be collected for acid-base evaluation. Most instruments used to measure pH and PCO_2 also determine PO_2, which can provide additional information related to the respiratory component of acid-base balance. Procurement of blood from the femoral artery of most dogs is not difficult. Whenever it is not practical to obtain arterial blood, free-flowing jugular venous samples usually provide reliable information.

If blood for acid-base evaluation is contaminated with air, falsely decreased PCO_2 and falsely increased PO_2 and pH values will result. Carefully filling the dead space of a syringe with heparin usually avoids contamination with air bubbles. It is best to do the analyses immediately. If the procedure must be delayed for more than 15 to 20 minutes, satisfactory results can still be obtained for up to 2 to 3 hours by placing the stoppered syringe into an ice-water bath.

Total CO_2 (TCO_2) concentration is included in many serum biochemical profiles. Since about 97% of TCO_2 is bicarbonate, the clinician should interpret TCO_2 as bicarbonate in the evaluation of acid-base disorders.

ANION GAP

Problem Definition and Recognition

The anion gap (AG) is a major tool used in evaluating acid-base disorders in humans, and its usefulness in veterinary medicine has been reported.[3,8,9] The formula most commonly used to estimate AG is

$$AG \ (mEq/liter) = (Na^+ + K^+) - (Cl^- + HCO_3^-)$$

With the common use of biochemical profiling, more veterinarians routinely determine serum Na^+, K^+, Cl^-, and TCO_2 (which can be substituted for HCO_3^- in the above formula) on clinical patients and can estimate AG. Normal AG for dogs is about 10 to 20 mEq/liter, and it is probably similar for cats.

Pathophysiology[2]

The term AG is a misnomer, because it implies that there is a gap between, or a difference in, plasma anion and cation concentration. This is certainly not the case because total plasma cation concentration must always be equal to total plasma anion concentration to maintain electroneutrality in body fluids.

It is helpful in understanding AG to derive another formula that more clearly states the true meaning of AG *in vivo*.[6] Since total serum cations equal total serum anions,

$$(Na^+ + K^+) + UC = (Cl^- + HCO_3^-) + UA$$

$$(Na^+ + K^+) - (Cl^- + HCO_3^-) = UA - UC$$

$$AG(\textit{in vivo}) = UA - UC$$

where UC is unmeasured cations in plasma and UA is unmeasured anions in plasma. Thus, whereas the AG is *estimated* from the concentrations of Na^+, K^+, Cl^-, and HCO_3^-, AG is actually *determined in vivo* by the concentrations of UA and UC in plasma.[7] Since plasma UA and UC in the patient do not change in the same direction in equal quantities simultaneously, "true" changes in plasma UA and UC can be accurately predicted by the following formula:

$$AG = (Na^+ + K^+) - (Cl^- + HCO_3^-)$$

Changes in AG can occur as a consequence of only three basic processes:

1. A change in plasma UA or UC in the patient
2. A gain or loss of water from plasma in the patient
3. Laboratory error in Na^+, K^+, Cl^-, or HCO_3^- measurement

Common causes of increased and decreased AG are shown in Table 63-3.

The most common change in AG is an increase; except for a few unusual situations, an increased AG is synonymous with an accumulation of acids, other than HCl, in the body (metabolic acidosis). However, anions—measured or unmeasured—are not acids. Acidosis is observed only when anions are accompanied by H^+ ions that dissociate from the anion and titrate buffers (*e.g.*, HCO_3^-), thus lowering the HCO_3^-/H_2CO_3 ratio.

Shown below are illustrations of the effects on AG of the accumulation of two different types of acids in the body.

1. H^+ lactate$^-$ + Na^+ HCO_3^- → Na^+ lactate$^-$ + H_2CO_3 → CO_2 + H_2O
2. H^+ Cl^- + Na^+ + HCO_3^- → Na^+ + Cl^- + H_2CO_3 → CO_2 + H_2O

TABLE 63-3. Causes of Abnormal Anion Gap*

Increased Anion Gap	Decreased Anion Gap
Increased unmeasured anions	Decreased unmeasured anions
Diabetic ketoacidosis	Decreased plasma albumin
Lactic acidosis	Acidosis, decreasing negative charge on
Azotemia	albumin
Increased plasma albumin	Dilution of extracellular fluid
Dehydration	Increased unmeasured cations
Alkalosis, increasing negative charge	Hypercalcemia
on albumin	Hypermagnesemia
Exogenous anions	Cationic proteins in multiple myeloma
Penicillin	
Carbenicillin	
Salicylate	
Ethylene glycol toxicity	
Dehydration	
Decreased unmeasured cations	
Hypoglycemia	
Hypomagnesemia	

*Laboratory error in the measurement of sodium, potassium, chloride, or bicarbonate will cause an erroneous anion gap.

(Cornelius LM, White NA, Becht JL: Principles of fluid therapy. In Anderson NV (ed): Veterinary Gastroenterology, 2nd ed, pp 103–133, Philadelphia, Lea & Febiger, 1992)

In example 1, the accumulation of lactic acid lowers the measured anion, HCO_3^-, and replaces it with the unmeasured anion, lactate. Therefore, AG increases in this example of metabolic acidosis. In example 2, the accumulation of HCl also lowers the measured anion, HCO_3^- but replaces it with another measured anion, chloride. Therefore, AG does not change in this example of hyperchloremic metabolic acidosis. Causes of metabolic acidosis with elevated and normal AG are shown in Table 63-4. An increased AG may be the only

TABLE 63-4. Selected Causes of Metabolic Acidosis*

Increased Anion Gap	Normal Anion Gap (Hyperchloremic Acidosis)
Diabetic ketoacidosis	Diarrhea
Azotemia	Renal tubular acidosis
Lactic acid accumulation (hypoxic tissues)	Addition of hydrochloride
Toxins	Ammonium chloride therapy
Ethylene glycol (antifreeze)	Methionine sulfate therapy
Salicylates	
Paraldehyde	

*Laboratory error in the measurement of sodium, potassium, chloride, or bicarbonate will cause an erroneous anion gap.

(Cornelius LM, White NA, Becht JL: Principles of fluid therapy. In Anderson NV (ed): Veterinary Gastroenterology, 2nd edition, pp 103–133, Philadelphia, Lea & Febiger, 1992)

laboratory evidence of acidosis in some patients with mixed metabolic acidosis and metabolic alkalosis.[6]

DIAGNOSTIC PLAN

Anion gap is estimated from serum sodium, potassium, chloride, and HCO_3^- (or TCO_2) and is used in the interpretation of acid-base balance.

REFERENCES

1. Cornelius LM: Fluid, electrolyte, acid-base, and nutritional management. In Bojrab MJ (ed): Pathophysiology in Surgery, pp 12–32. Philadelphia, Lea & Febiger, 1981
2. Cornelius LM, White NA, Becht JL: Principles of fluid therapy. In Anderson NV (ed): Veterinary Gastroenterology, 2nd ed, pp 103–133. Philadelphia, Lea & Febiger, 1992
3. Feldman BF, Rosenberg DP: Clinical use of anion and osmolal gaps in veterinary medicine. J Am Vet Med Assoc 178:396–398, 1981
4. Finco DR: Fluid therapy for profuse vomiting. J Am Anim Hosp Assoc 8:200, 1972
5. Makoff DL: Acid-base metabolism. In Maxwell MH, Kleeman CR (eds): Clinical Disorders of Fluid and Electrolyte Metabolism, pp 297–346. New York, McGraw-Hill, 1972
6. Narins RG, Emmett M: Simple and mixed acid-base disorders: A practical approach. Medicine (Baltimore) 59:161–187, 1980
7. Oh MS, Carroll HJ: Current concepts: The anion gap. N Engl J Med 297:814–817, 1977
8. Polzin DJ, Stevens JB, Osborne CA: Clinical application of the anion gap in evaluation of acid-base disorders in dogs. Comp Cont Ed 4:1021–1032, 1982
9. Shull RM: The value of anion gap and osmolal gap determination in veterinary medicine. Vet Clin Pathol 7:12–14, 1978
10. Welt LG: Agents affecting the volume and composition of body fluids. In Goodman LS, Gilman A (eds): The Pharmacological Basis of Therapeutics, pp 773–804. London, Macmillan, 1970

INDEX

The letter *f* after a page number indicates a figure; *t* following a page number indicates tabular material.

ISBN 0-397-51200-7

90000